AF619034

Hans G. Fassbender
Pathology and Pathobiology of Rheumatic Diseases

Dear MyCopy Customer,

This Springer book is a monochrome print version of the eBook to which your library gives you access via SpringerLink. It is available to you at a subsidized price since your library subscribes to at least one Springer eBook subject collection.

Please note that MyCopy books are only offered to library patrons with access to at least one Springer eBook subject collection. MyCopy books are strictly for individual use only.

You may cite this book by referencing the bibliographic data and/or the DOI (Digital Object Identifier) found in the front matter. This book is an exact but monochrome copy of the print version of the eBook on SpringerLink.

Springer-Verlag Berlin Heidelberg GmbH

HANS G. FASSBENDER

Pathology and Pathobiology of Rheumatic Diseases

Second Edition

With 308 Figures
and 12 Tables

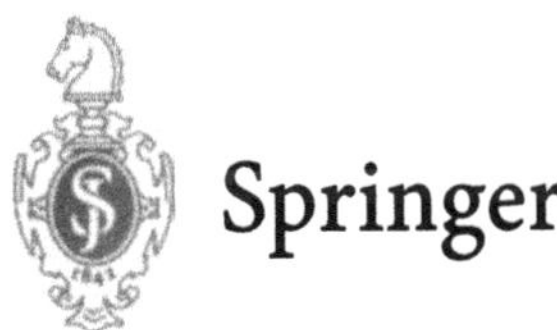

Springer

H.G. Fassbender, Prof. Dr.
Zentrum für Rheuma-Pathologie
Breidenbacher Straße 13
55116 Mainz, Germany

DOI 10.1007/978-3-662-04819-1

Library of Congress Cataloging-in-Publication Data
Fassbender, H.G. (Hans Georg), 1929- Pathology and pathobiology of rheumatic diseases / Hans G. Fassbender. p.; cm. Includes bibliographical references and index.

1. Rheumatism–Pathophysiology. I. Title. [DNLM: 1. Rheumatic Diseases–pathology. 2. Arthritis–pathology. WE 344 F249p 2002]
RC927.F38 2002 616.7'2307–dc21

This work is subject to copyright. All rights are reserved, whether the whole or part of the material is concerned, specifically the rights of translation, reprinting, reuse of illustrations, recitation, broadcasting, reproduction on microfilm or in any other way, and storage in data banks. Duplication of this publication or parts thereof is permitted only under the provision of the German Copyright Law of September 9, 1965, in its current version, and permission for use must always be obtained from Springer-Verlag. Violations are liable for prosecution under the German Copyright Law.

http://www.springer.de

© Springer-Verlag Berlin Heidelberg 2002
Originally published by Springer-Verlag Berlin Heidelberg New York in 2002
MyCopy version of the original edition 2002
The use of general descriptive names, registered names, trademarks, etc. in this publication does not imply, even in the absence of a specific statement, that such names are exempt from the relevant protective laws and regulations and therefore free for general use.

Product liability: The publisher cannot guarantee the accuracy of any information about the application of operative techniques and medications contained in this book. In every individual case the user must check such information by consulting the relevant literature.

Printed on acid-free paper.
SPIN 1062 8949 24/3130 ih - 5 4 3 2 1 0
www.springer.com/mycopy

In Memoriam *Gerald Loewi*

(31.10.1892–03.10.1977)

Foreword

Pathology and Pathobiology of Rheumatic Diseases glows with the uncommon precision of the pathologist, the clarity of the teacher, and the unswerving commitment of the investigator. Fassbender has produced a major contribution to the literature of rheumatic diseases. The practical experience and wisdom brought together in this book, substantiated by excellent examples of histopathology, produce a landmark for all who have made the study of rheumatic diseases their profession. The enormous achievements made in molecular biology, genetics, structural biochemistry, and clinical science have been assembled in this book to interact in a meaningful way with the anatomical histology of the rheumatic diseases.

It is not easy for any single investigator to paint the picture of a disease process, from its clinical description to its mechanisms, and then to a defined hypothesis, and finally an understanding. Nonetheless, Fassbender has done this in a clear and convincing way that integrates our current knowledge of this group of diseases.

Scientific discovery in medicine moves from the bedside to the bench, back to the bedside, and then back to the bench, etc. It is this iterative process of new observation and new discovery that has given us the achievements in medicine over the past century. The tools of modern science have allowed us to identify explicit cell types and functions, and the molecular tools have allowed us to look within cells to see how they operate and communicate with each other. These tools have given us an understanding of descriptive pathology in terms of basic molecular pathogenesis. In writing this book, Fassbender has demonstrated his mastery of the events, chronology, and outcomes of the pathogenetic processes involved in a very complex group of diseases.

The chapter on rheumatoid arthritis is by far the most lucid, visually convincing, and informative chapter on the topic that I have read. It should be read by every rheumatologist, and studied with intensity. Fassbender has examined many thousands of pathological samples and many more histological slides at the Zentrum für Rheuma-Pathologie in Mainz. As a result of this enormous experience, he has produced an integrated picture of the pathology of rheumatoid arthritis. His description of the proliferating synovial membrane lining cells in villous hyperplasia, and the way that this growing process evolves into synovial villi, constitutes a remarkable detective story in sorting out chronological events from multiple snapshots of the disease. In the extreme cases, he demonstrates the remarkable appearance of the proliferating synovial stroma, reminding us of the proliferation occurring in malignant tumors. He is able to use this extraordinary evidence to support his hypothesis that inflammatory processes are not the cause of joint destruction in rheumatoid arthritis, but rather it is excessive tumor-like proliferation of the synovial tissue that gives rise to expression of proteolytic enzymes and other generators of inflammation and destruction. The development of inflammatory processes in rheumatoid nodules and in non-articular tissues is also eloquently described in a cohesive way that allows one to appreciate the widespread systemic nature of this disease and to visualize its documentation in superbly presented histological samples.

Although the illustrations and photomicrographs presented tell a convincing story, the real jewel of this volume is the skillful way in which the author has managed to integrate the pathogenic process in time, space, and molecular context. All professional rheumatologists, as well as students of inflammation and connective tissue pathology, should read this scholarly work. Fassbender's earlier book, Pathology of Rheumatic Diseases, published in 1975, was a splendid documentation of rheumatic disease pathology. The current volume, almost entirely new in its format and content, reaches a new height and brings together a far greater knowledge and appreciation of those disease processes. It fits the context of our understanding of rheumatic diseases in the twenty-first century.

Summer 2001

J. Claude Bennett, MD
Birmingham, Alabama, USA

Preface

Whoever endeavours nowadays to write a book about the „Pathology and Pathobiology of Rheumatic Diseases" must realise that the term „rheumatic diseases" is a historical one. Concealed by, or rather within, this term is a host of entirely different diseases that are joined merely by the loose bond of a symptom of little significance, namely the „rheumatic" pain, particularly of the skeletal system.
The fact that over time several diseases emerged from this nebulous expression, diseases that do not share a common etiology, pathogenesis, pathology, or common clinical or immunological factors, must not least be credited to pathologists analysing the structures of the disease processes.
Quite a few members of this disease group emancipated themselves and won their own individuality. During this process, the name-giving manifestation in the skeletal system lost all but a marginal significance in many cases.
The specific task of the pathologist specialising in this group of diseases, however, is the detective-like identification of the etiology and the clarification of the pathogenesis. Such an elucidation is only possible using the substrate of the process. Clinical signs and symptoms and immunological phenomena can only provide clues and indicators.
Access to the structures of the disease process obviously depends on the availability of tissue samples and it requires the collaboration of pathologists and surgeons to be as close as possible.
It is with gratitude that I think of Kauko Vainio, Heinola, Finland, who introduced synovectomy as a treatment option for rheumatoid arthritis (RA) and, among the great number of physicians who collaborated with us, of Karl Tillmann, Bad Bramstedt, Germany; Norbert Gschwend, Zurich, Switzerland; Masuta Mori and Ryokei Ogawa, Kobe, Japan; and Ryoichi Kanie, Nagoya, Japan; but also of Alfred Swanson, Grand Rapids, USA; and Mack Clayton, Denver, USA. To the surgical methods these colleagues invented, established, and performed, I owe decisive insights into the pathological processes taking place in the synovial membrane as well as in cartilage and bone. They all have thus opened pathways to the structures of the „rheumatic" diseases. Their loyal co-operation enabled us to differentiate the various pathological mechanisms and to attribute them to the symptomatology of the different rheumatic diseases.
Thanks also to my surgically practising colleagues who were so kind as to conscientiously complete all the forms needed for our comprehensive documentation. By doing so, they have established the foundation for attributing structural processes to the respective nosological entities. Without their co-operation, this book could never have been written.

According to their particular importance, joint-destroying diseases, and, according to its clinical priority, RA, continue to be the focus of research of the Zentrum für Rheuma-Pathologie. For this, the amazing abundance of tissue material I am privileged to have at my disposal is – together with the relevant clinical information – an excellent basis.
Due to the almost life-long course of RA and other rheumatic diseases, single morphological findings are all but momentary and static images of a changeable process that is subject to several variables, such as age, duration of the disease, activity at a given time, and therapeutic efforts. Insights into the underlying process and its mechanisms do, therefore, require a very high number of tissue analyses.
The Zentrum für Rheuma-Pathologie is in the fortunate position to have at its disposal the greatest world-wide collection of tissue material taken from patients suffering from the different rheumatic diseases.
Therefore, we were able to detect the „signals" of the process proper among the „noise", as I often had the chance to follow the long-term course of different diseases by studying biopsies taken from the same patient at different stages.
The goal of our work has always been, and will remain, the understanding of structures and mechanisms of rheumatic diseases in the hope of defining them in such a way that they will become open to therapeutic attacks. Our morphological findings should also offer a basis for further immunological and biochemical investigations.
New – and unexpected – results of our work, above all those concerning RA, had to stand the test of being confronted with existing beliefs, and had to be discussed taking into account established opinions. In this respect I think, above all, of Claude Bennett, who admitted me to his Department of Medicine at the University of Alabama in Birmingham, USA, and Steffen Gay, Birmingham, Alabama, USA/Zurich, Switzerland. He took up my new and unusual concept of the synoviogenic joint destruction in RA and has been pursuing it in molecular dimensions. Bennett and Gay both succeeded in launching the initially painful change of paradigms in the concept of RA.
I owe important contacts in rheumatology and immunology to Ralph Snyderman, who made me a member of his department at Duke University, Durham, N.C., USA.
I also owe thanks to international protagonist rheumatologists, among them Eric G.L. Bywaters, Taplow; John T. Dingle, Cambridge; and – unforgettable – Gerald Loewi, Taplow, UK; Joseph Lee Hollander and H. Ralph Schumacher, Philadelphia, USA; Morris Ziff, Dallas, USA; and, not least, Fritz Schilling, Mainz, nestor of rheumatology in Germany.
I am grateful for the profit I gained from countless discussions with all of the above concerning my research results.
The decade-long stimulating co-operation with Elisabeth Stoeber, Garmisch-Partenkirchen, Germany, pioneer of the subspecialty of paediatric rheumatology, led to important insights into the problems specific to this field of study, which she and Barbara M. Ansell, Taplow, UK, have been developing since the 1950s.

I am indebted to Klaus E. Kuettner for welcoming me into his Department of Biochemistry at Rush University, Chicago, USA. My discussions about cartilage biochemistry with him, Eugene J.-M.A. Thonar, and the scientists at the institute turned out to be the most important basis for the pathology of osteoarthritis.
Pathology and Pathobiology of Rheumatic Diseases is a „one-man book". Yet it would never have been realised without the close and critical co-operation of my coworkers, all of whom identified with the project.
The author feels indebted to Tamara Hebert and Klaus-Dieter Martens for their dedicated literature research and for their discriminating editing, and to Carola Meyer-Scholten for going through countless specimens and selecting the appropriate ones for illustrations.
This book could not have been written without the incessant and devoted assistance of Ruth Gerhardt and Constanze Wolfert. I thank them for their tireless efforts, especially during the editing process that was first undertaken by Erzsébet Kuettner and Silvana Hess.
The translation into English was undertaken by M. Elisabeth Davies and Margaret Whittaker, Cambridge, UK, and Stephany M. Schneider, Düsseldorf, Germany. They were not only familiar with the subject but are also tied to our institute by friendship and mutual regard. Special author's thanks to all of them for their complex contribution that was essential to the project.
Thanks of a very special kind are given to a former student of mine, now a doctor, who has remained attached to my team and to me. We had to experience the failing of available treatments in the face of a particularly malignant course of RA as a result of destructive and necrotising processes. Thinking of the courageous Marion R. is, and will remain, a challenge for persisting in our research.
The author and his coworkers hope that this book may help attending physicians in their diagnostic and therapeutic decisions. On the other hand, we hope that it may also offer targets to pharmacological research that open up new tracks for therapy of severe rheumatic diseases.
Finally, I wish to thank Gabriele M. Schroeder, Stephanie Benko, Ingrid Haas, Martina Himberger, and Neil Solomon of Springer-Verlag for their infinite patience and supportive co-operation, especially with respect to their freely given generosity during the production stage.

August 2001

Hans G. Fassbender
Mainz, Germany

Contents

History of Rheumatic Diseases

The history of ways and side tracks of research in rheumatic diseases is printed by findings and hypotheses. Hippocrates (460–377 BC) took "Rheuma" and "Katarrh" to be synonymous with a process during which "mucous flux" left the brain for various foci in the entrails and also the joints, and there produced disease. It is understandable that the label "rheumatism", that perpetuated entirely erroneous concepts for decades, represented an obstacle to reliable research efforts.

Hippocrates: Katarrh

As recently as 1837 Schönlein lectured as follows: "The nature of this disease being more dynamic, explains the fact that few abnormalities of significance have been found at autopsy." Nevertheless, in the course of time, single strands have been disentangled from the bundle of confused ideas and definite nosological entities have been identified. Thus, increasing attention to the events at the actual level of the joint can be made out. Aretaeus (1st Century AD) having drawn attention to polyarthritis, i.e. involvement of several joints, Galen (129–199, AD) first speaks of arthritis as a collective term for joint inflammation. Rheumatism assumed an identity of its own through the work of the Parisian physician Baillou (1538–1616). He defined katarrh, a term still in use, as a disease of mucous membranes associated with inflammatory secretion and clearly separated from this "rheumatism" as marked by migratory pains.

Galen: Arthritis

Baillou: Rheumatism

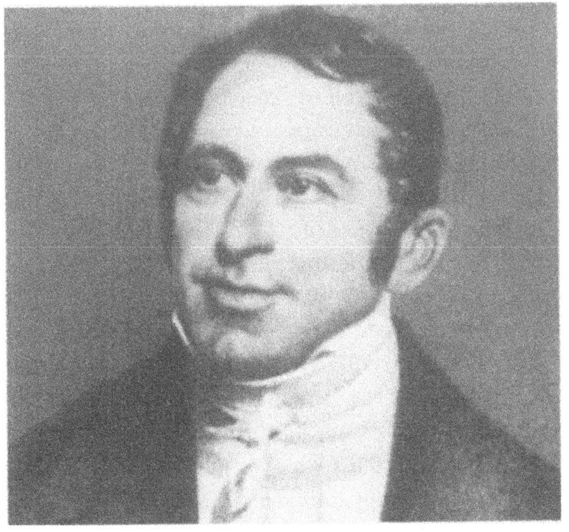

Johann Lucas Schönlein, 1793–1864
Physician in Berlin

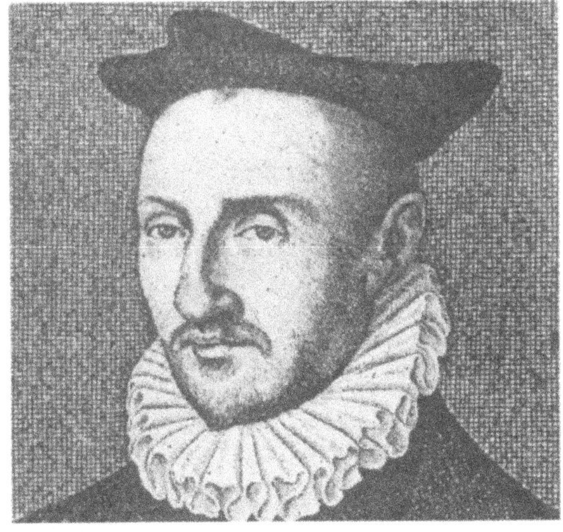

Guillaume de Baillou, 1538–1616
Physician in Paris

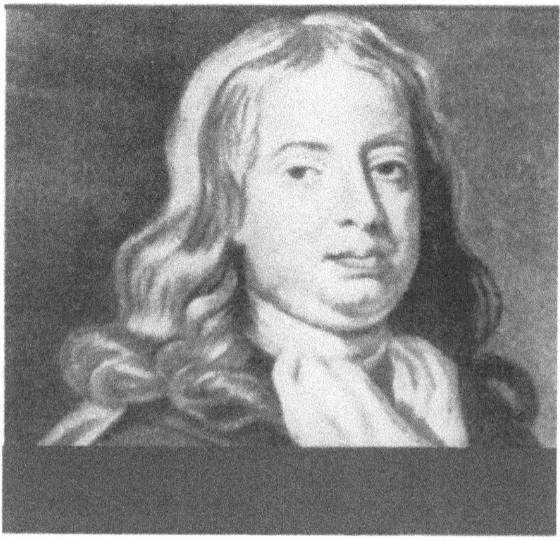

Thomas Sydenham, 1624–1689
Physician in London

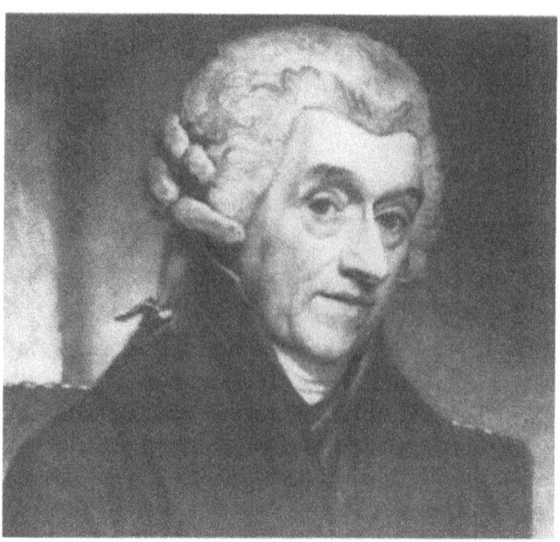

William Heberden, 1710–1801
Physician in London

Sydenham: Definition of gout

Pribram: Primary and secondary chronic arthritis

Bouillaud: Visceral focus of rheumatic fever

Fr. v. Müller: Arthrosis as a separate entity

Aschoff, Geipel: the "rheumatic granuloma"

Klinge: Cycle: fibrinoid-granuloma-scar

Thomas Sydenham (1624–1689) was the first to give a precise description of an attack of gout and distinguished this from chronic rheumatism as characterized by deformities of the fingers. Further precision was given to the concept of chronic arthritis by the work of Landrè-Beauvais (1800), Heberden (1802), and Haygarth (1805). It was Přibram (1901) who distinguished between primary and secondary arthritis. Bouillaud (1836) described the connection between acute rheumatism and endocarditis and pericarditis, and this marks the recognition of the importance of visceral involvement in rheumatic fever. Osteoarthritis was recognized as a distinct entity by Friedrich von Müller in 1913. Thus, in the course of more than 2000 years, when only the tools of clinical observation were available, a series of well-defined disease entities could be distinguished and replaced the vague collective term of "Rheumatism" which had only served to cover a series of phenomena. These entities comprised gout, acute rheumatism (rheumatic fever), and rheumatoid arthritis, which are solely connected by the symptom of "rheuma", i.e. the migratory pain. The morbid anatomical findings, which could have served to separate the various diseases further were still lacking. The turning point came with the discovery and description of the rheumatic granuloma by Aschoff (1904) and Geipel (1906) in the myocardium of patients dying of rheumatic fever. Aschoff regarded these cellular nodes as a primary reaction of adventitial cells to a putative virus. Geipel, Thorel (1915), De Vecchi (1910), and Talalajew (1924), on the other hand, considered this to be a granuloma following primary damage to fibres. To Klinge (1930) we owe the detailed description of the earliest tissue changes followed by maturation into an Aschoff body and finally into a collagenous scar based on his intensive histological studies of an unusually large amount of autopsy material. The first stage consists of swelling and homogenization of collagen fibres. This results in the fibrin-like appearance of the ground substance associated with the fibrils; the so-

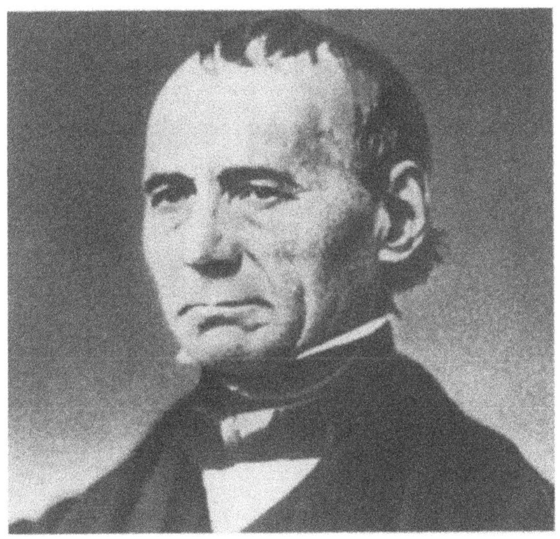

Jean-Baptiste Bouillaud, 1796–1881
Physician in Paris

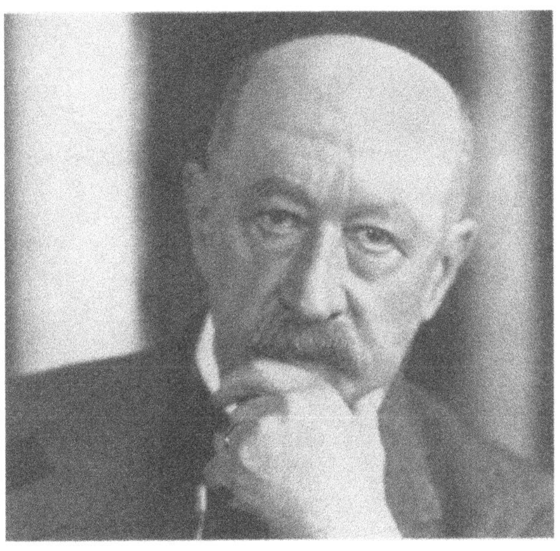

Friedrich von Müller, 1858–1941
Physician in Munich

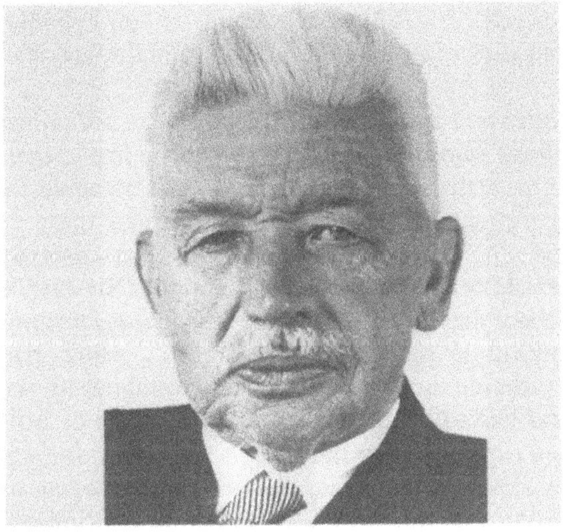

Ludwig Aschoff, 1866–1942
Pathologist in Freiburg

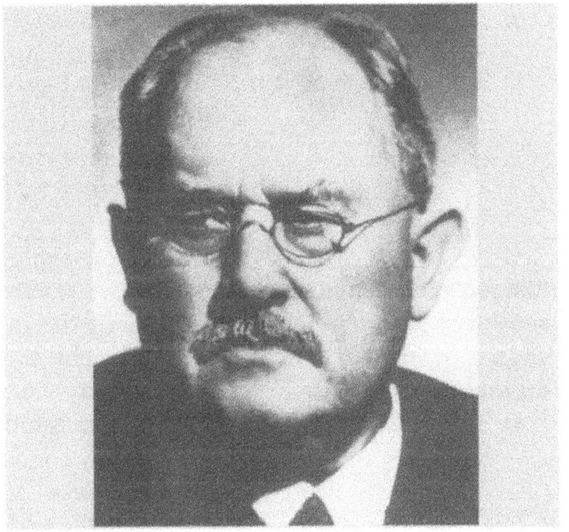

Paul Geipel, 1869–1956
Pathologist in Giessen and Dresden

called "fibrinoid". Klinge noted "an early rheumatic infiltrate"and he traced this into the later stages of granuloma and fibrous scar.

Misunderstandings

Apart from this sequence, fibrinoid-granuloma-scar, a second phenomenon influenced the pathogenetic concepts then prevalent. This was the rheumatic nodule. The attention of clinicians had quite early been drawn to these nodules, varying in size from a pea to a pigeon's egg and occurring in the proximity of joints. Fahr in 1918, and Swift (1924) considered these, in spite of great differences, to be analogous with the Aschoff node of the myocardium, a historical mistake, under which also Klinge was laboured. He regarded the fibrinoid centre of the different nodules, which he found by autopsy of patients aged 5–73 years with rheumatic fever as well as rheumatoid arthritis, to be the real

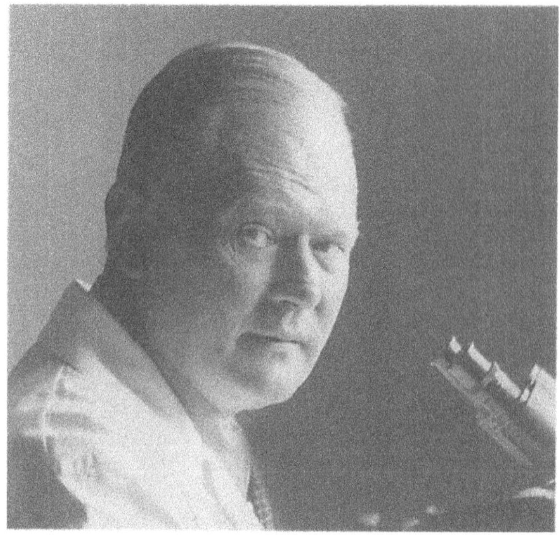

Fritz Klinge, 1892–1974
Pathologist in Münster, Strasbourg, and Mainz

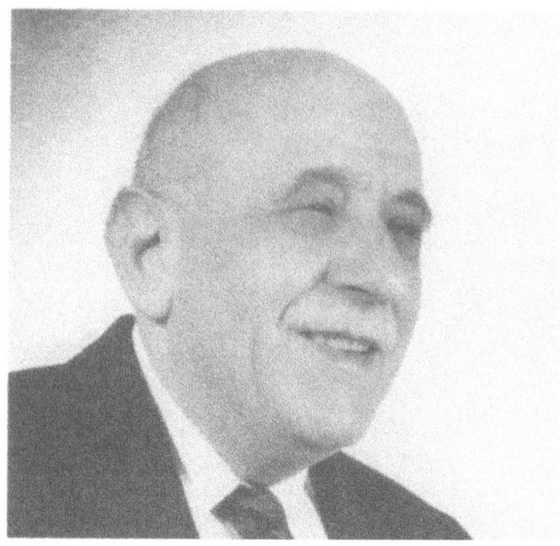

Paul Klemperer, 1887–1964
Pathologist in New York

"rheumatic" substrate. This is just one example of how hypotheses that have been allowed to leave the basis of solid findings lead to blind alleys.

Klinge: Experimental hypersensitivity to serum as an experimental basis for rheumatism research

In a series of extensive and very intelligently planned animal experiments, Klinge showed that by the use of the hypersensitization to serum, arthritis, vasculitis, and carditis could be induced in experimental animals and he regarded these as being analogous with "rheumatic" diseases. Klinge correctly appreciated the role of streptococci as an antigen. His special merit lies in the fact that he developed the morphology to complement the multitude of clinical observations which had already been gathered and that he firmly established the histopathological basis of "Rheumatism". In a series of brilliantly conducted experiments, Klinge was able to show the significance of hypersensitivity reactions in the pathogenesis of acute and chronic inflammatory diseases. In this way, he created a basis in experimental pathology upon which other experimental workers were subsequently able to expand and which later received an immunobiological superstructure by the identification of streptococcal antigens by Lancefield (1933) and the demonstration of rheumatoid factors by Waaler (1940) and Rose et al. (1948). In contrast to "fibrinoid" as a non-specific early change, the Aschoff node has not only retained its significance, but has come to be seen as a wholly specific feature.

Collagenous diseases

Research in rheumatology received a significant impulse by Paul Klemperer, pathologist at the Mount Sinai Hospital, New York, USA. He "liberated" the vascular connective tissue from its – until then – purely "serving" function and made it the central object of his research. Impressed by the fibrinoid swelling of collagen fibres, in the late 1930s of the twentieth century, he developed the concept of the collagenous diseases as result of intensive pathological studies. At first he counted Lupus erythematosus (LE) and sclerodermia among them (Klemperer et al. 1941;1942), later also rheumatic fever, rheumatoid arthritis,

and polyarteritis nodosa. He based his concept of autoimmune diseases on the discovery of the LE-phenomenon.
Klemperer was an excellent pathologist, indebted to the tradition established by Rokitanski and Virchow. The framework he constructed with subtle and elaborate efforts, provided the basis for creating increasingly stable pathogenetic concepts in rheumatology using the resources of morphology, immunology, and molecular biology.

1 Inflammation and Its Morphological Manifestation

1.1 Introduction

Flowing pain

Unspecific system

Rheumatic diseases are characterized by the commonplace symptom of flowing pain (ρειν=to flow). The cause of this pain in general is an inflammatory process. This inflammatory process, while it is definable, is also an unspecific system of cellular and molecular mechanisms. It is subject to regulations which adapt the composition of single factors to the respective pathologic demands.
The complex inflammatory process is unspecific and in fact qualitatively independent of the character of the rheumatic diseases, but it is subject to an individual imprinting by control of the special pathological situation.
The integrity of the human organism may be endangered by a multitude of harmful agents. The organism therefore attempts to maintain effective barriers against such noxious substances. If these barriers fail or if the body is attacked by any other means, the degree of damage is limited by humoral and cellular reactions, which together constitute inflammation.
Foreign material, altered "self", or damaged body cells stimulate afferent detection mechanisms. This stimulation leads, via a cascade of reactions, to the formation or activation of effectors which function to clear the tissue of such material. The tissue clearing is effected by cell lysis, phagocytosis, enzyme hydrolysis, and free-radical generating mechanisms. If removal or neutralization of the trigger substances is sufficient, inflammation ceases and a repair process takes over. The immune system may be involved in the inflammatory process. It allows for specific recognition and removal of complex substances alien to the body. The involvement of the immune system is dependent on the nature of the inducing agent and the duration of inflammation, its relative importance is, however, only recognized in the latter part of the inflammatory process. The inflammatory process constitutes a sequence of different reaction cascades which are very closely interconnected.

Three main phases

Inflammation has three main phases:
1. Exudation
2. Infiltration
3. Proliferation

The blood vessels play a central role not only in the inflammatory process as a transport system for the humoral and cellular defence mechanisms but also by activation of endothelial cells in the recruitment of inflammatory cells (Mojcik and Shevach 1997). Depending on the extent of the lesion, the organism responds via an alteration of the plasma constituents which is manifested by the "acute-phase response" (Baumann and Gauldie 1994).

„Acute-phase response"

The organism tries to adapt its defence processes against specific triggers, both qualitatively and quantitatively. This behavioural efficiency ensures that the border between the physiologically necessary regulation and the pathological inflammatory process is, as far as possible, not overstepped. As long as the reaction remains within a physiological framework a proportional balance between irritation and a defence reaction is maintained. The inflammatory process also has a tendency to self-limitation.
Pathogenicity overrides the inflammatory process if:
1. The quality, extent, and duration of the injury necessitate defence reactions which also destroy local host tissue.
2. The defence mechanism reacts against "self" because of an error in identification (autoimmune reaction).

1.2 Humoral Reactions

At the beginning of the inflammatory process, the humoral systems, i.e. complement, coagulation-fibrinolysis, and kinin-forming system, play a particularly important role (Proud and Kaplan 1988; Carroll 1998).

Coagulation cascade

The human plasma coagulation system consists of 15 different clotting factors whose activation is mediated by limited proteolysis. The coagulation cascade can be initiated both exogenously and endogenously. Both ways of activation lead finally to the formation of thrombin from prothrombin. Activated Hageman-Factor simultaneously catalyses the formation of kallikrein which leads to the formation of the vasoactive kinins bradykinin and kallidin. Thrombin cleaves fibrinogen at specific sites to release the fibrinopeptides A and B. Subsequently, the fibrin molecules aggregate forming a loose meshwork. Through the effect of Factor XIII intermolecular cross-links are formed which reinforce the meshwork. At the same time, fibrinolysis is activated by plasmin. The conversion of plasminogen to plasmin is catalyzed by both a tissue-type (t-PA) and an urokinase-type (u-PA) plasminogen activator. Activation of u-PA from the inactive pro-form is effected by kallikrein and plasmin. T-PA is primarily located in the endothelial cells and can be released by a variety of stimuli.

Complement system

The complement system is built up in a cascade-like fashion out of 20 plasma components. Its most important functions are the strengthening of antigen recognition by the immune system, facilitation of phagocytosis by opsonisation of particles, solubilisation of immune complexes and their transport to the phagocytic system, as well as the recruitment of leukocytes by leukotactic factors. The activation of C3 by the classical or alternative pathways initiates the formation of the membrane attack complex as an effector on the surface of cells, which leads to cell death. The activation of C3 leads simultaneously to the coating of particles and immune complexes with C3b. This opsonisation prevents precipitation of the immune complexes in the tissue and enables transport to the complement receptors on the cells of the mononuclear phagocytic system. C5a formed by cleavage of C5 produces a strong chemoattractant for macrophages and can also be generated by other proteases.

1.3 Cellular Reactions

In addition to the reactions of the humoral system, cellular reactions play an important role either via phagocytosis and/or by the secretion of mediators.
All cells, except erythrocytes, have the ability to synthesize prostaglandins, thromboxanes, and leukotrienes, which are arachidonate derivates, termed eicosanoids. These substances are not stored in the cell and have only a short biological half-life in the region of minutes. The first stage of their formation is the release of arachidonic acids by phospholipase as a result of stimulation or membrane damage. Prostaglandins and thromboxanes are produced in interim stages by the action of cyclo-oxygenase and the production of leukotrienes is initiated by the action of lipoxygenase. The amount and type of product is determined by the enzyme repertoire of the cells and tissues. Prostaglandins, leukotrienes, and thromboxanes influence the tone and permeability of the blood vessels and have, to some extent, a leukotactic action on other cells.

Chemotaxis and phagocytosis

The main characteristic of neutrophils is the ability for chemotaxis and phagocytosis. Important chemotactic factors for these processes are:
- C5a, C5, 6, 7, C3b
- Fibrin fragments
- Kallikrein
- Collagen fragments
- Bacterial cell wall components
- Leukotriene B_4 (LTB_4)

Neutrophils have the capability to ingest bacteria and other foreign bodies by phagocytosis and to digest them intracellularly. Phagocytosis is facilitated by opsonins (C3b and IgG) since recognition is via specific receptors for complement (CR1) and the Fc portion of the IgG molecule on the cell surface.

Free radicals

Hydrolytic enzymes

Furthermore, neutrophils can be activated by different signalling substances and react in two ways. On the one hand, they accelerate the oxygen consumption (respiratory burst) and generate oxygen-derived free radicals, which are extremely toxic for bacteria as well as being harmful to host tissue. On the other hand, degranulation leads to release of hydrolytic enzymes which effect tissue clearance in the surrounding area (Weiss 1989).

Macrophages

Macrophages become activated in response to cytokines from other cells or by contact with antigen or complement. Following an appropriate stimulus the macrophage is able to respond, releasing a number of secretory products such as lysosomal enzymes which are able to kill bacteria and degrade altered tissue.

Cytokines

The macrophage is also an important source of pro-inflammatory cytokines (IL-1, TNF, IFN etc.). Its most important function is phagocytosis of foreign or damaged material which is processed intracellularly and then presented to cells of the immune system.

Phagocytosis

Phagocytosis may be facilitated by opsonisation or, alternatively, as with neutrophils, may be accompanied by a respiratory burst resulting in release of oxygen free-radicals. The respiratory burst may also occur without simultaneous phagocytosis, being triggered by soluble factors (immune complexes, C5a). Parallel to this, release of arachidonic acid-oxidation products, such as TxA_2, LTB_4, LTC_4, occurs.

Lymphocytes

Lymphocytes are components of the humoral and cellular immune system. They are useful in manifold ways for the control of the immune response. B cells, after maturation to plasma cells, produce antibodies as components of the humoral immune system. T cells mature, after appropriate stimulation, to the respective effector cells which either attack directly cells as cytotoxic T lymphocytes or modulate the immune response as helper cells. The natural killer cells, a special type of lymphocytes, form the first barrier against attack and call in the mnemonic immune system. They have the capacity to regulate the activity of other cells, particularly cells of the immune system and, thus, serve as first defence against virus-infected cells. In contrast to macrophages, these effector cells of the immune system are not even distributed in the tissue but are localized in lymphoid organs (bone-marrow, spleen, lymph nodes). Some circulate in the lymph and blood.

1.4 Tissue Reactions

1.4.1 Exudation

The first event in the process of an inflammatory reaction is the detection of damage. The initial changes recognized morphologically are the reactions of the local capillary network and the post-capillary venules as a result of mediator release. The most important are histamine (from mast cells and basophils), serotonin (from platelets), bradykinin (through activation of coagulation), and arachidonic acid metabolites (from damaged or activated cells).

Reaction of micro-circulation

The first reaction of the micro-circulation is an increase in blood flow to the irritated area, which results in reddening and overheating of the tissue. Plasma enters the tissue via the enlarged gaps between the endothelial cells lining the capillaries (Fig. 1.1). The inflow of water caused by alteration of the osmotic balance leads to swelling.

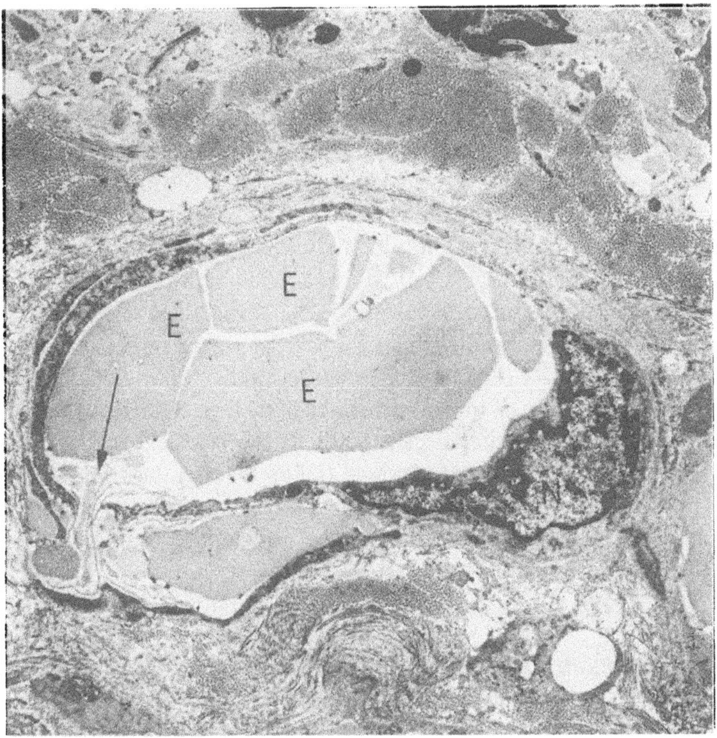

Electron micrograph of a venule within synovial tissue: plasma exudation between the extensions of two endothelial cells (*arrow*). *N*, endothelial cell nucleus; *E*, erythrocyte

Fig. 1.1

1.4.2 Infiltration

A new stage in the inflammatory reaction begins with cell infiltration into the irritated area.

Adhesion molecules

With increasing understanding of the part the adhesion molecules play in the inflammatory reaction, a considerable effect in leucocytic accumulation is assigned to the endothelium. According to the current conceptions, mediators stimulate the endothelial cells to express adhesion molecules which, in return, activate leucocytes and cause them to bind to the endothelium tube (Ziff 1991). Thereby an essential condition for the accumulation of leucocytes is achieved. The cells can then leave the vessel to follow the concentration gradient of leukotactic agents towards the focus of inflammation.

Endothelial cells

Neutrophils

The first cells to infiltrate the inflamed area are the neutrophils, followed in the second stage by the mononuclear cells (monocytes, macrophages, lymphocytes, and plasma cells). The infiltration of the tissue is controlled by the binding of cell surface receptors on lymphocytes (integrins) to ligands expressed on the surface of endothelial cells (adhesion molecules). Expression of integrins by leukocytes is augmented by antigen contact or under the influence of mitogens. The pattern of adhesion molecule expression on endothelial cells is controlled by cytokines. The combined effect of the resultant infiltration is therefore determined by the type of activation. For example, IFN-γ regulates the adhesion of lymphocytes and IL-1 promotes infiltration of neutrophils and lymphocytes.

1.4.2.1 Infiltration with Neutrophils

Simultaneous activation of the endothelium and slowing of blood flow through the capillaries and venules allow binding of neutrophils to the vessel walls. Attracted by chemotactic factors the neutrophils then migrate into the tissue through gaps between the endothelial cells.
The binding of neutrophils to the endothelial cell is mediated through the integrin CD 11b/CD18 (Mac-1). This binds to the intercellular adhesion molecules ICAM-1 (inducible) and ICAM-2 on the endothelial cell surface. Further binding of neutrophils is given by ELAM-1 (endothelial leukocyte adhesion molecule) following activation of the endothelial cell by IL-1, TNF, or LPS. The activation of endothelial cells leads to the synthesis of colony-stimulating factors which induce the production and release of further neutrophils from the bone-marrow. Long-term stimulation results in reduced ability of the neutrophils to adhere and the infiltration phase terminates.

1.4.2.2 Infiltration with Lymphocytes

The inflammatory process acquires a new dimension by the switching-on of the cell-mediated response, morphologically represented by the accumulation of monocytes, T and B lymphocytes, and plasma cells. The infiltration of the tissue by lymphocytes begins with the expression of corresponding adhesion ligands on the activated endothelial cells. The expression is initiated by IL-1, IL-4, TNF, and IFN-γ, appears later than with neutrophils, and is longer lasting. The interactions between lymphocyte function antigen-1 (LFA-1) with ICAM-1 and ICAM-2 as well as between very late activation antigen-4 (VLA-4) and vascular cell adhesion molecule (VCAM) are well-known.
Further binding occurs following induction of ELAM-1. Additional control of lymphocyte circulation is effected by interaction of homing receptors on the lymphocyte with addressins, the corresponding ligands.

Processing of antigens

A turning point and critical step in the infiltration stage is the processing of antigens by MHC Class II positive cells. Macrophages and B cells contribute to this step but other cells (endothelial cells, fibroblasts, chondrocytes) can also be stimulated by IFN-γ to express MHC Class II. An important role is attributed to the dendritic cells (Cella et al. 1997). Foreign substances are phagocytosed and processed within the cell. Small peptide fragments are presented by MHC class II at the cell surface to T lymphocytes for recognition by the T cell receptor. Upon antigenic stimulation, T lymphocytes respond by the secretion of mediators (including IL-2) which stimulate other lymphocytes to proliferate and become effector cells.

Plasma cells

Plasma cells develop from B lymphocytes and produce antibodies. Following proliferation, other subset of B cells differentiate into resting antigen-reactive cells which serve as an immunological memory. T lymphocyte proliferation produces cytotoxic T cells which are capable of destroying the body's own cells. The secretion of migration inhibition factor

(MIF) and macrophage activating factor (MAF) promotes the recruitment of further macrophages to the irritated area.

1.5 Pathophysiological Aspects of Inflammation

Time-limited and self-limiting process

From a pathological point of view, inflammation is a time-limited and self-limiting process with the aim of reestablishing the disturbed integrity. This corresponds to the term "acute inflammation".

"Chronic inflammation"

So-called chronic inflammation, although an established term, is, however, pathologically incorrect if it is simply based on evidence of mononuclear cell infiltration into the synovial tissue.
It is important to make a distinction between genuine inflammation and the chronic immunological process because both processes require different therapeutic treatment. This is well demonstrated by the fact that conventional anti-phlogistic therapy, whilst suitable for the true inflammatory stage, is totally ineffective during the subacute chronic phase. It is a common misinterpretation to conclude that monocytic infiltration is proof of "chronic inflammation" as, for example, in the use of the term "chronic synovitis". In this process, the synovial membrane manifests infiltration by cells morphologically characteristic of an immune reaction. As the studies of Hanly et al. (1990) show, the infiltrating cells in patients with rheumatoid arthritis (RA) consist of up to 92% CD4+ lymphocytic memory cells (see p. 67).
Systemic immunological diseases such as RA are characterized by episodic inflammatory bursts which are triggered from time to time by the systemic immune process. Our observations show that during the intervals between these episodes the infiltration of tissues by lymphocytes and plasma cells is indicative of an expression of the continuing basic immunological process.
The fact that with all kinds of joint diseases mononuclear infiltrates (monocytes, lymphocytes, plasma cells) are found after a short time, especially in the synovial villi, confirms that fundamentally:

- The inflammatory process never occurs without immunological participation.
- The synovial membranes, especially the synovial villi, are particularly suited for the local immune reactions.
- Lymphocyte and plasma cell infiltration is not specific for a special disease.

Consequently, the inflammatory reactions can be viewed as having two different aspects.

1. As a physiological, localized, and self-limiting mechanism which is required for self-preservation of the organism.
2. Although the time-course over which this physiological reaction occurs is short, severe reactions are still capable of causing extensive structural damage.

If the control of antigenic and non-antigenic stimuli requires an increase in both qualitative (neutrophils, elastase, collagenase) and quantitative (macrophages, fibroblastic proliferation) activity, then biological tolerance will be broken, particularly if the immune process manifests itself in episodic bursts. As a consequence, the primarily physiological inflammatory process becomes pathological in nature, requiring the corresponding therapeutic intervention, in particular if the defensive motivation is lost, as is the case with chronic immune diseases.

Chronic immune diseases

The inflammation itself tends to destroy its trigger, whatever it may be, enzymatically and by way of resorption, in order to repair any damage as fast as possible. By producing and releasing numerous growth factors, the migrating macrophages pave the way for the development of granulation tissue that promotes resorption and repair. Over time, the granulation tissue consists of less cells and more fibres. TGF-β and PDGF are particularly fibrogenetic and capable of triggering fibroblast proliferation and stimulating the production of connective tissue. The result of this scarring phase is permanent evidence of the inflammation having taken place (Martinet et al. 1986; Assoian et al. 1987; Kovacs 1991).

In concert, the cell elements involved in the inflammatory process (neutrophils, basophils, eosinophils, macrophages, lymphocytes, plasma cells), together with the complement cascade and the secondarily triggered cell proliferation (of the synovial membrane) constitute an impressive arsenal of defence mechanisms. However, they also represent weapons which not only damage localized structures but can also endanger life under certain conditions.

2 Rheumatic Fever*

2.1 Definition

Rheumatic fever (RF) is a widespread inflammatory disease that occurs as a delayed sequel to pharyngeal infection caused by β-haemolytic streptococci of group A. The clinical manifestation is characterized by an acute painful polyarthritis of the large joints. But the illness can also attack the heart, blood vessels, serous membranes, and the nervous system.

2.2 History

RF was first described by Sydenham in 1666 (Pechey 1701). According to Mathew Baillie (1797), it was Pitcairn (1696) who gave the first account of the cardiac abnormalities found in a patient with valvulitis. The joint manifestations were described very much later by Fahr in 1921.

It was only by the discovery of the characteristic myocardial nodes by Aschoff (1904) and Geipel (1906) that RF obtained a morphological hallmark and thus attracted so much attention by successive generations of pathologists.

Morphological hallmark

The precise histological studies of Klinge (1933) brought an understanding of the evolution of events in the connective tissue, since Klinge described the cycle: early fibrinoid lesion – Aschoff granuloma – scar. Fowler (1880) was the first to suspect a pathogenetic relationship between RF and preceding tonsillitis.

---

* *Synonym:* Streptococcal rheumatism

Glover (1930) noted a convincing connection between epidemic waves of RF and streptococcal infections occurring 3 weeks earlier.

"Acute rheumatism licks the joints but bites the heart"

Lasègue's dictum (1864) "Acute rheumatism licks the joints but bites the heart" still characterizes the significance of cardiac involvement in RF, predominantly in children. The bite can, however, as is now known, strike at different structures and in varying ways and thus have different clinical manifestations.

2.3 Epidemiology

In contrast to earlier times, RF has become progressively rarer in Europe and the USA since the end of the 1930s, however, in the countries of the third world it occurs with undiminished frequency.

The decline of RF in the more highly civilized countries is predominantly due to improved hygienic conditions and early treatment with antibiotics. However, an alteration in the pathogenicity of the infective agent may also be a factor.

Host factors

Host factors, many of which may possibly be genetic, could account for an innate susceptibility within individual patients. Extensive histocompatibility testing in many parts of the world thus far have not been able to relate distinct HLA phenotypes to actual RF susceptibility. However, studies originally reported by Patarroyo and coworkers (1979) appear to link the occurrence of B cell alloantigen 883 with the occurrence of or susceptibility to RF and subsequent rheumatic heart disease. It is still not clear whether the 883 B cell alloantigen is related to the DR/DS Ia-like system or whether it represents an entirely new marker somehow linked to RF susceptibility (Williams 1986).

2.4 Etiology

Pharyngeal mucous membrane

Since the investigations of Lancefield (1933) there is no doubt about the causal role of the β-haemolytic A-streptococcus. In addition to the nature of the infecting agent, the pharyngeal mucous membrane appears to have a decisive function as the place of entry. Thus, RF does not occur following streptococcal infections at other sites, such as skin, wounds, puerperal sepsis, or pneumonia. It seems that the structure of the pharyngeal mucous membrane and the tonsils provides a favourable culture site for the colonization of the A-streptococci and a sufficient persistence for an immunisation. There is a general relationship between the severity of the pharyngeal streptococcal infection, the attack rate of RF, and the degree of the streptococcal antibody response.

2.5 Clinical Features

Acute oligo- or polyarthritis

Two to 3 weeks after a pharyngeal infection with β-haemolytic A-streptococci there usually develops an acute, persistent, and painful oligo- or polyarthritis of the large joints. This involves predominantly the knee, foot, shoulder, and elbow joints. Localization and intensity of pain change in a few days, thus the arthritis is, in general, transient. The arthritides are more clearly pronounced in adolescents and adults, whereas in children the heart complications are predominant. This clinically significant cardiac involvement is, however, in no way limited to the first acute attack but can recur periodically and thus cause progressive and irreversible damage to the structure of the myocardium, endocardium, and pericardium.

Intermittent fever up to 104°F (40°C) can occur for many weeks. In children (particularly girls), an involvement of the central nervous system can manifest itself as Sydenham's chorea, almost unvariably associated with concurrent cardiac involvement. Occasionally in children, subcutaneous nodes appear in mechanically stressed sites, especially in the scalp after minor traumas, but disappear again after a few weeks. In the skin of the upper arms as well as of the thorax of children, an erythema marginatum can occur in 1%–5%. At first glance, RF appears to be an illness with a distinct profile, characterized by three distinguishing features:

Sydenham's chorea

Subcutaneous nodes

Erythema marginatum

1. A-streptococcal pharyngitis
2. Fever, joint pain, myocardial symptoms
3. Aschoff granuloma in the myocardium

Variations

The disease phenomena caused by the A-streptococcal pharyngitis show, however, the following variations:

1. Subacute course with fleeting arthritides and myocardial symptoms which disappear again after a few weeks; no endocarditis, and no resulting valve damage.
2. Subacute course with fleeting arthritides and myocardial symptoms which disappear again after a few weeks; but in addition, an endocarditis occurs with resulting valve damage.
3. Highly acute course with fatal myocardial insufficiency.
4. Chronic, subclinical late form with previously occurring rheumatic valve defect; possible insidious myocardial insufficiency.

2.6 Pathogenesis

The systemic clinical picture of RF is the result of a complex of toxic and immunological influence of the germ as well as of still little-known host factors.

It might be supposed that the variations are simply quantitative differences of one unified mechanism, but the intervention of other pathogenetic factors arising from the indisputable fact of the primary A-streptococcal infection, must also be taken into account in RF.

Role of streptococcal toxin

Evidence of direct streptococcal infection is lacking, but a direct effect of streptococcal toxin (streptolysin S) particularly on the heart structure cannot be ruled out. Streptolysin S is one of the most potent biologic poisons on a microgram basis that ever has been characterized and studied. Direct injections of streptolysin S into cardiac structures of experimental animals can in some instances produce histological lesions somewhat similar to those seen in acute rheumatic carditis. The fact that the latent time between streptococcal pharyngitis and RF is not reduced in later recurrences, which would be expected if it were a secondary immune response (Stollermann 1985), argues therefore that RF is not exclusively caused immunologically.

Immunological aspects

Primary consideration should, however, be given to the immunological aspects of the above:

- Streptococcal antibodies have no direct cytotoxic effect on the host structures.

Cross-reactions

- On the other hand, cross-reactions between streptococcal antibodies and human tissue are known since it has been shown in animal experiments that rabbit antisera against certain group A-streptococci react with human heart preparations in the immunofluorescent test (Kaplan 1963; Kaplan and Suchy 1964). Meanwhile, a series of streptococcal antigens have been discovered which may have cross-reactions with human tissue (Table 2.1).

Molecular mimicry

A very promising insight into the pathogenesis of RF offers the concept of molecular mimicry, whereby bacterial antigens present on the infecting group A-streptococcus evoke an immune response in the host. The host reaction then induces cross-reactivity with autologous host tissues that are similar to the antigens originally present in the infecting group A-streptococcus. Experimental demonstration has been provided by several groups of cross-reactions between human heart muscle structures and group A-streptococcal cell walls as well as heart muscle sarcolemmic membrane material. Also different cross-reacting determinants between streptococcal M protein and human heart muscle membranes gain more and more importance (Williams 1986). M proteins play a decisive role in the pathogenesis of RF. The cell wall has a complex structure. The murein layer, which provides the cell with stability, is firmly

Table 2.1. Streptococcal antigens cross-reacting with human tissues (Williams 1986)

Streptococcal antigen	Human tissue	Possible result of cross-reaction
Group A cell walls	Human myocardium	Carditis
Group A membranes	Human myocardial sarcolemmal membranes	Carditis
Group A polysaccharides and glycoproteins	Human heart valve glycoproteins	Valvulitis and endocarditis
M-protein polypeptides	Human myocardial sarcolemmal membranes	Carditis
Group A streptococcal membranes	Human neuronal cytoplasmic antigens in caudate nucleus	Chorea
Group A streptococci	Cardiac myosin subunits	Carditis

connected with the cytoplasmic membrane. Next to it is a polysaccharide layer that consists of substance C and is linked to the murein layer by covalent bonds. Next to this layer, there is a protein layer that exhibits several antigens, among them the M antigen, the chemistry of which allows the group A streptococci to be classified into 55 subtypes. The protein layer has anti-phagocytic properties as has the loosely structured, non-immunogenic, hyaluronic acid capsule, which in some strains is located adjacent to the protein layer. A large amount of M proteins can be extracted from the rheumatogenic strains, which facilitates their identification. After untreated pharyngitis, rheumatogenic strains strongly induce type-specific antibodies. Some serotypes have been clearly associated with epidemics of RF. M5 is the most common type, and M3, 6, 14, 18, 19, 24, and a few others are well represented (Stollermann 1997). The structure of the very large M protein molecules on the surface of rheumatogenic strains is relevant to the pathogenesis of RF. The M-associated surface protein extractable from virulent throat strains associated with RF has an epitope distinguishable from that of the M-associated proteins of non-rheumatogenic serotypes (Bessen et al. 1989). Interesting, however, is Dale's and Chiang's finding (1995) of epitopes that are cross-reactive with heart tissues, synovium, and brain on an area on the M molecule proximal to the type-specific epitopes of the N-acetyl amino terminus. The deposition of heavy antigenic load of such epitopes in pharyngeal lymphoid tissues, already hypersensitized during childhood by repeated previous streptococcal infections, may cause a break in immune tolerance that can lead to the various signs of the disease (Stollermann 1997). The susceptibility of rheumatic hosts to recurrences of RF might result from an acquired autoimmune response that is amplified by subsequent bouts of infection with additional rheumatogenic strains that contain the same cross-reactive epitopes.

Autoantibodies

▸ Thus, the serum from patients with RF contains autoantibodies to many tissues. Of greatest significance are heart antibodies, γ-globulin with specificity for cardiac components, primarily sarcolemma membranes. It is possible that the smouldering myo-aggressive granulomata, which we found in the myocardium of deceased as well as in the auricular appendages of clinically healthy persons, can thus be explained.

As, however, of course not only rheumatic, but also traumatic and ischaemic heart damage lead to the formation of these autoantibodies, Stollermann (1985) queried whether heart antibodies in rheumatic carditis are the result or the cause of the tissue damage.

Accordingly, different pathogenetic routes may exist between the A-streptococcal infection and the various manifestations which result.

2.7 Pathology

Aschoff granuloma

As a general concept, the heart process in RF is characterized by fibrinoid swelling and Aschoff granuloma. This unitary concept is in opposition to the different clinical courses which cannot be explained solely as quantitative variations.
We had the opportunity to investigate the tissue from ten patients who had died from acute RF and from one patient with subacute RF who had died from an intercurrent infection. In addition, there were available to us 36 heart auricles from patients who had had a commisurotomy performed for a defective rheumatic heart valve (Fassbender 1963).

2.7.1 Myocardium

Three different types of morphological changes

Light-microscopic analysis of the myocardial changes revealed three qualitatively different pathological processes: classical rheumatic myocarditis of the Aschoff type, acute diffuse exudative myocarditis, and chronic lingering myo-aggressive rheumatic myocarditis.

Classical rheumatic myocarditis of the Aschoff type

The myocarditis of RF involves exclusively the perivascular connective tissue of the heart muscle. The first phase, occurring about 14 days after the onset of RF, consists of oedema of the connective tissue fibrils. Small, homogeneous, highly refractile foci occur, in which no fibrils are recognizable by conventional

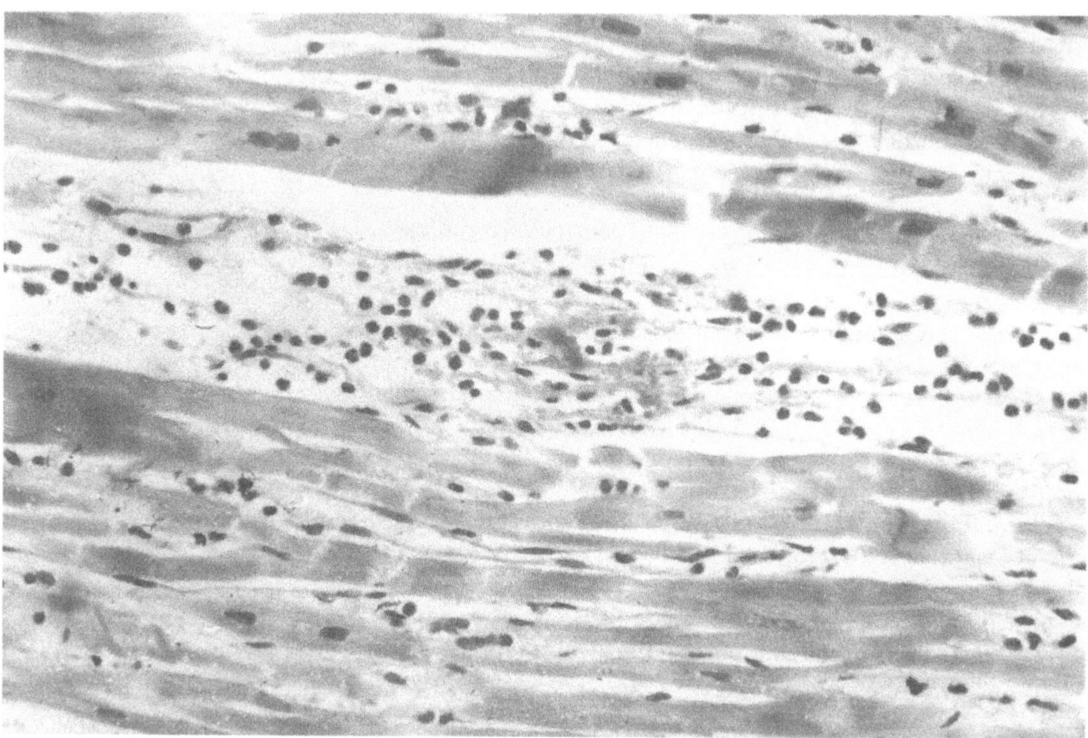

Fig. 2.1
Rheumatic fever

Myocard. Fresh fibrinoid in perivascular tissue surrounded by macrophages, lymphocytes, and neutrophils

stains. In the earlier stages, these lesions can be stained by methods which demonstrate fibrin. The fibres can, however, be shown by silver impregnation methods. Klinge (1930) named these appearances "the early rheumatic infiltrate". Following Neumann's (1880) nomenclature, the term "fibrinoid" was applied, purely as a descriptive name (Fig. 2.1).

"Fibrinoid"

Little can be added to the voluminous and detailed observations of Klinge. Fibrinoid makes its first appearance within the collagen bundles and only later spreads to the inter-collagenous spaces. The fibrinoid masses become coarser and distinct. As explained above, the term fibrinoid merely indicates a group of light-microscopical phenomena covering different chemical compositions according to the associated disease.

Fibrinoid of RF contains fibrin and γ-globulin. The focal exudation must be presumed to follow increased permeability of a damaged capillary wall. This event is of significance in the further pathogenetic evolution of RF. Capillary injury and exudation signify the starting point in rheumatic myocarditis. The appearance of fibrinoid in perivascular connective tissue is tem-

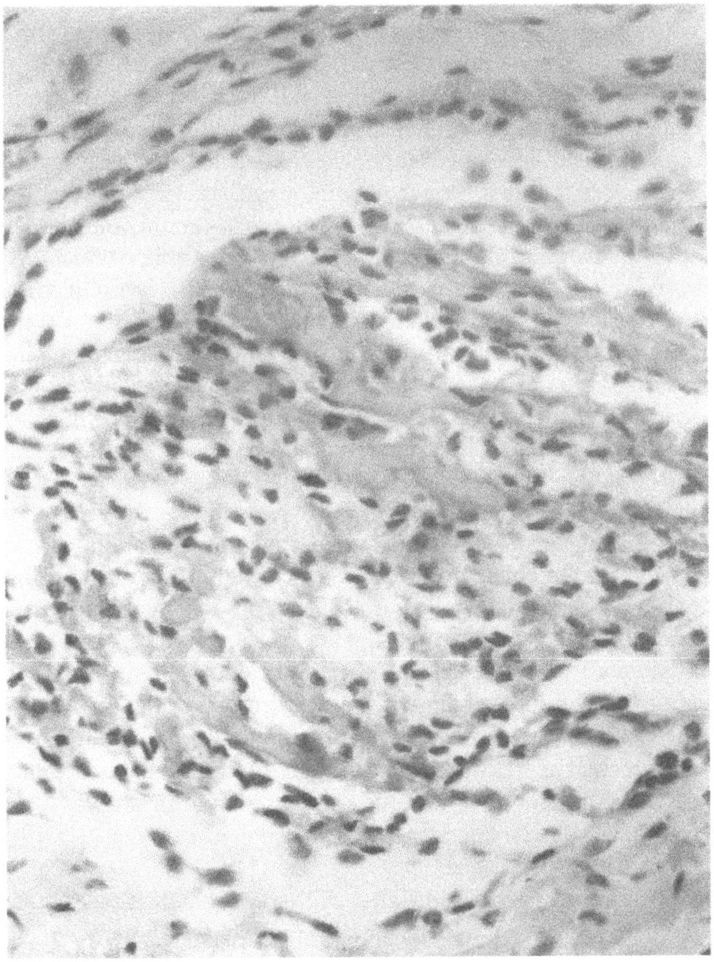

Myocard. Fibrinoid of longer standing and the beginning of cellular resorption by macrophages and fibroblasts

Fig. 2.2
Rheumatic fever

porally related with pericardial, pleural, and occasionally peritoneal fibrin exudation: a pointer to widespread involvement of capillaries. The presence of exudate leads to appearance of fibroblasts and macrophages presumably associated with absorption of the material. Fibrinoid of the early infiltrate is associated with small unimpressive cells but with ageing of fibrinoid, cells begin to swell and proliferate (Fig. 2.2). By the end of the 2nd week of the illness, Klinge was able to observe a small number of giant cells associated with a few lymphocytes and neutrophils. After the 4th week, proliferation of the connective tissue cells already imparts the typical appearance of the Aschoff granuloma (Fig. 2.3). Localization, shape, and cell composition of the Aschoff node are entirely characteristic of RF. They are most frequently seen in the interstitial tissue of the myocardium of the left side of the heart and the septum as well as in the subendocardial tissue. The Aschoff body, as the preceding fibrinoid, is strictly localized to the perivascular connective tissue. The early granuloma, in particular, shows a remarkably close relationship to the vessels (Fig. 2.4). McEwen (1932), who was a collaborator of Klinge, observed 49 nodes in successive serial sections and only in five cases failed to find such close contact. There are adventitial cells which swell and become separated, and participate in the formation of the granuloma (Fig. 2.5). The main constituents of an Aschoff node are large macrophages with one or two plump nuclei with a heavy content of chromatin. Electron-microscopy shows a well-developed endoplasmic reticulum. These macrophages are the most important and also characteristic constituents of an Aschoff body. They are grouped around the initially readily recognizable remnant of fibrinoid, sometimes forming a rosette (Fig. 2.6). More peripherally, an occasional lymphocyte or mast cell is found, especially in an early granuloma. In an active granuloma, the cells are initially in a loose arrangement imparting a round or oval shape to the node, whereas later, they assume the characteristics of fibroblasts and come to lie in a parallel arrangement. The granuloma becomes spindle-shaped and the cells lie with their long axes parallel to the muscle and connective tissue fibres (Fig. 2.7). With increasing age, the argyrophil material of the granuloma decreases together with an increase of newly formed collagen fibres. In this way, the Aschoff node, becoming less cellular and more collagenous, changes into a permanent scar. Occasionally, a small oval scar surrounds a centrally situated blood vessel. In most cases, one or two myocardial fibres can be recognized within the scar tissue (Fig. 2.8). While the Aschoff node is unrecognizable to the naked eye, the oval perivascular scars can be made out on incision of the heart muscle as small light grey dots, the size of a pin's head (Fig. 2.9). The characteristic scars persist as evidence of past rheumatic carditis forever.

Aschoff granuloma

Recurrent granulomata

Fibrous scars are often the sites of rheumatic recurrences in the form of newly formed Aschoff granulomata. These recurrent granulomata are clinically latent, i.e. symptom-free, and are only discovered in post-mortems of patients who have died of non-rheumatic illnesses (see Fig. 2.8).

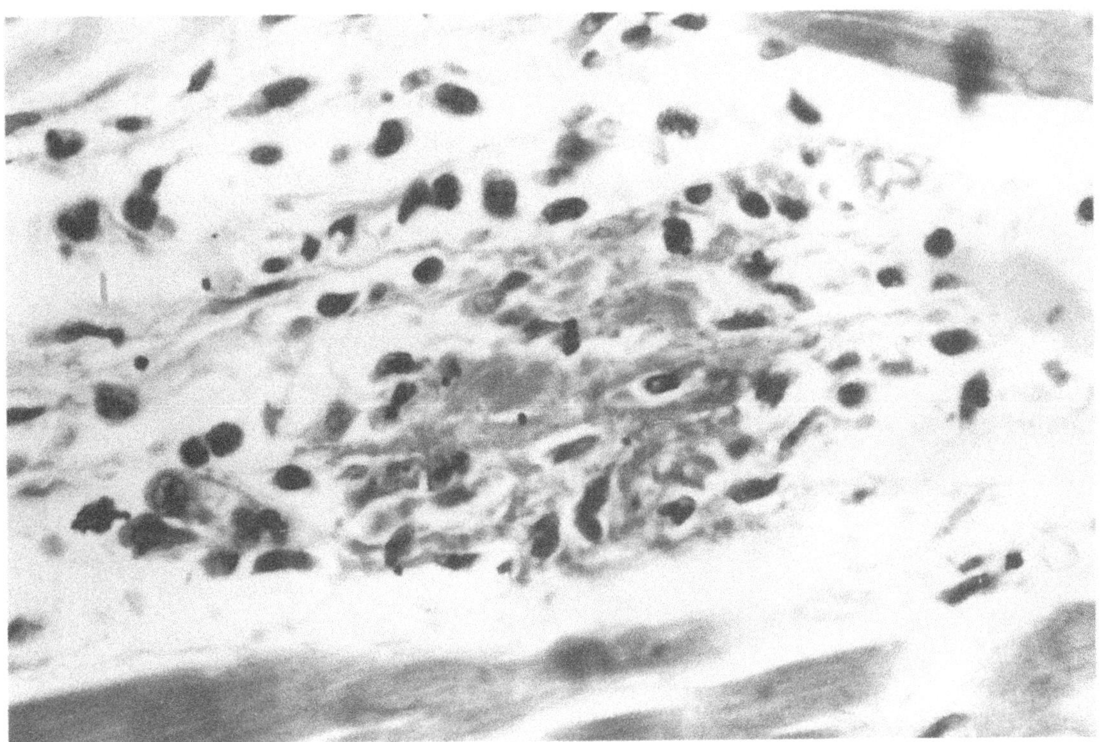

Myocard. Long standing fibrinoid and birth of the Aschoff granuloma

Fig. 2.3
Rheumatic fever

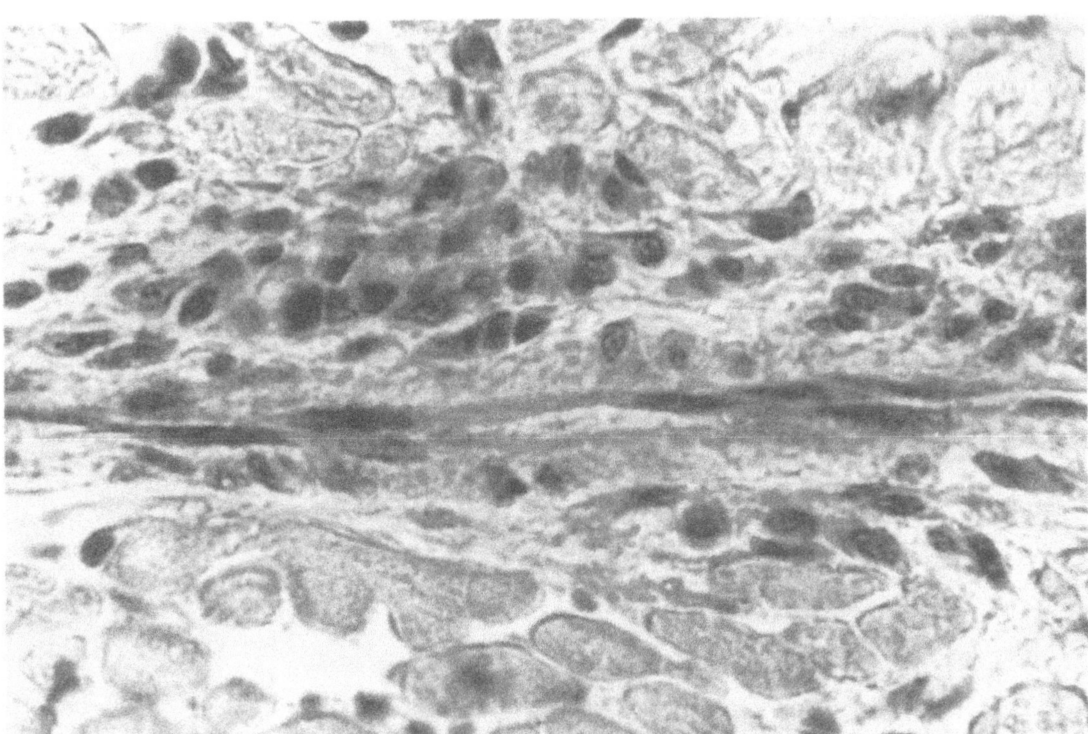

Myocard. Formation of an Aschoff granuloma in close contact with a blood vessel

Fig. 2.4
Rheumatic fever

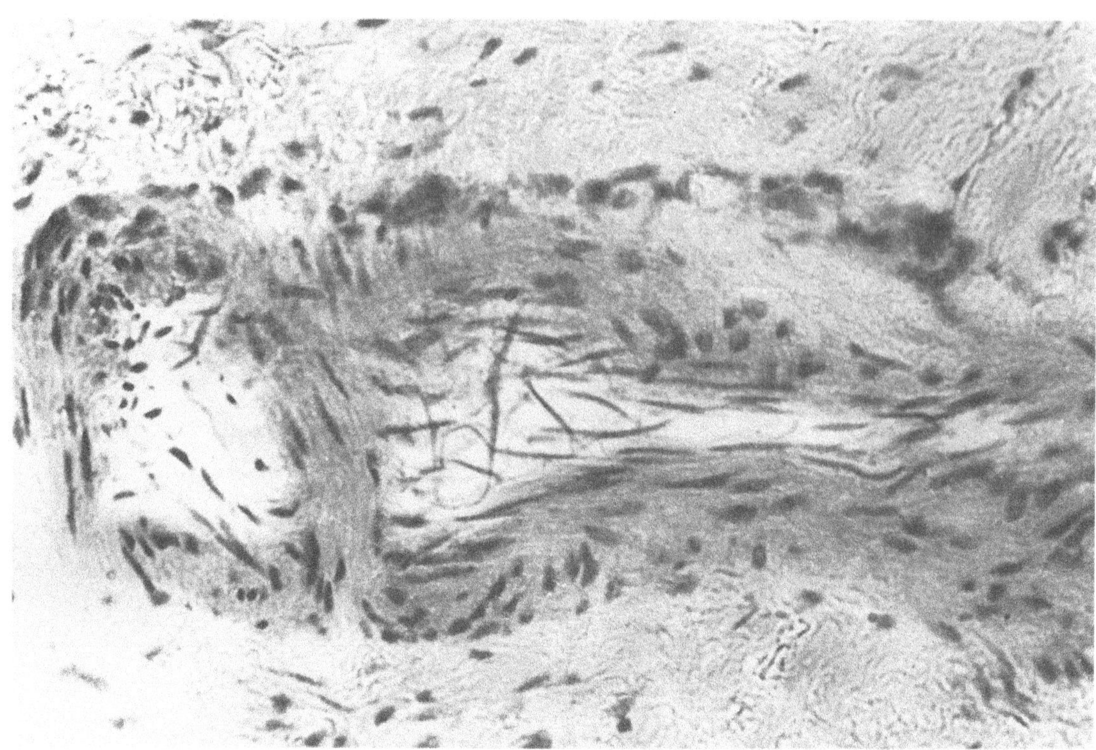

Fig. 2.5
Rheumatic fever

Myocard. Advanced swelling and early dissolution of adventitial cells of a coronary artery branch

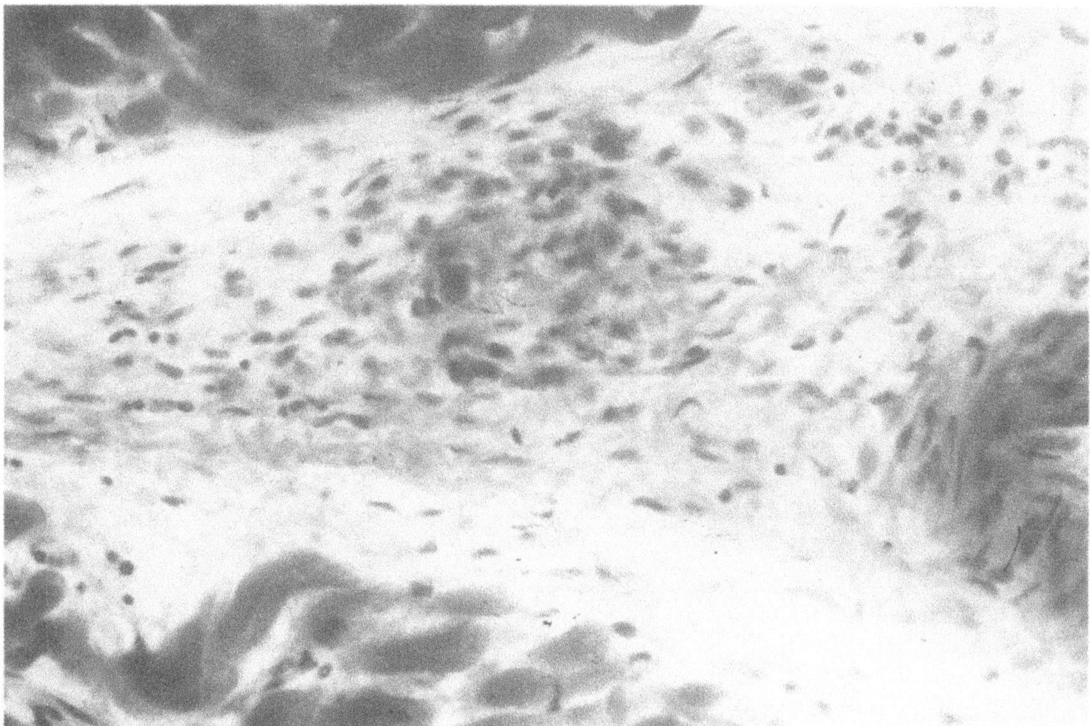

Fig. 2.6
Rheumatic fever

Myocard. Fully developed Aschoff granuloma with central fibrinoid remnants

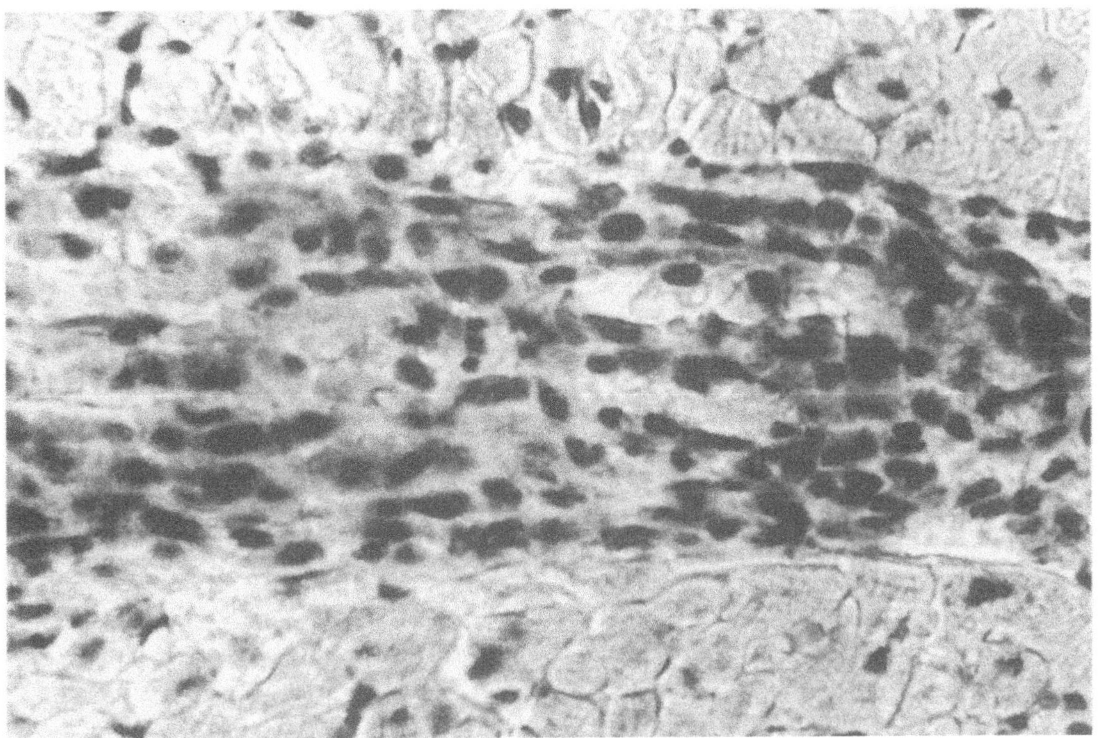

Myocard. Older Aschoff granuloma predominantly consisting of fish draught-like arranged fibroblasts

Fig. 2.7
Rheumatic fever

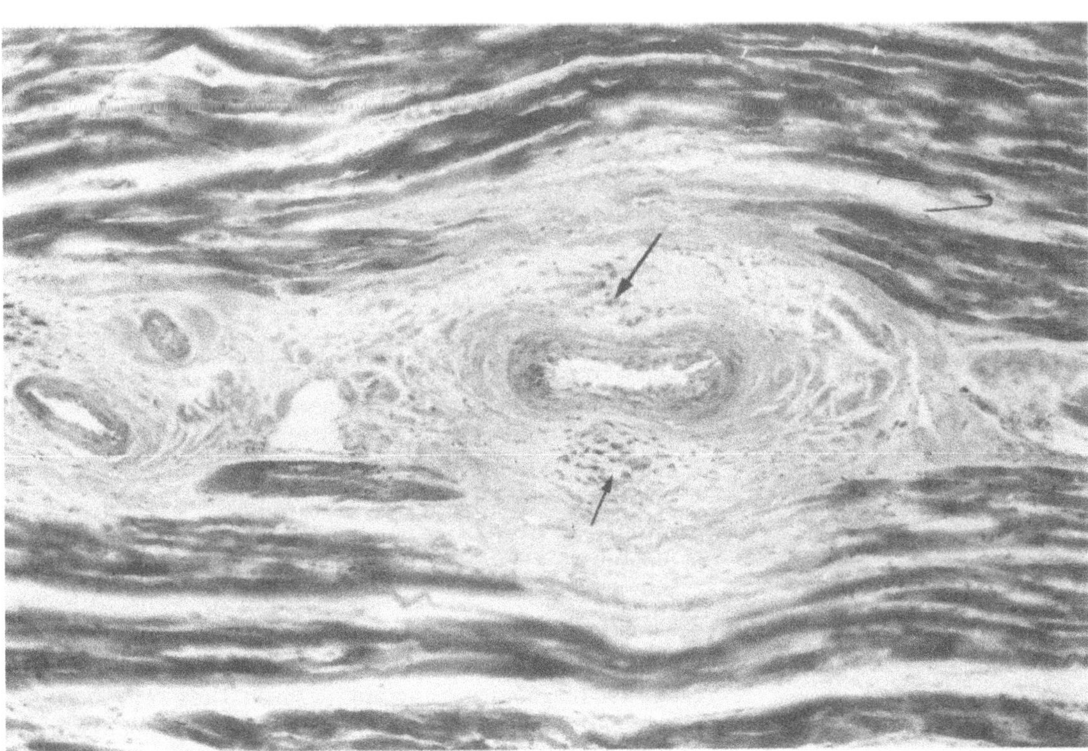

Myocard. A typical spindle-shaped (lemon-like) scar following rheumatic carditis. Some surrounding muscle fibres have undergone destruction and replacement by collagen. Above and below the coronary branch, there are small residual granulomata (*arrows*)

Fig. 2.8
Rheumatic fever

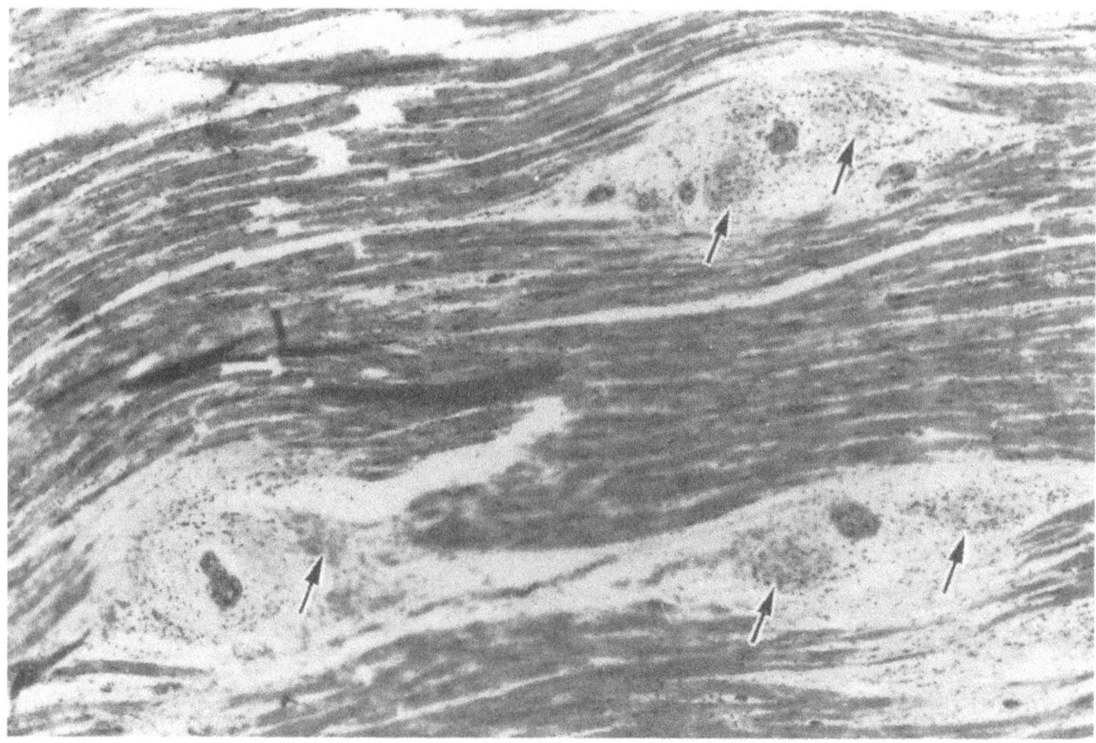

Fig. 2.9
Rheumatic fever

Myocard. Three typical spindle-shaped perivascular scars following rheumatic carditis. Some small remnants of the granuloma are present (*arrows*)

Biological significance of the Aschoff granuloma

The Klinge-cycle "fibrinoid – granuloma – scar" unquestionably expresses the course of the tissue processes encountered in the majority of the cases of the disease in adolescents and adults. The significance of this classic myocardial process for the continuing quality of the heart musculature, however, is of only a minor degree as the granulomata are exclusively in the heart connective tissue and never in the musculature itself (see Fig. 2.8). The destruction of a few neighbouring muscle fibres is not significant in the total mass of the myocardium.

Acute diffuse exudative rheumatic myocarditis

The rheumatic process, especially in the case of children, can run such a severe course that the death from heart failure may occur within a few weeks. In such rare cases, the pathological signs are impressive but the characteristic changes may be absent. Instead

Fibrinous exudate

of discrete foci of fibrinoid necrosis there is diffuse fibrinous exudate which penetrates from the interstitial tissues into the myocardium (Fig. 2.10). Large numbers of neutrophils and occasional lymphocytes are present (Fig. 2.11). Without clinical and serological evidence, the morphological picture would hardly suggest rheumatic carditis, particularly in the absence of a single Aschoff body. These myocardial changes have no similarity to the classical cycle "fibrinoid – granuloma – scar". They are rather concerned with a qualitatively and quantitatively quite different process, in which, in contrast to the interstitially occurring Aschoff granuloma, the heart musculature itself is affected. It might be possible that this is a direct effect of streptolysin. In our autopsy

Coronary arteritis

investigations, there was a simultaneous presence of severe coronary arteritis with a fibrinoid necrosis of the vascular wall.

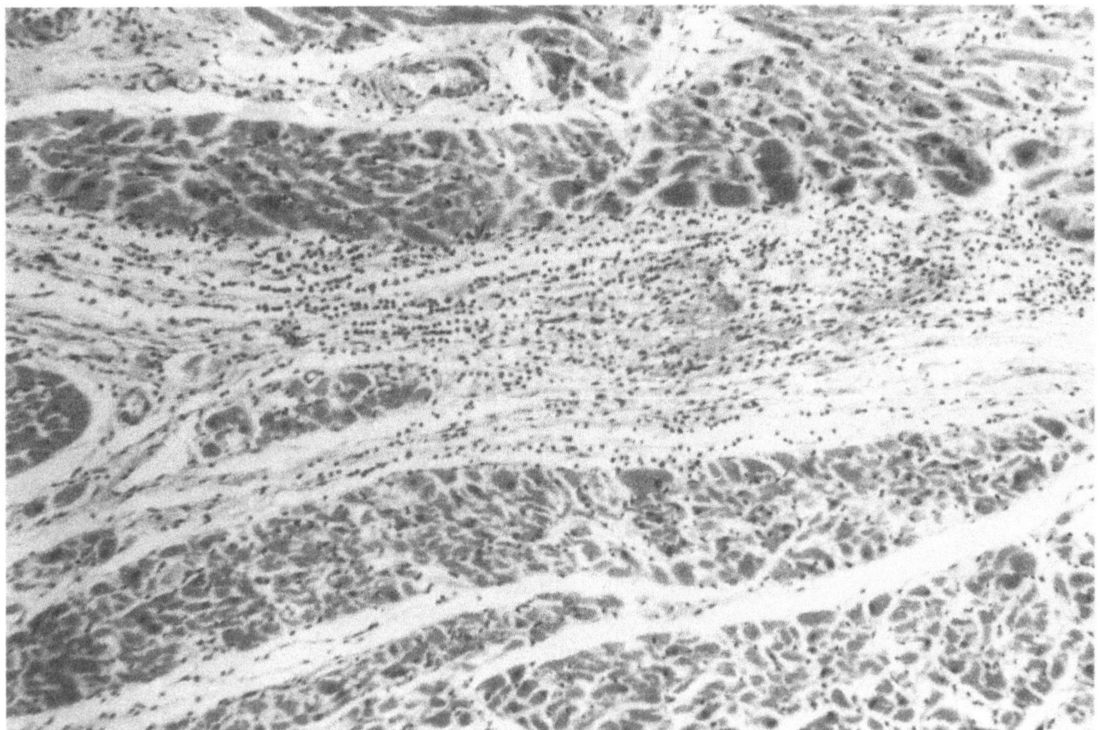

Diffuse exudative myocarditis. Interstitium and muscle fibres are soaked in fibrin and infiltrated by neutrophils

Fig. 2.10
Rheumatic fever

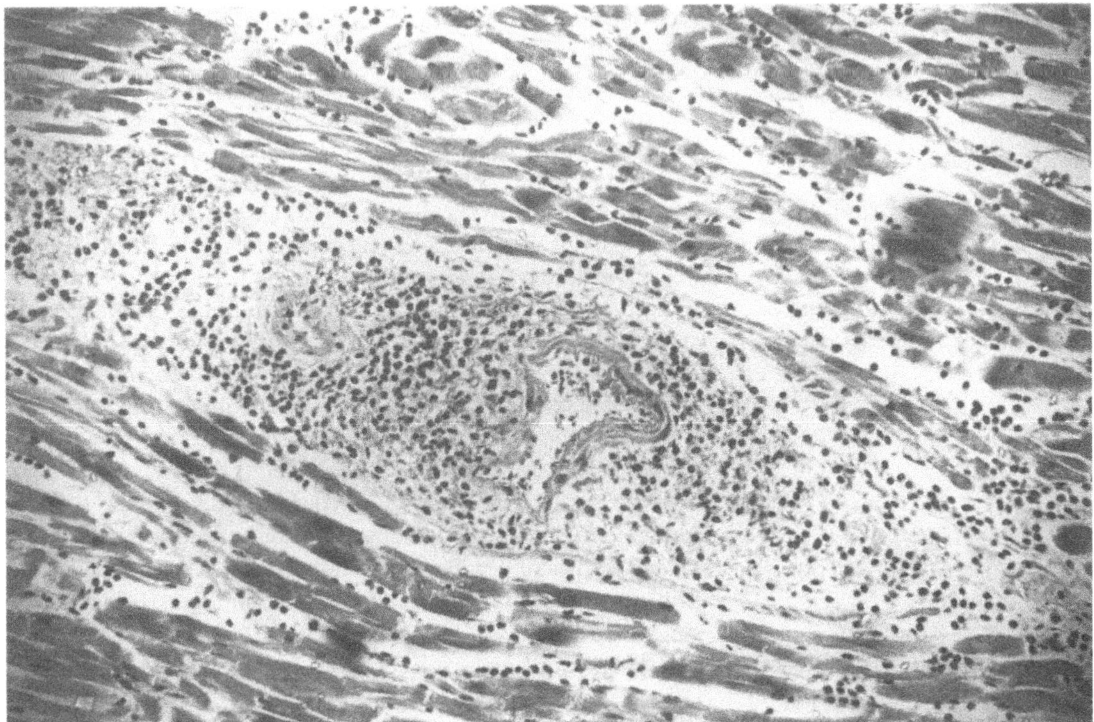

Diffuse exudative myocarditis. Perivascular tissue. Myocardium and the wall of a coronary vessel are infiltrated by fibrin and neutrophils

Fig. 2.11
Rheumatic fever

Fatal course

The grade of severity and extent of these diffuse exudative processes correspond to the stormy course and fatal outcome of this type of carditis.

Chronic lingering myo-aggressive rheumatic myocarditis

Our knowledge of pathological anatomy was entirely based on autopsy material until the middle of the last century, but since then biopsy material obtained at cardiac surgery has produced material from patients who, at the time of surgery, showed neither clinical nor laboratory evidence of active rheumatic carditis.

Granulomata in cardiac auricles

The finding of granulomata in operatively removed auricles of the left atrium was therefore a matter of considerable surprise, especially because it concerned patients who did not show any clinical hallmarks of RF. They were regarded from the first observers as typical Aschoff granulomata patients.

Our own considerable material showed the following features:

- The granulomata are found in the loose subendothelial tissue in the neighbourhood of fine muscle fibres. Such fibres are destroyed (Fig. 2.12).
- No fibrinoid was seen but only small muscle fragments.
- The granulomata contain histiocytes as well as cells of myogenic origin (Fig. 2.13).

All three criteria distinguish these granulomata sharply from Aschoff granuloma, which occurs exclusively in vascular connective tissue. We have termed these granulomata "myo-aggressive granulomata" (Fassbender 1963).

Myo-aggressive granuloma in fatal cases

This has led us to a search for such bodies in the myocardium of patients dying from RF. We found this type of lesion in three cases of recurrent activity. It is noteworthy that we have not seen this type of lesion in association with typical Aschoff nodes. Whilst in typical rheumatic myocarditis the lesions occur exclusively in perivascular connective tissue and at most involve a few peripheral myofibrils, the heart muscle itself is spared (see p. 15). The "myo-aggressive granuloma", on the other hand, spares the connective tissue but is found in the myocardium itself (Figs. 2.14, 2.15).

Fatal myocardial insufficiency

If these diffuse myocardial granulomata destroy a considerable part of the contractile substance, a fatal myocardial insufficiency is understandable (Figs. 2.16, 2.17).

Myo-aggressive granuloma in animal experiment

As early as 1906, Geipel described nodules both in connective tissue and in the myocardium. Von Albertini (1953) also referred to the occurrence of myocardial granulomata. Of the many efforts to produce an experimental model of rheumatic myocardial lesions only those of Murphy (1952) were attended by any semblance of success. However, the lesions found in rabbit hearts following repeated injections of killed group A-streptococci do not resemble the Aschoff body but are lesions of heart muscle: a primary necrosis of heart muscle is followed by a secondary formation of granuloma ("myo-aggressive granuloma"). It has been generally recognized that this experimental picture does not represent the equivalent of the classical lesions seen in RF.

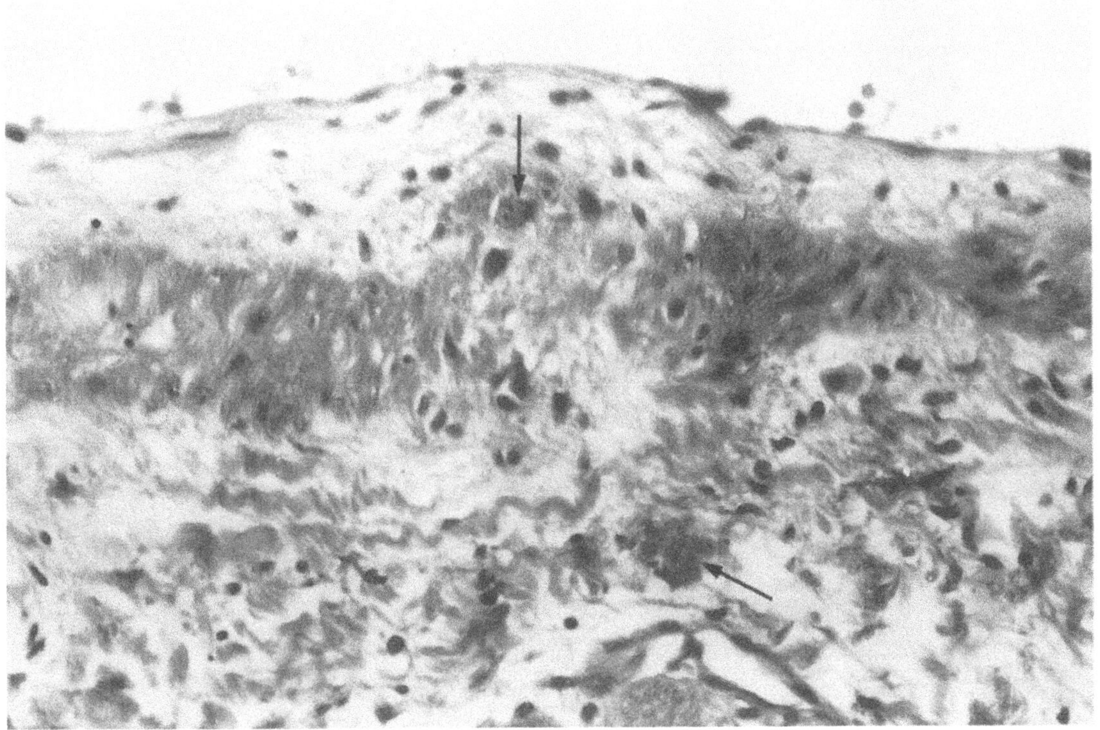

Myo-aggressive granuloma in the left auricle. The subendothelial muscle layer has been destroyed. In the granuloma, several myogenic giant cells (*arrows*)

Fig. 2.12
Rheumatic fever

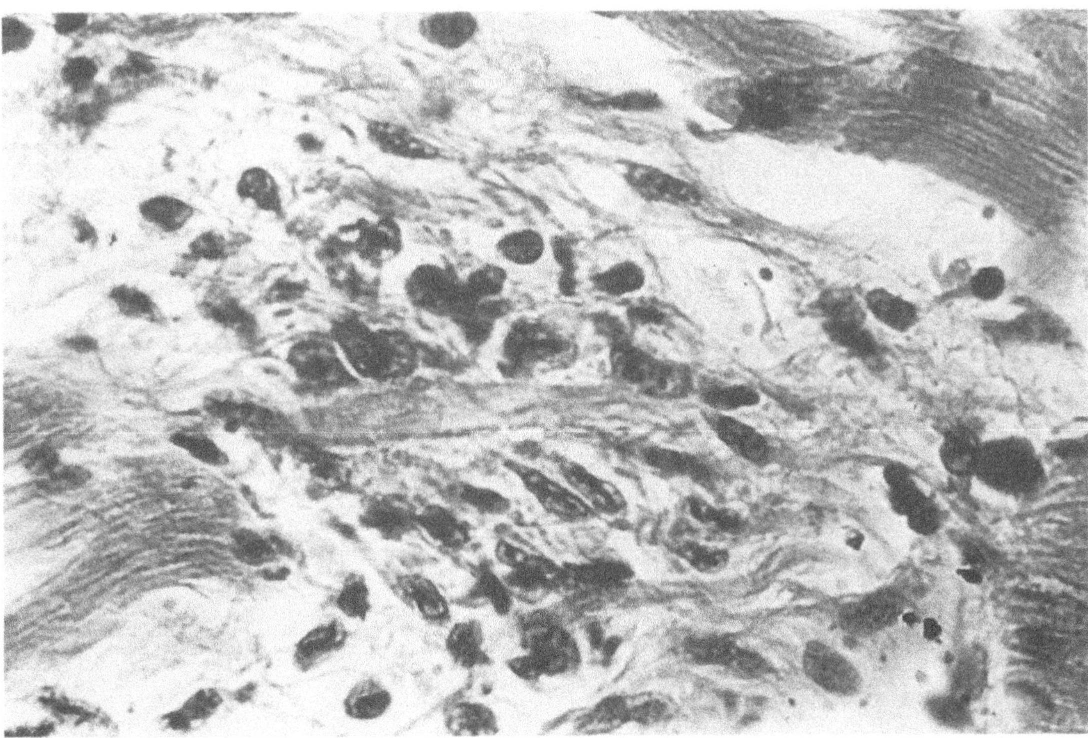

Myo-aggressive granuloma. A necrotic fragment of heart muscle is surrounded by macrophages and myogenic giant cells

Fig. 2.13
Rheumatic fever

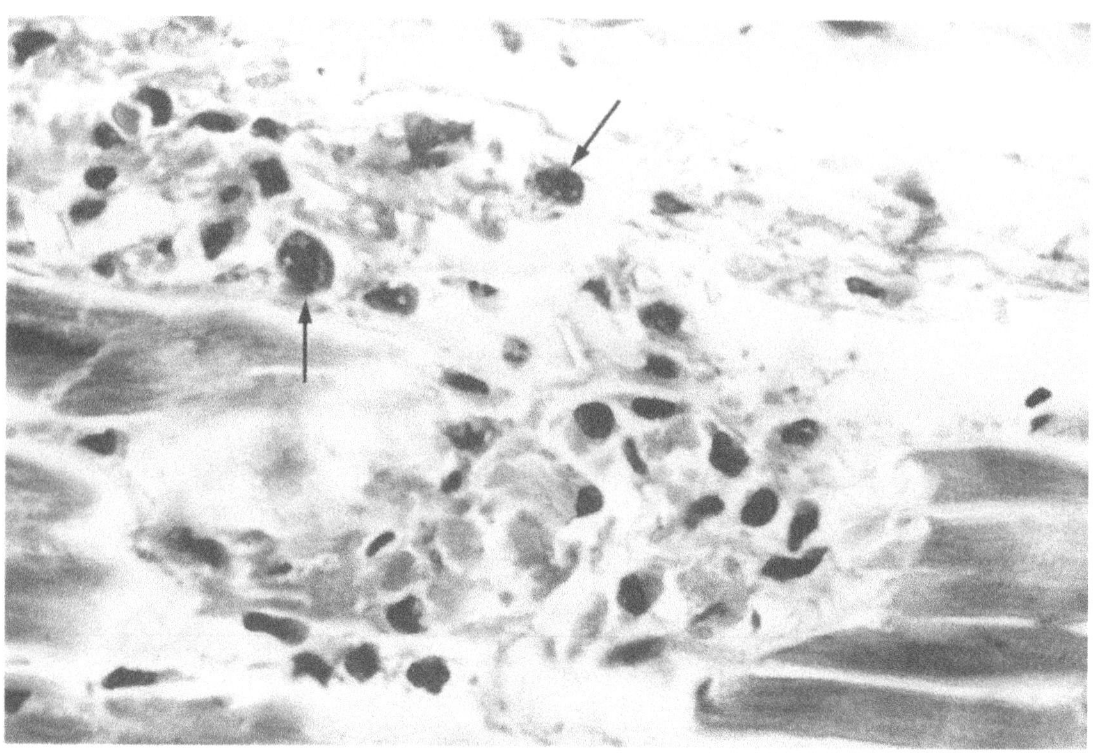

Fig. 2.14
Rheumatic fever

Myo-aggressive granuloma showing destruction of several myofibre bundles. Some myogenic giant cells (*arrows*)

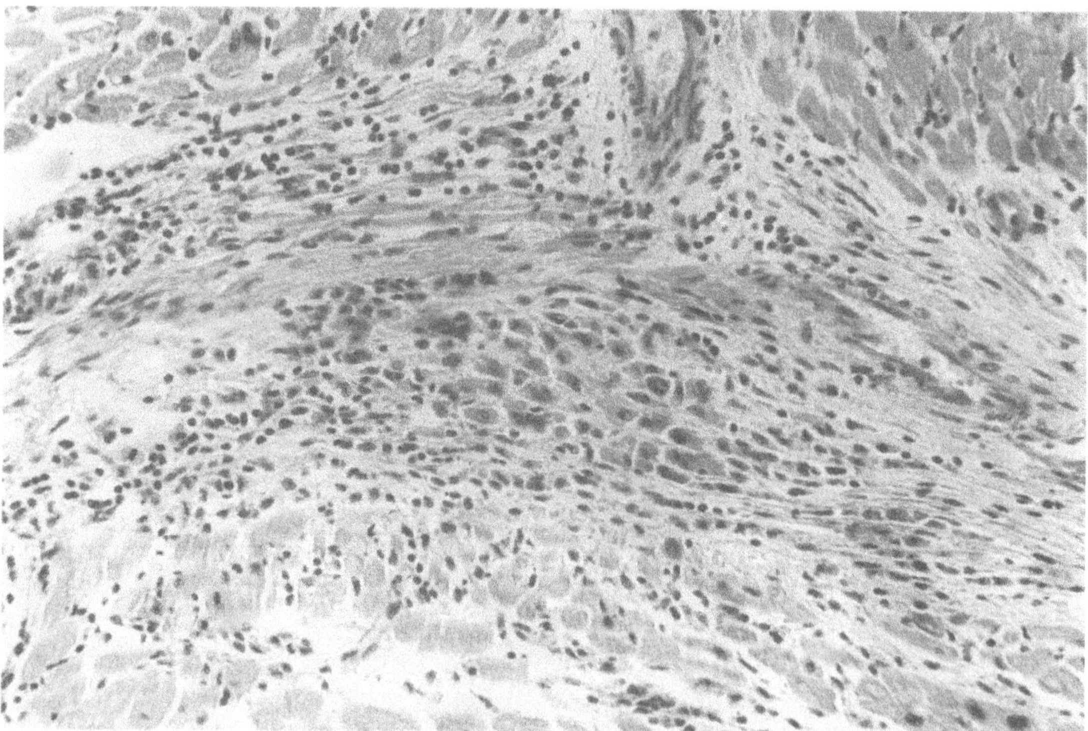

Fig. 2.15
Rheumatic fever

Myo-aggressive granuloma of long standing, consisting predominantly of myogenic cells. Extensive destruction of the myocard

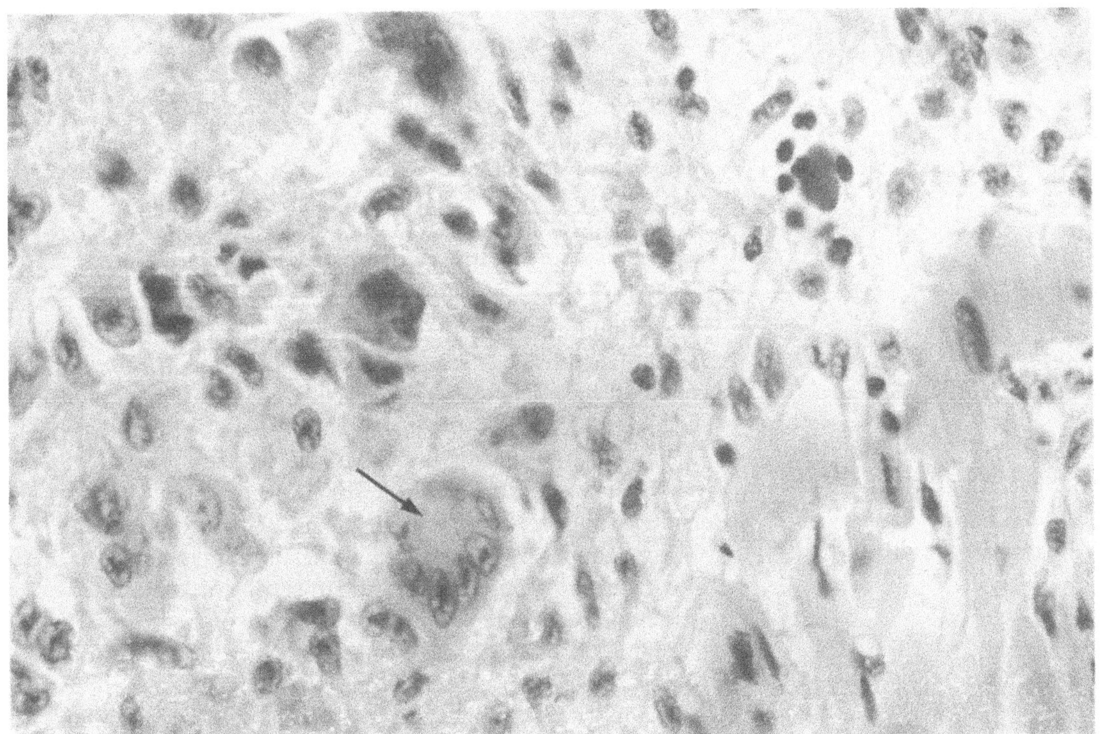

Myo-aggressvie granuloma with multi-nucleated myogenic giant cells (*arrow*), macrophages, and lymphocytes. *Bottom right*, remnants of muscle fibres

Fig. 2.16
Rheumatic fever

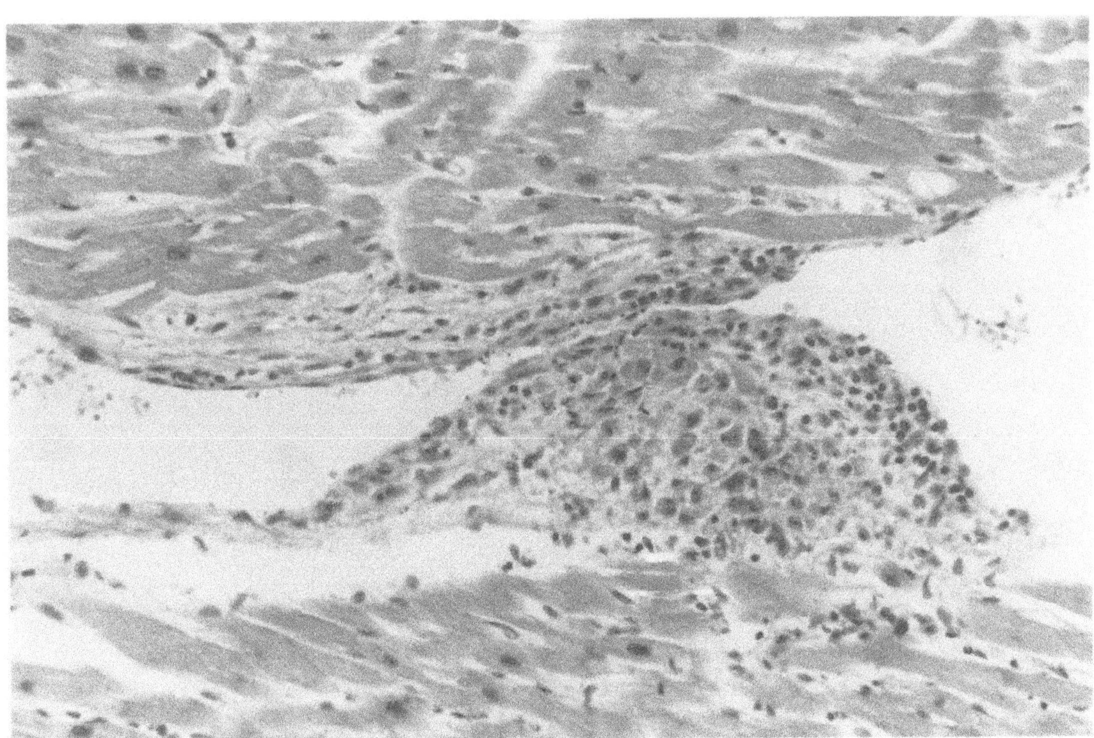

A myo-aggressive granuloma is narrowing the lumen of a small coronary vein

Fig. 2.17
Rheumatic fever

2.7.2 Endocardium

The main clinical interest in RF concerns the endocardial involvement and its consequences.

Structure of endocardium

The structure of the endocardium corresponds largely to that of the intima of the blood vessels. A flat, single-staged endothelial cell layer forms the contact surface with the blood-stream. The endothelium lies upon a basement membrane. External to this, a loosely structured, avascular layer of fibres is attached. As the heart valves are reduplications of the endocardium, they generally show the same structure as the parietal endocardium and are normally free of blood vessels. In its florid stage, the inflammation of the parietal endocardium is clinically insignificant. It can be life-threatening if the branches of the His' bundle are affected, as Aschoff (1904) observed in an unusual case. The inflammatory process of the valve endocardium, however, is of great clinical importance.

Inflammatory process

The inflammatory process in the endocardium is similar to that in the myocardium and pericardium. It is somewhat modified by the structure of the endocardium. While in the case of myo- and pericardium, fibrinoid change results from increased permeability of capillaries of perivascular connective tissue, plasma components enter the endocardium from the intracardiac aspect. Influx of fibrinogen and fibrinoid damage occur diffusely over a large area of subendothelial tissue. With a large accumulation of fibrin, in a recent case, some neutrophils occur, while fibrinoid change as such is rarely associate with neutrophil infiltration (Fig. 2.18).

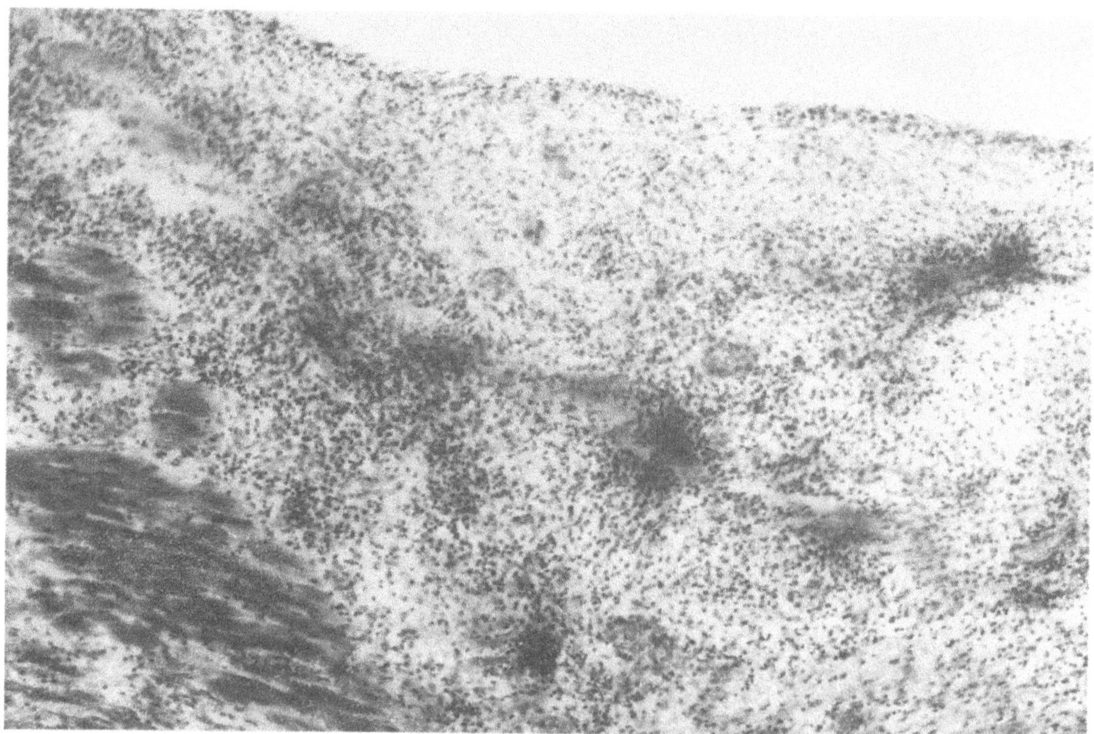

Fig. 2.18
Rheumatic fever

Parietal endocarditis with small fibrin remnants and extensive infiltration by neutrophils and lymphocytes

In the heart valves, appearances differ from those in the general endocardial layer: fibrinoid is deposited focally rather than in a more diffuse arrangement. According to position and size of these foci, such surface deformity may result that warty fibrinoid vegetations can be distinguished superficially. Subendothelial fibrinoid foci are far less common here than beads of fibrin which are commonly situated at the margins of cusps where they meet on closure. The topography of the subendothelial morbid process is inadequate to account for occurrence of these vegetations.

Heart valves

We found from light-microscopical investigations of heart valves derived from autopsy two distinct processes which are responsible for the valve damage:

Two different processes of rheumatic endocarditis

1. Fibrinoid nodules and Aschoff granulomata can develop in the interior of the heart valves and in the chordae (Fig. 2.19). This acute stage is followed by an induration. The sequel of resorption of the exudative events and granuloma formation in the endocardium differs from those seen in the myo- and pericardium. Fibroblasts of varying size as well as lymphocytes, and plasma cells appear around the streaks of fibrin (Fig. 2.20). Giant cells with multiple nuclei are rarely seen. This variety of connective tissue reaction is morphologically nonspecific. There are, however, also focal areas of fibrinoid change in association with collagen fibres which are surrounded by medium-sized to large fibroblasts: here, the appearances largely correspond to those of Aschoff nodes in the myocardium.

   Valve shrinkage

   With time, the valvular scar undergoes progressive shrinkage. Calcification may follow. Thus, the normally mobile valve components may turn into a hard, immobile rigid structure which not only restricts blood flow but also allows for regurgitation. The result is valvular insufficiency (Fig. 2.21).
2. At the rim of the valve cusps, a different process can occur: The cells of the valvular endocardium are normally single-layered and flat (Fig. 2.22). In patients who had died of acute RF, we found instead a marked proliferation of the endothelial cells which had become high-cylindrical in shape. These large, cylindrical cells have dark, oval nuclei and are arranged in the form of a dense palisade thus producing a brush-like superficial structure (Figs. 2.23, 2.24). This coarse surface furthers the deposition of fibrinous clots (Fig. 2.25). At the free rims of the valve cusps, there occur the grey, shiny little growths which after a time fuse with the valve cusps rims. The situation is quite different in the valve commissures. Here, the fibrin deposits lead to an adhesion of the opposing valve cusps rims and a permanent fibrous adhesion results (Fig. 2.26). This process explains the progression to a valvular stenosis with its clinical consequences (Fig. 2.27).

   Palisade-like transformation of endocardium cells

   Fibrous adhesion

   Valvular stenosis

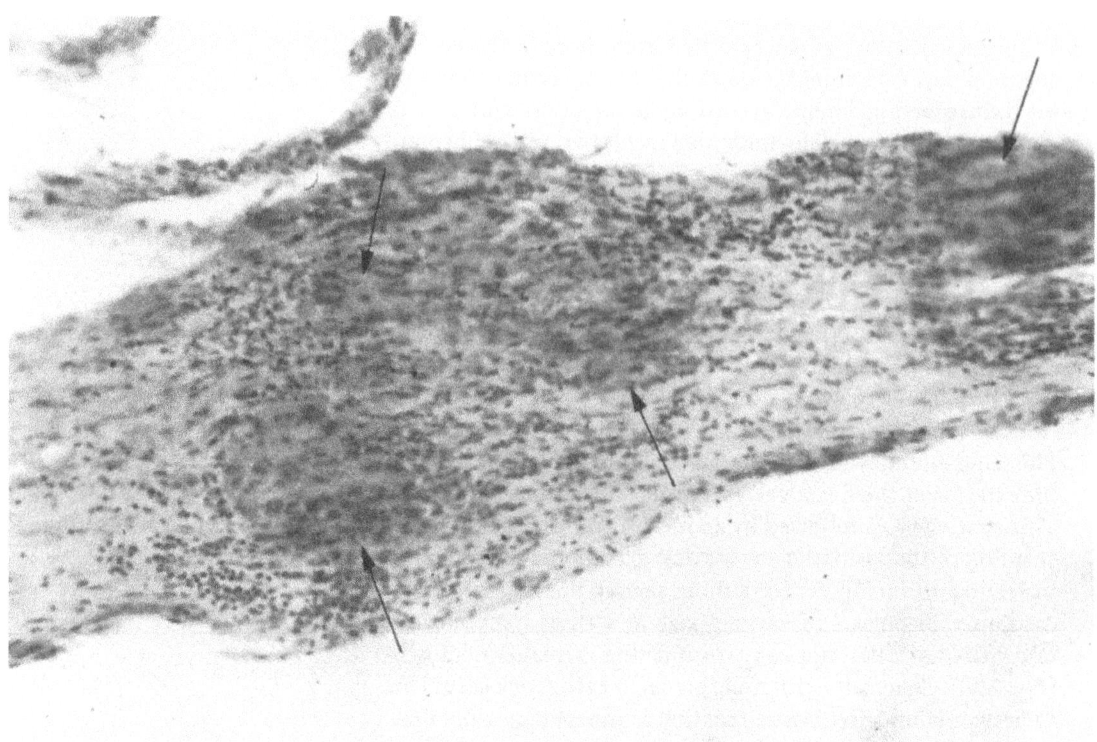

Fig. 2.19
Rheumatic fever

Several Aschoff granulomata (*arrows*) in a mitral valve

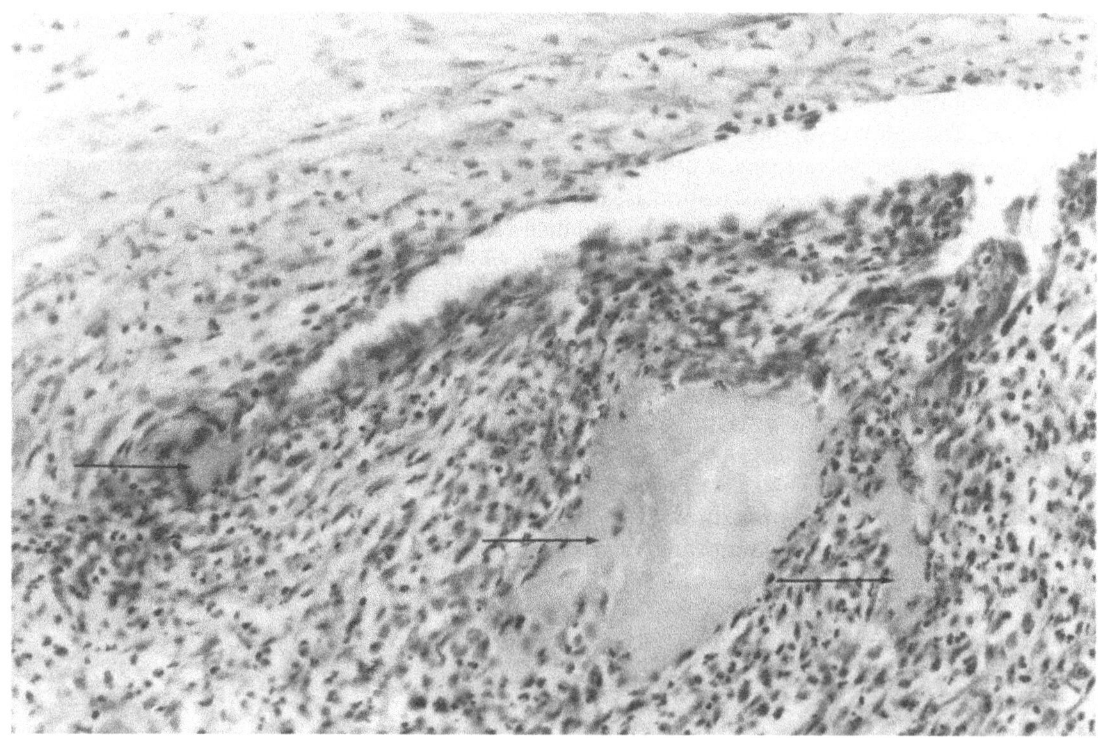

Fig. 2.20
Rheumatic fever

Endocarditis affecting the junction of an aortic valve cusp. Fibrin (*arrows*) has been deposited within the granulating endocardium. In the *left corner*, there is some freshly deposited fibrin. Lining cells are swollen

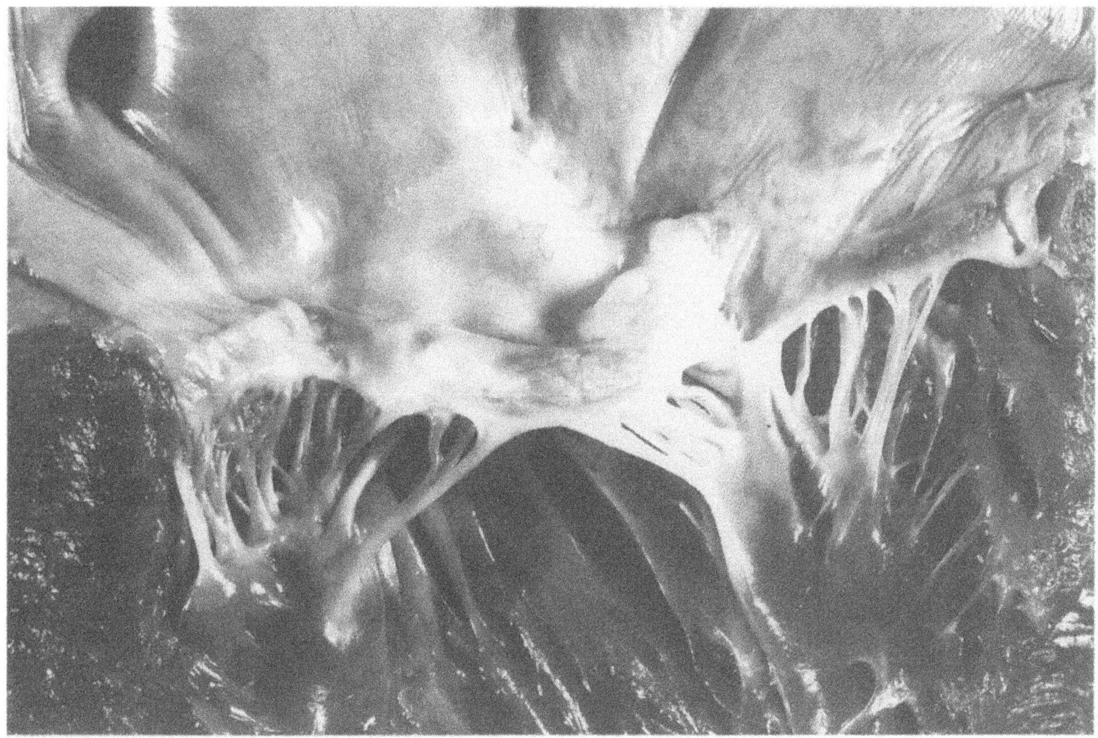

Shrinkage and deformity of the mitral valve with thickened and shortened chordae

Fig. 2.21
Rheumatic fever

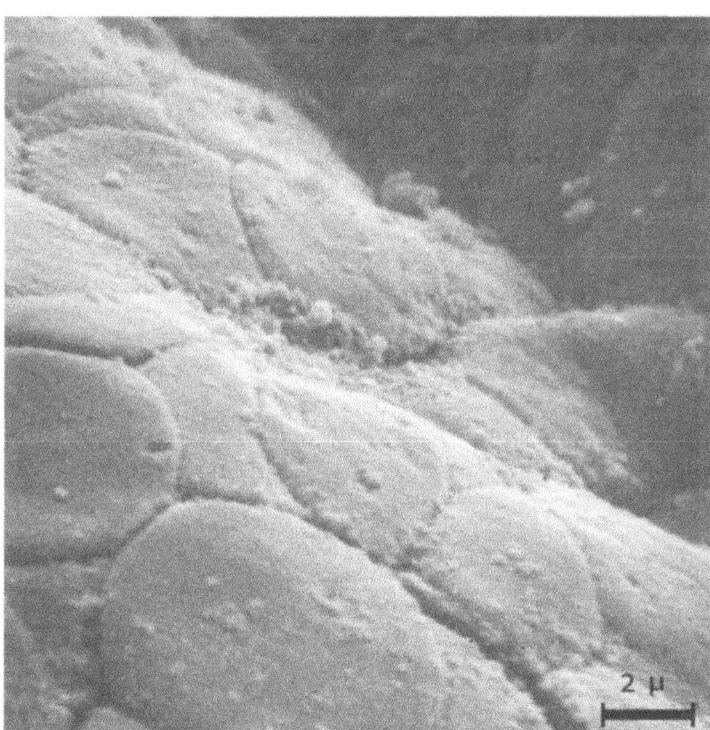

Normal endothelium of a bicuspidal valve. The endothelial cells form a pavement and have a smooth surface (scanning electron micrograph)

Fig. 2.22
Rheumatic fever

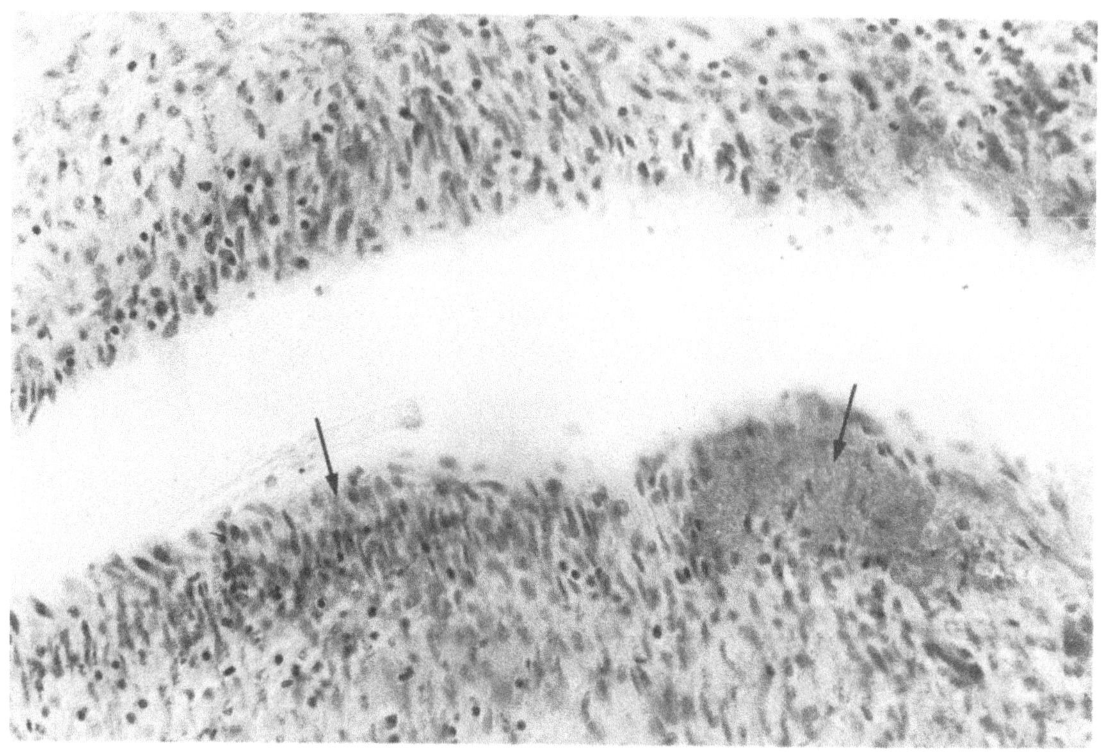

Fig. 2.23
Rheumatic fever

Brush-like transformation of the cells of the endocardial lining of two opposing cusps. Fibrin deposits (*arrows*)

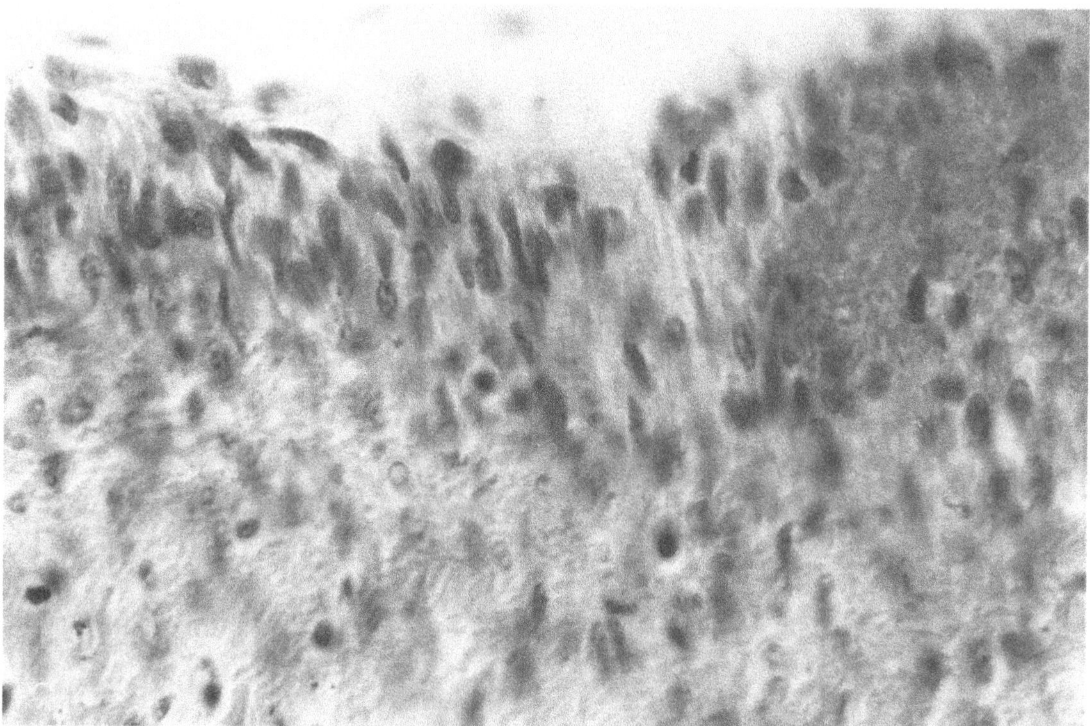

Fig. 2.24
Rheumatic fever

Endocard. Enlarged section of Fig. 2.23. The proliferated endothelial cells have formed a palisade. On the *right*, adherent fibrin

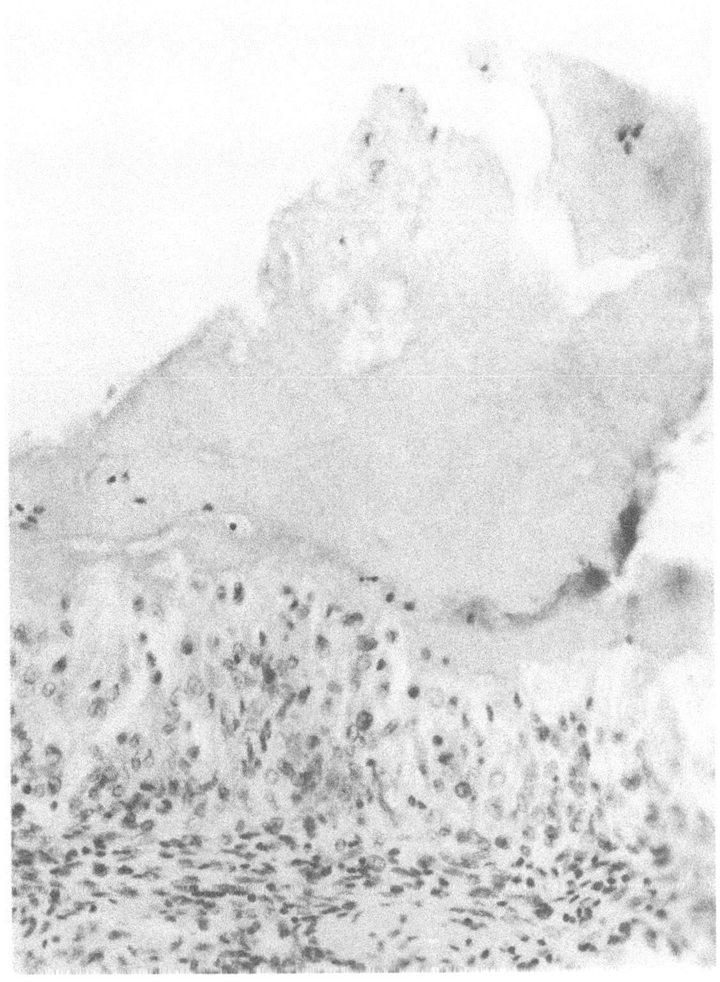

Deposition of a fibrinous clot on top of brush-like transformed endothelium of the mitral valve

Fig. 2.25
Rheumatic fever

Thus, it is shown that two different rheumatic mechanisms lie behind the valvular insufficiency and -stenosis: shrinkage of the valves, resulting in incompetence, is caused by a proliferative process with formation of granulomata inside the valvular stroma as well as in tendinous fibres. After the fading of granulomata, the shrinkage of the valves starts. The valves and tendinous fibres become too short and the valves incompetent.

Opposed to that, it is a case of palisade-like proliferation of the valvular endothelium (see p. 27) which causes the valvular stenosis. A brush-like surface develops and thus deposition of fibrin masses can occur. These fibrin plates lead to adhesion and finally to coalescence of the valvular margins among themselves. The valvular orifice becomes thus restricted and this results in the valvular stenosis (Fassbender 1975).

Minimal remnants following endocarditis

Careful examination of heart valves at death shows, in direct proportion to age, an increasing incidence of minimal adhesions of commissures of the aortic valve and of the chordae and cusp edges of the mitral valve (Fig. 2.28). These findings are so inconspicuous that they may easily be missed and are without functional

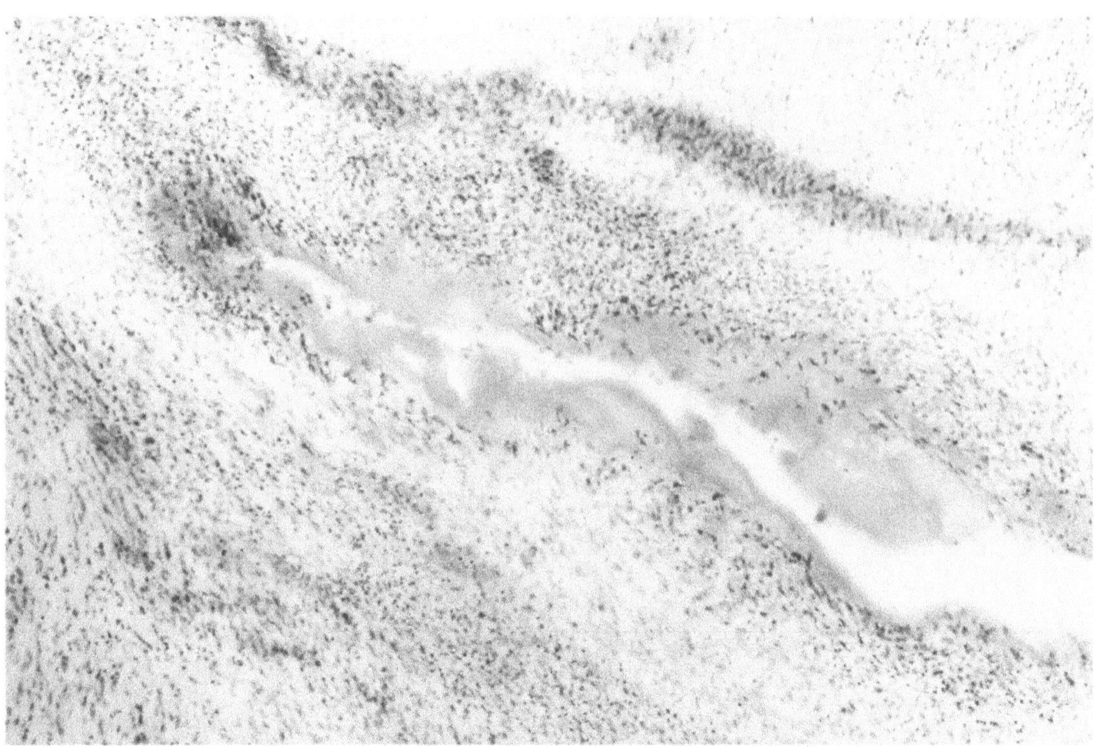

Fig. 2.26
Rheumatic fever

Fibrin adhering to the surface of a commissure of a bicuspidal valve. Both surfaces are covered with fibrin and this forms a stage preceding adhesion

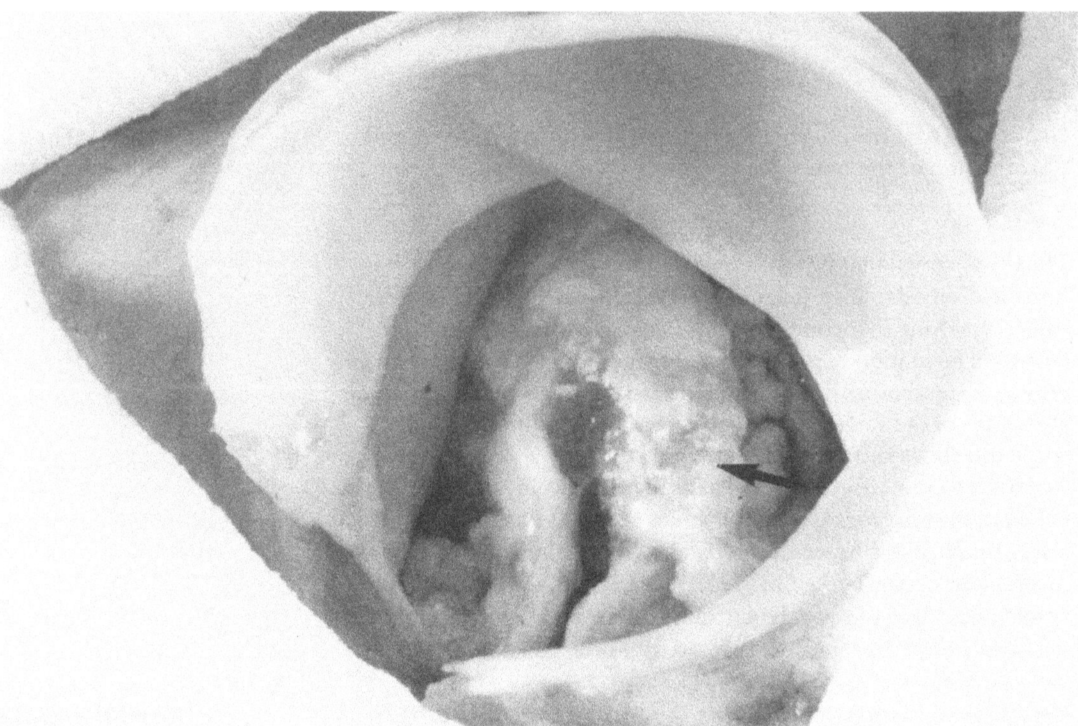

Fig. 2.27
Rheumatic fever

High-grade aortastenosis with partial calcification of the valve (*arrow*)

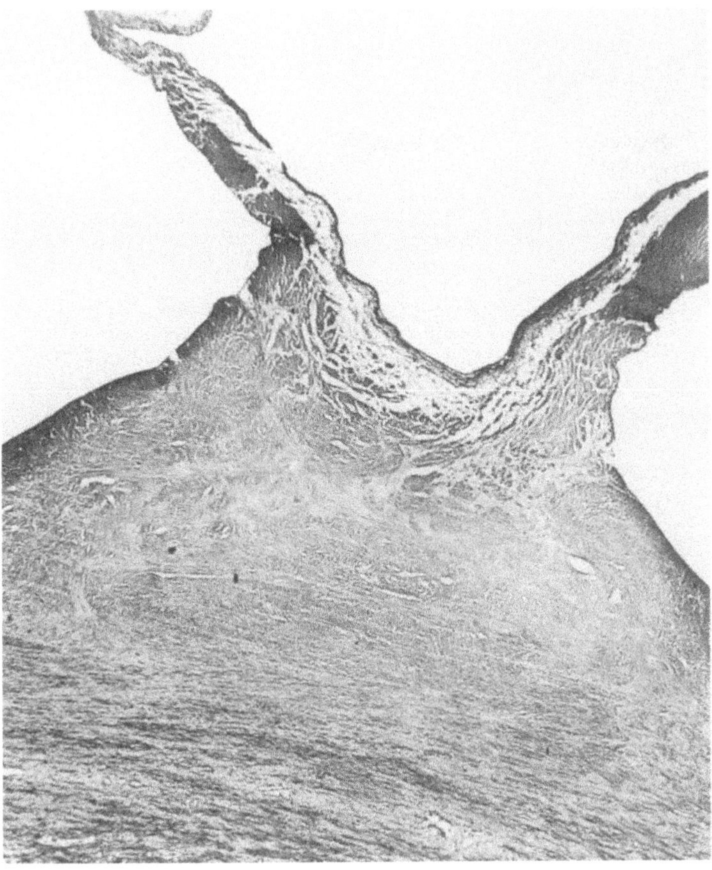

Long standing minimal adhesion representing the remainder of an old endocarditis affecting the commissure of the aortic valve without functional significance

Fig. 2.28
Rheumatic fever

significance. The question whether this represents the remains of a past attack of minimal rheumatic carditis remains open. In the absence of other characteristic scars of healed RF, it is more probable that an endothelial lesion of different etiology has led to fibrin deposition.

Vascularisation of heart valves

During the phase of subendothelial activity in the endocardium, angioblasts are found in the valve stroma, presumably as part of connective tissue cell proliferation; these are the basis for the formation of small blood vessels. Thus, an originally avascular valve may become vascularized as a sequel to rheumatic endocarditis (Fig. 2.29). Those vessels may, in the course of subsequent rheumatic activity as in the case of the pericardial scar, allow for exudation of fibrinogen. It has also been suggested that they may be instrumental in the occasional sequel of bacterial infection.

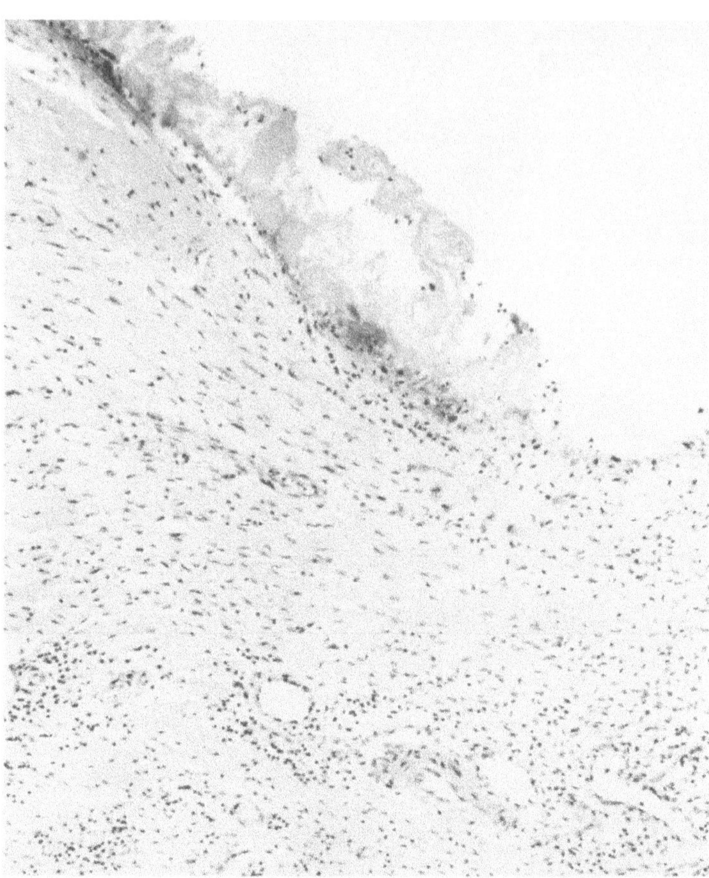

Fig. 2.29
Rheumatic fever

Relapsing endocarditis in a previously damaged valve. The newly formed arteries and veins are surrounded by lymphocytes and fibroblasts. Fresh fibrin on the surface

2.7.3 Pericardium

Exudate formation in mesodermal spaces

As in other mesodermal cavities, effusions collect in the pericardial sac. Fibrinogen as well as proteolytic enzymes are present which may serve to attack the cohesion of mesothelial cells. The formation of exudate is evidence of capillary damage in the submesothelium. The situation of capillaries in the tissue of the pericardium is comparable to that existing in the synovial membrane. In both cases, there is a network of capillaries which is not separated from the mesodermal cavity by a layer of epithelium. There is, however, in the pericardium and pleura, as distinct from synovium, a basement membrane beneath the superficial cell layer. In both cases, a serous dialysate flows from the capillaries into a cavity which has a negative pressure. This may explain the similar reaction shown in both systems to a general systemic process as witnessed in RF and rheumatoid arthritis (RA), similar in nature and sometimes in timing. A plasma dialysate may be readily resorbed into lymphatics: when, however, through capillary damage, fibrinogen has exuded and its fibrin polymer product is present, then resorption, if it takes place, requires the participation of large numbers of macrophages and fibroblasts in the exudate.

The fibrin is sequentially compressed and stretched by cardiac action. Since cardiac motion differs for different sections of the heart, fibrin covers the left chamber in the form of a net, while parallel wavy lines are formed over the right ventricle at right angles to the outflow-tract (Fig. 2.30). This configuration is particularly marked if the pericardium still contains some fluid. If this is lacking, the two fibrin layers come together in diastole and are pulled apart in systole. This mechanism accounts for the "bread and butter"-pericarditis (Fig. 2.31). After a lapse of several days, macrophages, fibroblasts, and some neutrophils appear in large numbers. These changes correspond to the course taken by inflammatory exudates of serous membranes in general, and possess characteristic properties of RF. In addition, there are focal fibrin deposits in submesothelial tissue as well as fibrinoid degeneration of some collagen bundles.

Characteristics of rheumatic pericarditis

Granuloma of the Aschoff type in pericarditis

When a granuloma of the Aschoff type succeeds fibrinoid change, this may be considered to be characteristic for RF. These granulomata are, however, much less frequent in the epi- than in the myocardium. Indeed, they are rarely seen in the pericardium and are more variable in size and form and usually smaller than in the myocardium.

Scarring in pericarditis

If pericarditis predominantly affects the submesothelial tissue and little fibrin is deposited in the cavity, only a white, glistening area of scarring remains in the epicardium. If, however, too much fibrin has been laid down in the cavity for complete resorption to take place, then the visceral and parietal layers become attached to one another. Fibroblasts and capillaries enter from both sides, granulation tissue forms and eventually collagen fibres attach the two layers together. This pericardial scar tissue contains large numbers of vessels, particularly veins, and fat cells are sometimes seen in the interfibrillar spaces.

Formation of new interstitial layer

As the scar tissue is formed around the constantly pulsating heart, a loose connective tissue network of spongy consistency results, differing by a considerable degree of plasticity from the usual collagenous scar tissue. In accordance with this, the newly formed vessels follow a tortuous course, allowing for adaptation to cardiac movements. Thus, the heart is still enabled to pulsate with the necessary degree of freedom. Epicardial adhesions may be locally limited to individual fibre bundles or form a complete layer.

Residual infiltrates of lymphocytes and plasma cells

Even after the subsidence of an actual pericarditis, lymphocytes and plasma cells may persist in the loose scar tissue for a considerable period, either diffusely or perivascularly located. Lymphocyte foci or densely packed collections of plasma cells are also found. The duration of the persistence of these infiltrates cannot be deduced from examination of autopsy material, since it is not usually possible to date the preceding acute attack of RF.

Relapse of rheumatic pericarditis

The pericardium usually becomes re-involved with a recrudescence of rheumatic activity.

When rheumatic pericarditis has terminated, there is no residual calcification in the scar tissue ("armoured heart"), in contrast to the tuberculous pericarditis.

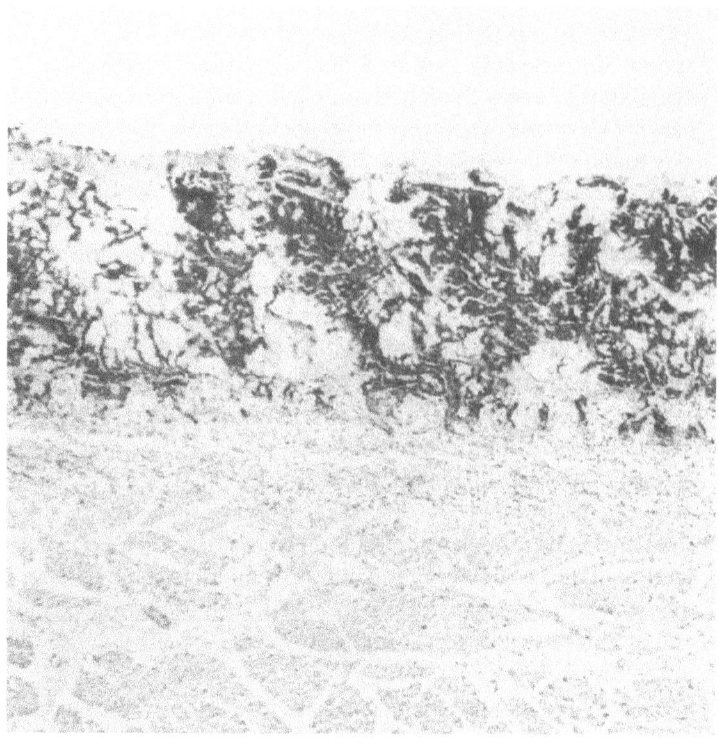

Fig. 2.30
Rheumatic fever

Pericarditis. Fibrin deposition on the epicardial surface showing early organization

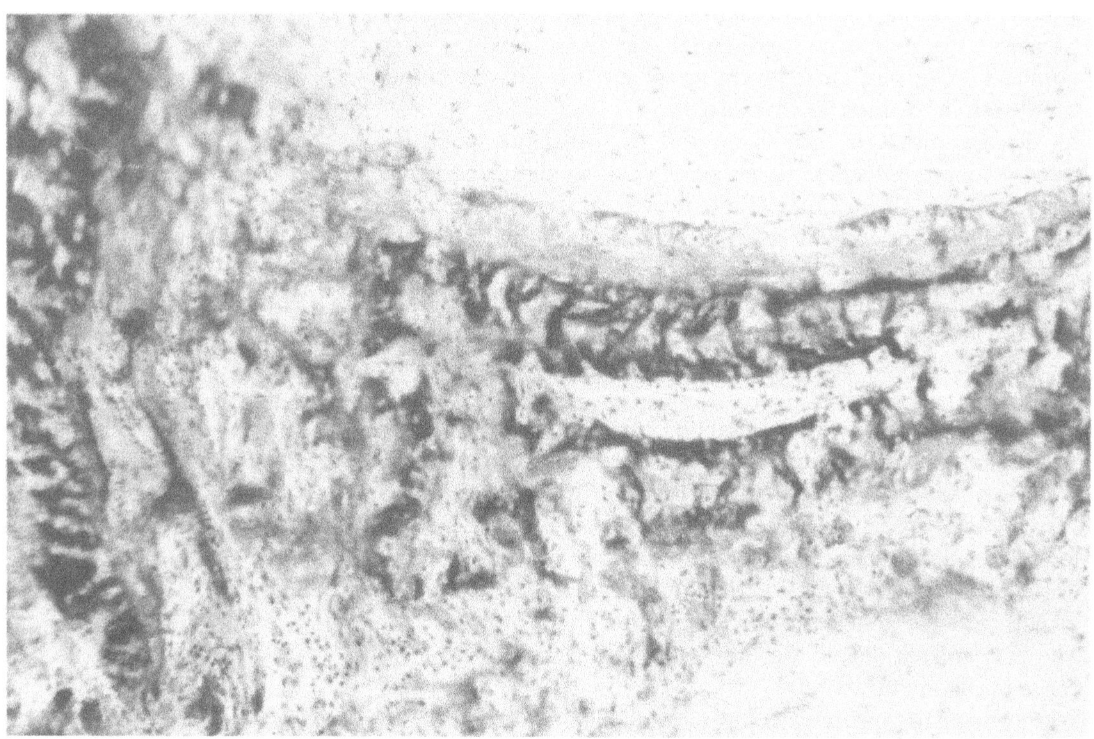

Fig. 2.31
Rheumatic fever

Fibrinous pericarditis. The two layers have become adherent and to the left of the figure, epicardium and pericardium show continuity

2.7.4 Blood Vessels

The arteries and veins are affected by RF in a manner analogous to that of the heart, a fact which becomes readily explicable when the similarity of structure in the form of the three layers is considered.

First systematic investigation

Klinge (1930) made a systematic post-mortem study of the localization, manner, and frequency of vascular involvement. He concluded that in RF, the tissue of vessels shows a more frequent involvement than the joints and may be more severely affected than the heart. It has to be remembered, however, that Klinge's assessment was based on material obtained at death from acute or recurring cases of RF. This does not permit an assessment of vascular involvement in cases of lesser severity without fatal outcome. Nevertheless, the findings of Klinge are of basic interest since they give some insight into the pathogenetic mechanisms of RF.

Rheumatic aortitis

Lesions are found particularly at the branch points of the aorta, the abdominal part, in contradistinction to syphilis, being more frequently affected than the thoracic portion. The vessels may show two different processes: adventitia or media may be involved by the way of the vasa vasorum or the intima may be affected directly. In the aorta, where structural differences are especially well-marked, Klinge was able to study this extensively.

Adventitia

The earliest phase in the adventitia consists of hyperaemia, oedema, and perivascular infiltration with lymphocytes with a smaller proportion of neutrophils. Such small foci sometimes contain-

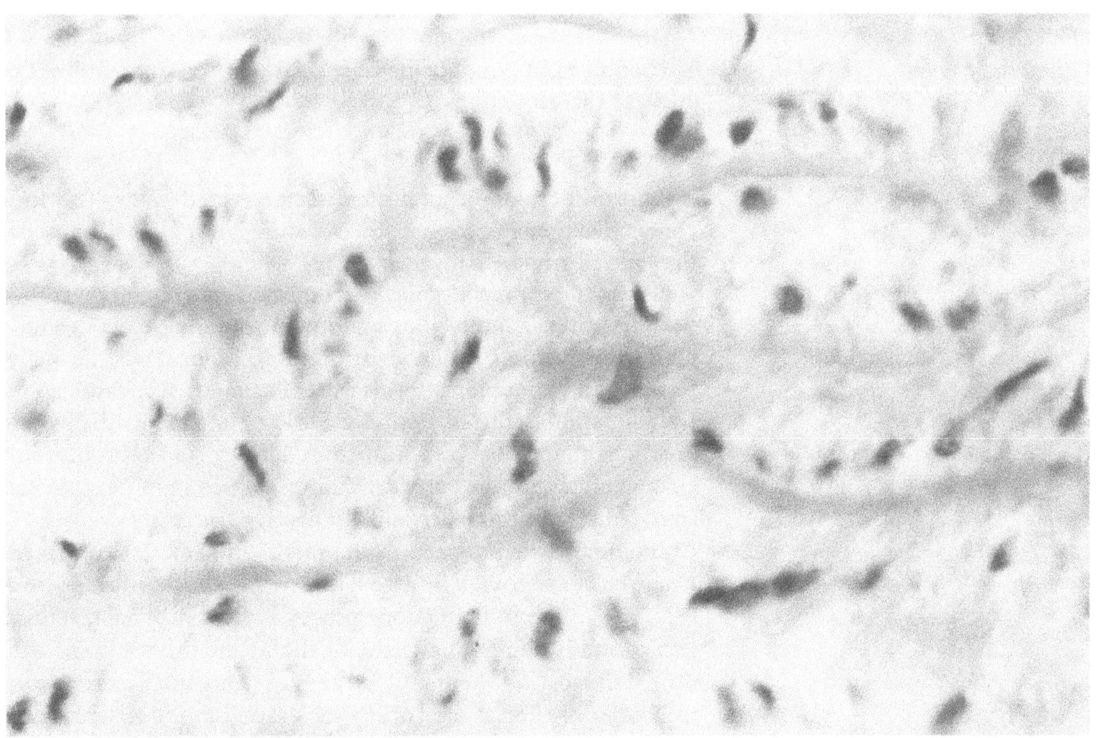

Fig. 2.32 Rheumatic fever

Aortic media. Oedema and swelling of fibres with reactive proliferation of local fibroblasts

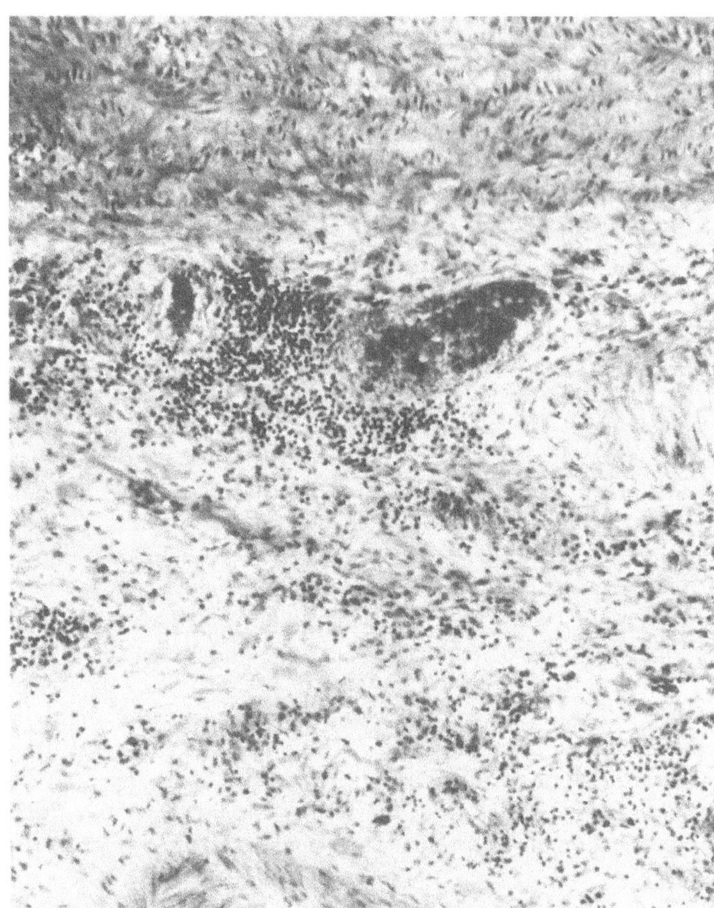

Fig. 2.33
Rheumatic fever

Aortic adventitia. Fibrinoid swelling and marked infiltration of neutrophils and lymphocytes, especially in the surroundings of the vasa vasorum

ing fibrin, develop around small arteries and veins. The local connective tissue fibres become separated, fragmented, and may undergo fibrinoid change (Fig. 2.32).
However, the compact typical Aschoff node is only rarely seen in the adventitia. Lymphocytes surround the granulomata in a rather diffuse fashion, while neutrophils disappear as the active phase of inflammation subsides. A collagenous scar results.

Media

Inflammation in the adventitia may reach into the media by progressing along the vasa vasorum. Linear zones of fibrinoid change affect bundles of elastic fibres, which later become surrounded by macrophages and connective tissue cells (Fig. 2.33). Granulomata are not seen in the media but rows of connective tissue cells are found in association with elastic fibre necrosis (Fig. 2.34). The inflammatory process results in small, collagenous scars in the elastic tissue of the media. Klinge coined the term "mesaortitis rheumatica" ranging from small perivascular infiltrates of the vasa vasorum to a rarely found extensive destruction of the media.

„Mesaortitis rheumatica"

Intimal lesions

The intimal lesions are analogous to those of the heart valves. As in heart valves, fibres may undergo a local or rarely a more widespread fibrinoid change (Fig. 2.35). During the further stage of

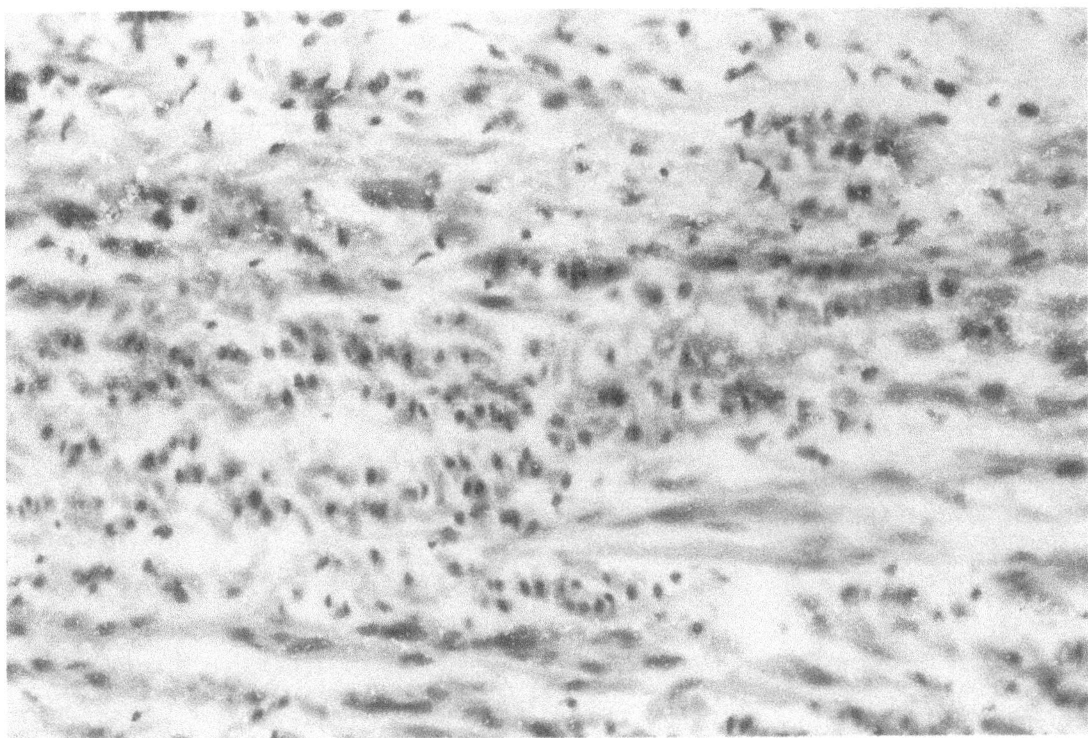

Aortic media. Neutrophils and fibroblasts surrounding focal swollen fibres

Fig. 2.34
Rheumatic fever

the process, there is a diffuse or more rarely focal proliferation of intimal cells with the addition of some lymphocytes and plasma cells and an occasional neutrophil. This may be indistinguishable from the granulation tissue and may transgress into the media and destroy it (Fig. 2.36). Healing of these intimal lesions results in foci of intimal sclerosis presenting as broad plaques of yellowish-white appearance. Klinge (1930) shows a picture of the abdominal aorta of a 21-year-old patient who died after a recurrence of RF. The intima is covered by sclerotic plaques. Thus, as in the case of the heart, all three layers of the great vessels may become involved.

Coronary arteritis

Lesions in small muscular vessels, such as the coronary arteries, are of special interest. Here, too, although all layers may become diseased, separate histological assessment of the structural components is not possible (Fig. 2.37). Usually, the whole thickness is involved, but intima and media are preferentially affected by fibrinoid change (Figs. 2.38, 2.39). This deposition of fibrin in the wall may be extensive enough to cause stenosis of the lumen (Fig. 2.40). Thus, acute changes of this nature may lead to fatal coronary occlusion. Scarring occurs in less severe cases depending on the extent of the preceding changes.

Coronary occlusion

Differences of arteritic processes in RA and RF

The arteritis in RA differs from the arteritic process in RF as follows: In contrast to RF, the crucial point of the vascular changes in RA occurs in the media; only in rare cases, the lumen is occluded and there are no neutrophils nor lymphocytic infiltrates. In contrast, the necrosis of the vessel wall in RA is surrounded by a more or less well-marked palisade of connective tissue cells (see p. 117).

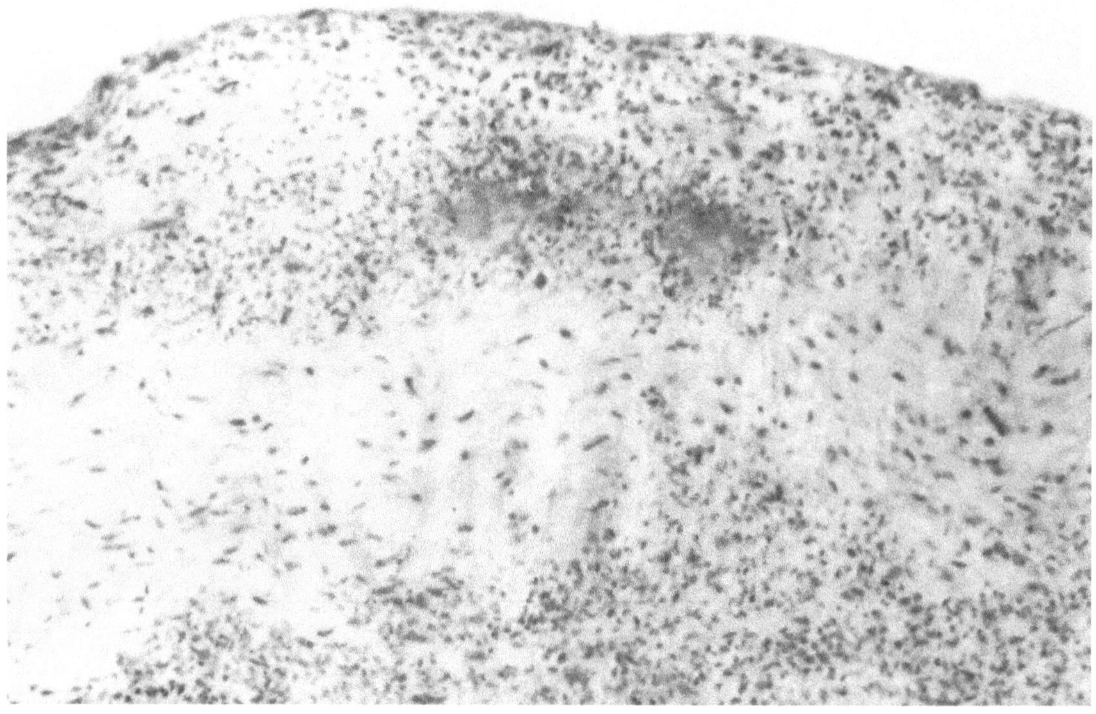

Fig. 2.35
Rheumatic fever

Aortic intima. Foci of fibrinoid swelling. Dense neutrophil and lymphocyte infiltrates invading the media from the intima

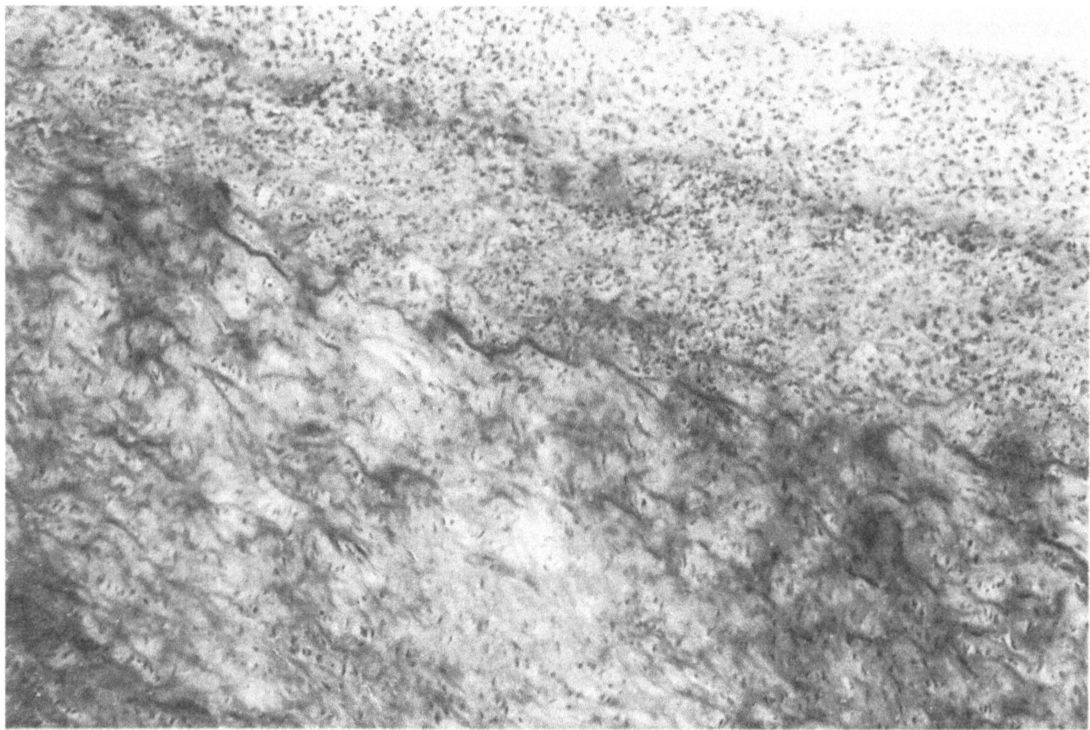

Fig. 2.36
Rheumatic fever

Severe aortitis involving intima and media. Neutrophil infiltration and fibrinoid swelling of the internal elastic membrane. There are foci of swollen and proliferated local fibroblasts in the media

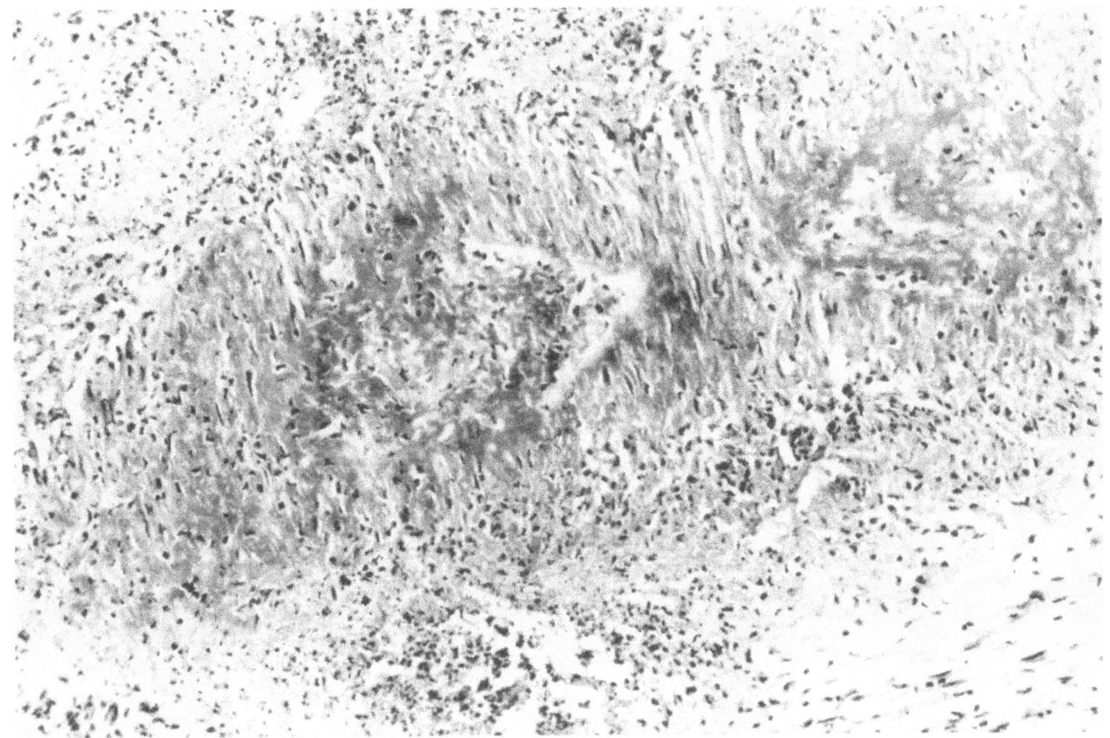

Coronary artery. Fibrinoid swelling extending through the wall with marked perivascular exudation of fibrin and neutrophil infiltration

Fig. 2.37
Rheumatic fever

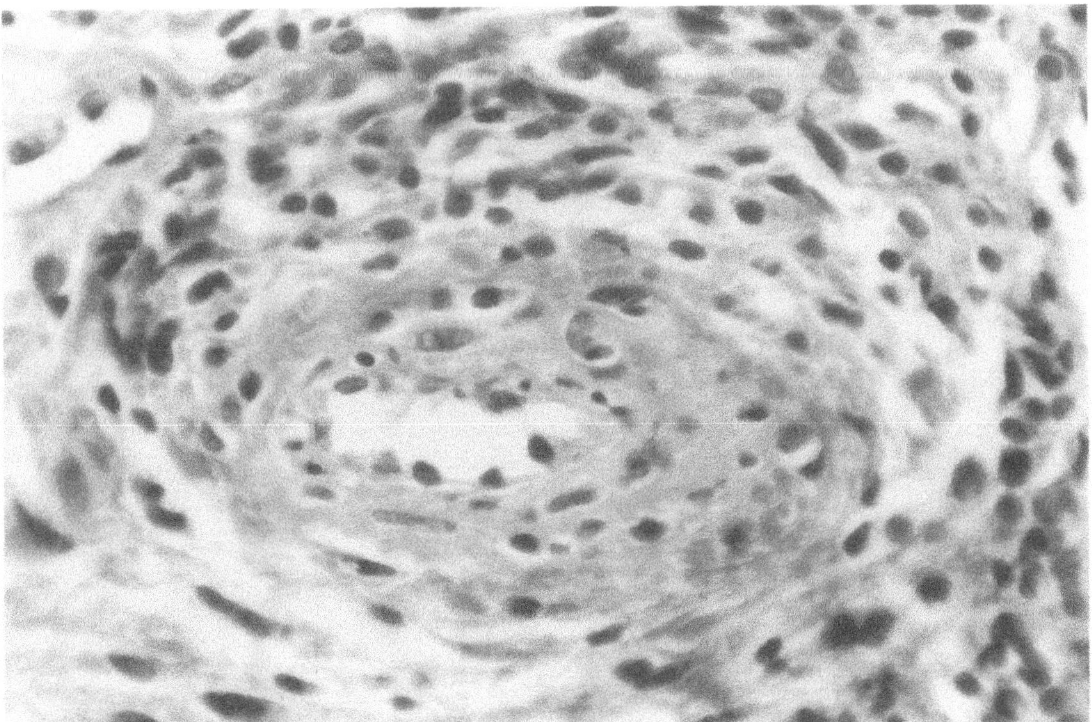

Coronary artery. Marked fibrinoid swelling of the media with proliferative reaction and lymphocyte infiltration

Fig. 2.38
Rheumatic fever

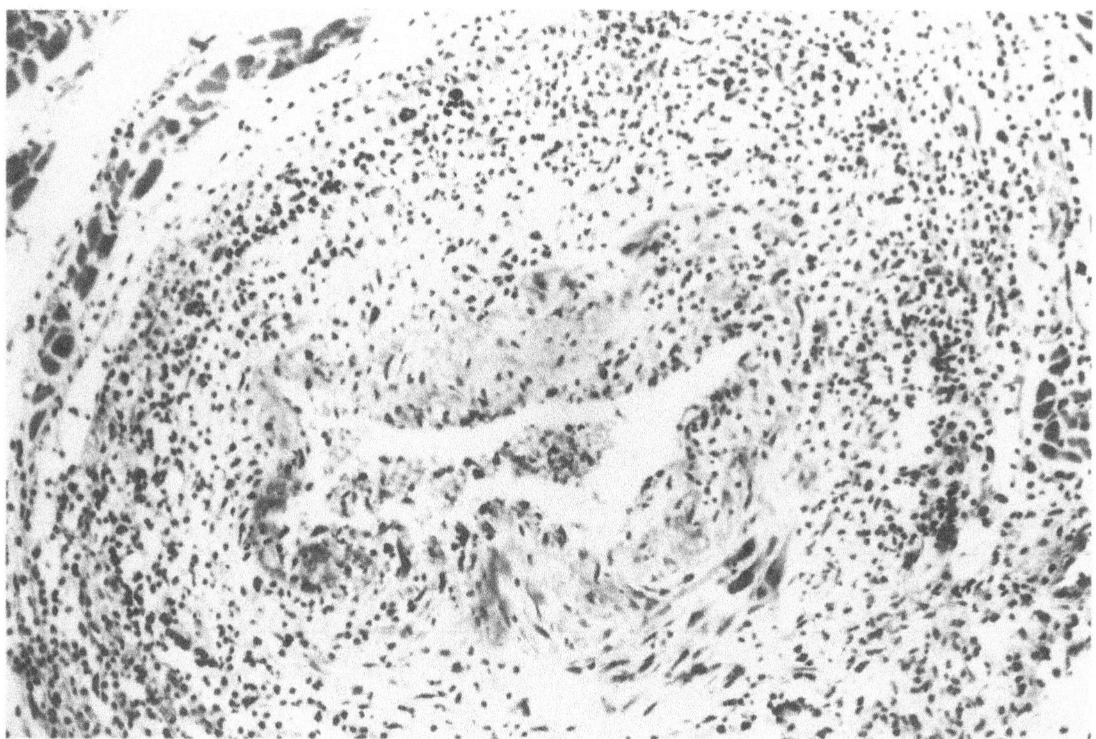

Fig. 2.39
Rheumatic fever

Coronary vein. Exudative inflammation mainly limited to the media and adventitia

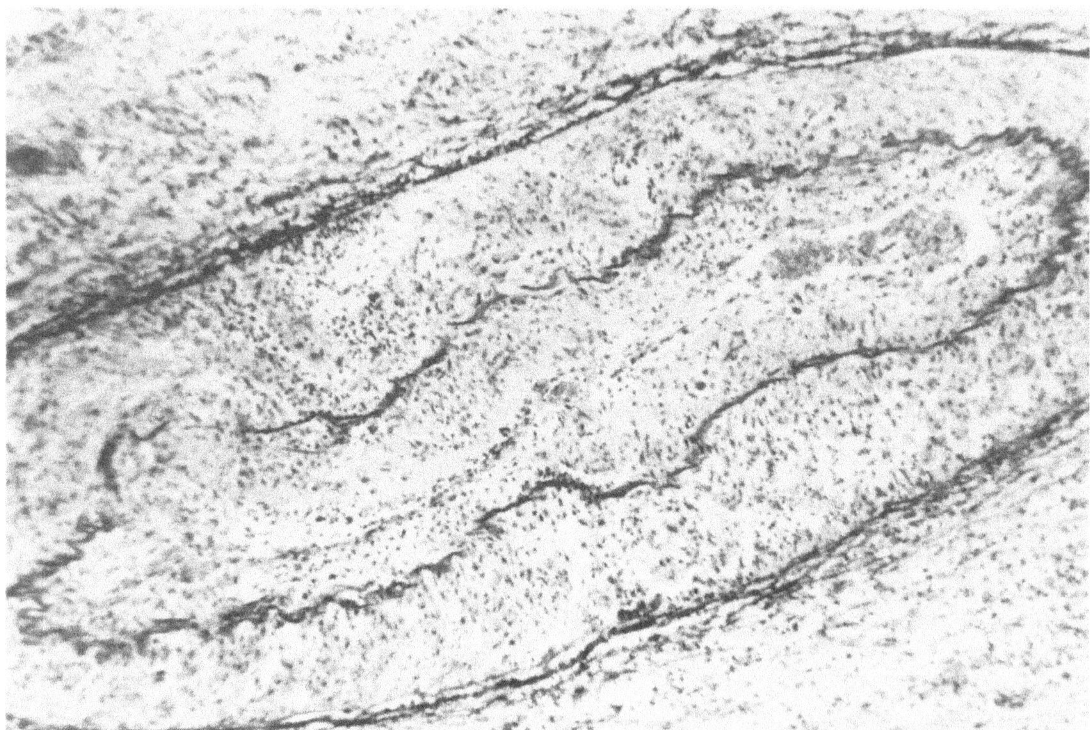

Fig. 2.40
Rheumatic fever

Coronary artery. Completely occluded lumen by intimal fibrinoid swelling with extensive proliferated reaction of fibroblasts and some loss of the internal elastic membrane

2.7.5 Joints

Immune complexes

It seems probable that circulating immune complexes are responsible for the involvement of joints as well as of serous surfaces in RF. Although the symptoms of arthritis receive primary clinical significance in RF and were the basis of the original German term of acute "Gelenkrheumatismus"(joint rheumatism), severity of symptoms and pathological changes are altogether different from those of RA. Neither cartilage destruction nor the resulting functional impairment are characteristics of RF.

Macroscopic findings

Macroscopic inspection of the joints is unimpressive and only the most acute cases show oedematous synovial villi. There is an increased amount of synovial fluid containing small particles of fibrin but showing no turbidity. Nevertheless, some 7,000–10,000 cells may be found per ml of fluid consisting mostly of degenerated neutrophils with some cells shed from the synovial surface layers. If the disease persists for a few weeks, lymphocytes may also appear. There is some hyperaemia of the synovial surface with occasional adherence of fibrin. Vessels are most prominent along the cartilaginous rim. Even with RF persisting for several weeks, the articular cartilage is macroscopically unchanged.

Microscopic findings

Klinge in his studies of post-mortem material (1930) reported microscopic findings which were similar in finger, toe, ankle, wrist, knee, elbow, shoulder, and hip joints. The synovial membrane shows moderate synovial hyperplasia, partly with clumsy villi. The villous stroma is oedematous and loose. Lymphocytic

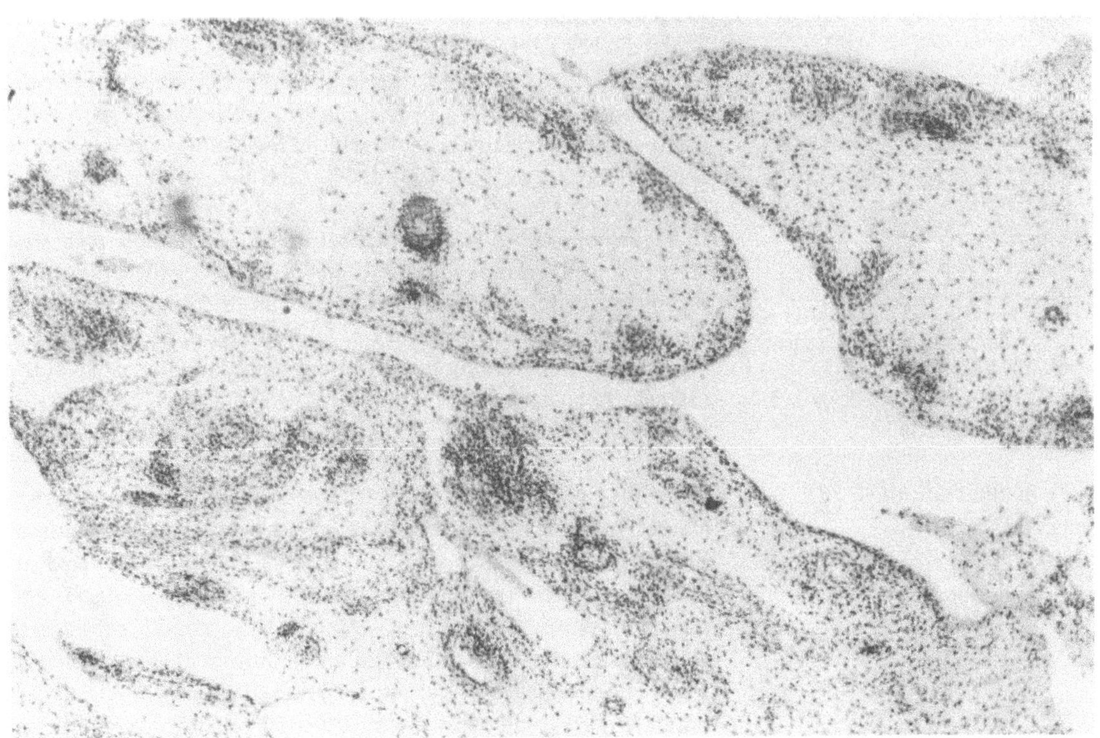

Fig. 2.41 Rheumatic fever

Villous hyperplasia of the synovial membrane. Low-grade swelling of lining cells. Oedema of the stroma. Accumulation of lymphocytes surround small blood vessels

foci around small blood vessels lie inside, a discrete or slight fibrin film has been deposited on the surface, there is loss of lining cells (Fig. 2.41). The fibrin contains occasional neutrophils or nuclear remnants. After an interval of a few days, cells of the synovial surface regenerate. Thus, in some cases, a multi-staged lining cell layer is formed. The surface cells, depending on the duration of the process, may be columnar in shape, have nuclei with prominent chromatin and differ in shape and size. In RF, as opposed to RA, the cells of the synovial stroma undergo no changes and we have never observed a tumour-like proliferation (tlp) as in RA (see p. 75) neither has this been described by Klinge or other observers. The changes are only the stigmata of non-specific inflammation as may be observed in other immunological conditions and which are dictated by the special morphology of the joint components. Inflammation is limited to the synovial surface and results from increased local capillary permeability.

Non-specific inflammation

Fibrinoid swelling

The characteristic feature of RF is found more deeply in the fibrous capsule as fibrinoid change of collagen fibres. The small elongated foci sometimes lie parallel to the joint cavity (Fig. 2.42). These foci of fibrinoid, irrespective of their localization, correspond basically to the "fibrinoid" in the heart, only they are here markedly wide-spread. The cells of the local connective tissue only begin to show microscopically recognizable changes in response to the fibrinoid deposit after an interval of 1–2 weeks (Klinge). Cellular aggregates surround the fibrinoid and these resemble, to some extent, the cardiac Aschoff node. However, while this constitutes a small compact body in the heart, the cell aggregate in the synovial stroma is loosely formed, has no definite outline, and is usually larger than the cardiac one. The component cells are fibroblasts and macrophages with some multi-nucleated giant cells. Newly formed blood vessels in the synovial stroma keep surrounded by lymphocytes for a long time (Fig. 2.43).

Aschoff node

Healing

In RF, as opposed to RA, synovitis undergoes complete recession after one or even repeated attacks of RF. Cells of the granuloma disappear. Following increased formation of collagen fibres, the number of fibroblasts decreases. Some fibrosis of the synovial stroma may thus remain but morphological characteristics of the disease are lacking.

Articular cartilage

Microscopic changes of cartilage, again in contrast to RA, are absent.

Late manifestations – Jaccoud's arthritis

Jaccoud's arthritis or chronic postrheumatic fever arthropathy is a rare, indolent, and slowly progressive process which deforms fingers and sometimes toes. Some cases following repeated attacks of RF show peculiar changes of metacarpophalangeal and interphalangeal joints, as first described by Jaccoud (1869) and to which Bywaters, in an important contribution, drew attention in 1950. The hallmarks are ulnar deviation, flexion of the metacarpophalangeal joints, and hyperextension of the proximal interphalangeal joints just as in RA, but without the arthritic pain, heat, and swelling. No true erosions are radiographically detectable (Fig. 2.44).

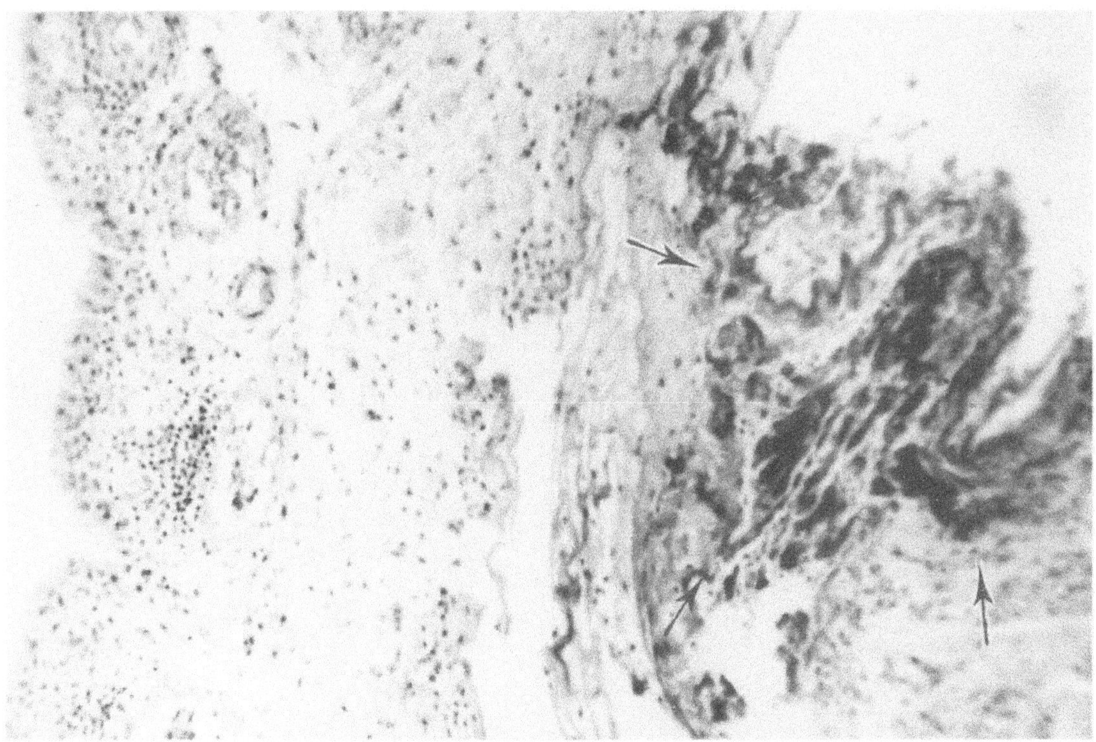

Fibrinoid swelling at the junction between synovial membrane and fibrinoid capsule (*arrows*)

Fig. 2.42
Rheumatic fever

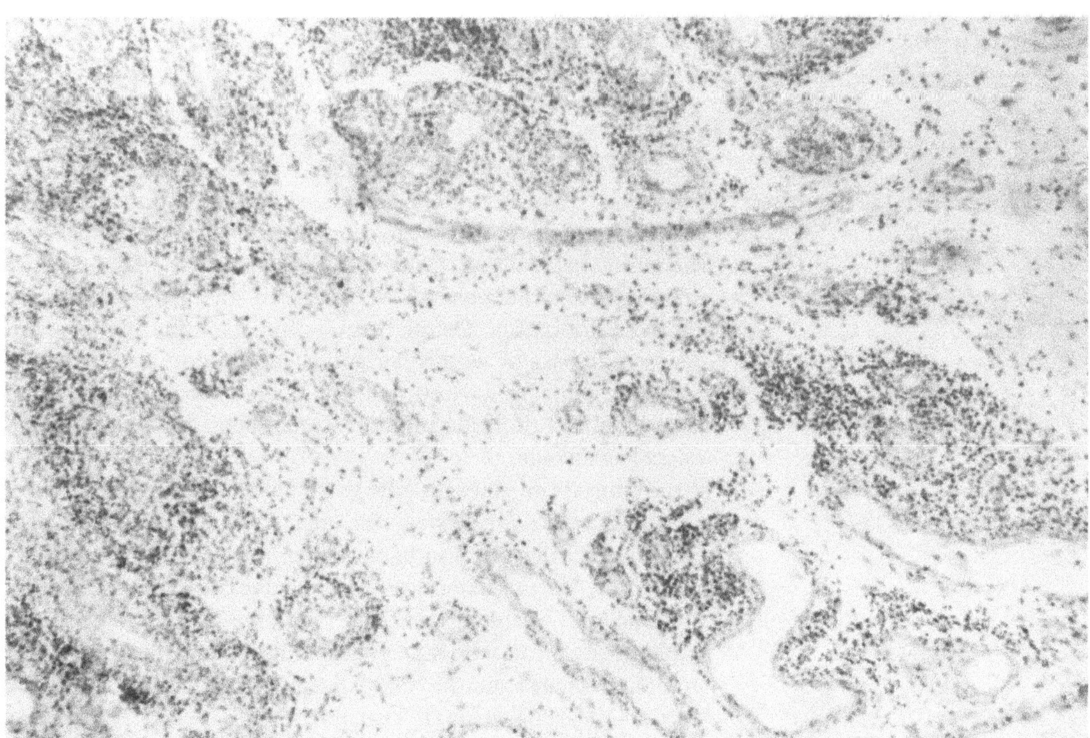

Late stage of synovitis. Newly formed blood vessels are surrounded by large numbers of lymphocytes

Fig. 2.43
Rheumatic fever

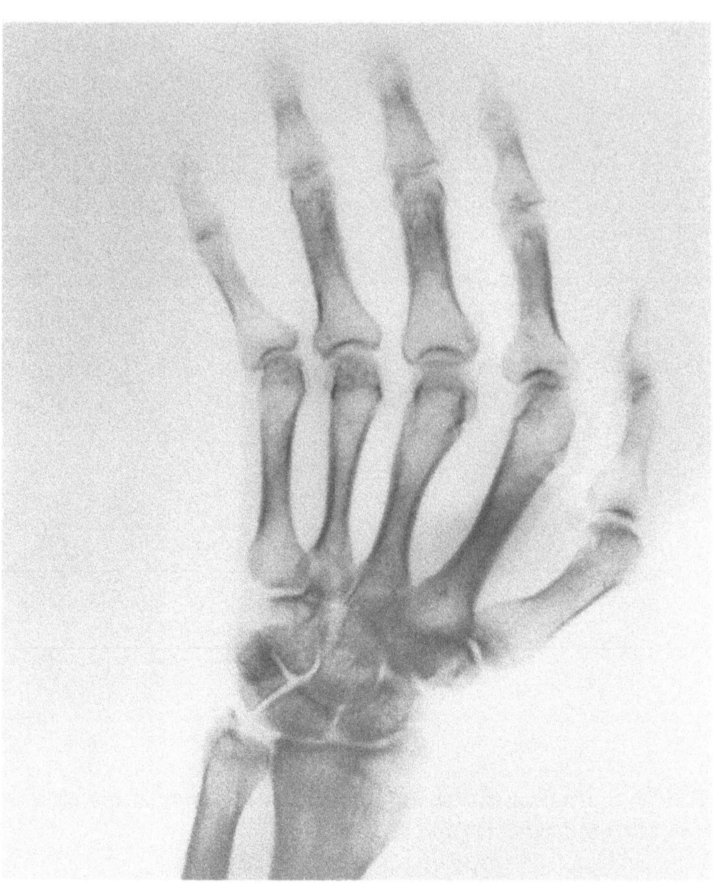

Fig. 2.44
Rheumatic fever

Jaccoud's so-called chronic postrheumatic fever arthropathy with ulnar deviation of the fingers

Shrinkage of joint capsule tissue

The term "arthritis" is incorrect insofar as the deformities are due neither to a primarily articular process nor to a synovitis. The cause lies rather in a chronic shrinkage of joint capsule tissue. This process of shrinkage courses clinically parallel to severe rheumatic heart disease, whereas the erythrocyte sedimentation rate (ESR) remains normal. We see herein an analogy to the unexpected findings of rheumatic granulomata in the auricular appendices in patients with rheumatic heart failures. Both processes course clinically asymptomatic and smouldering with neither morphological nor inflammatory components but lead to fibrosis and shrinkage.

It is important to state that the extremely painful synovitis even after weeks does not destroy the affected joints. RF shows sheer paradigmatically that non-bacterial, for instance immunological, synovitides do not endanger the articular cartilage. As in other non-bacterial purulent arthritides, too, local inhibitors succeed in paralyzing proteases and cytokines, developing during inflammation. Lasegue's dictum "acute rheumatism licks the joints but bites the heart" is correct! The remaining damages at Jaccoud's deformation are, in contrast, results from rheumatic inflammatory processes coursing in periarticular collagenous capsule tissue.

Periosteal changes

While in rheumatoid arthritis the juxta-articular bone shows erosions, bone destruction is not recognized in RF. Periosteum, by contrast, frequently shows foci of fibrinoid. Klinge reported the case of a 22-year-old man who died of pancarditis during a recurrence of RF. There were large numbers of such foci in the periosteum in the proximity of joints. This was especially marked in zones of mechanical stress, such as elbows, patella, and talus. The fibrinoid centre may be so prominent as to be macroscopically visible.

Tendons and fasciae

The lesions of RF in the most severe cases can also affect tissues such as tendons and fasciae.

Skeletal muscle

Focal necrosis of myofibrils was first described by Geipel in 1909 as occurring in three cases of RF with myocardial involvement; the lesions were found in the gastrocnemius, quadriceps, and sternomastoid muscles.

We reached the conclusion that, as in cardiac muscle, the manifestations of RF in skeletal muscle may occur in one of two different ways:

Primary inflammatory process in interstitium

1. A process analogous to that in the myocardial interstitium (see p. 15) may occur in muscular connective tissue. In contrast to myocardium, the process in skeletal muscle may be diffusely distributed and spread over large areas, particularly in the pharynx.

   Fibrinous infiltration

   This process is marked by diffuse fibrinous infiltration and fibrinoid change of collagenous fibres (Fig. 2.45). In this way, skeletal muscle fibres are much more severely affected than cardiac muscle in which isolated foci occur in the more loosely textured perivascular connective tissue. Analogous to the process in the cardiac tissue, a cellular reaction with involvement of macrophages and fibroblasts follows an exudative phase.

   Aschoff granulomata

   Granulomata of the Aschoff type can develop also in skeletal muscles (Fig. 2.46). This course of process corresponds to the morphological primary type of RF which, however, is modified by the local situation. The structure of the skeletal muscle grants, so, in contrast to the myocardium, a more diffuse spreading of the exudative-proliferative process (Fig. 2.47).

Primary necrosis of muscle

2. The alternative mode of muscle damage originates as a primary focal muscle fibre necrosis. The observable changes range from an appearance of homogenization of the muscle fibre to total necrosis. Such foci become surrounded by macrophages and fibroblasts. This gives rise to an appearance which we have already described as the muscle aggressive granuloma in the case of the myocardium (see p. 22). From the point of view of pathogenesis, it is of interest that we have only seen this variety of primary muscle necrosis in cases which also showed cardiac muscle granulomata.

   Antibodies against muscle

   This leads us to propose the hypothesis that necrosis of skeletal muscle as well as cardiac muscle necrosis may be effectively associated with antibodies against muscle.

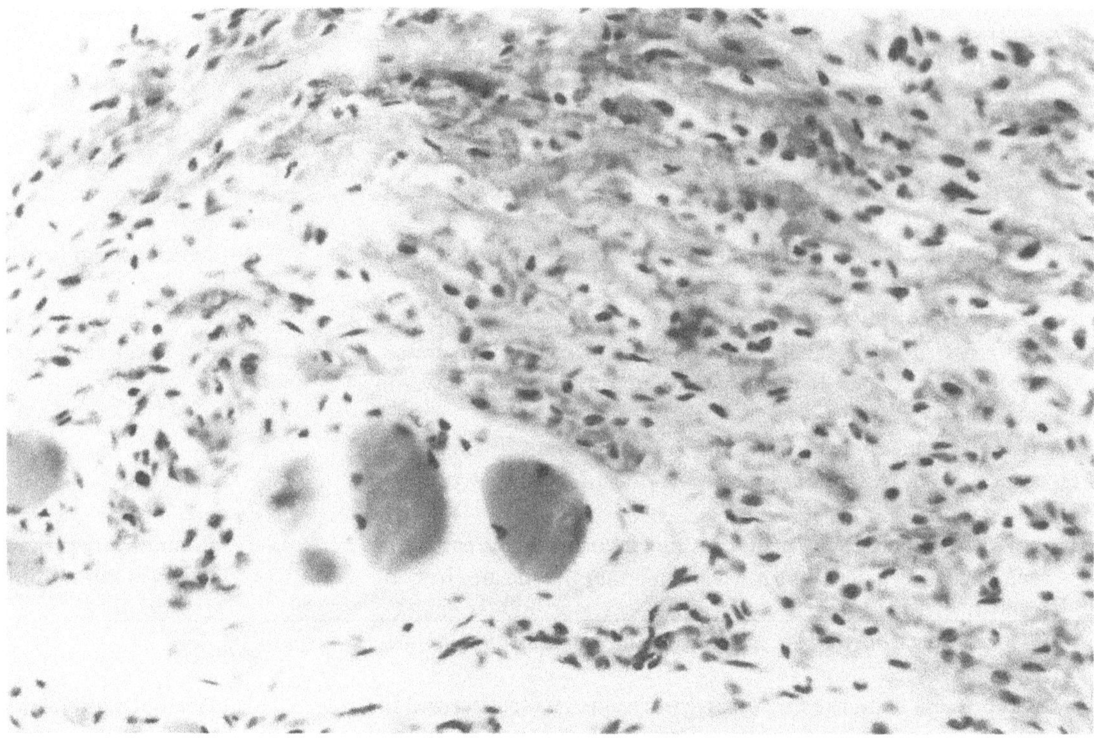

Fig. 2.45
Rheumatic fever

Skeletal muscle. Extensive fibrinoid strands in the perimysium with local cell reaction and a few neutrophils

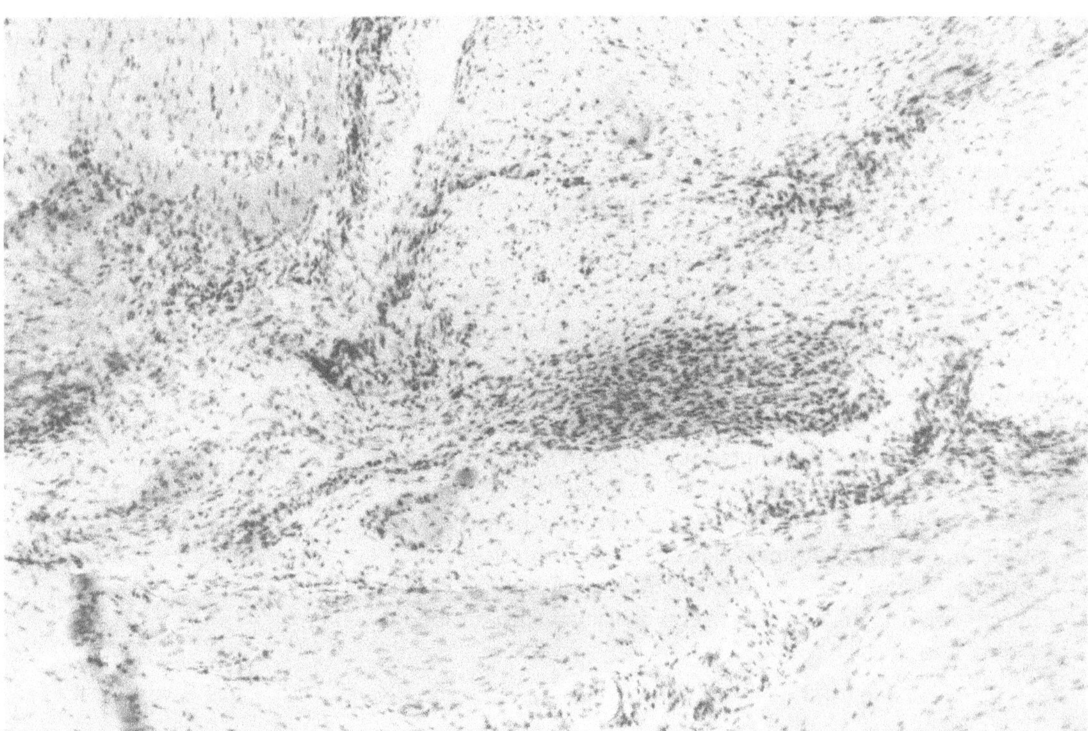

Fig. 2.46
Rheumatic fever

Skeletal muscle. A very cellular granuloma lying in a direction parallel with that of the muscle fibres

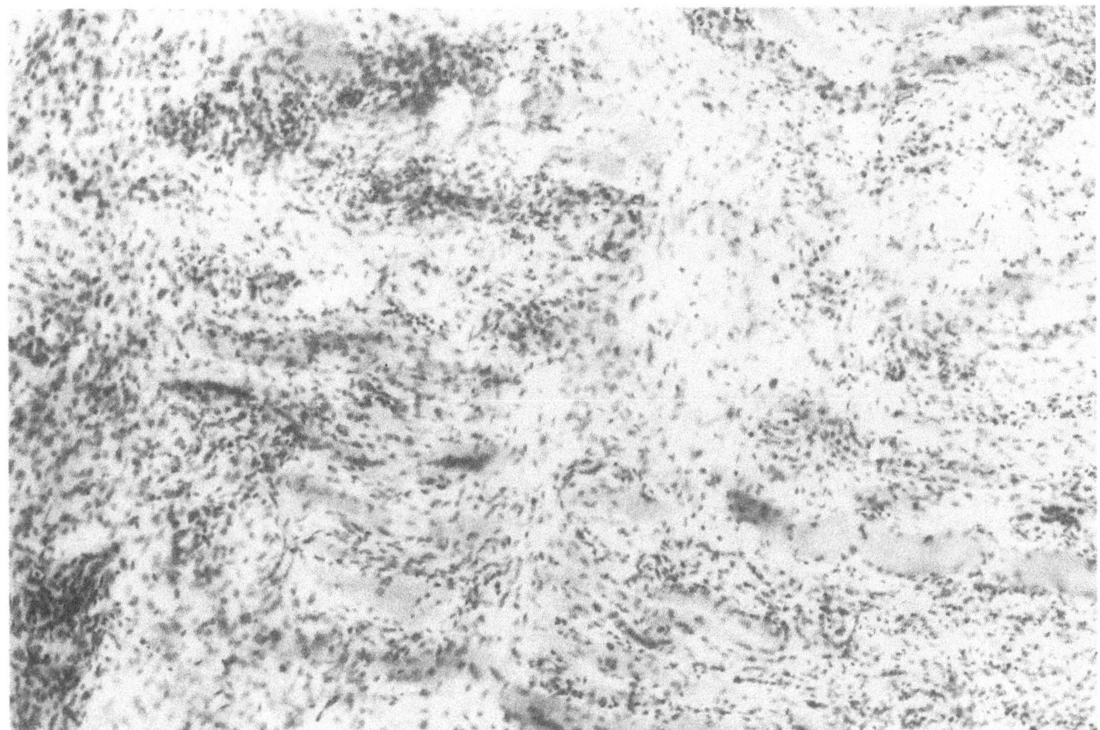

Skeletal muscle. Myositis with partial destruction of muscle fibres. Reactive proliferation of local fibroblasts and infiltration by macrophages, lymphocytes, and only a few neutrophils

Fig. 2.47
Rheumatic fever

2.7.6 Lung

The pulmonary capillaries are another tissue component that may become involved early in the course of RF, and the explanation may well reside in the circulation of immune complexes. However, descriptions of the lung lesions show considerable variation.

Haemorrhagic pneumonia

Coburn (1931) and also Klinge (1933), in their survey of a large amount of necropsy material, found foci of haemorrhagic pneumonitis in cases of RF. No granulomata or other characteristics of RF were seen.

Rheumatic pneumonia

Masson and coworkers (1937) were the first to describe a special "rheumatic pneumonia". Fibrin is deposited in bronchioles overlying the muscular wall and may be aspirated into the alveoli. Fibrin is attached to the lining which it may cover in the form of a continuous coating. This shows a striking resemblance to hyaline membrane disease of the new-born (Fig. 2.48). Connective tissue cells may migrate into the fibrin and thus form the so-called Masson-body (Uehlinger 1959). Here again, the histology lacks specificity for RF. The clinical significance of these membranes is not clear.

"Masson-body"

Blood vessels in pulmonary hypertension

In cases which show persistence of myocardial or valve injury, the lung may become secondarily involved. Thus, the pulmonary hypertension of mitral stenosis becomes associated with hypertrophy of the muscle layer of pulmonary arteries. In analogy to the events in systemic arterial hypertension, arterioles of the lung may similarly show necrosis in the course of RF.

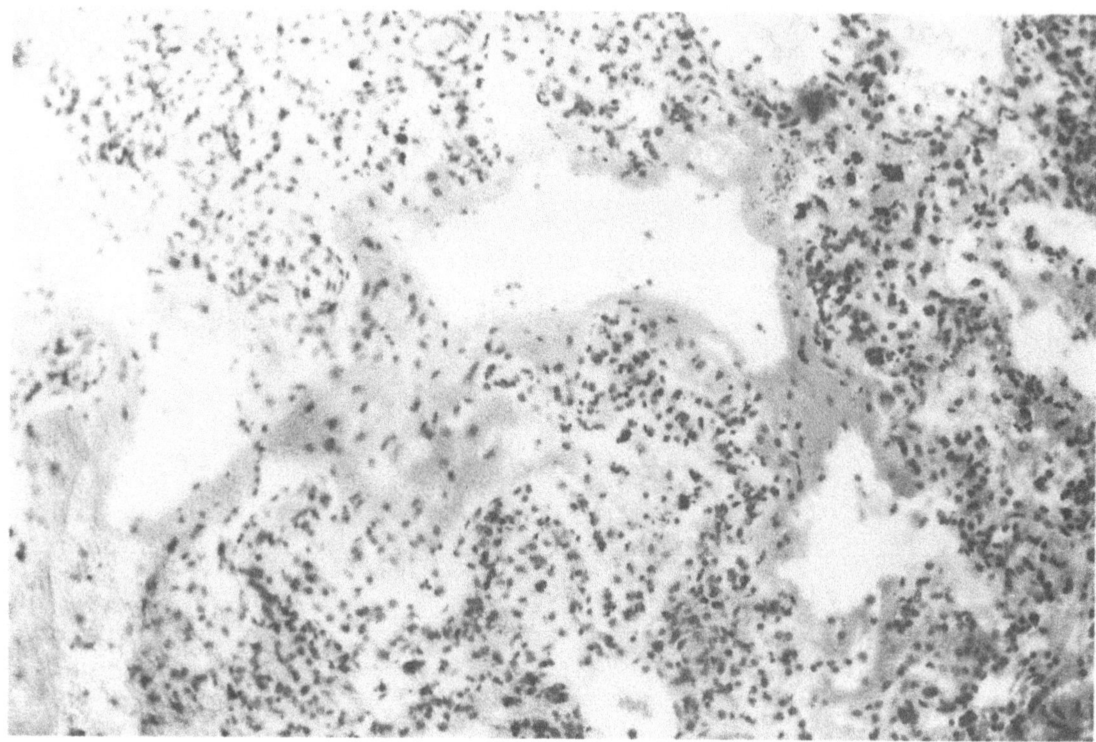

Fig. 2.48
Rheumatic fever

Eosinophil pulmonary membranes

Pleura

In principle, the pleura, since it resembles a mesodermal cavity like the pericardium, may be affected in the same way. Pleuritis is, however, rarely encountered in RF.

2.7.7 Skin

RF nodes

In parts of the body where friction occurs, such as elbows and the back of the head, painless nodes may occur subcutaneously usually some weeks after the onset of RF, especially in childhood. They indicate the appearance of a rheumatic carditis. Diameter varies from 0.5 to 2.5 cm. Unlike the rheumatoid nodule which is of long duration, the RF nodule is evanescent and disappears with the subsidence of the arthritis.

Histological structure of cutaneous nodules

The histological picture is not reminiscent of that of RA. The fibrinoid centre is of loose texture and, in contrast to the rheumatoid nodule, contains a lot of fibrin which is deposited in the form of lines or small lakes between the collagen fibres. Again unlike the nodule of RA, no palisade of cells surrounds the central fibrin deposit. A few macrophages and fibroblasts are loosely arranged at the margin without any sharp division, as seen in RA (Fig. 2.49). In RF, cells enter the fibrin at the margin, while the necrotic centre of a nodule in RA is sharply walled off after the fashion of a sequestrum, showing a strict boundary between dead and viable material.

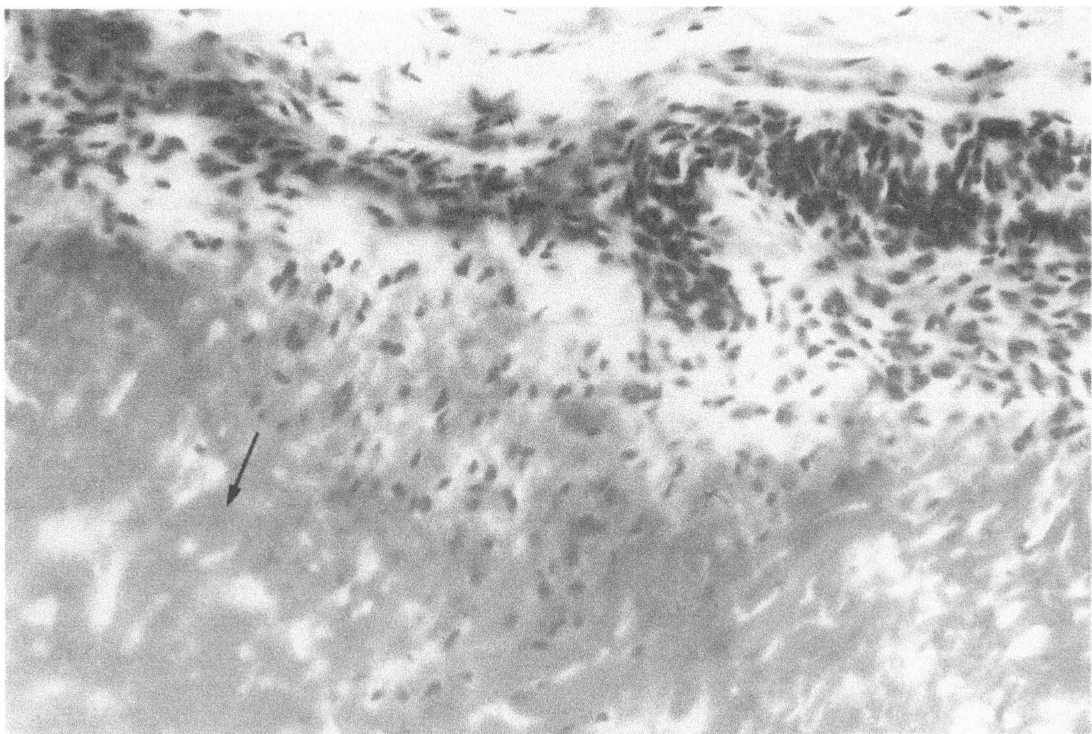

Rheumatic nodule. The fibrinoid centre (*arrow*) is not surrounded by a cell palisade. A few fibroblasts and macrophages are seen to be invading the fibrinoid material

Fig. 2.49
Rheumatic fever

Cutaneous nodules of Still's disease

It should be noted that cutaneous nodules in children with Still's disease (see p. 175) do not show the typical features of the adult rheumatoid nodule but resemble largely the picture seen in RF. We may well recall that children with Still's disease usually lack rheumatoid factors, while the adult rheumatoid nodule is almost invariably associated with rheumatoid factor-positive serology. The rheumatoid nodule in RA is a manifestation of local necrosis; the RF and Still's disease's nodules are dependent upon local inflammatory exudate formation, somewhat analogous to events in the cardiac perivascular tissues and synovium.

2.7.8 Synopsis of the Pathological Processes

If one reviews the colourful panorama of pathological processes hidden behind the term RF, a multi-layered picture of the disease is revealed showing diverse qualitative variations in quantitative graduations.

The disease can be acutely fatal, limited in time, with and without resultant damage, but persisting latently. It is difficult to imagine how this periodic, qualitative, and quantitative diversity can result directly from an A-streptococcal pharyngitis. A comparison of experimentally proved mechanisms and morphologically established damage provides an arsenal of possible pathomechanisms which could explain the various manifestations (see

p. 12). If, however, the variations in structural damage are taken as the basis, then the following logical connections appear:

Sub-acute, productive form (standard process)

The sub-acute standard process of RF (classical rheumatic myocarditis of the Aschoff type) is characterized in the heart muscle by the cycle "fibrinoid – Aschoff granuloma – scar". The same process can occur in the stroma of the heart valves without involvement of the valve rims. An analogous process in the mesodermal-mesothelial cavities (synovial membrane, pericardium, and pleura) results in fibrin exudation and in the skin in fibrin insudation. RF is defined by this standard process. The central event is the capillary damage which initiates an insudation in the vascular connective tissue of the heart and an exudation at the surface of the synovial membrane, pericardium, and pleura. It suggests that this systemic vascular damage is caused by the immune complexes emerging at the end of the sensibilisation process. The uncomplicated RF standard process itself leaves behind no clinical consequences in the myocardium since it takes place in the interstitium. In the heart valves, it can, however, lead to a valve shrinkage and a contraction of the chordae.

In the pericardium and pleura, residual fibrinous adhesions result in persisting scars, while the joint process, in general, heals without trace.

Acute exudative form

The acute, fatal form of RF (acute diffuse exudative rheumatic myocarditis) is characterized by a diffuse infiltration and impregnation of the myocardium and interstitium. A large number of neutrophils are scattered between the damaged muscle fibres. In the interstitium, there are small areas of fibrin. While the exudative phase of the classic cycle manifests itself solely in the discrete form of the fibrinoid, in the acute, fatal form it becomes excessive. We believe that here, too, the circulating immune complexes play a role and this is also supported by the high content of neutrophils. In this form, we also always saw severe fibrinoid swellings of the coronary vessels. The severity of the diffuse myocardial damage explains the fatal outcome.

Chronic lingering "myo-aggressive" form

While the acute and sub-acute forms of RF progress in a clinically impressive way, the myo-aggressive process (chronic lingering myo-aggressive rheumatic myocarditis) eludes clinical observation. In contrast to the Aschoff granuloma, the specific substrate, the "myo-aggressive granuloma", causes focal destruction of the contractile substance of the heart and also of the skeletal muscles. The "myo-aggressive granulomata" were found in the heart auricles as well as in the heart musculature itself even in patients without rheumatic manifestation (Fassbender 1963). All these patients had, however, experienced a sub-acute RF with participation of the heart valves some years before. The long interval and the fact that at the time of the histological investigation, there was no longer an indication of A-streptococcal infection, points primarily to the role of the autoantibodies against the heart musculature which, over a time, had developed and led to an insidious, clinically silent destruction of the myocardium. The fact that in myo-aggressive granulomata muscle fibres stand in the focus is most likely explainable by the direct influence of streptolysin A.

The standard process triggered by circulating immune complexes can continue as an isolated phenomenon but it can also become complicated by the interfering of cross-reacting antibodies against streptococcal antigens on valvular endothelial cells (rheumatic endocarditis; see above). The standard process triggered by immune complexes and the endocarditis caused by cross-reacting A-streptococcal antibodies can in combination characterize the picture of acute RF. These cases heal completely, leaving heart valve defects behind. The combination is, however, not invariable; in adults the involvement of the endocardium is markedly rarer than in children.

Endothelial reactions of heart valves

3 Rheumatoid Arthritis

3.1 Definition

The term rheumatoid arthritis (RA) in reality hides a complex systemic disease that although it predominantly affects joints and tendon sheaths may also involve other structures such as tendons, pericardium, myocardium, pleura, lung, skin, sclerae, blood vessels, as well as the cervical spine and may progress under certain circumstances to a life-threatening condition.

Table 3.1. The American College of Rheumatology (ACR) 1987 revised criteria for the classification of rheumatoid arthritis (Arnett, Edworthy, Bloch et al. 1988)

Criterion	Definition
1. Morning stiffness	Morning stiffness in and around the joints lasting at least 1 h before maximal improvement
2. Arthritis of three or more joint areas	At least three joint areas have simultaneously had soft-tissue swelling or fluid (not bony overgrowth alone) observed by a physician; the 14 possible joint areas are right or left PIP, MCP, wrist, elbow, knee, ankle and MTP joints
3. Arthritis of hand joints	At least one joint area swollen as above in a wrist, MCP or PIP
4. Symmetric arthritis	Simultaneous involvement of the same joint areas (as in 2) on both sides of the body (bilateral involvement of PIPs, MCPs or MTPs is acceptable without absolute symmetry)
5. Rheumatoid nodules	Subcutaneous nodules, over bony prominences, or extensor surfaces, or in juxta-articular regions, observed by a physician
6. Serum rheumatoid factor	Demonstration of abnormal amounts of serum 'rheumatoid factor' by any method that has been positive in less than 5% of normal control subjects
7. Radiologic changes	Radiologic changes typical of rheumatoid arthritis on PA hand and wrist roentgenograms, which must include erosions or unequivocal bony decalcification localized to or most marked adjacent to the involved joints (osteoarthritic changes alone do not qualify)

PIPs, proximal interphalangeal joints; *MCPs,* metacarpophalangeal joints; *MTPs,* metatarsophalangeal joints; *PA,* posteroanterior.

An attempt has been made by the American College of Rheumatology (ACR) to establish criteria for the diagnosis, especially to introduce some consistency of patients in clinical trials in RA. Originally 11 criteria were used, reduced to 8 in 1970 and then to 7 criteria after a further revision (Arnett et al. 1988; Table 3.1).
For classification purposes, a patient shall be said to have RA if he/she has satisfied at least four of the above seven criteria.
Criteria 1–4 must have been present for at least 6 weeks. Patients with two clinical diagnoses are not excluded. Designation as "classic", "definite" or "probable" is not to be made.
Just as the onset of RA already shows significant differences, the disease is capable of taking many different courses. In general, all joints may be affected, characteristic, however, is the tendency to symmetrical involvement of the interphalangeal, metacarpophalangeal, and metatarsophalangeal joints which, with exacerbations over decades, leads to joint destruction, deformities, and invalidism.
On the other hand, RA may resolve after the first attack with variable residual damage. The different manifestations make scepticism about the nosological purity of RA understandable. Until

there is evidence to the contrary, it is recommended, however, to consider the condition as a defined systemic illness with various disease subsets.

3.2 Historical Background

The first description of RA is attributed to Augustin-Jacob Landré-Beauvais, who in Paris in 1800 described nine women suffering from what he considered to be a variation of gout. He called the disease "goutte asthenique primitive". Landre-Beauvais felt that the illness primarily affected persons who had been weakened through poverty, whereas true gout typically affected more robust individuals (an error that was later rectified by Charcot 1889).

In 1813, Benjamin C. Brodie described a slowly progressive disease that not only affected tendons but also bursae and tendon sheaths. He recognized that the illness began with synovitis and then progressed to involve the cartilage of the joint.

Jean-Marie Charcot (Paris 1889) was the first to succeed in distinguishing between gout, rheumatic fever (RF), RA, and osteoarthritis (OA). However, he assumed that all these diseases were attributable to the same cause. He, too, considered RA to be an illness that primarily affected women of the lower classes .

Alfred B. Garrod gave the disease the name "RA". In 1892, he wrote: "The study of articular affectations some 30 years ago led me to the conclusion, that the majority of cases, then called "rheumatic gout", were related neither to true gout nor true rheumatism and that they had an independent pathology of their own and if such is the case, the term "rheumatic gout" was doubly wrong. I propose the name "rheumatoid arthritis", a name which does not imply any error, but assumes the disease having some external characters of rheumatism..."

Subcutaneous and intrabursal nodules clearly associated with RA were described by Robert Adams (1857). The fact that subcutaneous nodules were a well recognized feature of RF gave support to the assumption that RA was a variant or the chronic form of RF. After a detailed study of these nodules, Fahr (1918) as well as Swift (1924) felt that despite some differences they were analogous to the Aschoff bodies found in the heart of patients with RF.

In a large study of post mortem material, Klinge (1930) demonstrated that the Aschoff granuloma (body) was preceded by a swelling and homogenisation of the collagen fibre bundles, during which the ground substance within the fibres took on a fibrin-like appearance. In this "fibrinoid" appearance, which he could reproduce in animal experiments, Klinge saw a comparison (tertium comparationis) between the tissue lesion in RF and the rheumatoid nodule in RA.

From the historical point of view it is interesting that this interpretation of the collagen lesions in two completely different diseases could lead to an unitary concept, whereby RA was seen to be the chronic form of RF.

The meaning of "fibrinoid" was further developed by Klemperer et al. in 1941: the "fibrinoid degeneration" was considered to be a characteristic histopathological feature common to a group of "collagen diseases". Of course, these diseases have other totally different features in common apart from the enigmatic "fibrinoid". RF, RA, polyarteritis nodosa (PAN), systemic lupus erythematosus (SLE), Libman Sacks syndrome, dermatomyositis (DM), and serum sickness are probably best defined as "systemic connective tissue diseases" with an immunological etiology. It were the studies of Collins (1937) and Bennett and colleagues (1940) that permitted their ultimate histological differentiation and nosological classification of those skin manifestations.

In 1896, G.A. Bannatyne demonstrated the joint destruction of RA in one of the first radiographs. However, it was the discovery of rheumatoid factors by methods developed by Waaler (1940) and Rose et al. (1948) that proved decisive for the characterization of RA. The latex-fixation test of Singer and Plotz (1956) is technically easier, but less specific.

Since various poly-articular diseases can occasionally mimic RA, the demonstration of rheumatoid factors by means of the Waaler-Rose test can be an important feature in its differential diagnosis (see p. 60).

3.3 Epidemiology

It is estimated that the worldwide prevalence of RA in the general population lies between 0.3% and 2.0%. The incidence is thought to be 0.9–1.5/1,000 per year (Lawrence and Shulman 1984). However, the prevalence and incidence are higher in the urban black population in South Africa and among certain North American Indians.

RA affects women to men in a ratio of 2–3:1. The peak incidence of the adult form of RA corresponds with the third and fourth decades of life. But RA can also occur in the second decade and as late as in the eighth or ninth.

3.4 Etiological Considerations

Much work has been undertaken in trying to enlighten the cause of RA, characterized as a complex and life-long condition. After the failure to find evidence of obvious infection, during the 20s and 30s the importance of immunological mechanisms was suggested for the first time by the results of animal studies performed by Rössle (1933) and Klinge (1927).

Klinge: "fibrinoid swelling"

Klinge (1930) regarded the "fibrinoid swelling" of the collagen fibres as a specific sign of an immunological reaction. This led inevitably to the widespread expression "rheumatism". Klinge wrote in 1933: "Rheumatism" in the broadest sense means, based on particular immunological conditions producing an allergic-hyperergic reaction with the result of a fibrinoid swelling of the connective tissue and all the consequences. Klinge, thus, replaces the pathogenesis (pathogen specificity) with morphological appearance (reaction specificity).

Confirmation brought the inclusion of RA and RF in the expression "collagen diseases" coined by Klemperer et al. in 1942. In that respect, the inflammatory alterations of the connective tissue ground substances of the entire organism were united as a whole body reaction. Articular rheumatism is contrasted with a visceral rheumatism. In this concept, visceral rheumatism may dominate the clinical feature or may accompany polyarthritis as a minor component.

Klemperer: "collagen diseases"

In the ensuing period until the present, very different immunological mechanisms for RA have been hypothesized. One should bear in mind, however, that although RA has a specific nosological and morphological profile, the immunological processes known to date are by no means specific but belong to the general inflammatory and defence mechanisms of the organism. They therefore offer no explanation for the uniqueness of the RA process.

Unspecific immunological phenomena

Numerous studies have shown an increased association between RA and HLA-DR4. Twin studies, however, have failed to show a clear indication of strong genetic influence (Engleman et al. 1983; Lawrence and Shulman 1984).

Role of HLA-DR4

However, the importance of HLA-DR4 is not to be overlooked. Thus, the studies of Gran and colleagues (1983) and Calin and colleagues (1989) show a significant association of HLA-DR4 with seropositive RA (65% or 69%, respectively) and with seronegative RA (55% or 60%) in comparison with the frequency in healthy individuals (27% or 36%, respectively).

Besides, HLA-DR4 seems to play a pathogenetic role for joint destruction in RA.

As, in the final analysis, these immunopathological hypotheses fail to provide an adequate explanation, pathogens such as mycoplasmas, clostridia, and viruses have been proposed as possible triggers for RA (Alarcon 1986). The proof of virus antigens, virus genomes or viral products make a slow virus infection more likely than a conventional virus infection (Ziegler et al. 1989).

Role of bacteria and viruses

The search for etiology and pathogenetic associations in this disease leads to a complicated "criminal investigation", in which one is confronted by a mass of clues that have to be critically analysed in terms of the likelihood of pathogenetic "guilt".

3.5 Phenomenology of RA

The numerous phenomena ("clues") observed in RA may be divided into three groups:

1. Clinical features
2. Immunological phenomena
3. Structural components

The clinical diagnosis may be based on a number of features, which in general suffice to identify RA. These features are:

Clinical features

- Predominance of female sex.
- A preference for symmetrical involvement of interphalangeal and metacarpophalangeal joints of the hands and metatarsophalangeal joints.

- Presence of rheumatoid factors: latex-fixation test positive in 60%–80%. Waaler-Rose-haemagglutination test positive in 40%–50% of cases.
- Typical early radiological changes of the juxta-articular bone structure.

Immunological phenomena

The investigator's task is to consider all the disease phenomena and decide in how far they are consistent with the specific profile of RA or whether they are merely non-specific features of an inflammatory process.

Rheumatoid factors

The characteristic immunological phenomenon is the presence of rheumatoid factors. These are antibodies with affinities for epitopes in the Fc part of the IgG. The dominant isotope, however, is IgM, although IgG and IgA rheumatoid factors are also observed. Only few patients show rheumatoid factors at the beginning of the illness, but the rate increases to 75% as the illness progresses.

Rheumatoid factors may also occur during long-lasting bacterial or viral infections and even in healthy individuals. The prevalence in a normal population is 3%; 10% of the B lymphocytes are able to secrete antibodies with rheumatoid factor activity. As in many other inflammatory disorders, the presence of a variety of different antibodies against intracellular antigens and components of the connective tissue may be proven in RA patients. For example, antibodies against nuclear factors (ANA), against perinuclear antigens (APF) as well as against intermediate filaments may be found (Osung et al. 1982). Antikeratin antibodies, which may allegedly be proven before the manifestation of the illness (Kurki et al. 1992), show a high tendency for RA (95%). Ninety percent of all seropositive RA patients have antibodies against an antigen associated with RA (RANA), which is identical to particles of the Epstein-Barr virus (Venables 1988). However, none of the phenomena are specific to RA. Nevertheless, the rheumatoid factors possess a certain pathognomonic and prognostic importance.

The complete profile of RA is characterized by three different mechanisms: inflammation, destruction (see p. 83), and primary necrotization.

Although neither the inflammatory nor the destructive process is bound to the presence of rheumatoid factors, the appearance of RA-necroses (RA-granuloma) is bound to the presence of IgM rheumatoid factors. This primary necrotization process, whose "key fossil" is the subcutaneous rheumatoid nodule, can damage various structures of the organism, like tendons, myocardium, pericardium, vessel walls, and sclerae (see p. 112). Hence it follows that there are considerable qualitative and prognostic differences between the seropositive and seronegative process of RA.

Structural components

As RA is characterized by damage and destruction of various tissues, a systematic examination of the morphological process is required. Therefore, joint tissue from patients with different rheumatic diseases should be compared by the following morphological features:

- Fibrin
- Granulation tissue

- Lymphocytes
- Lymph follicles
- Plasma cells
- Neutrophils
- Siderophages
- Lining cell proliferation
- Villous formation
- Giant cells
- Stromal cell proliferation
- Tumour-like proliferation (tlp)
- Joint destruction
- Rheumatoid necroses
- Fibrous stratum

To gain a specific profile of RA, the morphological features of RA need to be compared to the morphological features of OA (see p. 339), seronegative spondarthritides (SSA; see p. 178), or bacterial arthritides (BA; see p. 386).

This process leads to a marked reduction in the number of "clues". What is clear is that the above illnesses share many morphological features with RA. Thus, only a few features remain which are associated with the specific profile of RA and they may be thought of as "characteristic features" and have a role in a pathogenetic process.

Specific profile of RA

3.6 Synopsis of RA

RA is a chronic systemic illness with an episodic course, marked by inflammatory exacerbations. The disease is variable in the extent of joint involvement and in the speed of progression. However, it is characterized by the pattern of involvement, its chronicity, and the type of structural destruction found in joints and tendon sheaths. A specific feature is the development of primary necroses in structures of collagen type I. To summarize, in its nosological core, RA is a well-defined condition although the disease may be variable in time, course, and extent of involvement.

Structures involved in RA

The primary structures involved in RA are:

- Joints
- Tendon sheaths

Secondary structures include:

- Lungs, pleura, pericardium, myocardium, and peritoneum
- Subcutis, tendons, and sclerae
- Bursae
- Blood vessels
- Cervical spine

Three different mechanisms

The expression of RA is determined by three different mechanisms:

- An exudative-inflammatory process
- A proliferative-destructive process
- A primary necrotizing process

These mechanisms operate in the following tissues:
- Exudative-inflammatory process:
  - Synovial tissue
  - Tendon sheaths
  - Bursae
  - Pleura, pericardium, and peritoneum
- Proliferative-destructive process:
  - Joints
  - Tendon sheaths
  - Cervical spine
- Primary necrotizing process:
  - Subcutis
  - Joint capsule
  - Tendons
  - Lungs
  - Pleura, pericardium, and myocardium
  - Sclerae
  - Blood vessels
  - Bursae

3.7 Joint Process in RA

3.7.1 Structural Components of the Synovial Process

The processes occurring in the joint in RA are initiated from the synovial tissue. The normal, unchanged synovial membrane has the following characteristics:
- The surface is folded but has only a few villi.
- The lining cell layer is single-staged and comprises flattened lining cells.
- The synovial stroma consists of a loose collagen fibre network sparsely populated with cells. The few fibroblasts are spindle-shaped, with small dense nuclei. Occasional macrophages may be found.
- Blood vessels are thin-walled and sparse.

Lining cells

The most sensitive components of the already very reactive synovial membrane are the lining cells, which are functionally differentiated mesenchymal cells. Several introductory remarks may aid in the understanding of this topic.
Since the investigation of Barland, Novikoff, and Hamerman (1964) we differentiate between:
1. The phagocytizing A cell, enriched with lysosomes and vacuoles
2. The B cell, which is similar to fibroblasts and secretes hyaluronan, proteins, procollagen, α-2-globulin, fibronectin, and other plasminogen activators (Fig. 3.1)

The A cell shows electron-microscopically all the qualities of a macrophage. The cell surface is considerably enlarged due to many evaginations (filopodia). The cytoplasm is rich in lysosomes, which, due to their high basic phosphatase activity, are easy to identify. In RA, the lysosomes of the A cell are, compared

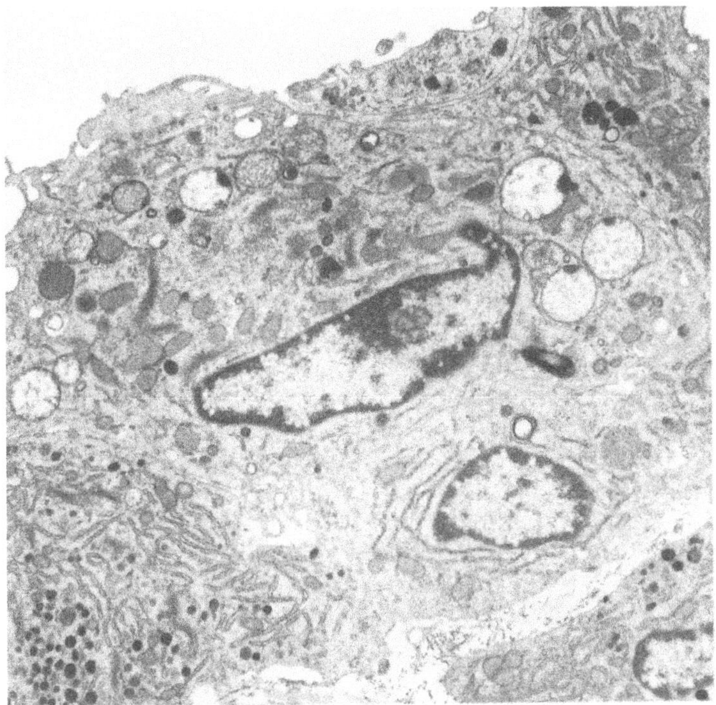

Lining cells. In the middle, an A cell with vacuoles and phagolysosomes, on both sides B cells with rough endoplasmic reticulum. (Electron micrograph)

Fig. 3.1

to the norm, multiplicated and larger. Moreover, the cytoplasm contains granular structures with a diameter of 0.4–3.2 μm. These "residual bodies" show a changing content of electron-dense material. Occasional remnants of fibrin may be seen in phago-lysosomes.

The B cells have a relatively smooth surface. The cytoplasm shows rough endoplasmic reticulum. These cells synthesize and secrete both the formed structures and the amorphous components of the ground substance. The formation of mucopolysaccharide polymers is essential for the proper functioning of the joint.

According to observations of Ghadially and Roy (1967), the percentage of B cells in synovitis of patients with RA is increased in comparison to the normal population. This is in contrast to studies of Stofft and colleagues (1988) who found in patients with RA an increase of A cells to 50.36% in comparison to the normal population of 34.73%. The amount of rough endoplasmic reticulum is increased in the B cells; additionally we find swollen abnormal mitochondria and lipid droplets.

From the point of view of joint function, different roles are assigned to the two different cell types. It is reasonable to assume that even in the normal joint undergoing mechanical stress, debris would be produced during the course of normal movement. It is the task of the A cells to remove and catabolize such material. Should fibrin appear in the course of synovitis this too will be phagocytozed. The electron-dense material appears in the cytoplasmic phagosomes. This corresponds light-microscopically

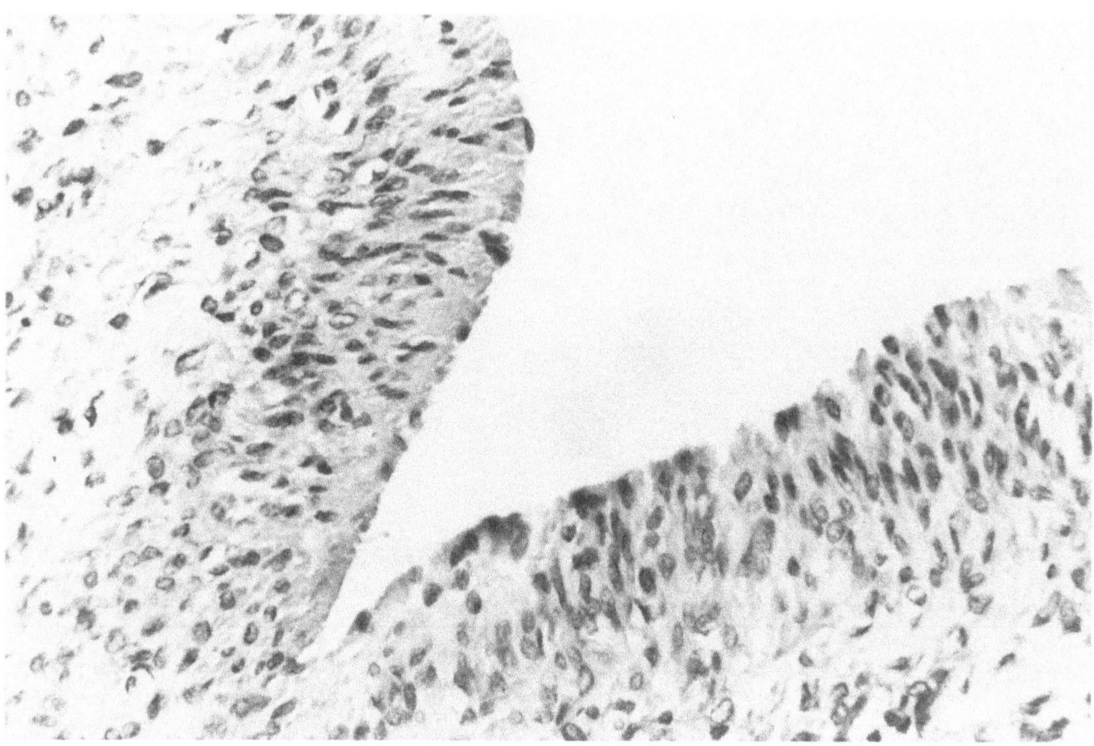

Fig. 3.2
Rheumatoid arthritis

Synovial membrane. The lining cells are cylindrical and multilayered

with the diagnosis of fine eosinophilic particles in the most superficial layer of synovial cells as seen in exudative synovitis.
While in a latent state, the lining cells are flat and single-layered. In response to various stimuli, generally to exudates, the lining cells increase to a cubic or cylindrical shape and become multilayered if the stimulation is prolonged (Fig. 3.2). At this stage, polynuclear synoviogenous giant cells are seen, also in contact with the lining cell layer (Fig. 3.3; see p. 71). Although these occur frequently in RA, they may also be found in synoviotides of other genesis. The lining cells may return to their original flat shape when the stimulus ceases (Fig. 3.4).

Polynuclear synoviogenous giant cells

While one could assume that the origin of the A cells is found in bone marrow, new findings negate this: according to the investigations of Stofft and coworkers (1988), A cells are peroxidase-negative and OKM-1-negative. Also the inability of the A cells to bind lectin disproves their monocyte character (Zschäbitz and Stofft 1988). However, it is probable that monocytes may also encroach the synovial membrane in the course of a synovitis.
A third type of cells is also found among the lining cells. The ultrastructural characteristics of these cells deny their classification as either A or B cells.
Today it seems to be probable that all three cell types are morphologically and functionally differentiated forms of mesenchymal synovioblasts.

Villous formation

The reaction velocity and power of proliferation of the lining cells is impressively demonstrated by the ability of the synovial

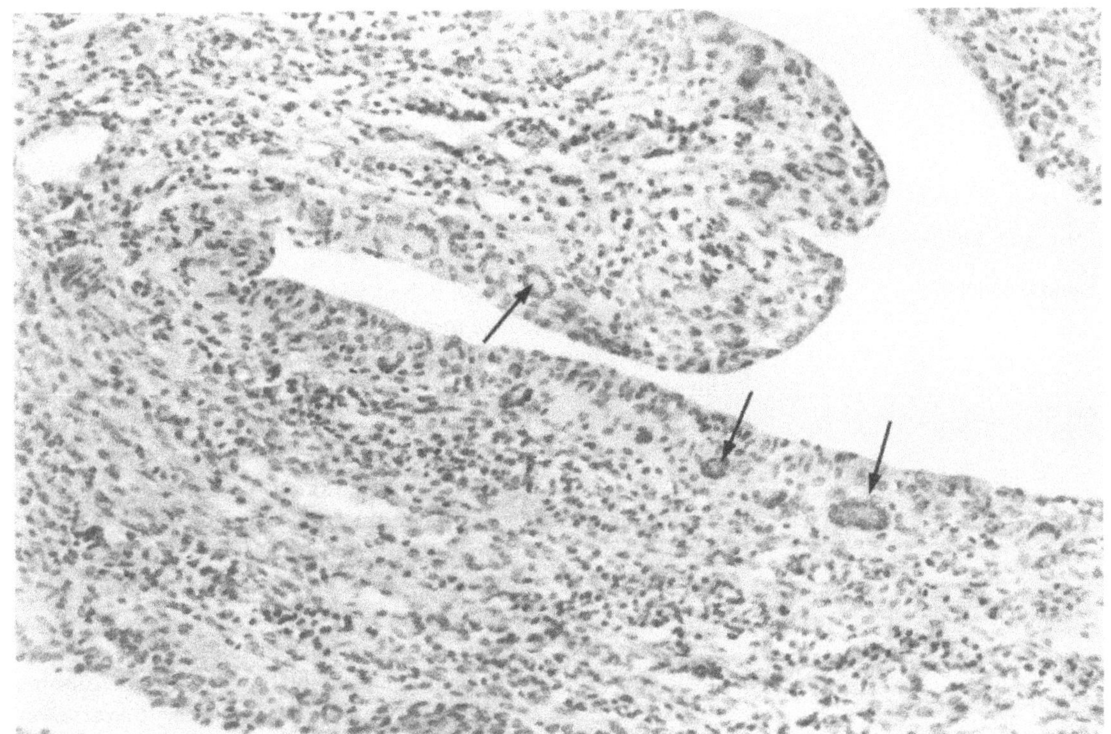

Numerous polynuclear synoviogenous giant cells (*arrows*) in the proliferating synovial membrane

Fig. 3.3
Rheumatoid arthritis

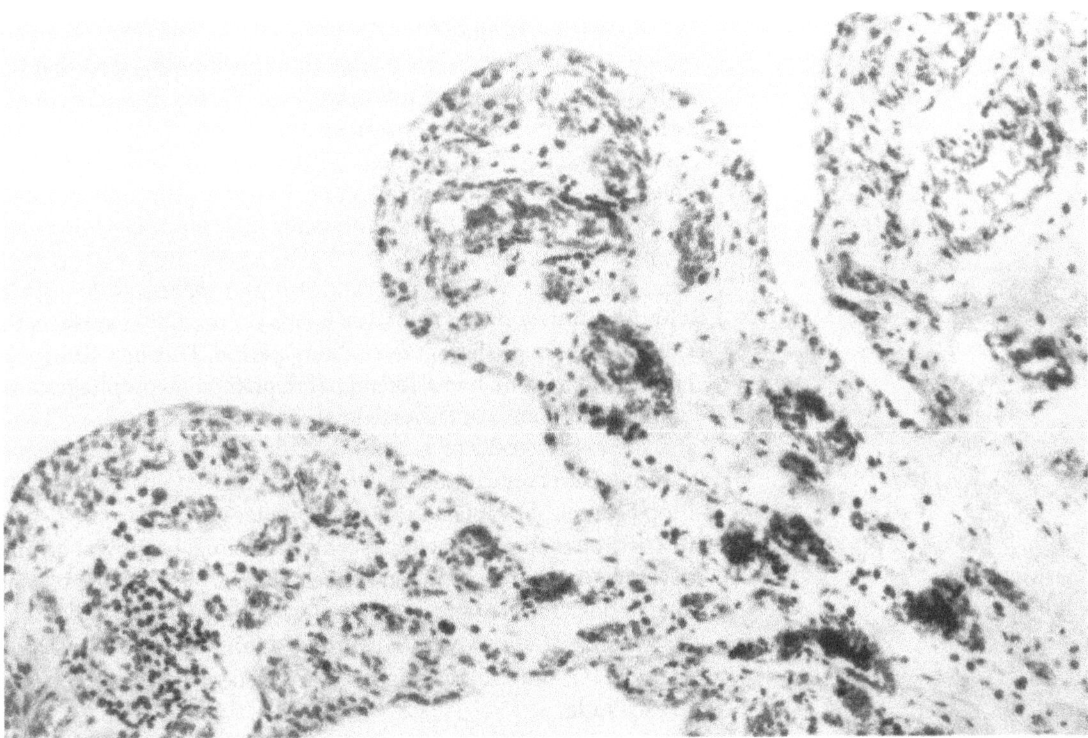

Flat lining cell layer in latent stage

Fig. 3.4
Rheumatoid arthritis

membrane to turn into a villous hyperplasia. The synovial membrane shares with the surfaces of other mesothelial membranes like pleura and peritoneum the feature to create polypous structures, but they are nowhere else so excessively marked. Starting point of the villous hyperplasia is the protrusion of delicate lining cell buds, at first compact without stroma and blood vessels. These branch in later and, thus, the growing process of the typical synovial villi begins.

Synovial villi

The distinction of these villous polypose proliferations may vary in size and shape. The most extreme case is the villous hyperplasia following a continued existing accompanying synovitis in OA, in which the villi are, in contrast to RA, usually very plump (see p. 339). In SSA and psoriatic arthritis (PSA), the villi are usually long, slender, and not as numerous. The lining cell layer of the villi mirrors the momentary irritation of the synovial membrane and is uncharacteristic. In contrast, the structure of the villi gives clues about the approaching illness. In RA, e.g., the stroma has few fibres and is moderately dense, in OA, it has a dearth of fibres and is transparent (glass villi; see p. 340).

The functional importance of villi formation is primarily an enlargement of the absorbing surface of the synovial membrane, which is aided by either a previous exudation or the accumulation of detritus matter.

Fibrin

However, only a structurally intact synovial membrane is prerequisite for the formation of villi. For example, in bacterial synovitis, the architecture of the synovial membrane is destroyed and is replaced by granulation tissue. In this case, a flat surface free of villi is observed (see p. 390).

As impressive as the villous hyperplasia of the synovial membrane in RA and other synovitides is, it must be stressed that impairment of the cartilage has never, even during intimate contact with synovial villi, been observed.

Sparse exudate fibrin deposits in RA are not, as with BA, dissolved by neutrophil enzymes and absorbed through granular tissue (see p. 390). Fibrin remnants are enmeshed into the synovial membrane.

Synovial cells equally migrate through deposits of fibrin. Although a new lining cell layer forms on the fibrin surface, the fibrin core remains intact over a long period. This new lining cell layer is, on the one hand, formed of deposited macrophages and, on the other hand, of traversed genuine lining cells.

It is only after weeks or months that the base of the fibrin deposit comes into contact with the vessels of the synovial membrane. Blood vessels, fibroblasts, and macrophages grow into the deposit. The fibrin core is slowly resorbed and a new synovial stroma develops under the lining cell layer. In this manner, fibrin exudate deposits in RA and other non-bacterial arthritides are integrated into the synovial membrane maintaining a functional synovial structure that again may be the stage for another exudative episode.

Joint mouse

In this manner, for example plump villi with a densely hyalinized nucleus (old fibrin) can detach themselves from the base and lie as free bodies in the joint space.

Synovial stroma cells

Normally, the synovial stroma shows cell deficiency. The loosely structured collagen fibre frame contains only a few dispersed fibroblasts with relatively small elongated nuclei. In RA, however, excessive proliferation of the stroma cells may occur, which we never observed in other arthritides (see pp. 75).

Inflammatory cells in rheumatoid synovitis

Essentially, lymphocytes and plasma cells are in no way specific for RA. They may be found to a variable extent in all types of synovitis, from RA to post-traumatic synovitis.
Lymphocytes are principally found in groups, which, in patients with RA, consist up to 92% of CD4+ memory cells (Hanly et al. 1990).
According to Natvig and colleagues (1988), the distribution of "inflammatory cells" in rheumatoid synovitis is as follows (Table 3.2):

Table 3.2. Inflammatory cells in rheumatoid arthritis (Natvig, Førre, Randen, Steinitz, Thompson and Waalen 1988)

Dendritik cells (2%-4%)

- CD45+, HLA-DR, DP, DQ+
- Antigen-presenting cells
- Induce mixed lymphocyte reactions (MLR)
- Make clusters with T-cells

T-cells (70%-80%)

- Mostly CD4+ T-helper cells, but also CD8+ T-suppressor cells
- T-cells activated in vivo, HLA-DR+, IL-2R+, TfR+ (20%-40% positive for these activation markers)
- Spontaneously produce and consume interleukins (IL-2)
- T-help augmented, T-suppression decreased

B-cells (10%-15%)

- Activated in vivo, develop into plasma cells
- Spontaneously produce Ig and antibodies (e.g. RF)
- Immune complex formation from antibodies (e.g. IgG RF) with activation of complement cascade

Macrophages (5%-10%)

- Activated in vivo with phagocytosis of IgG and IgM complexes and ADCC type cytotoxic reactions
- Antigen processing and presentation
- Collaboration with dendritic cells (?)

IL-2R, interleukin-2 receptor; *TfR*, transferrin receptor.

Lymph follicles

In contrast, plasma cells are scattered and only occasionally found in aggregates. Focal concentrations of lymphocytes, at times lymph follicles with germal centres, are preferably found in the synovial villi (Fig. 3.5). Klimiuk and colleagues showed in different stages of lymphocyte infiltration (i.e. diffuse and follicular) in the synovial membrane of 21 patients with RA different cytokine profiles (1997). It should be emphasized that this follicle formation is in no way specific. In our experience, follicle formation is also quite frequently seen in synovitis accompanying OA. It should also not be considered as a characteristic feature for continuing inflammation, but rather as the expression of the immunological reaction of the organism to antigenic material. These lymph follicles can persist for years.

As little as lymphocytes in RA and OA (and other synovitides) differ light-optically from each other, nevertheless, the challenge remains to search for immunological or molecular-biological criteria possibly specific for RA and OA or other disorders which can give insight into their pathogeneses. The field of cell typing is continously developing. A report about the progress is given for example by Fox (1997). In the synovial membrane in RA, T cells are mostly T helper/inducer cells while cytotoxic/suppressor T cells occur in the synovial membrane in OA only sparsely. The equipment of the synovial membrane in OA with immunocompetent cells is an expression for an immunological reaction with cartilaginous antigens occurring in the course of cartilage and bone destruction, from which one may draw the conclusion that it may influence the further progress of OA (Johnell et al. 1985; Fassbender and Zwick 1995).

Neutrophils

Neutrophils appear during the exudative phase and, in contrast to lymphocytes, rapidly migrate through the synovial membrane, which lacks a basement membrane, penetrating into the synovial fluid where in RA 2,000–75,000 leukocytes may be found. More than 50% of these cells are neutrophils (Schumacher 1985).

Neutrophils do not belong to the synovial process in RA, as Bywaters and Ansell already pointed out (1965).

Bacterial infection

If, however, an accumulation of neutrophils in the synovial membrane in RA is present, they are indicative of a superimposed bacterial infection. This we could prove in 13.5% in the tissue samples of patients with RA (see p. 395).

Siderophages

When synovitis is prolonged, most of the time the synovial membrane contains a number of siderophages (Fig. 3.6). Small groups of macrophages laden with haemosiderin can be demonstrated in the deeper part of the synovial membrane at the border of the fibrous capsule around small blood vessels. In contrast to these findings, in villonodular synovitis (VNS) siderophages are dispersed through the whole synovial membrane (see p. 419). On the other hand, with joint haemorrhage, siderophages are found almost exclusively in the cytoplasm of the lining cells.

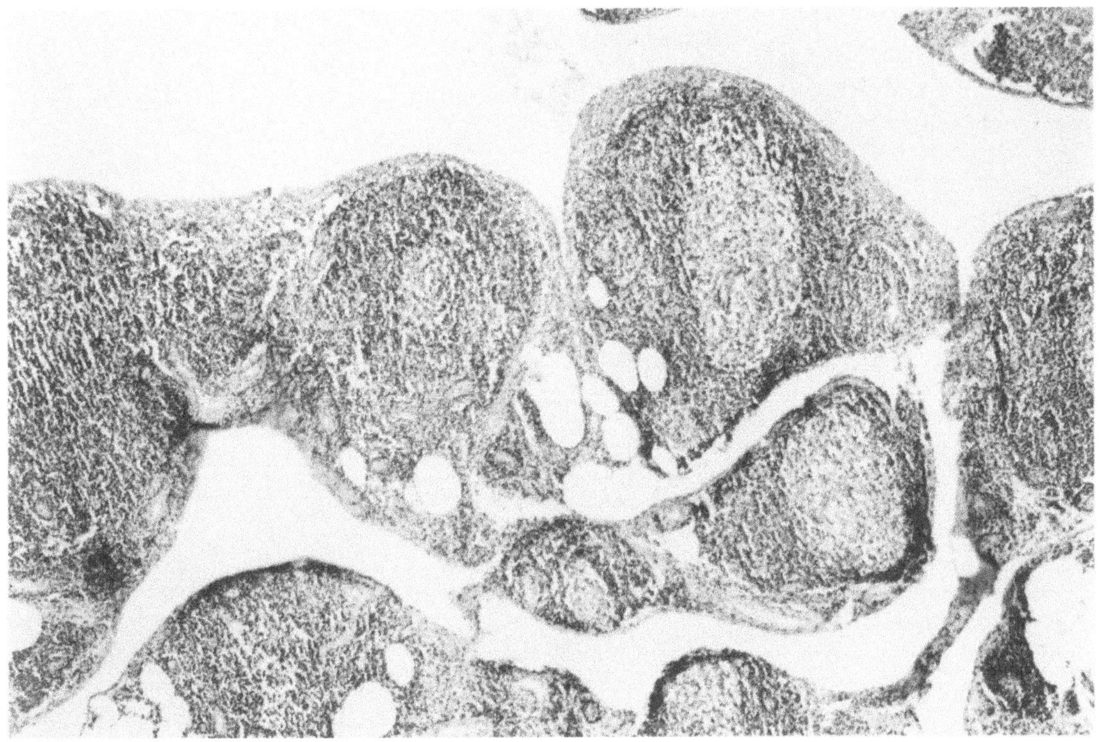

Lymph follicles with germal centres in synovial villi

Fig. 3.5
Rheumatoid arthritis

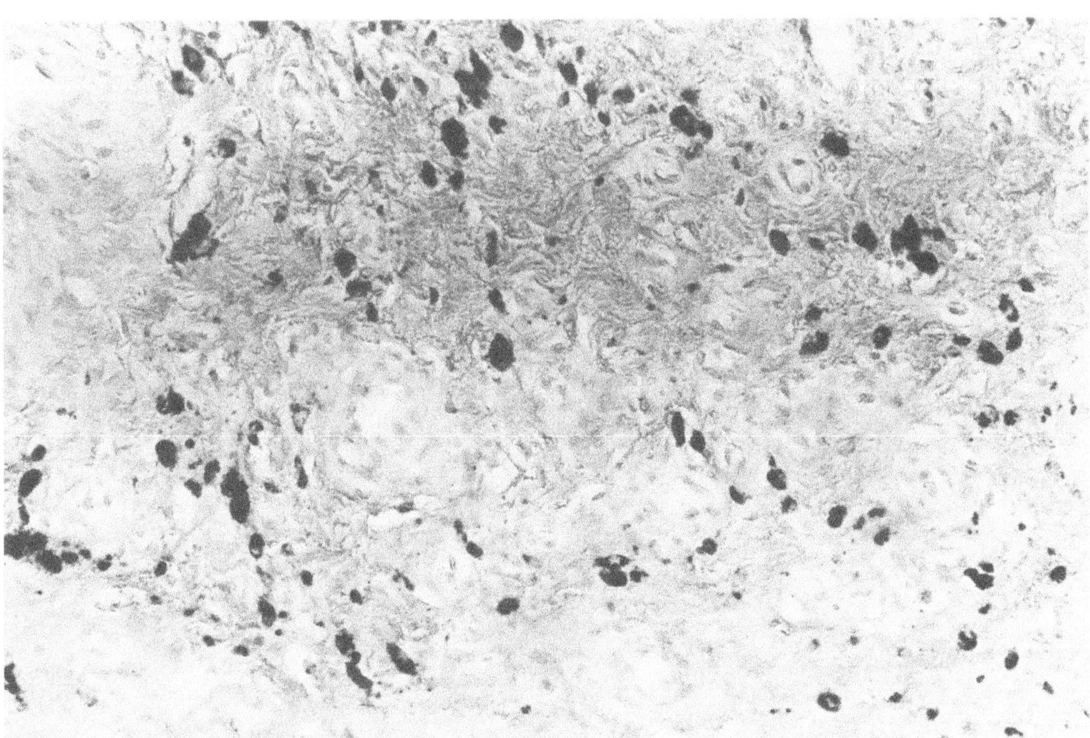

Numerous siderophages in the synovial membrane

Fig. 3.6
Rheumatoid arthritis

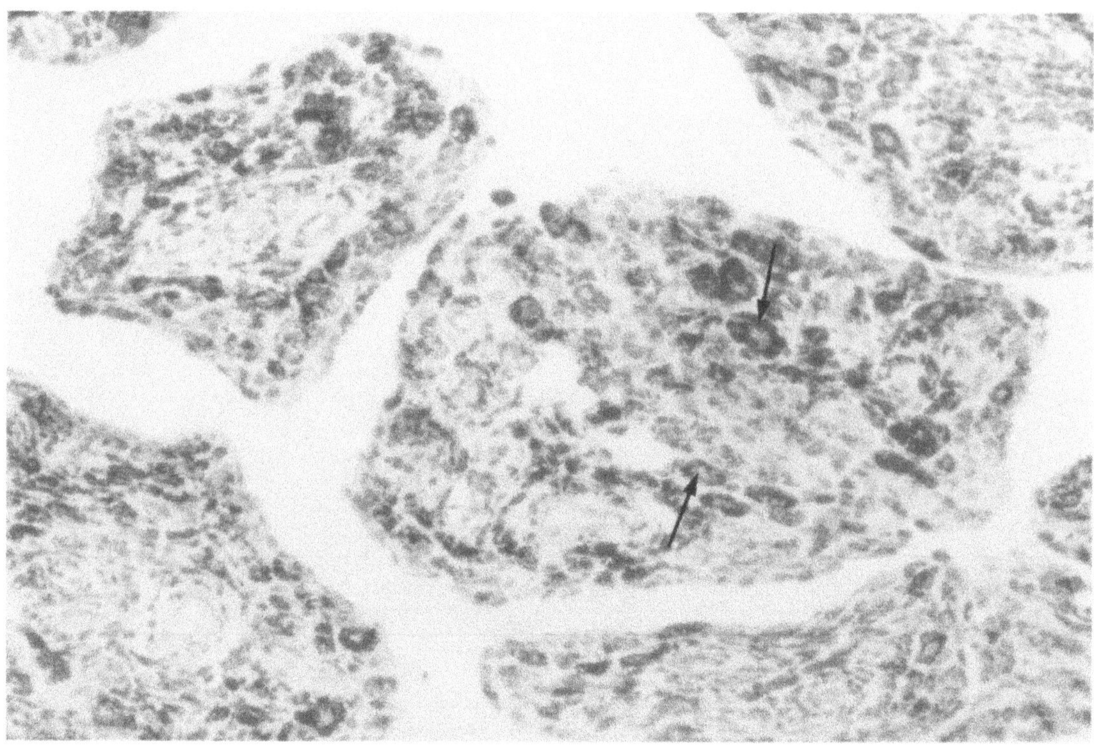

Fig. 3.7
Rheumatoid arthritis

Giant cells with bifringent foreign bodies (*arrows*) in the synovial membrane

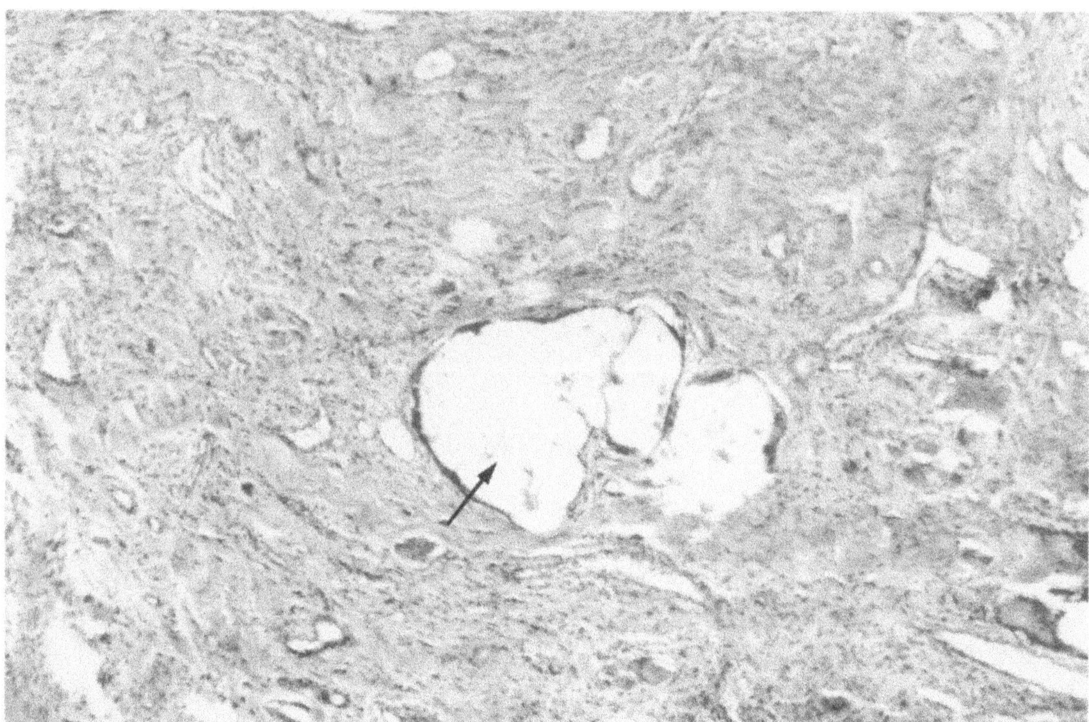

Fig. 3.8
Rheumatoid arthritis

Cement particles (*arrow*) in the region of an endoprosthesis

Giant cells

Numerous synovial-derived giant cells are seen not infrequently especially in RA in the area of the proliferating lining cell layer mainly after fibrin exudation. These giant cells do not contain any foreign bodies. Compared to the multinuclear Langhans' giant cells seen in tuberculosis and with foreign body giant cells, they only contain a few nuclei. Further differentiating points are the oval form of the nuclei and their unarranged position. Although they are commonly seen in RA and according to Grimley and Sokoloff (1966) more frequently in seropositive than in seronegative patients, they are, however, also found in synovitis of other etiology. The same type of giant cell is a characteristic feature of VNS (see p. 419).

Foreign body giant cells

Following operations, particularly after prosthesis implantation, foreign body giant cells may be seen in great numbers. Their cytoplasm contains foreign material, which sometimes may be bifringent depending on the nature of the foreign material (Figs. 3.7, 3.8).

Bone and cartilage fragments

With preceding joint destruction, especially in RA, the mainly fibrotic transformed synovial membrane contains small, rarely large cartilage and bone fragments. Depending on the duration of deposition, they may be surrounded by macrophages and giant cells or, later, by fibrosed scar tissue, which is not capable of any reaction. The cartilage fragments are often still alive, in contrast to the already dead bone fragments.

Fibrous stratum

The fibrous stratum plays no part in either the exudative or proliferative process. Occasionally, a mild perivascular lymphocytic infiltrate can be evident. On the other hand, in seropositive patients, the fibrous stratum can be the site of RA necroses (see p. 112).

Unlike the fibrous stratum, the synovial membrane rarely contains RA-necroses.Upon reaching the surface, these can soften and resemble fibrin deposition.

3.7.2 Dynamics of the Synovial Process in RA

A photomicrograph entitled "RA synovitis" could suggest the conception of a definitive picture characteristic or even specific for RA and thereby of a stationary process. In reality, a more or less dramatic process occurs in the synovial tissue, especially in RA but also in other arthritides, with a changing scenario which reflects the dynamics of the patient's individual course of disease. The photographic reproduction of lymphocyte and plasma cell infiltrates, lining cell proliferation, and villi formation could be not only a "snapshot" of RA synovitis but of other non-bacterial joint diseases. [Only the reproduction of an RA-necrosis, which is rarely seen in the synovial membrane, is specific for RA (see p. 109).]

In the same way that one chord cannot represent a Mozart symphony, a single histological "snapshot" cannot represent the synovial process in RA. The systemic illness moulds and directs the synovial process.

In this way, the synovial membrane proves to be an extremely variable stage. Three components are involved:

Three components

1. Fibrin exudation
2. Cellular infiltration
3. Cellular proliferation

Any of these three components may dominate the respective current picture. The capacity of the synovial membrane for a voluptuous exophytic surface hyperplasia [a particular characteristic of the synovial membrane (see p. 66)] as well as the stroma fibrosis and new vascularisation lead to a remodelling of the synovial membrane and can give information about the length and intensity of the synovial process.

The dynamics of RA are reflected in the phasic nature of the morphological processes.

The synovial process in RA may essentially be divided into four different stages, which during the course of the disease merge into each other and which may be repeated after every exacerbation: Exudative-infiltrative stage, proliferation stage, transition stage, and quiescent stage.

Exudative-infiltrative stage

The exudative-infiltrative stage courses as follows:

1. The synovial surface is either smooth or contains villi resulting from a previous fibrinous phase.
2. The synovial surface elaborates discrete fresh deposits of fibrin (Fig. 3.9). In contrast to BA, the fibrin is sparse, has no lamellar structure, and only contains occasional neutrophils.
3. In the area of fibrin deposition, the lining cell layer is disintegrated (Fig. 3.10).
4. The synovial stroma demonstrates variable cell density due to hypertrophy and hyperplasia of the synovial fibroblasts. During this phase, lymphocytes and plasma cells numbers can vary between sparse to moderate, with the appearance of occasional macrophages (Figs. 3.11, 3.12). Neutrophils, if seen at all, are found singly in contact with the fibrin deposits.

Usually, the exudation of fibrin is followed by formation of granulation tissue which afterwards transforms into collagenous scars. In the joint cavity, such a process would lead to destruction of the synovial architecture. This, however, only occurs in the course of bacterial arthritis because of the exudation of huge masses of fibrin. In RA and other non-bacterial, mostly immunological synovitides, the exudation of fibrin is sparse and, thus, does not result in formation of granulation tissue and scarring. Therefore, regeneration of the synovial surface is not prevented. With this background, the uniqueness of the synovial reaction in RA and other non-bacterial arthritides becomes clear. In these conditions, the process is as follows:

After the exudation of plasma, fibrinogen polymerizes to fibrin on the synovial surface. The lining cells underneath die. The synovial stroma fails to react with the formation of granulation tissue but instead reacts with the proliferation of homogeneous, oval synovial cells with large nuclei. These cells penetrate and migrate through the overlying fibrin and form a new lining cell layer on the fibrin surface. By avoiding the formation of scar tissue, limited deposits of fibrin are thus integrated into the genuine structure.

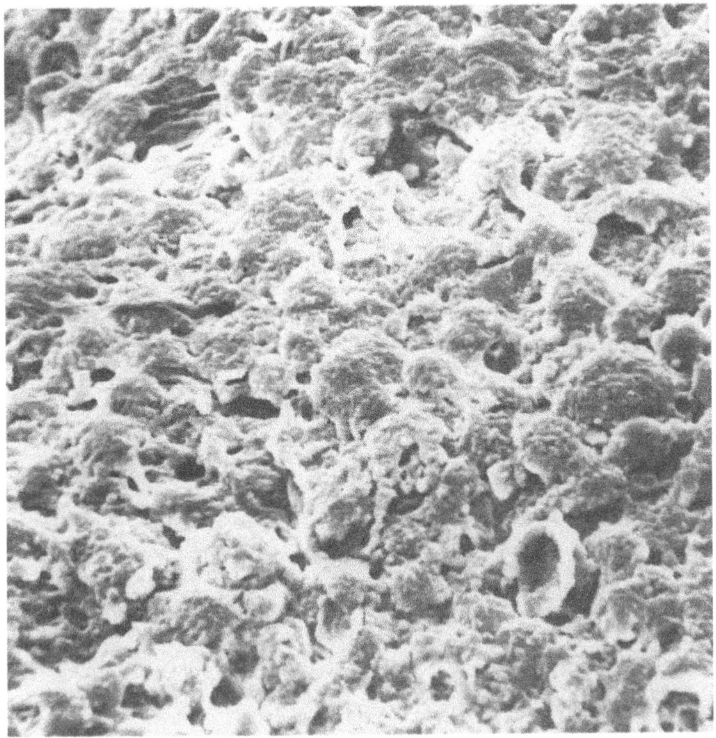

Proliferation of lining cells of the synovial layer beneath the network of fibrin. (Scanning electron micrograph)

Fig. 3.9
Rheumatoid arthritis

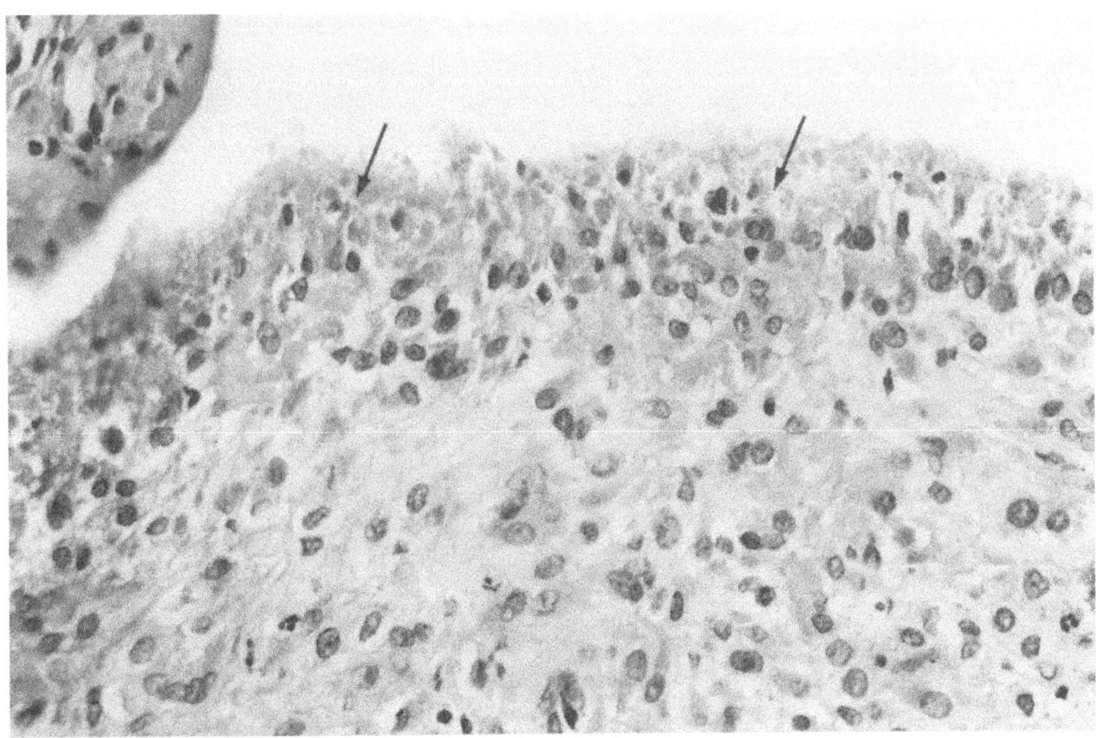

Exudative-infiltrative stage: fresh fibrin exudation (*arrows*). The lining cell layer is disintegrated

Fig. 3.10
Rheumatoid arthritis

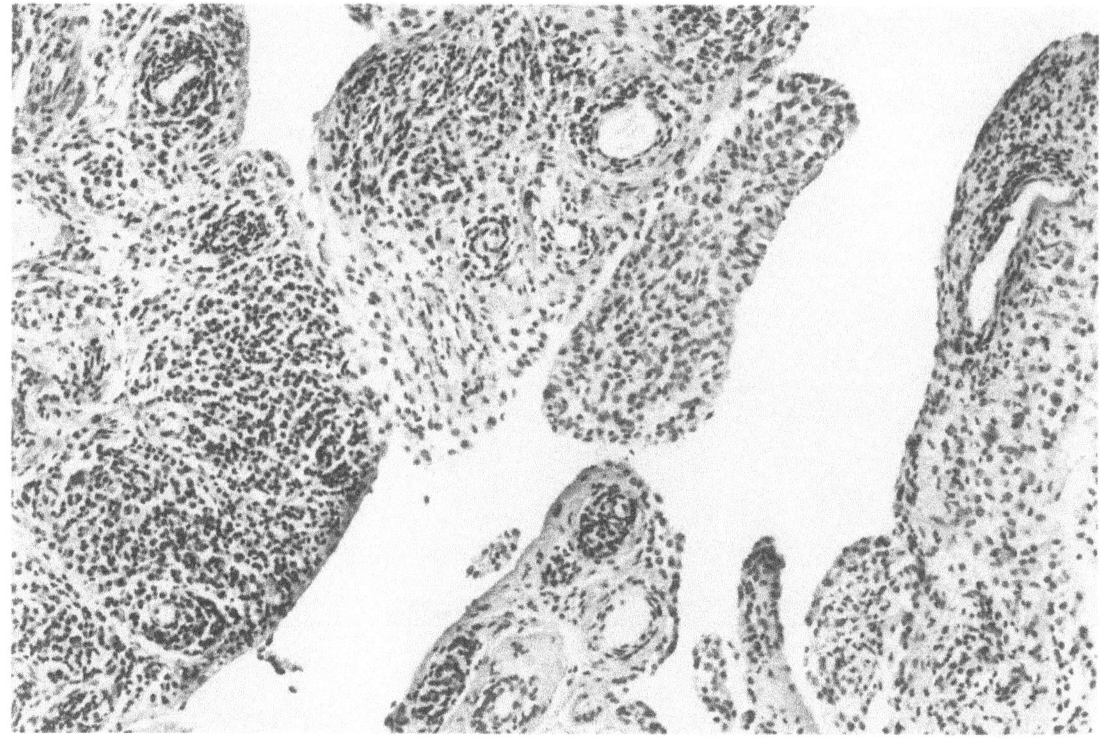

Fig. 3.11
Rheumatoid arthritis

Exudative-infiltrative stage: no fibrin. The lining cell layer is regenerated. The synovial stroma shows numerous lymphocytes, plasma cells, macrophages, and fibroblasts. Low-grade formation of villi

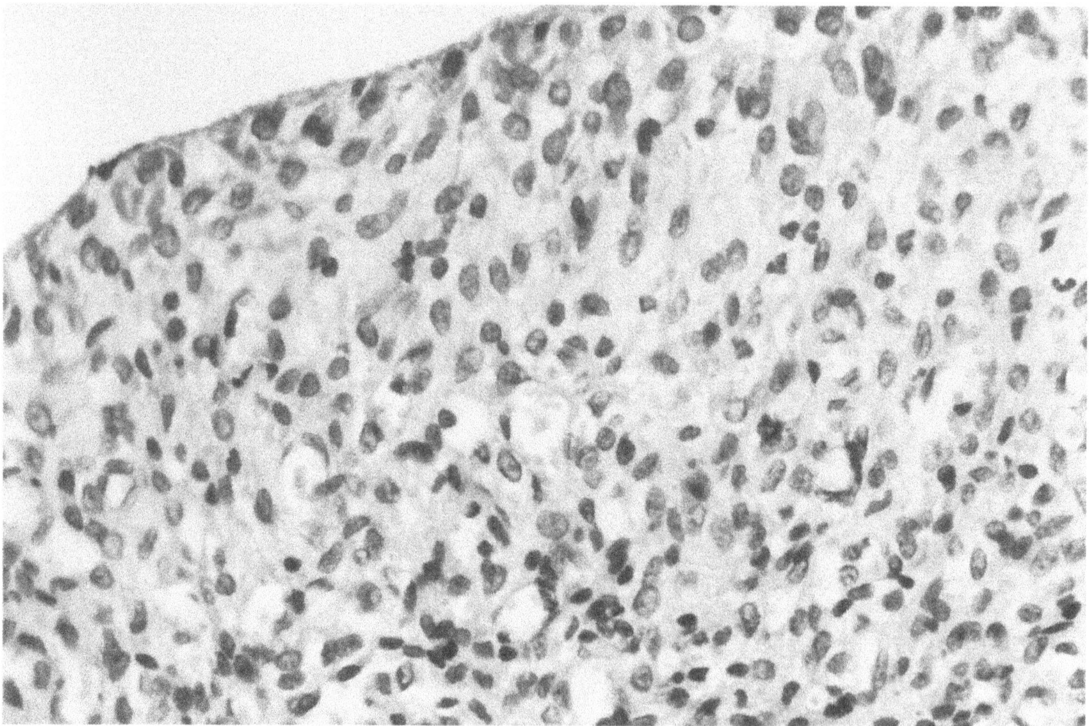

Fig. 3.12
Rheumatoid arthritis

Exudative-infiltrative stage: segment from Fig. 3.11

The assumption for this structure maintaining process is based on the fact that, in comparison with the fibrin masses occurring in BA, fibrin exudation in RA and other non-bacterial arthritides is minimal.

The inflammatory fibrinous exudate is a hallmark of clinical exacerbation of the underlying systemic immunologic process in RA. The response of the mesenchymal cell elements to the acute exudative phase is one of proliferation in the following sequence:

Proliferative stage

1. The synovial surface shows a new formation of villi.
2. The lining cell layer is dispersed with sparse membranous deposits of fibrin.
3. The lining cell layer is partly multi-graded, the regenerated cells are either cuboidal or high-cylindrical in shape (Fig. 3.13). Bud-like outgrowths of the lining cells can be seen. In the synovial tissue, frequently multi-nuclear synoviogenous giant cells, occasionally seen in large numbers, lie in close contact with the lining cell layer. These giant cells do not contain foreign bodies (see p. 71).
4. The synovial stroma appears to be extended. Areas are seen in which the synovial fibroblasts (synoviocytes) are hypertrophied, markedly increased in numbers and densely packed (Fig. 3.14). On the margin of these proliferative zones, a few lymphocytes may be found together with occasional widely dispersed macrophages. No neutrophils are evident.

Synoviocyte proliferation may be focal or may involve large areas or all of the synovial membrane.

Tumour-like proliferation

Proliferation of the synovial stroma cells may take on excessive proportions. At the peak of the proliferative stage, the demarcation line between the lining cell layer and the synovial stroma disappears.

In extreme cases, the proliferation of the synovial stroma is such that one cell lies next to another. This appearance can be very similar to that seen with malignant tumours (Figs. 3.15–3.17). In agreement with the "Deutsches Krebsforschungszentrum" (German Cancer Research Centre) in Heidelberg and the "Abteilung für Krebsforschung am Pathologischen Institut der Universität Zürich, Switzerland" (Department of Cancer Research at the Institute of Pathology of the University of Zürich, Switzerland), we have called this phenomenon "tumour-like proliferation" (tlp; Fassbender et al. 1980; see p. 89).

The normally unremarkable synovial stroma cells in their quiescent stage are oval to spindle-shaped. Similarly, the nucleus is elongated to oval in form, relatively small and stains darkly with haematoxylin. With increasing degrees of proliferation, the cells become progressively rounded, with the nucleus/plasma ratio increasing.

The nuclear structure becomes less dense, the nuclei are round, vesicular, with one or two nucleoli. At this stage, mitoses are also found (Figs. 3.18, 3.19). Occasional macrophages may solely be evident at the edges of the zone of proliferation.

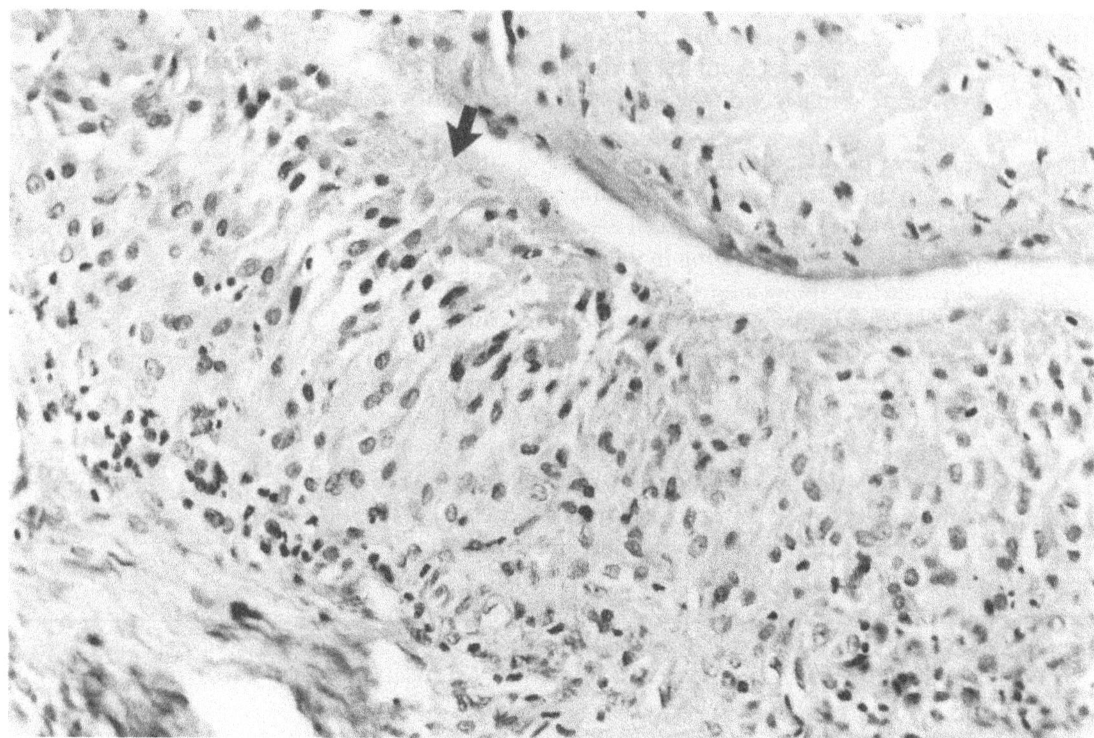

Fig. 3.13
Rheumatoid arthritis

Proliferative stage: remnants of fibrin on the surface. Multi-layered proliferation of cuboidal and cylindrical lining cells. Beneath beginning proliferation of synovial stroma cells (*arrow*)

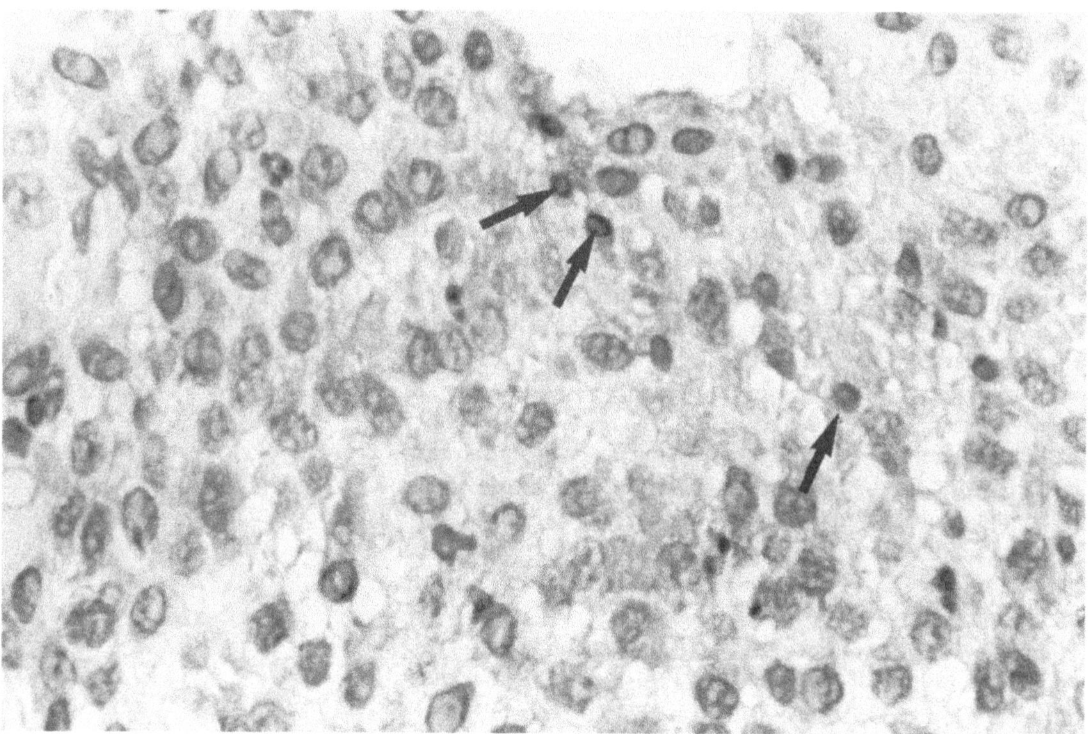

Fig. 3.14
Rheumatoid arthritis

Proliferation of synovial stroma cells. In between, only few lymphocytes (*arrows*)

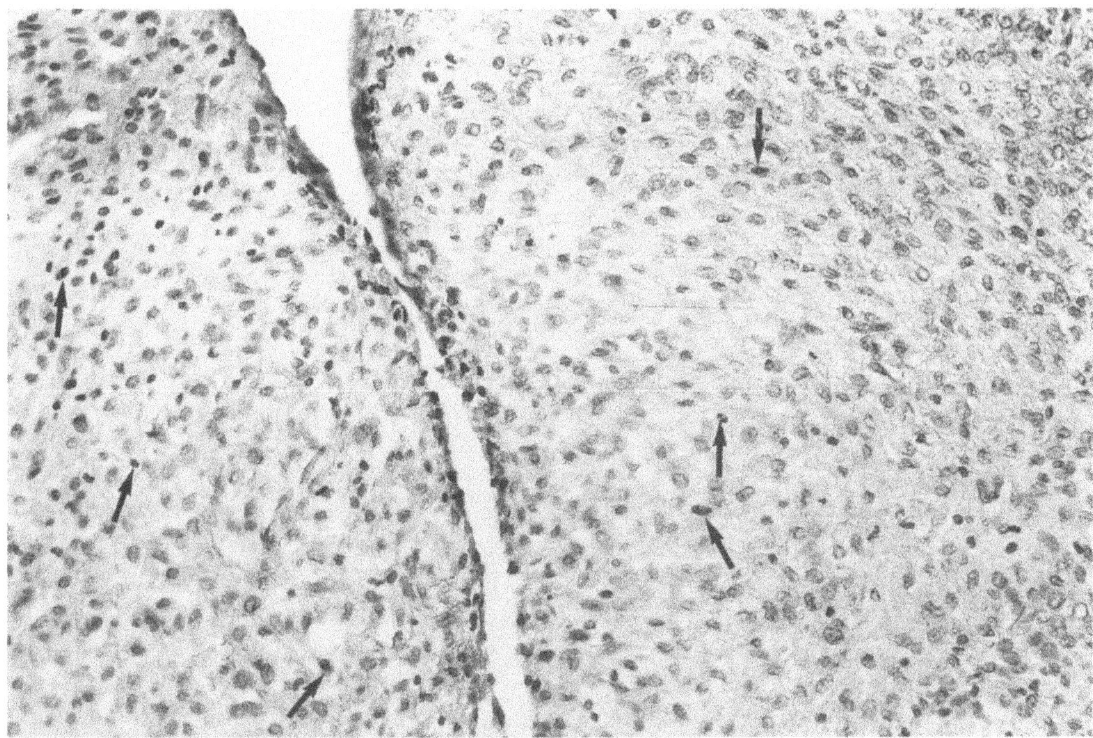

Extreme proliferation of synovial stroma cells. Tumour-like proliferation (tlp). Scarse mitoses (*arrows*)

Fig. 3.15
Rheumatoid arthritis

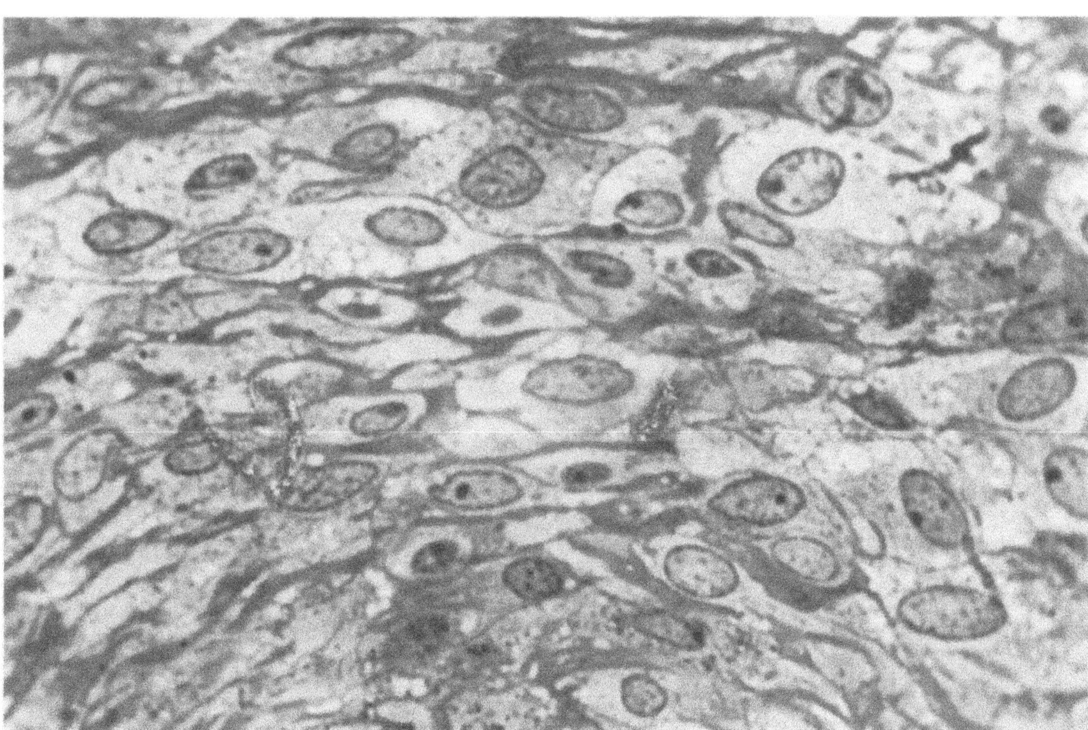

Compact tumour-like proliferation (tlp). The nuclei are uniformly sized and vesicular. The cells show a broad cytoplasmic fringe and are densely packed in an homogenous formation (semi-thin section)

Fig. 3.16
Rheumatoid arthritis

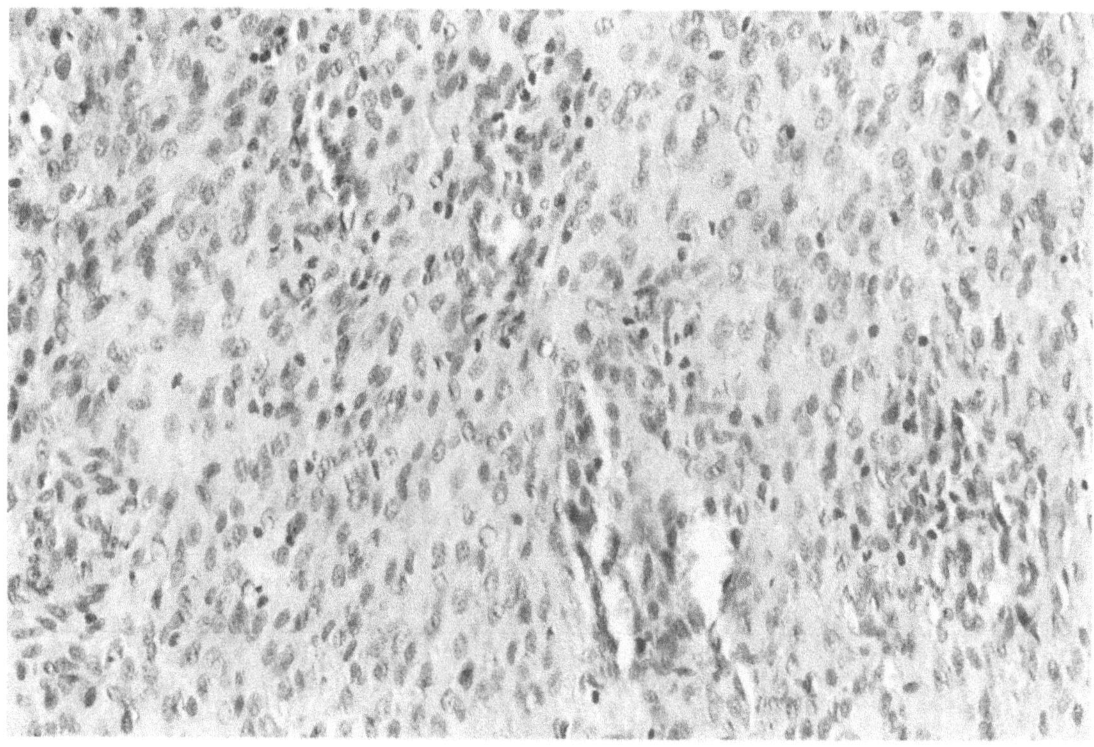

Fig. 3.17
Rheumatoid arthritis

High-grade, almost homogenous tlp formation without blood vessels. Big-sized, uniform, oval nuclei

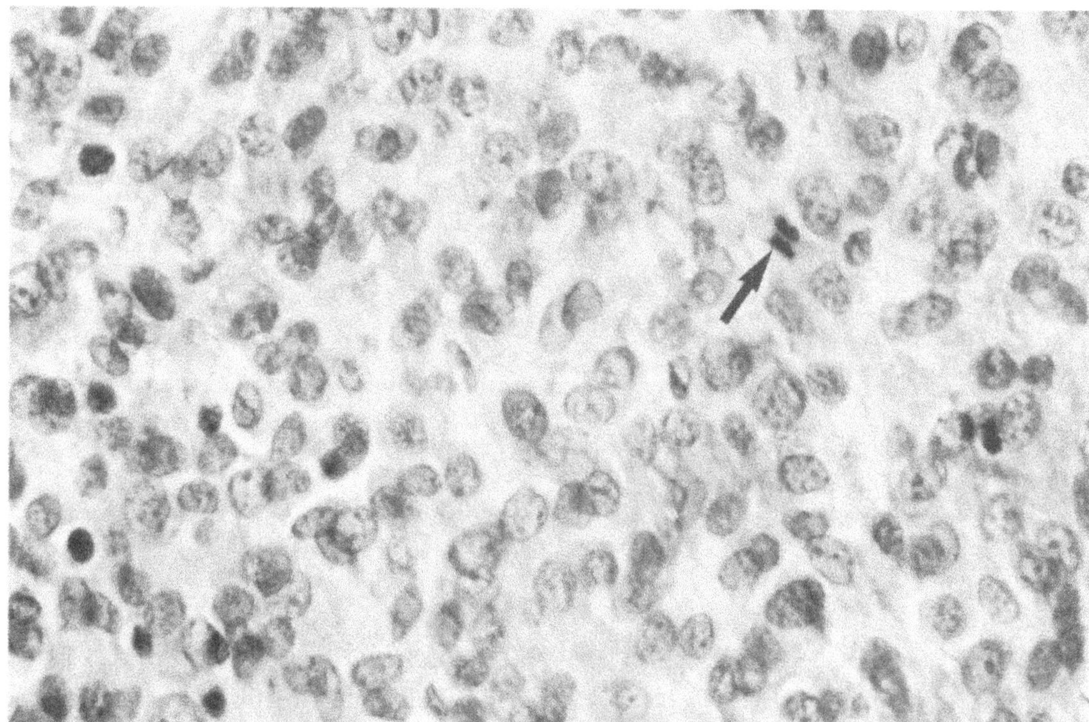

Fig. 3.18
Rheumatoid arthritis

Homogenous tlp formation with some mitoses (*arrow*). One recognizes vesicular, oval nuclei and only shadow-like cytoplasm

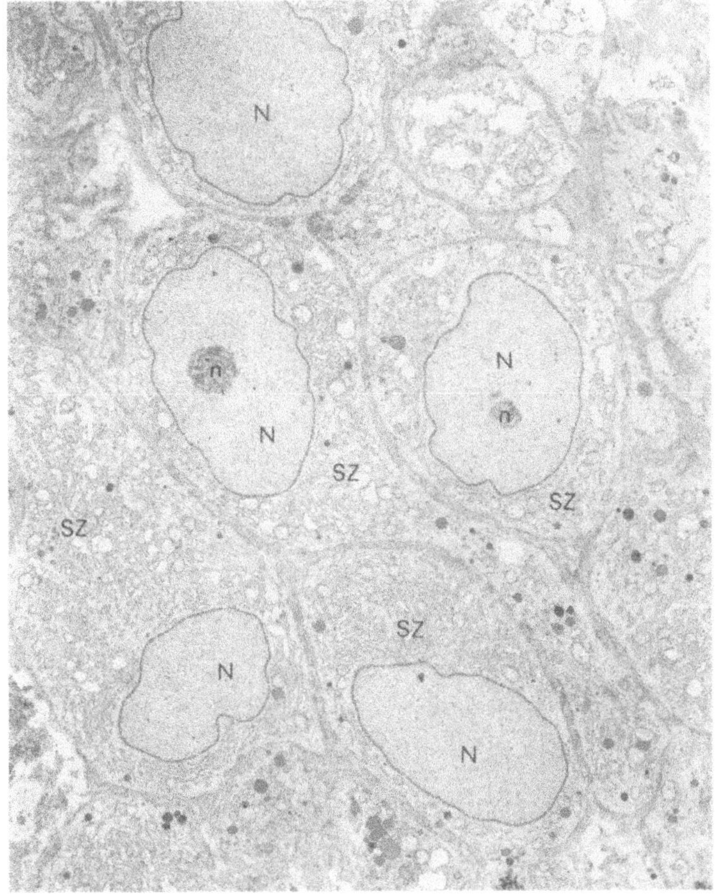

Compact synovial cell formation (tlp) with predominantly rough endoplasmic reticulum. Large vesicular nuclei with singular nucleoli. *SZ*, synovial cells; *N*, nuclei; *n*, nucleoli. (Electron micrograph)

Fig. 3.19
Rheumatoid arthritis

The endothelial cells of the arterioles and venules also participate in the proliferation process (Fig. 3.20). In the region of the tlp, the lymphocytic and plasma cell infiltrates largely or completely disappear. These infiltrates, however, tend to persist in the synovial villi which rarely or to only a small extent participate in the high proliferation process.

Oncogene expression

The evidence that inflammatory processes – although clinically impressive – do not cause the joint destruction in RA, but an excessive tumour-like proliferation (see p. 89) is responsible, has led to include proteins, which are associated with proliferation, adhesion, intercellular communication, and expression of lytic enzymes, in the discussion of the pathogenesis of RA. In collaboration with Gay and coworkers, we were able to find proof for the overexpression of c-myc, c-ras, and c-fos in the synovial tissue of patients with RA, which had previously been classified as tlp (Gay et al. 1989).
As the proliferation of synovial cells appears to be a very early step in RA, Trabandt et al. (1992) examined the expression of the early response gene egr-1 in RA. Egr-1 was significantly upregulated in RA-synoviocytes (Trabandt et al. 1992) and in long-term

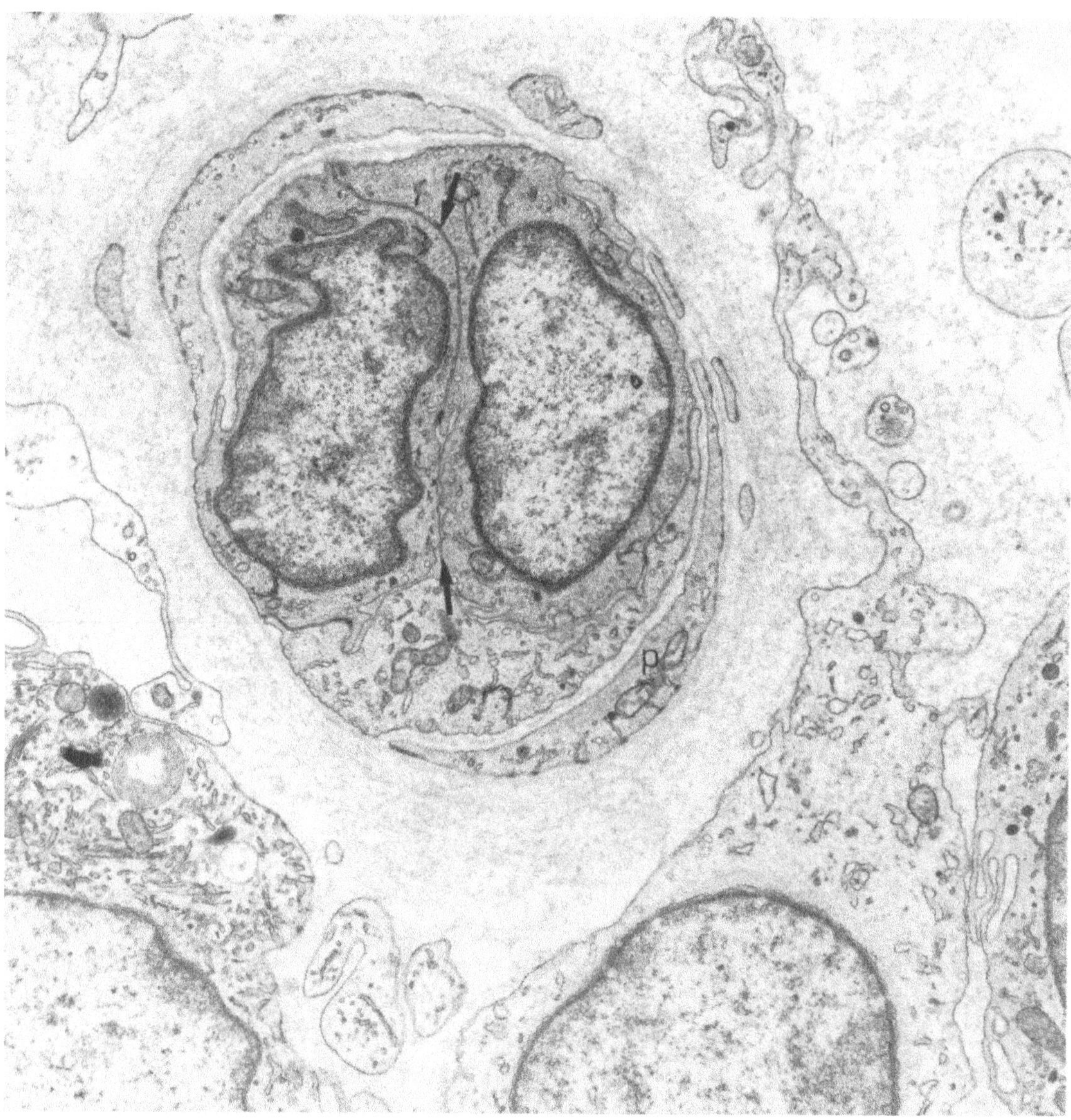

Fig. 3.20
Rheumatoid arthritis

Venule in the stage of extreme synovial proliferation. High-grade hypertrophy of the endothelial cells with occlusion of the lumen

culture this elevated transcription of egr-1 persisted (Aicher et al. 1994). Egr-1 regulates the expression of oncogenes like ras and sis, which were also overexpressed in RA synovial tissue (Trabandt et al. 1990). Therefore, it may be one of the initial steps in the pathogenesis of joint destruction in RA.
Expressed oncogenes are responsible for the proliferation on the one hand, on the other for the activation of degrading molecules such as collagenase (Schönthal et al. 1988) and stromelysin (Mauviel 1993).
In this context, also the colocalization of ras and myc with cathepsin B and L emphasizes the role of oncogenes in the upregulation of cysteine proteinases in the synovial membrane in RA. Cathepsin L seems to be the major ras-induced protein. Cathepsin B and L have an important function in degradation of cartilage collagen types II, IX, and XI (Maciewicz et al. 1990). The role

of oncogenes, particularly fos, jun, and the AP-1 complex, is subject of intensive research and becomes increasingly elucidated (Müller-Ladner et al. 1995; Firestein and Manning 1999).

Beyond that, there are some details pointing to a dysregulation of oncogenes – resulting in altered apoptosis – presumably being a major pathologic pathway in RA, since it possibly causes a prolonged lifetime of destructive synovial cells in RA.

Retroviral infection

Retroviral infection associated with subsequent transcription of oncogenes after genomic incorporations is well established. A transforming retrovirus can contribute a promoter oncogene (host) sequence that enhances the transcription of gene sequences of the host as well as its own transcription (Hayward et al. 1981; Payne et al. 1982). Based on the observation that synovial hyperplasia and especially tlp in RA is associated with a transformed appearing phenotype of the synovial proliferating cells expressing ras and myc oncogenes (Gay et al. 1988), we searched for evidence of transforming factors, especially retroviral antigens in the synovial membrane in RA. Immunohistology showed reactivity with antibodies against HTLV-I p19 and p24 in the synovial tissue, but, as the same patients were seronegative for HTLV-I, we concluded that antigens cross-reactive with or related to these HTLV-I constituents were present in the synovial membrane (Ziegler et al. 1989). In addition, studies from Aicher and coworkers have shown that synovial cells derived from rheumatoid tissue exhibit reverse transcriptase activity (Aicher et al. 1991), and, thus, enhance the possibility that a hitherto unknown retrovirus may play a part in the pathogenesis of RA (Table 3.3).

Table 3.3. Hypothesis for the etiopathogenesis of rheumatoid arthritis (modified from Gay et al. 1993)

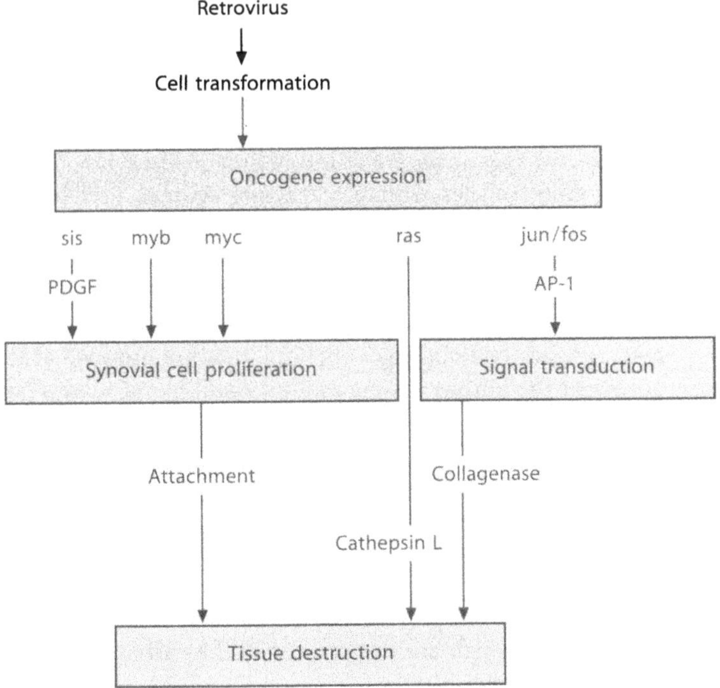

The fact that the nuclear oncoproteins myb, myc, and fos have immortalizing activity rescuing primary cells from senescence and the ability to cooperate with an activated ras gene in the transformation of primary cells, indicates that these oncogenes are associated with the tlp cells found at the site of joint destruction in RA (Gay et al. 1989).

Transition stage

Our extensive studies on a large number of synovial specimens from patients with well documented, clinically typical RA has led us to the conclusion that the changes seen in the synovial membrane represent a dynamic process corresponding to the exacerbations and remissions characteristic of the clinical disease course. And so, the tlp phase of the stroma cells is followed by a waning of the extremely proliferated synovial cells and the transition into a resting phase for the synovial membrane. This transition stage is characterized by the following features:

1. The lining cell layer regenerates; the cells vary between flat to cuboidal in shape.
2. The tlp cells decrease in size and number. They lose their round form, and there is a reduction in the nucleus/plasma ratio. Single giant cells are only seen very occasionally.
3. Lymphocytes and plasma cells reappear together with macrophages and a small number of mast cells.
4. Newly-formed, small calibre blood vessels are found in the stroma and there is a slight increase in collagen (Fig. 3.21). This long-lasting phase is consequently the one most extensively documented by photography.

Quiescent stage

The ensuing quiescent stage is characterized by the lack of exudative and proliferative activity:

1. On the surface, numerous villi are found with a non-compact fibrosed stroma and few newly-formed blood vessels. There is no fibrin deposition.
2. The lining cell layer is single-graded; the cells are flattened. No giant cells are seen.
3. The synovial stroma is moderately fibrosed and contains newly-formed blood vessels, predominantly venules. Only a few slender fibroblasts are evident. In contrast, large numbers of lymphoctye aggregates are found mainly in the synovial villi, also lymph follicles with pale germal centres. Perivascular plasma cells may be found occasionally. They are more diffusely spread and very seldom forming in dense aggregates. No neutrophils are to be seen!
4. The subsided exudative-proliferative phase leaves iron-laden macrophages (siderophages) behind, that are grouped at the border of the fibrous stroma around small blood vessels (see p. 68).

Due to the, in contrast to the proliferative stage, prolonged persistence of the transition stage, it is understandable that most studies cited in literature are concerned with the synovial membrane in this late stage. This is evident also from the reported findings of macrophages and blood vessels in the synovial stroma, both of which are not present in the early proliferative and aggressive stage.

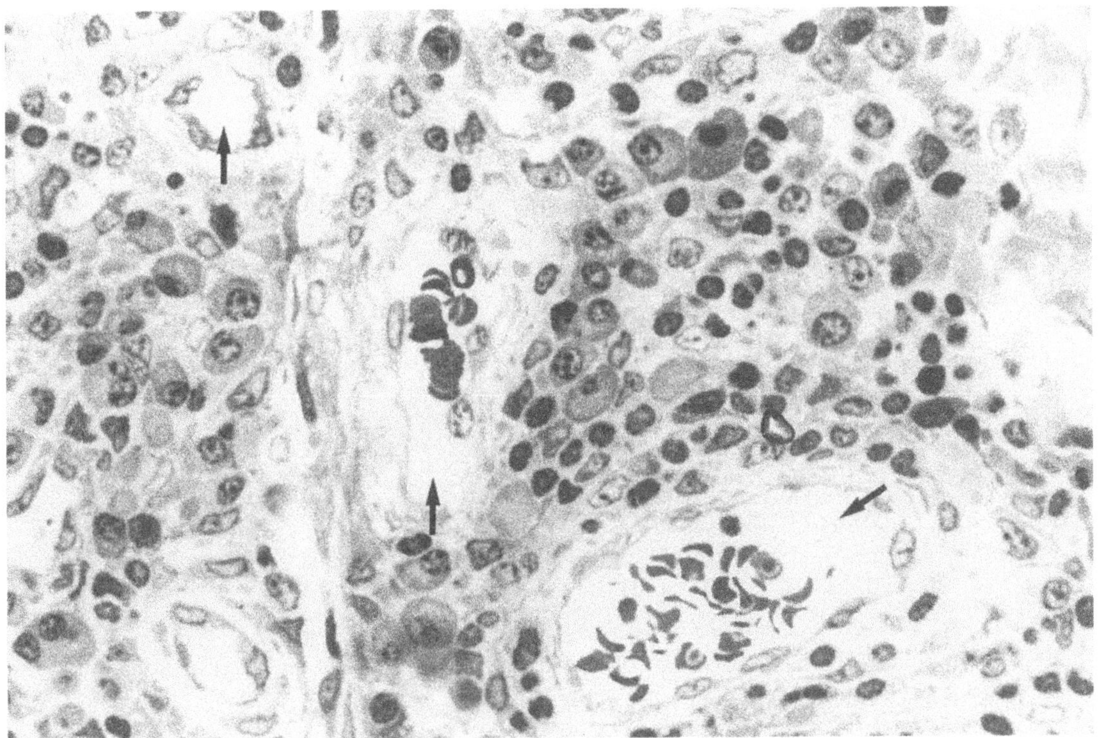

Transition stage: newly formed blood vessels (*arrows*) surrounded by lymphocytes and plasma cells (semi-thin section)

Fig. 3.21
Rheumatoid arthritis

It is understandable from the episodic nature of RA that the remnants of the local processes summate with every single exacerbation of the disease. In this way, villous formation, fibrosis, accumulation of siderophages, and the formation and size of blood vessels increase with each flare.

3.7.3 Joint Destruction in RA

Basically, it seems plausible that joint destruction in RA is the deed of joint inflammation that has been well documented clinically, immunologically, and biochemically. However, this concept is not compatible with the experience that although pain and inflammation can be controlled with the available arsenal of steroids and non-steroidal anti-inflammatory agents, the process of joint destruction as evident on the radiograph is not influenced. When considering the possible pathogenetic mechanisms, it must be borne in mind that the destructive process not only involves the articular cartilage, but preferentially cortical bone, as our investigations have shown (see p. 96).

Different hypotheses

At present, different hypotheses with regard to joint destruction in RA are being considered:

Neutrophils

The possible leading role of neutrophils with regard to joint destruction in RA is being discussed (Weissmann 1971; Mohr and Menninger 1979; Kitsis and Weissmann 1991; Chatham et al. 1993; Gauger and Mohr 1995). There can be no doubt that collagenases and elastases of the neutrophils are able to degrade hyaline articu-

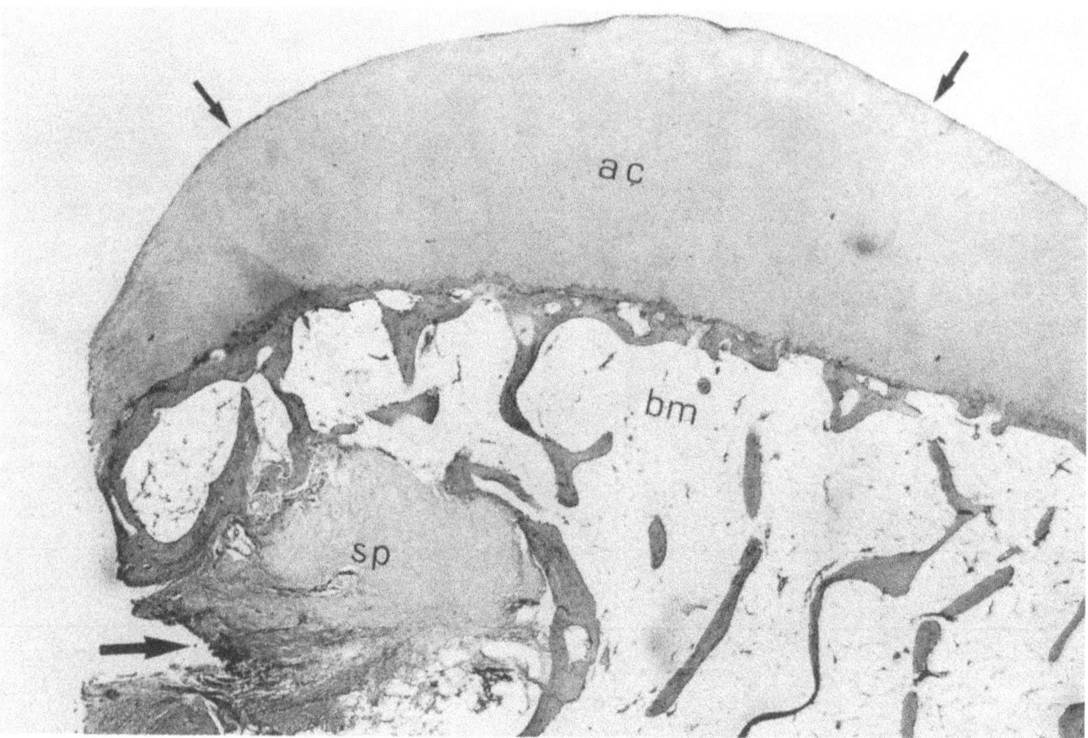

Fig. 3.22
Rheumatoid arthritis

Proximal metatarsophalangeal joint after months of high-grade synovitis. The articular cartilage (*arrows above*) is completely intact. Fibrous scar in the cortical bone following the invasion of tlp cell masses (*arrow on the left*). *Ac*, articular surface; *bm*, bone marrow; *sp*, scar pannus with cartilage fragment

lar cartilage as is the case in septic arthritis, in contrast to RA where the amount of neutrophils is lower. In BA (see p. 386), masses of neutrophils are found in the synovial fluid whose concentration of proteolytic enzymes can digest whole sequesters of the joint surface.
According to our observations, neutrophil occurrence is a very rare finding in synovial membranes in RA, as Bywaters and Ansell pointed out as early as in 1965. As previously mentioned, the occurrence of a high number of neutrophils in the synovial fluid of patients with RA suspects the presence of a superimposed bacterial infection (see p. 68).
If, hypothetically, there would be an influence of neutrophil enzymes on articular cartilage also in RA, destruction all along the joint convexity that has come into contact with synovial fluid could be expected, as it is the case in septic or BA.Consequently, the articular surface in RA would be destroyed extensively. Under no circumstances could we expect the simultaneous existence of an intact cartilaginous surface and a destroyed cortical bone (Fig. 3.22), as we were able to show in 49% of evaluated 288 capitulae from patients with RA (see p. 96).
In RA, the amount of neutrophil enzymes released does not exceed the capacity of the inhibitors in the synovial fluid.
The majority of studies regarding the collagenolytic activity in the synovial fluid in RA reveal that the active enzyme is found only in few patients.

But even in these positive cases, the enzyme activity amounted only to 0.2%–0.5% of the overall enzyme activity. This is due to the suppression through enzyme inhibitors; their most important part appears to be the α2 macroglobulin. This large molecule is present in the plasma and, so, in inflammatory effusions. In the synovial fluid, the always present lower molecular glycoprotein TIMP (tissue inhibitor of metalloproteinases) can be observed in higher concentration than in the plasma, which points towards a local synthesis (Firestein and Paine 1992; Ishiguro et al. 1996).

α2 macroglobulin

TIMP

Macrophages and cytokines

Of special interest is a possible immunologically mediated activity of macrophages for the destruction of articular cartilage. One can reckon with interactions between antigen-presenting cells, T lymphocytes, and B lymphocytes.

Lymphocytes lead to a release of cytokines that stimulate macrophages in the synovial tissue. Whether or not the presence of activated T cells and their products is necessary to sustain the synovial macrophages in a stimulated state remains a controversial point. Of major importance, however, is the fact that these cells appear to secrete or release both IL-1 and TNF-α that could be able to drive the process of tissue destruction (Chu et al. 1991).

IL-1 and TNF-α

IL-1 and TNF-α are two pure inflammatory cytokines. Cytokines are proteins synthesized by many cell types which bind to receptors on several cells and exert a variety of biological effects.

Thus, fibroblasts and chondrocytes are stimulated to produce collagenases and other neutral proteinases (Arend and Dayer 1990).

TNF-α was abundant in macrophages in RA synovium, both in lining cells and perivascular distribution in the synovium (Chu et al. 1991). TNF-α-containing cells also were localized at the cartilage-pannus-junction in these studies, suggesting production near the site of tissue destruction.

We have to take into consideration that the release of IL-1 and TNF-α is a non-specific process that takes place in every inflammatory episode in general but especially in arthritides, thus, also in OA.

In this context, the occurrence of soluble TNF-receptors in patients with infectious or other inflammatory diseases gains special attention. In the circulation of RA patients and also in the synovial fluid were elevated levels of soluble TNF-receptors present (Cope et al. 1992; Barrera et al. 1993; Chikanza et al. 1993).

The levels of soluble TNF-receptors were higher in the synovial fluid than in the sera of patients with RA, suggesting local production in the joint (Cope et al. 1992). These soluble TNF-receptors appear to be inhibitory as indicated by the lack of biologically active TNF-α in the serum and synovial fluid samples containing high levels of measurable TNF-α protein.

Therefore, it appears that the articular cartilage is protected against proteases as well as against cytokines via an inhibitory system. Here we find an explanation for the fact that non-bacterial, generally immunologically induced synovitides do not destroy the articular cartilage (see p. 72).

In BA, however, the disintegrating neutrophils release proteases to such a high extent that the dykes of the inhibitory system breach and, so, the articular cartilage can be destroyed in a short time (see p. 385).

Immune complexes

Two observations lead to the assumption that immune complexes are important factors regarding the destruction of cartilage: immune complexes are proven to be found only in articular cartilage free of pannus and not in the area underneath the pannus; macrophages from the pannus, which border on the cartilage, have taken in IgG (Shiozawa et al. 1980).

Storage of immune complexes in the joint cartilage was also said to play a role in the possible conditioning of the macrophages and was therefore attributed as important to the joint destruction. Already in 1975, Cooke et al. proved the existence of immune complexes in articular cartilage near to the surface predominantly in RA but also in OA patients. Antibodies against collagen type II and rheumatoid factors were identified in RA (Mannik and Person 1994). However, the presence of immune complexes near the surface as well as serum constituents may also be proven in normal articular cartilage.

We have examined articular cartilage of 12 patients with RA, 14 with PSA, 10 with OA, and 2 with ankylosing spondylitis (AS) on the presence of immune complexes (Lühr 1997). We found IgG, IgM, and IgA as well as C1q and C3c in 11 of 12 patients with RA, and IgA, C1q, and C3c in 13 of 14 patients with PSA. IgG, IgM, IgA as well as C1q were also found to be present in the articular cartilage of all ten OA patients. IgG, IgM, IgA, and C1q were also found in both AS patients. We agree with other authors that there is no doubt that the storage of immune complexes and serum constituents is an unspecific accompanying phenomenon of the inflammatory process. On the one hand, circulating serum antibodies are not unusual; on the other hand, however, the avascular articular cartilage seems to be predetermined for storage, although a certain previous mechanical damage, as is to be expected in most adult patients, seems necessary because it is difficult to understand how the macromolecular immune complexes find their way into a completely intact cartilage.

It has to be emphasized that immunologically caused non-bacterial inflammations occur not only in RA but also in reactive arthritis (REA) as well as in RF without destroying the cartilage. As macrophages belong to the tools of every inflammation one cannot expect any explanation about the specific destructive mechanism in RA only from their proof in the joint.

RA has its own specific clinical and morphological profile which is characterized with regard to quality and quantity. Especially the preferred destruction of the cortical bone in RA can hardly be explained by the action of macrophages. On the contrary, in accordance with Bromley and Woolley (1984), we have found single macrophages and some mast cells scattered in the region of the subchondral bone destruction in RA, but only in a relatively late stage, i.e. when vascularisation had taken place.

The question about the role of macrophages in cartilage destruction was further settled by immunohistological investigations of Petrow et al. (1997). Proliferating cells from the area of the cartilage invasion in RA patients were double labelled with the macrophage specific marker CD68 and the proliferation marker KI-67. It turned out that the KI-67-positive cells were negative for CD68, indicating that the proliferating cell population consists of synovial stroma cells.

Chondrocytic chondrolysis

Based on the studies of Dingle et al. (1979), chondrocytic proteases are also being held responsible for the destruction of articular cartilage (Jasin 1987; Arend and Dayer 1990). There are numerous in-vitro analyses on chondrocytic chondrolysis, especially with regard to the genesis of OA (Aydelotte et al. 1986). Occasionally, we were able to prove a minimal circular degradation of the territorial matrix in OA and RA, but these minor changes cannot be spatially connected to joint destruction. Furthermore, radiographic analyses of Mohr and Hummler (1986) demonstrated that the chondrocytes morphologically and functionally remain intact until they come into contact with the site of invasion by synoviogenous cell masses. From the quantitative point of view, the possible destructive role of chondrocytes should be doubted considering the fact that the cartilage cells form only 0.1% of the total cartilage substance (Vignon et al. 1977). With regard to the destruction of cortical bone substance, the hypothetical role of chondrocytes being involved becomes irrelevant.

Osteoclasts

Many authors (e.g. Salisbury et al. 1987; Leisen et al. 1988) ascribe the collapse of the cortical bone in RA to osteoclasts. We, however, never found osteoclasts in the region where the destructive attack by synoviogenous cell masses takes place. In a study on 100 capitulae of metatarsal and metacarpal joints from patients with definite RA showing florid destruction of bone, no more than 12 showed single osteoclasts which were found exclusively in the area where dead bone fragments were located and where remodelling was in progress (Fassbender 1986a).

"Chondroclasts"

In accordance with Bromley and Woolley (1984), we detected single "chondroclasts" in the region of the breakthrough of the subchondral osseous lamella underneath a yet intact articular cartilage. In this region, scattered "chondroclasts" in subchondral "pockets" could also be found (see p. 97). But this represents a relatively late stage already with cell deficiency and numerous blood vessels which marks the beginning of scar pannus formation.

Tumour-like synovial cell masses

As long as granulation tissue or pannus at variable stages was the sole finding in the area of destruction in RA, there was understandably room for various hypotheses, all based on the premise that the destruction was secondary to inflammation.

Kauko Vainio's concept

In the 1950s, Kauko Vainio in Heinola (Finland) developed synovectomy as a therapeutic principle in RA. He considered the removal of the proliferated synovial tissue to be analogous to the elimination of a malignant destructive tumour (Vainio 1967). The removal of the damaging, "aggressive" synovial tissue is based on the perception that the joint destruction is not caused by inflammatory processes but rather by synovial aggression. But this concept was forgotten for years.

We could prove this concept in 1972, as we described for the first time the appearance of compact groups of cells in the normally loose and relatively acellular synovial tissue in patients with RA

(Fassbender 1972). At the same time, we could pursue a stepwise change in the qualitative and quantitative behaviour of the synovial fibroblasts (synoviocytes; mesenchymoid transformation; see p. 75).

Tumour-like transformation

The synoviocytes, normally lying scattered and sparsely, increase dramatically in number and lose their original spindle shape. They become oval and then round up. This process can progress to such an extent so as to give rise to a compact, homogeneous mass of cells, which lie in contact with one another, like in an epithelial tumour. At this stage, the round to polyhedral cells are large and rich in cytoplasm. The cell nuclei are similarly large, pale, and vesicular with a loose structure and contain one to two nucleoli. At this time, a moderate number of mitoses can be demonstrated.

Electron-microscopical findings

In 1980, we were able to document electron-microscopically the transformation of the normal synovial cell into the proliferating and actively secreting tlp element (Fassbender et al. 1980). The RER is strongly developed, the cisternae similarly as in plasma cells are layered in a parallel mode. In the cytoplasm, free ribosomes are present. The increased cell activity is also expressed in an increase in number and size of the Golgi-complexes.

Later, the cisternae of RER break down through vesiculation and fragmentation into cysts of varying size. In their place, numerous small primary lysosomes are formed. The nucleus reacts with an increase in volume and a lightening of the karyoplasm by hydration. The consequent large pale nuclei are signs of highly active cells and by light-microscope are distinctive marker for the highly active tlp cells.

In two studies of synovial tissue in 100 (Botzenhardt 1975) and 265 patients (Misskampf 1984) with clinically defined RA, we demonstrated that this proliferation of synovial cells corresponded with a flaring of the disease and an increase in ESR. Afterwards, the synoviocytes return to a fibroblastic form.

Synoviogenous joint aggression

We succeeded in reaching the decisive stage in the explanation of joint destruction, however, when in 1978 we observed the continuous aggression of such a compact synoviogenous cell mass from the synovial membrane along the "bare" area of bone onto hyaline articular cartilage (Fig. 3.23).

Contrary to the "pannus" known until this point, this was a compact, homogeneous cell mass, which contained no fibres and importantly, no blood vessels! The cells and their nuclei demonstrate all characteristics of immaturity in form and structure: the cells are round to polyhedral and their nuclei are large and vesicular. Numerous nucleoli and scattered mitoses can be observed. The cells correspond to the formerly described mesenchymoid transformation in the synovial membrane (see p. 75).

The lining cells themselves, however, do not play any role in the development of tlp formations. This was confirmed by immunohistological investigations of Petrow and his team (1997) on the invasion front as well as in synovial biopsies of RA patients. The proliferation marker KI-67 was predominantly detected in fibroblast-like stroma cells whereas only single lining cells expressed this marker.

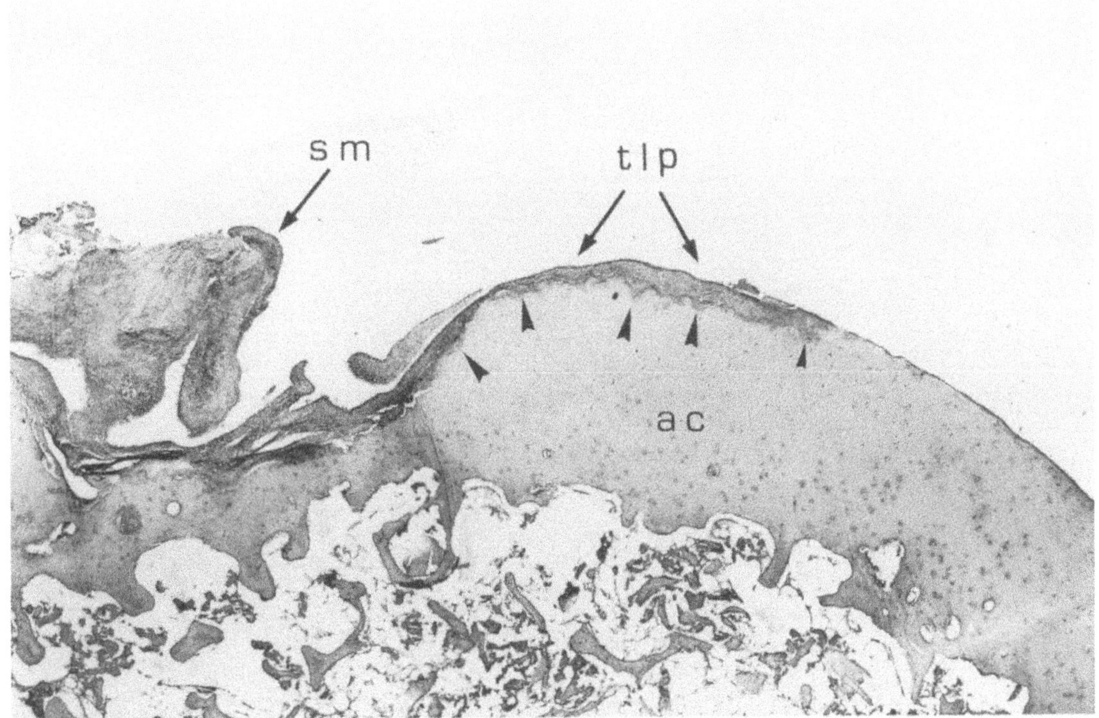

Metacarpophalangeal joint. Attack of the aggressive synovial cell masses from the synovial recess onto the articular surface. One can recognize the start of the invasion into the cartilaginous matrix. The subchondral bone lamella has already been destroyed by previous attacks. *Arrowheads*, site of invasion; *tlp*, tumour-like proliferation; *ac*, articular cartilage; *sm*, synovial membrane

Fig. 3.23
Rheumatoid arthritis

Invasion of compact synoviogenous cell masses

We could clearly demonstrate and document the penetration of the compact synoviogenous cell masses into the cartilage matrix (Fassbender et al. 1980; Fassbender 1983). These were the same large nucleated cells that we had described in the tlp of the synovial tissue (see p. 75). Lymphocytes, plasma cells or macrophages are not detectable in this homogeneous mass.

Cartilage destruction

With invasion in the cartilage, the first step is degradation of the aggrecans; the denuded collagen fibres remain intact, but with further progression they are also enzymatically destroyed. The cells can be observed adopting a radial formation at the invasion front as they penetrate between the fibres. The neighbouring chondrocytes remain intact until they are also caught-up in the destructive process (Figs. 3.24–3.27).

"Tumour-like proliferation" (tlp)

We have termed these immature, destructive cell masses "tumour-like proliferation" (tlp; see p. 75).

Size and nuclear structure of the densely packed cells are indicative of high metabolic activity. As may be expected, these compact cell masses have only a very short life-span as they are avascular and the partial pressure of oxygen in synovial fluid in RA is low, thus, because of inefficient supply of oxygen and lack of blood vessels these cell masses lack equivalent life conditions on the joint surface and consequently the cells rapidly die.

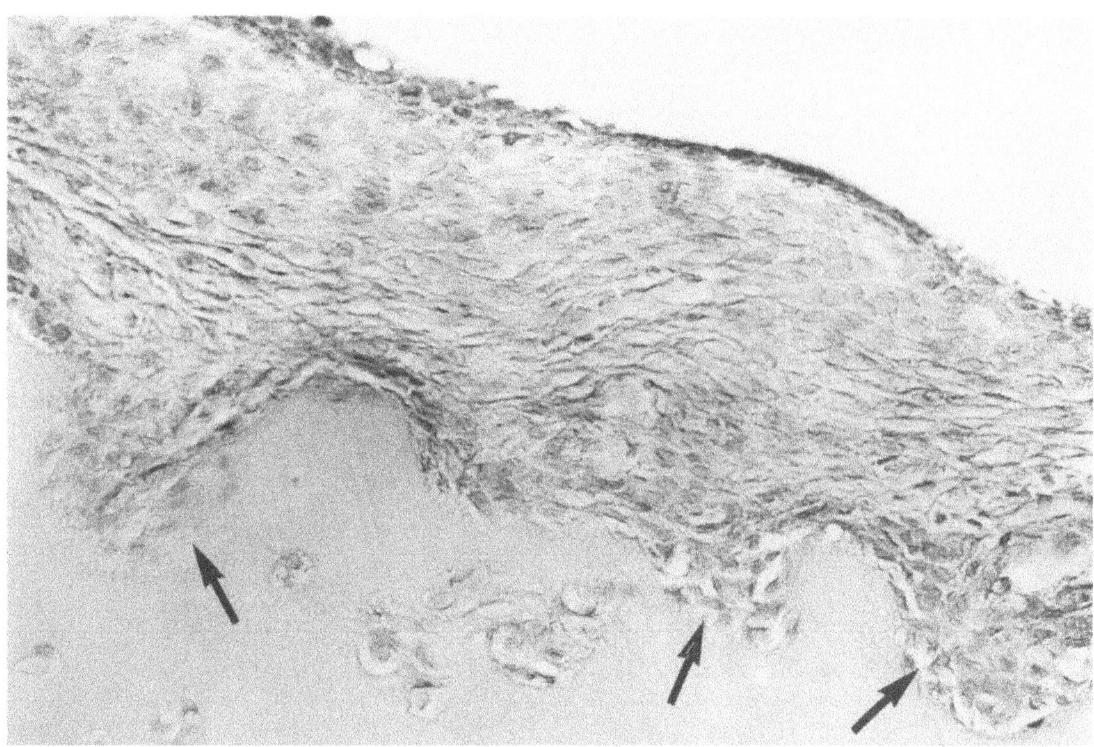

Fig. 3.24
Rheumatoid arthritis

Metacarpophalangeal joint. The *arrows* mark the invasion of the avascular, homogenous, macronuclear synovial cell masses (tlp). Segment from Fig. 3.23

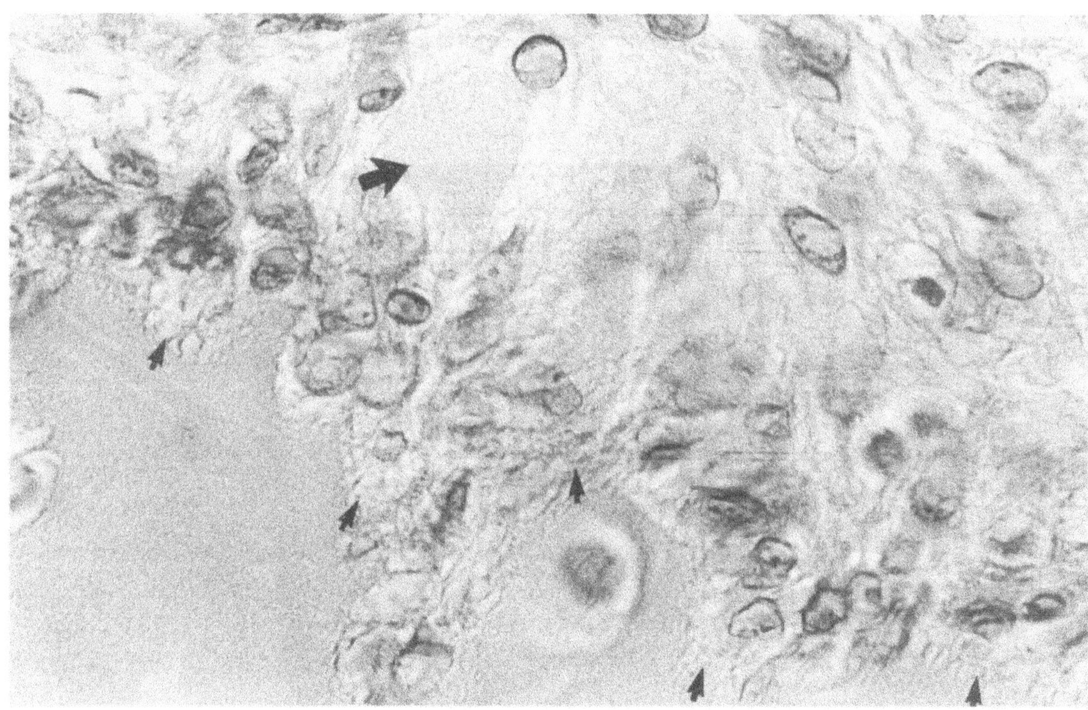

Fig. 3.25
Rheumatoid arthritis

Proximal interphalangeal joint. Invasion of the macronuclear synovial cell masses (tlp) into the articular cartilage. One recognizes the denuded collagen fibres after proteoglycan depletation by enzymes of the tumour-like cells (*arrows*). *Bottom middle*, preserved chondrocyte. *Big arrow*, cartilage remnant

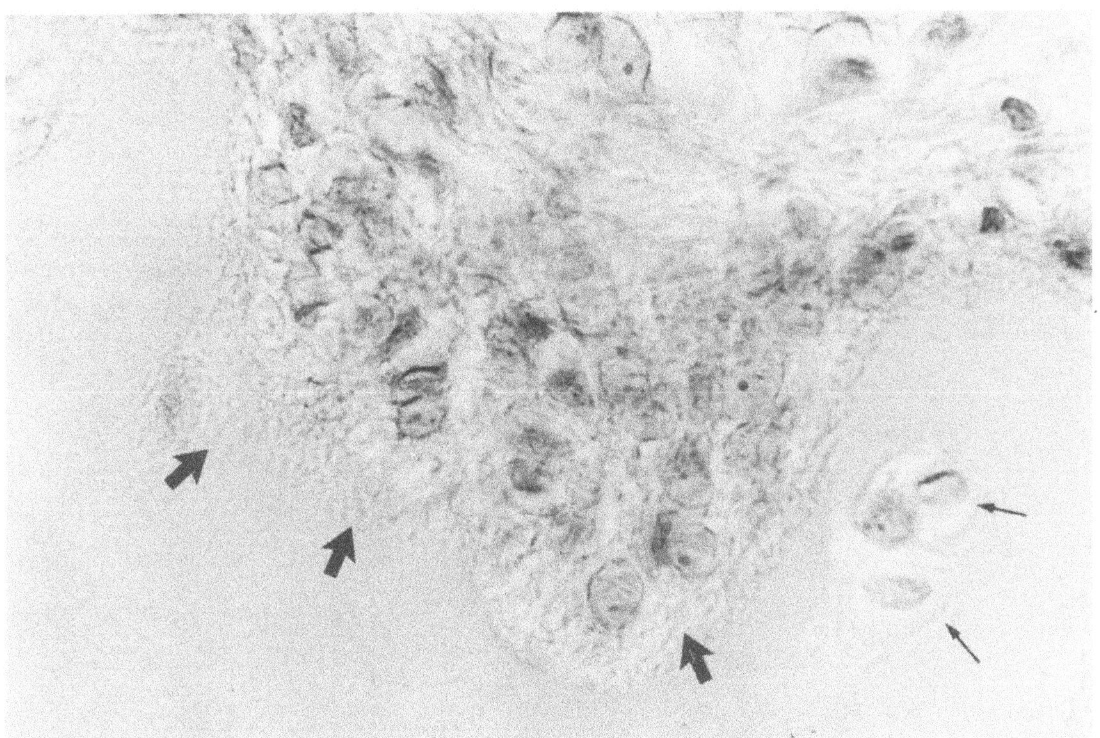

Proximal interphalangeal joint. Denudation of collagen fibres after proteoglycan depletion by the enzymes of the invading tumour-like cells (*large arrows*). *Bottom right*, preserved chondrocytes (*small arrows*)

Fig. 3.26
Rheumatoid arthritis

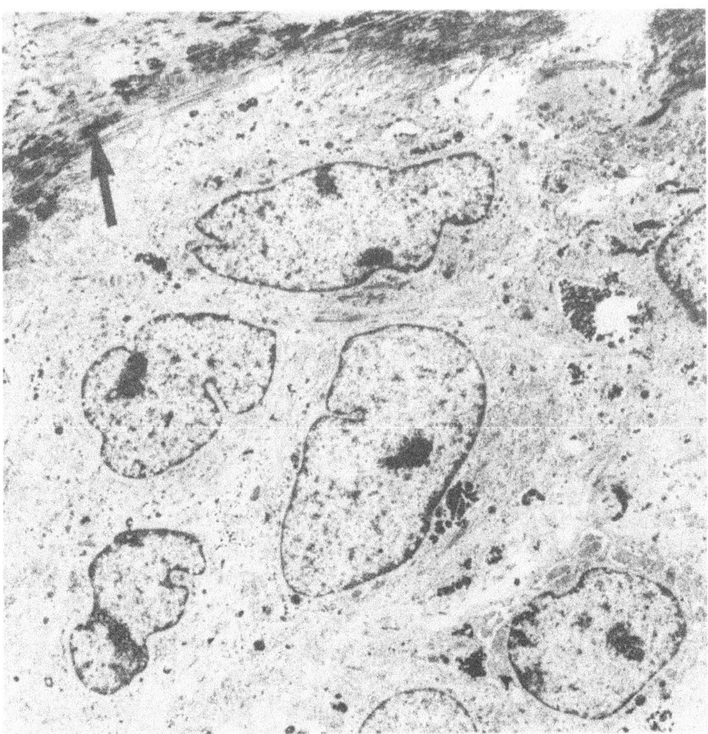

Invasion of aggressive tumour-like cells into the articular cartilage. Light nuclei with 1–2 nucleoli. *Arrow*, articular cartilage. (Electron micrograph)

Fig. 3.27
Rheumatoid arthritis

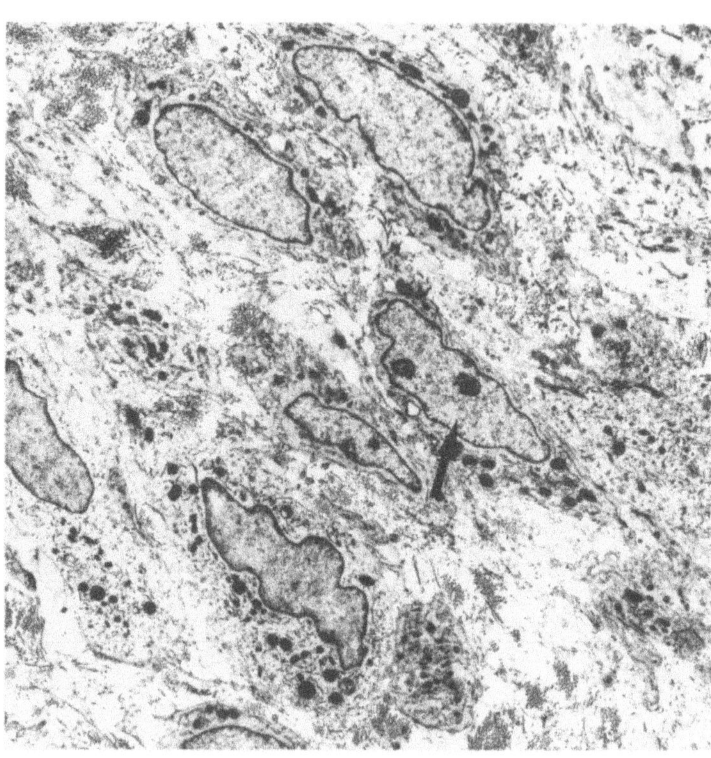

Fig. 3.28
Rheumatoid arthritis

Collapse of tlp formation: fibroblastic modulates with still large nuclei showing 1–2 nucleoli (*arrow*). The beginning of procollagen secretion is the hour of birth of the "pannus" (Electron micrograph)

Also the possibility has to be discussed if the collapse of the tlp cells is caused by apoptosis. The first occurrence of macrophages in this stage would correspond to this.
The short life-span explains the very difficult detection of the tlp phase. It is a problem to hit on it.

Collapse of tlp formation

We could demonstrate the remnants of dead tlp cells using electron-microscopy. The majority of the surviving cells show modulation to fibroblasts, although cell shape, nucleus, and the presence of one to two nucleoli betray their origin as tlp cells. In between, single tlp cells are observed with their original form and structure (Fig. 3.28).

Intermediate phase

On light-microscopy, it is possible to detect in this intermediate phase now a few branched in small blood vessels and macrophages as well as occasionally single lymphocytes and mast cells. Those cells in contact with the invasion front are now mainly lying parallel to the cartilage surface, in contrast to the tumour-like phase during which the cells penetrate between the collagen (type II) fibres of the cartilage (Fig. 3.29). The macrophages that have appeared concurrently with the blood vessels are only engaged in a "clearance operation". We have never been able to demonstrate the penetration of macrophages into cartilaginous tissue in the region of the invasion front.

"Pannus"

In this intermediate phase, it is possible to recognize for the first time the synthesis of collagen fibres by the fibroblast-like modulated cells (Fig. 3.30). This represents the beginnings of later pan-

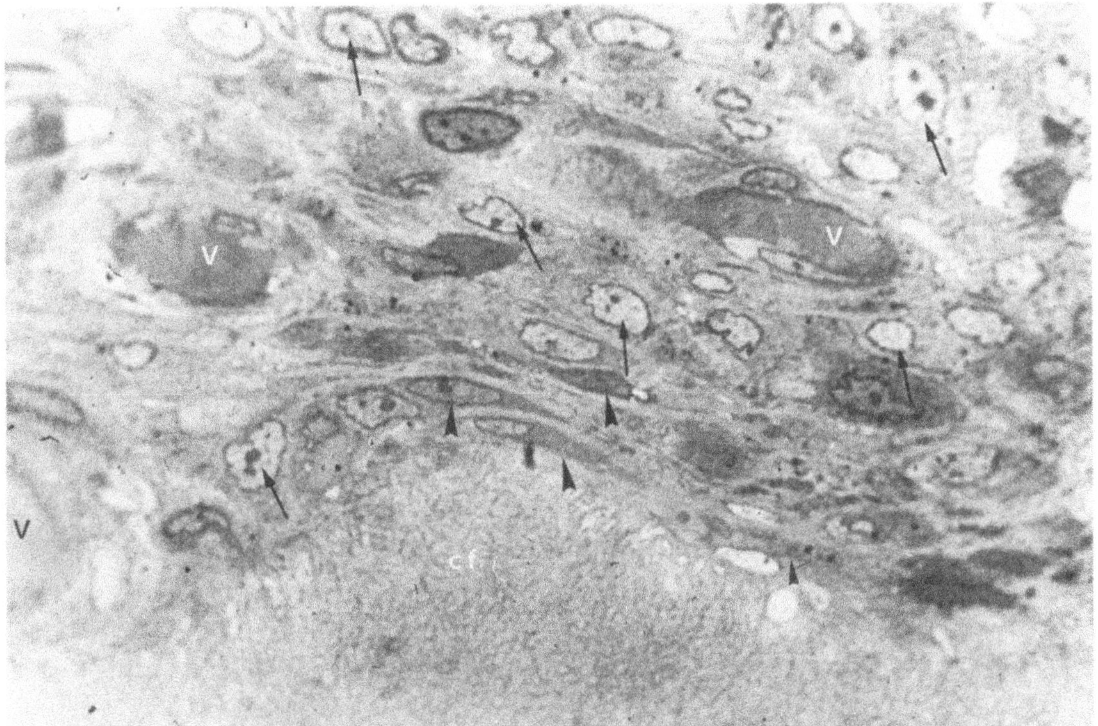

Intermediate phase: tumour-like cells partly with typical light nuclei (*arrows*), partly fibroblastic modulated with narrow dark nuclei. The fibroblast-like cells (*arrowheads)* are lying parallel to the cartilage surface in contrast to the attack position of the tlp formation. At the invasion front denuded collagen fibres (*cf*) of the articular cartilage are distinctly recognizable. Between the cells, some newly formed blood vessels (*v*, semi-thin section)

Fig. 3.29
Rheumatoid arthritis

nus formation. This development is characterized through increasing deposition of collagen fibres (type I) and a decreasing cellular content (Fig. 3.31).

"Pannus" (lat. cake) is a completely uncharacteristic, cell-deficient, collagenous scar tissue – a remnant whose structure no longer reminds of its development from the synoviogenous tissue with high cell density. The pannus does not damage the articular cartilage. It seems more likely that it acts as a shield to protect the underlying cartilage from further synovial invasion (Fig. 3.32).

Bone destruction

In the region of the "bare area", between the start of the synovium and the border of articular cartilage, the tlp tissue is able to invade into the cortical bone, penetrate into the neighbouring marrow space and destroy the bone trabeculae (Fig. 3.33). This penetration into bone corresponds to the radiological finding of the marginal erosion (Fig. 3.34).

Bone repair

The region of bone invasion by synoviogenous cell formation is soon surrounded by newly formed bone trabeculae, the point and the way of penetration becomes filled by collagenous scar tissue after the tlp tissue has died away and remains recognizable.

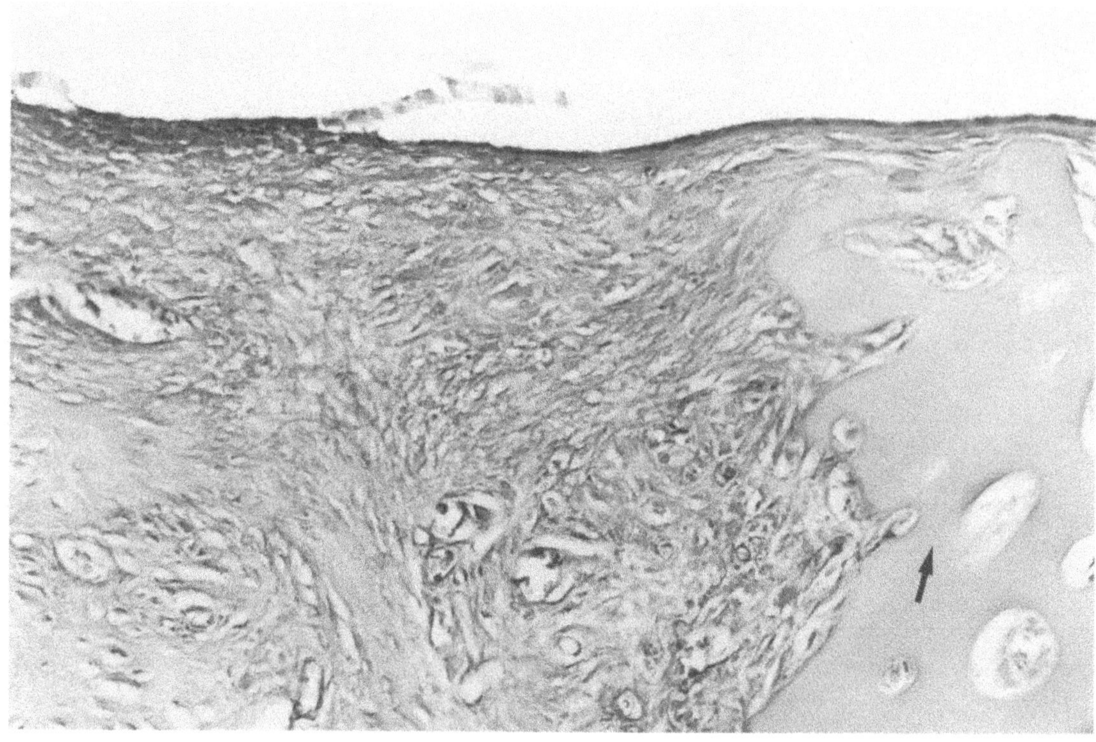

Fig. 3.30
Rheumatoid arthritis

Proximal interphalangeal joint. Intermediate phase: scar tissue with increasing fibrosis but still numerous cells. Newly formed blood vessels between relics of articular cartilage (*arrow*)

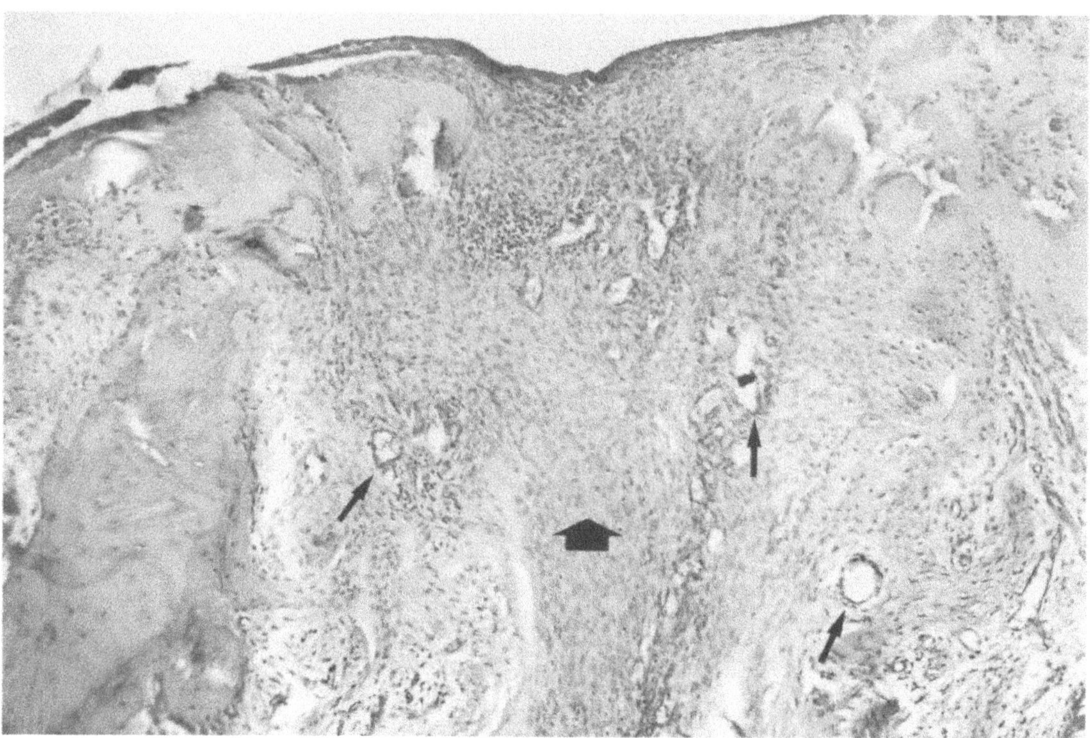

Fig. 3.31
Rheumatoid arthritis

Proximal interphalangeal joint. Intermediate phase: in the middle still compact tlp formations (*large arrow*). In between branched in blood vessels (*small arrows*). At the margins, increasing fibrosis

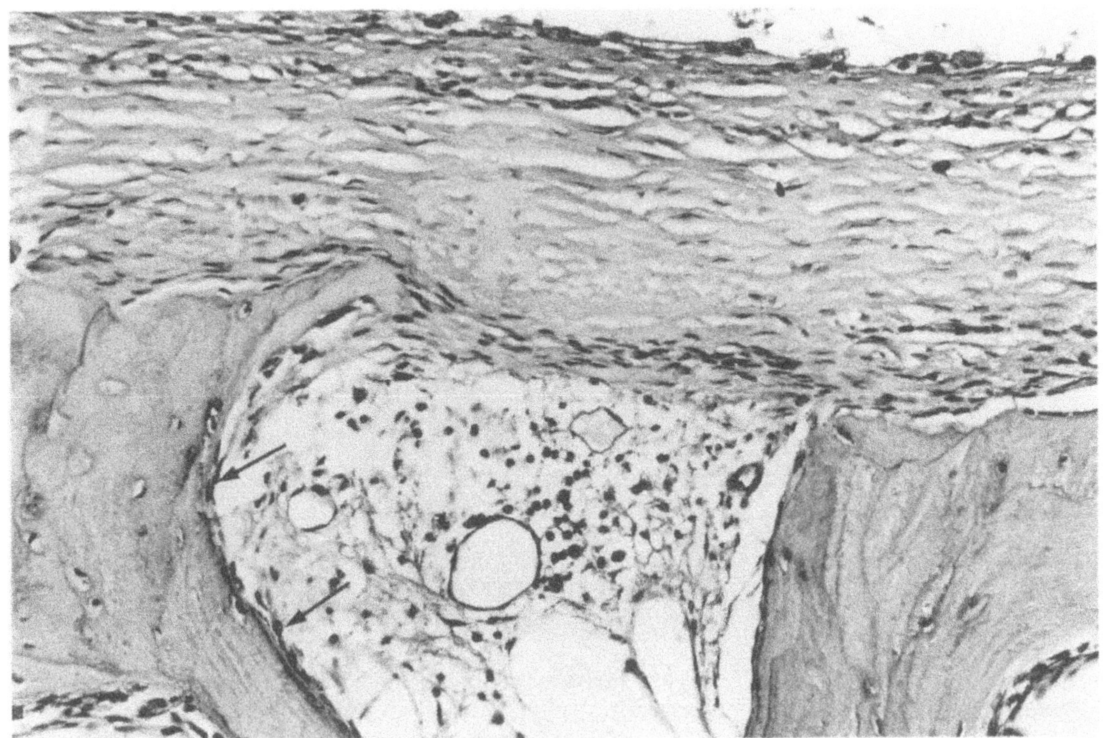

Metatarsophalangeal joint. Totally developed collagenous scar tissue ("pannus") in the region of the destroyed articular cartilage and the subchondral bone. Osteoblast activity at the bone

Fig. 3.32
Rheumatoid arthritis

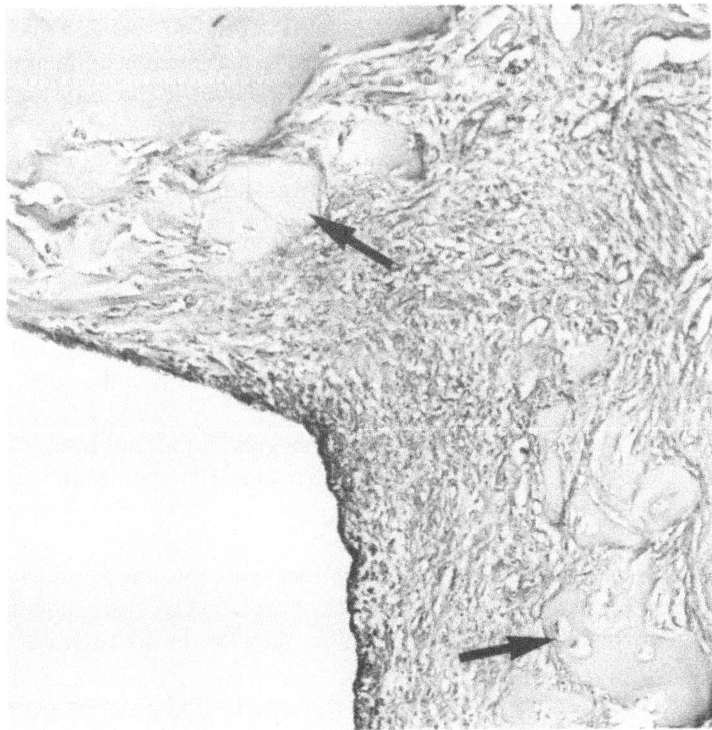

Proximal interphalangeal joint. Marginal break-through of tlp formation into the marrow space with destruction of cortical bone. *Arrows*, remnants of bone

Fig. 3.33
Rheumatoid arthritis

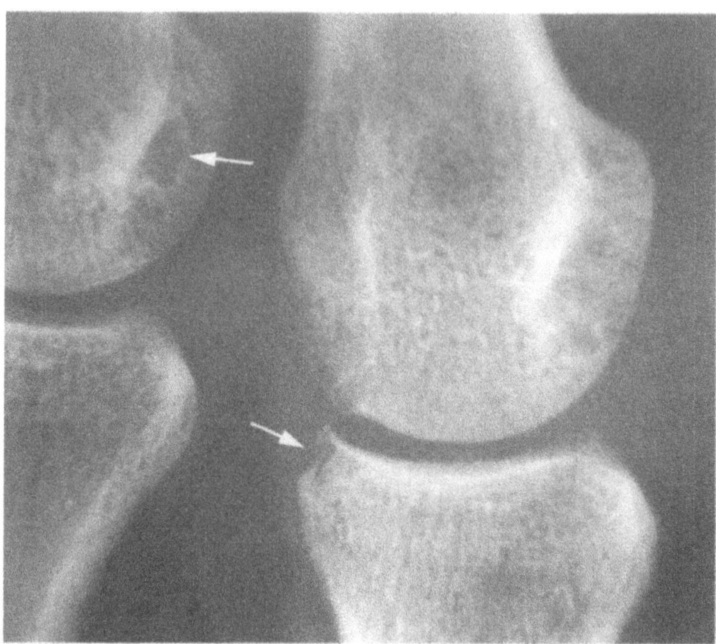

Fig. 3.34
Rheumatoid arthritis

X-ray. Metacarpophalangeal joint with marginal erosions (*arrows*)

According to the conventional concept of "inflammatory" destruction of the joint in RA, interest is focused on hyaline articular cartilage.
However, with the experience of examining a large number of joint resection specimens (predominantly metacarpal and metatarsal heads), we gained the impression that the non-inflammatory tlp cell masses chiefly attack cortical bone in the "bare area" between the synovial membrane and the cartilage.
Therefore, we examined the different pathways leading to joint destruction by studying 219 metatarsal and 69 metacarpal heads obtained during surgery from patients with definite RA (Fassbender et al. 1992).
The evaluation of the specimens revealed three pathways of aggression:

- Pathway A: in 15% aggression onto the articular cartilage only.
- Pathway B: in 49% direct invasion exclusively into the cortical bone.
- Pathway C: in 36% a "pincer-like" aggression, a combination of A and B in which the joint is attacked from both sites (Table 3.4).

In contrast to the hitherto conventional concepts, the findings of this study reveal a clear preference of the synovial aggression for the cortical bone (pathway B) rather than for the articular cartilage.

Expansion of invasive synoviogenous cell masses

After destruction of the zone of contact, the tlp formation penetrates into the structure of the joint in the following ways:

- Starting at the cartilage surface:
  - Marginal cartilage destruction with centripetal expansion following the subchondral bone lamellae.

Table 3.4. Proportional distribution of ways of aggression of synovial cell masses on articular cartilage and bone of 306 metatarsal and metacarpal heads (Fassbender and Gay 1988)

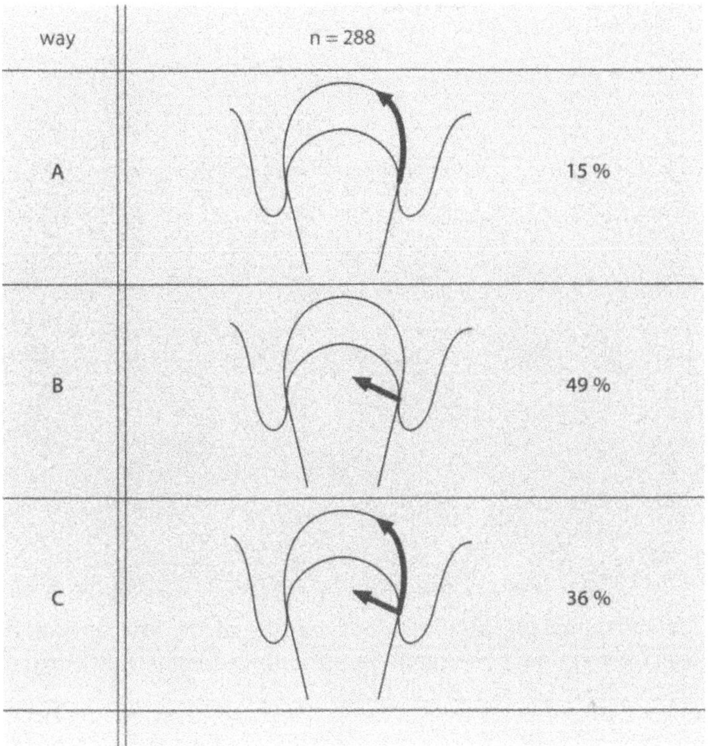

way	n = 288	
A		15 %
B		49 %
C		36 %

- ▸ Marginal cartilage destruction with destruction of the subchondral bone lamellae and rupture into the marrow space with undermining of the joint cartilage (Fig. 3.35).
- ▸ Starting at cortical bone:
  - ▸ Expansion of subchondral "pincers" (together with the point above).
  - ▸ Spread into adjacent marrow space (Figs. 3.36, 3.37).

The tlp cell masses are only demonstrable a short time, the persisting scar tissue, however, remains as a permanent mark of synovial aggression (Figs. 3.38, 3.39).

Subchondral "pockets"

Although the invasive tlp cell masses, corresponding to their short life, are only seldom found in the marrow space, we sometimes observe little subchondral "pockets" of newly-formed blood vessels together with a variety of cells including fibroblasts, occasional tlp cells, macrophages, a few mast cells, and a few multinuclear giant cells ("chondroclasts"; Bromley and Woolley 1984; see p. 87) and collagen fibres during the intermediate phase. Rarely, occasional lymphocytes and neutrophils are also seen. The ratio of cells to the newly formed collagen fibrils is soon altered in favour of an increasingly dense fibre net. This smouldering subchondral process persists for a while after the tlp phase has subsided. Its destructive potential is, however, minimal.

Cycle of tumour-like proliferation

The transition of destructive tlp tissue to well-recognized scar pannus (over cartilage and bone) may be divided into three stages:

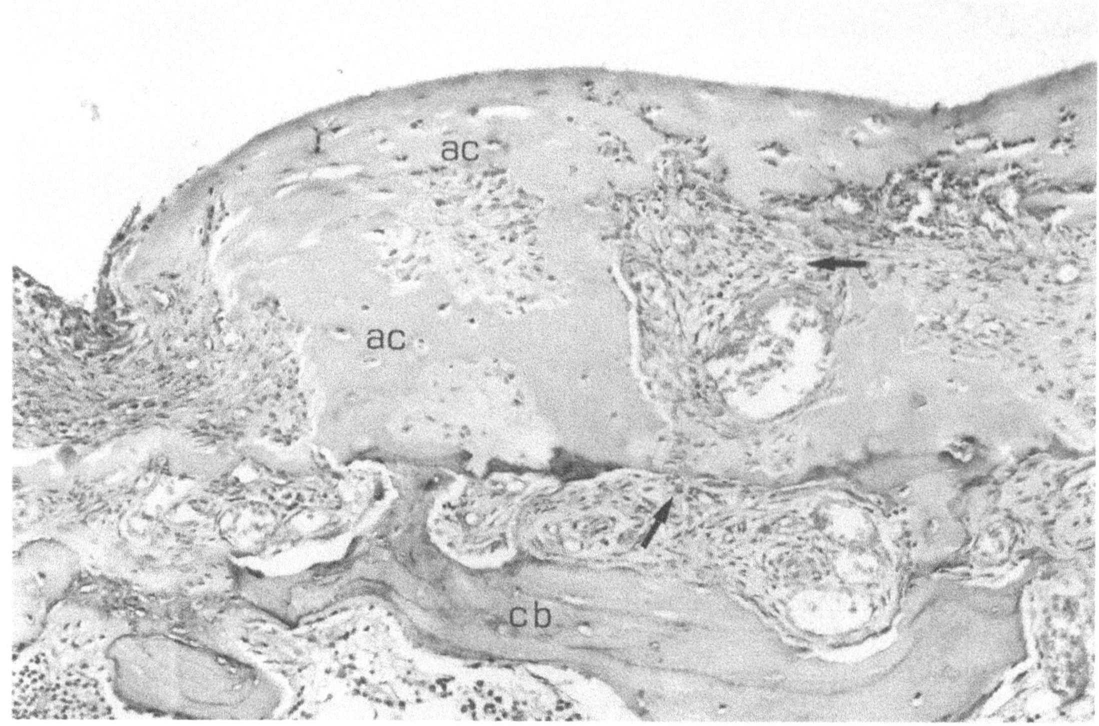

Fig. 3.35
Rheumatoid arthritis

Metatarsophalangeal joint. Undermining of the articular cartilage by marginal penetrated tlp formations (*arrows*). *AC*, articular cartilage; *CB*, cancellous bone

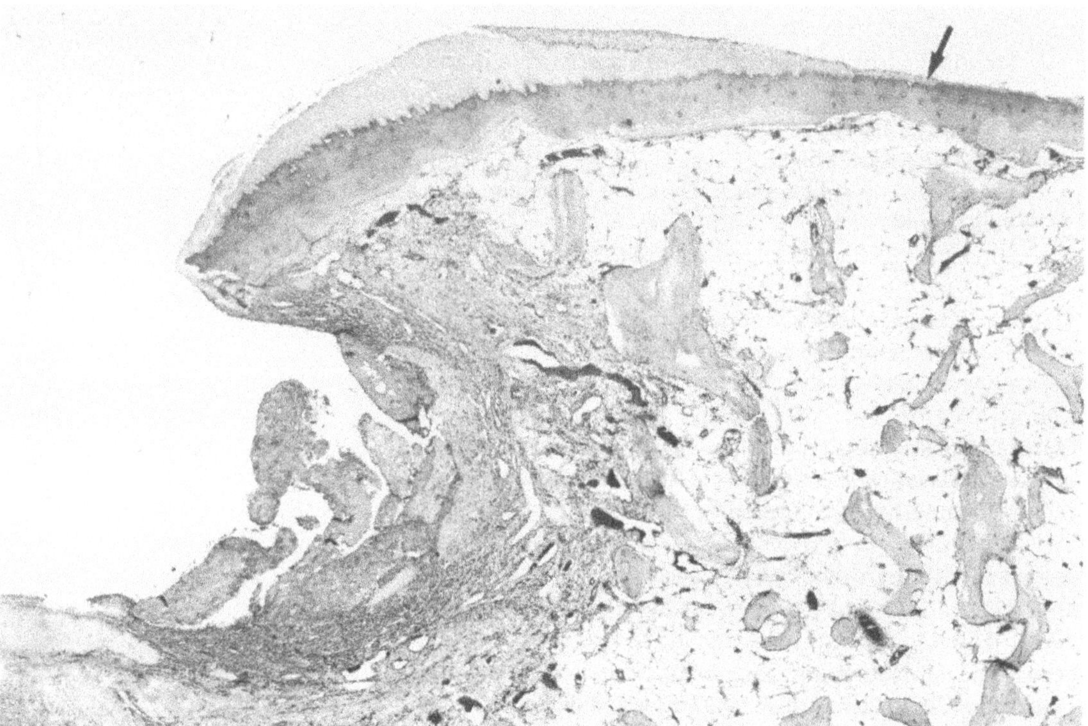

Fig. 3.36
Rheumatoid arthritis

Metatarsophalangeal joint. Older marginal penetration of tlp formations in the subchondral bone with mechanical abrasion of the articular cartilage (*arrow*)

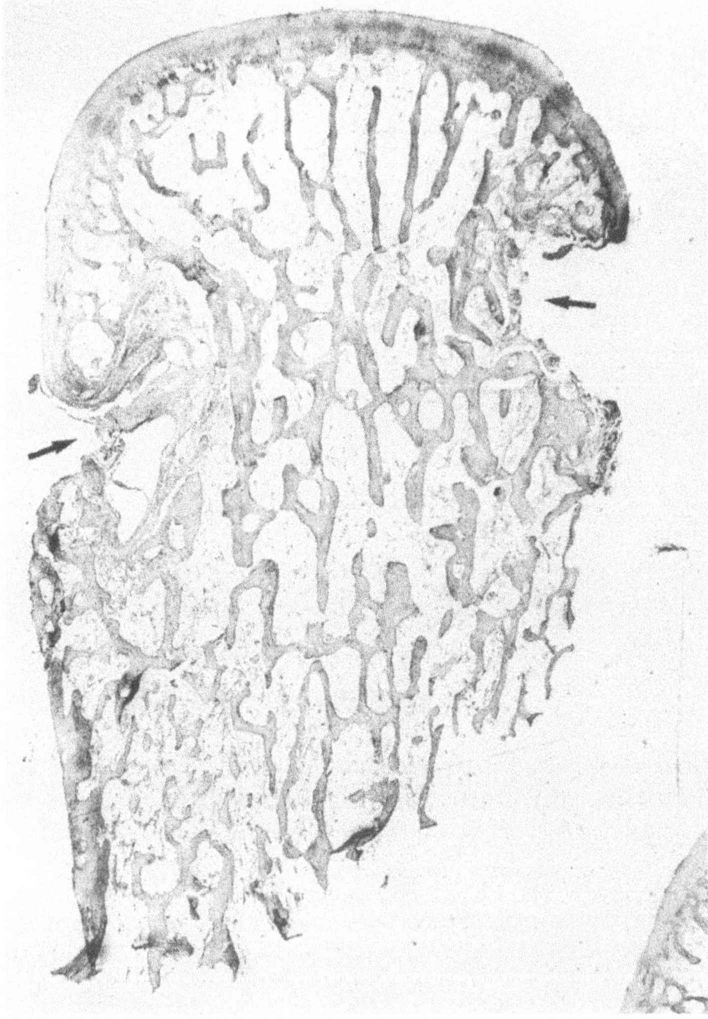

Metatarsophalangeal joint. Traces of former tlp invasions with marginal destruction of cortical bone (*arrows*). Secondary mechanical abrasion of the articular cartilage and osteoporosis

Fig. 3.37
Rheumatoid arthritis

Stage I: tlp Phase

Characteristic features:

- Dense, homogeneous cell formation
- Avascular
- Cells round to polyhedral, large blister-like nuclei
- The cells penetrate perpendicular to the invasion front, between the enzymatically denuded collagen fibres (see p. 88)

Stage II: Intermediate Phase

Characteristic features:

- Loose tissue
- Occasional, newly-formed, small caliber blood vessels
- Mixed cell population of fibroblasts, occasional tlp cells, macrophages, lymphocytes, and mast cells. This phase is characterized by phagocytosis and collagen fibre synthesis
- Cells lie flat on the cartilage surface and not in an invasive formation

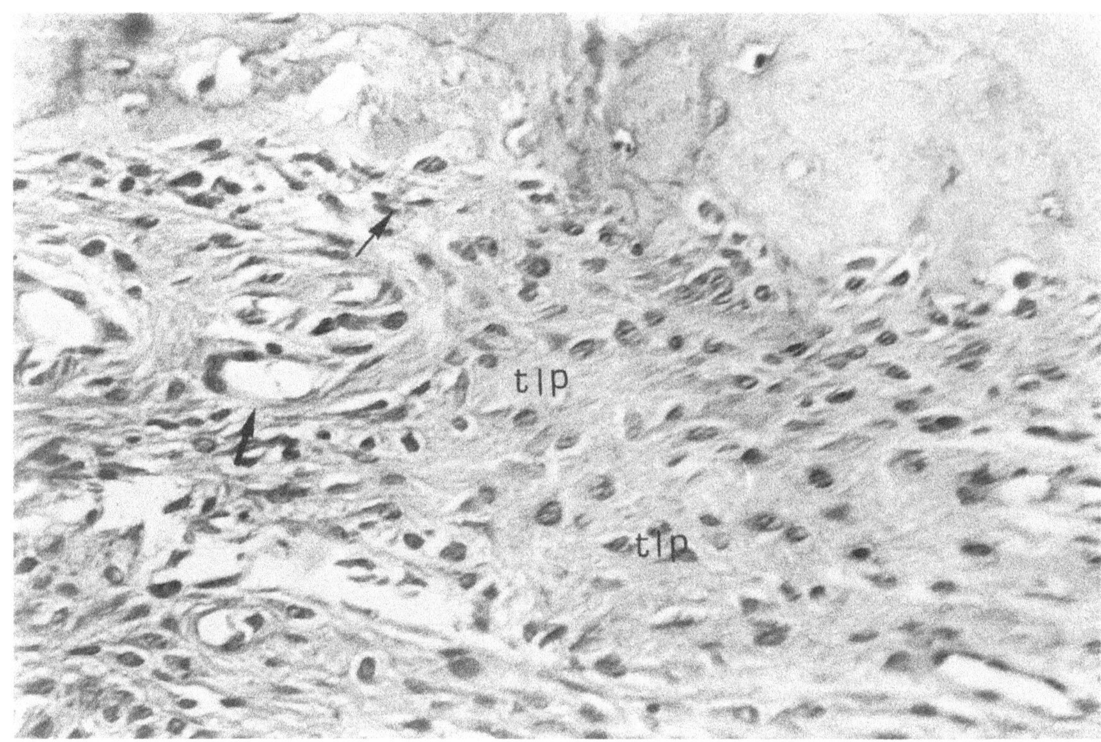

Fig. 3.38
Rheumatoid arthritis

Undermining and destruction of the articular cartilage by *tlp* formations after penetration of the cortical bone. *Left margin*, starting fibrosis and new formation of blood vessels (*arrows*)

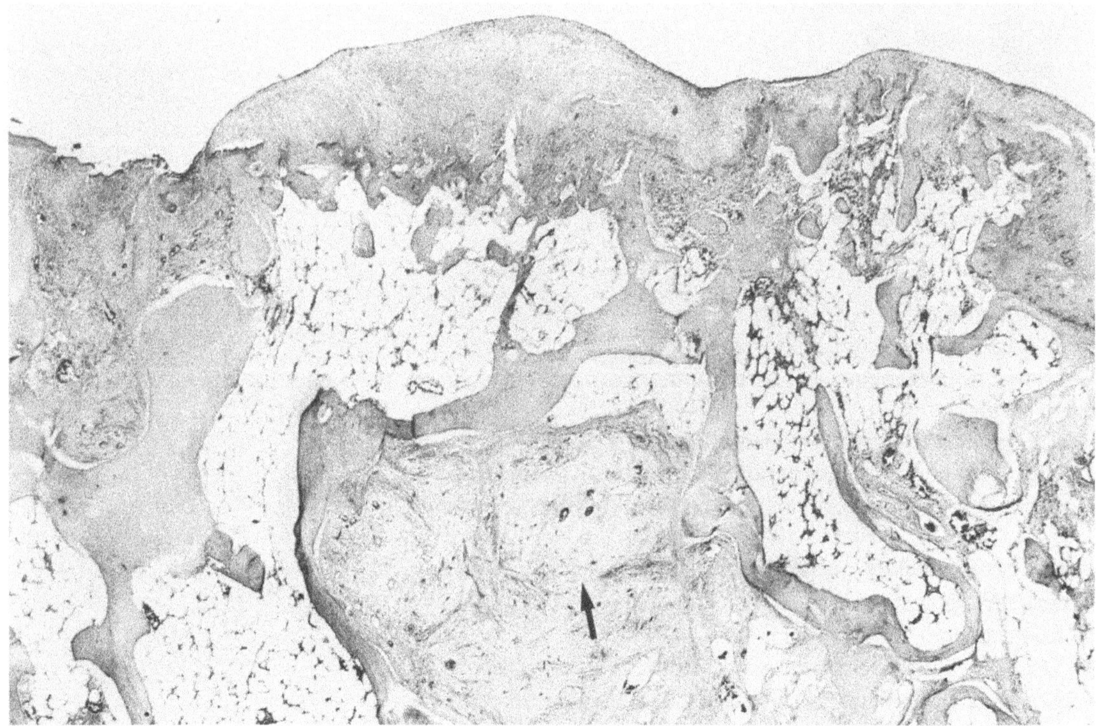

Fig. 3.39
Rheumatoid arthritis

Metatarsophalangeal joint. Devastation of articular cartilage and subchondral bone by the old central and marginal tlp invasions. *Bottom*, large scar area (*arrow*)

Stage III: Persistent "Pannus"

Characteristic features:

- Compact collagenous scar tissue (fibre density related to its age)
- Numerous newly formed blood vessels
- Occasional fibroblasts and sparse lymphocytes (cell content inversely related to the age of the scar tissue)

The scar tissue consisting of collagen type I is closely intertwined with the collagen type II-fibre scaffold of the cartilage. The area of contact between scar tissue plate and cartilage does not show reactive changes.

Role of macrophages in joint destruction

As the tlp phase is very short (see p. 89), the intermediate phase lasts many times longer and the pannus persists, accordingly the probability is higher to obtain and then examine biopsy tissue from the long-lasting phases (see p. 92). It also seems plausible that from the evidence of macrophages in the joint tissues of RA one concludes that they play a certain role in joint destruction (Sack et al. 1994; Yanni et al. 1994; Mulherin et al. 1996; Burmester et al. 1997). Macrophages are undoubtedly instrumental to destruction in RA, even if they do not belong to the actual aggressive "troop" but to its followers. The investigations of Müller-Ladner and his team (1995) using the macrophage marker CD68 confirm the innocence of macrophages in the destruction itself. According to him, the "fibroblast-like synoviocytes" (tlp) in the area of invasion were, in contrast to other tissue segments, nearly invariably CD68-negative (Müller-Ladner 1995).

Task of the macrophages, equipped with collagenases, stromelysin, and elastases, is to phagocytize the dead cell elements and the debris in the invasion area. This solves also the discrepancy stating that a macrophage attack on healthy endogenic tissue is relatively improbable.

Ectopic synovial membrane

Epithelial formations have the ability to encroach onto the neighbouring tissues from the margins of the surface they cover (for example cervix uteri, tonsillar crypts). This corresponds with the epithelial layer's ability to spread horizontally and to close defects. In contrast, the lining cell layer of the synovial membrane regenerates itself vertically from the depth of the synovial stroma. The distinguishing characteristic of the vital synovial membrane is the ability to form villi from lining cell buds. Under pathological conditions, the synovial membrane borders on protrusions of the joint capsule, such as the "Baker's cyst" or other synovial herniae. Here, both surfaces are in direct contact. However, in contrast to the epithelial layer, the borders of synovial membrane rest distinctly demarkated. This means that the surfaces of the synovial herniae, for example of the "Baker's cyst", are not lined by a synovial membrane, but by a single- or multilayered smooth macrophage lining without villous formation.

Therefore, we were surprised to find synovial islands with regular synovial stroma containing often lymphocytes and typical, frequently abundant villi vegetations on the scar pannus formed after cartilage destruction on the joint's surface (Figs. 3.40–3.42). Thus, we searched in 180 surgically removed joint heads (fingers and toes) for the presence of synovial villi on the scar pannus.

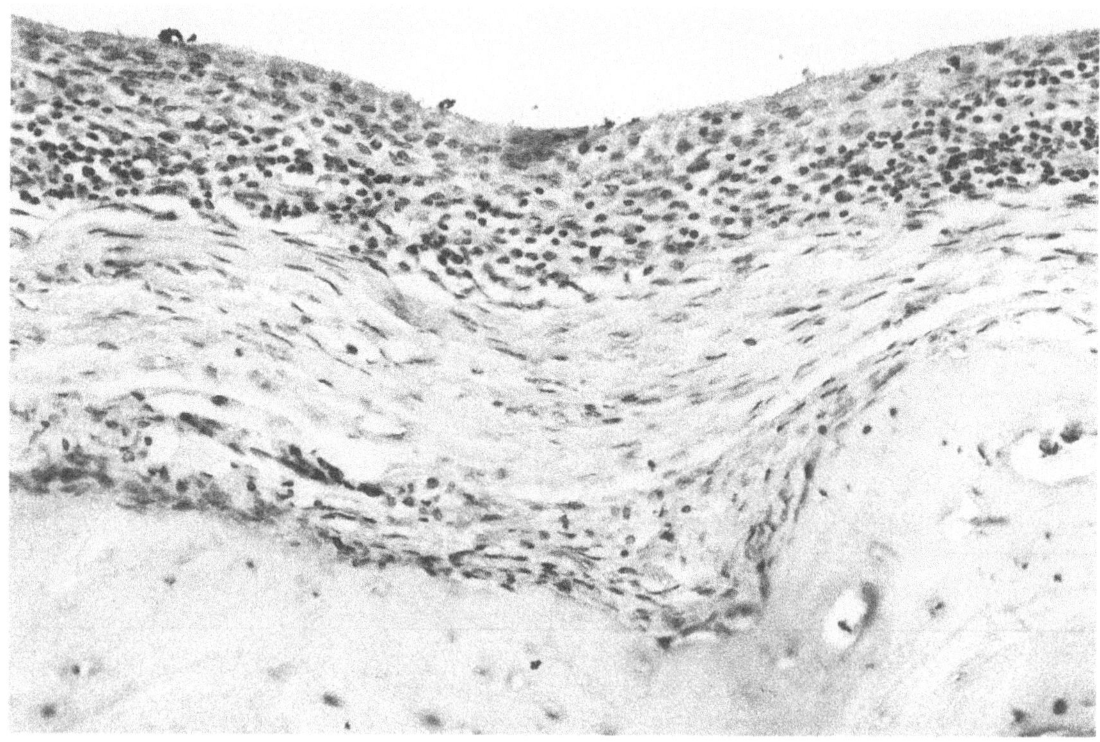

Fig. 3.40
Rheumatoid arthritis

Metatarsophalangeal joint: the destroyed articular cartilage is replaced by old scar tissue. Above newly formed proliferated synovial tissue with infiltration of lymphocytes

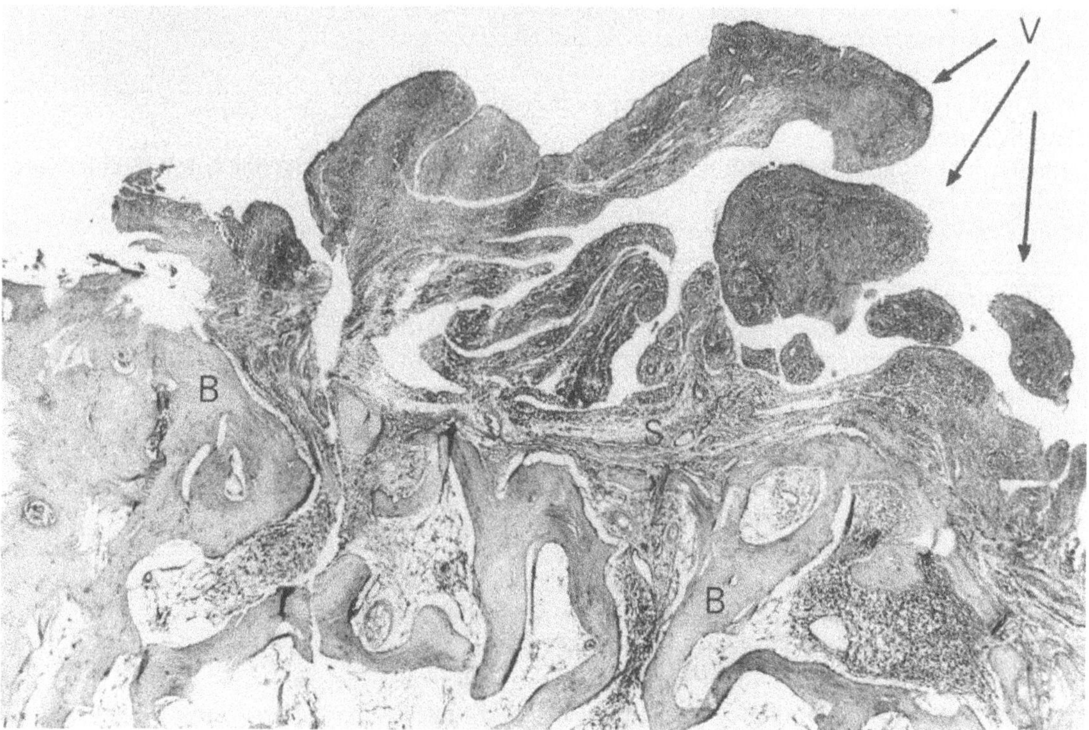

Fig. 3.41
Rheumatoid arthritis

Metacarpophalangeal joint. Newly formed vegetation of villi *(v)* in the region of a previous joint destruction. *S*, collagenous scar; *B*, bone

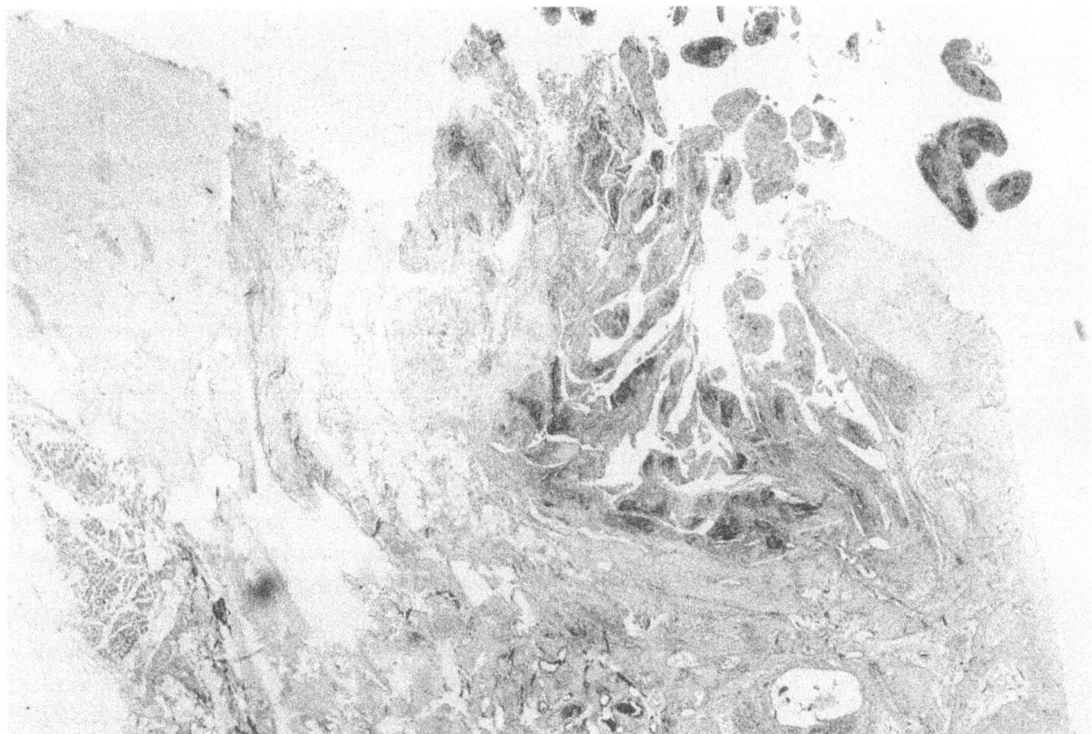

Metatarsophalangeal joint. Exuberant vegetation of villi on newly formed synovial membrane, originated out of old scar tissue

Fig. 3.42
Rheumatoid arthritis

The tissues removed came from 90 patients with clinical clear RA, 30 with OA, 30 with PSA, and 30 with SSA. (The cases were examined non-selectively in the order of their receipt.) In 41 cases (23%), we found villi formation above the scar tissue. Ninety percent of these 41 were RA patients, 2 cases each PSA and OA (Adamicek 1998). These villi vegetations above the scar pannus are an indication of the synoviogenous origin of the scar tissue, which has kept the qualities of an autochthonous synovial membrane.
This is a supplementary proof that the pannus is a relic of the synovial invasion (tlp) and not the remnant from inflammatory granulation tissue.
We have no explanation for the villi in the two cases of OA and PSA, respectively. If RA can be definitively excluded, an attachment of villi in a bone crater would be conceivable. Nevertheless, the fact that in RA synovial villi grow from nearly every second scar pannus (41%) is an indication of the previous synoviogenous invasion.
In occasional cases, we have observed that this ectopic synovial membrane can threaten the remaining cartilage in that tlp tissue may form from these ectopic "outposts" and then invade neighbouring cartilage that is not covered by scar pannus.

Hyperplasia and apoptosis

It is a matter of course that, when discussing a disease like RA, characterized by cell proliferation and hyperplasia, the role of apoptosis has to be considered. For hyperplasia and proliferation a disturbed tissue homeostasis is the prerequisite.
In RA, two processes are characterized by a disturbed balance between the formation and the death of cells: the hyperplasia of

the lining cells, leading to villi formation, and the excessive hyperplasia, the aggressive and invasive tlp, whereby the villous hyperplasia of the synovial membrane is by no means specific to RA, as it occurs in other joint diseases, too. Causes may be found in either new cell formation or in a reduction of the programmed cell death (apoptosis). Attempts to make one or the other mechanism responsible for this imbalance have, until today, not arrived at a clear conclusion. The production of cytokines such as TGF-1β and IL-1β promoting the proliferation of synoviocytes and inhibiting the susceptibility to apoptosis, are accused (Kawakami et al. 1996; Tsuboi et al. 1996). For apoptosis, at present, Fas-L und TNF-α are the best characterized inductors. On the other hand, TNF-α is able to induce both cell death as well as cell formation. Kriegsmann and his team (1997) came according to their studies using the proliferation marker KI-67 on the synovial tissue in RA patients to the conviction that hyperplasia of the lining cell layer in RA is due to a reduced rate of apoptosis rather than in situ proliferation of the lining cells.
Akkoc and coworkers (1997) observed, opposed to it, an increased proliferation rather than an increased apoptosis after a Fas antigen stimulation of human fibroblasts. The studies of Firestein and coworkers bring into one's mind also the role of p53 in RA (Firestein et al. 1995). According to these studies, mutations of the suppressor gene can lead to disturbance of apoptosis and, thus, synovial hyperplasia gets out of control.
As unclear as the importance of apoptosis for the hyperplasia of the lining cells and the resulting villous formation is, as important may be the role of apoptosis in the development of tlp. The number of mitoses in this compact, avascular, rapidly growing cell formation is in contrast to the excessive hyperplasia of the synovial cell elements surprisingly small. The apoptosis mechanism may also play a role for the short life-span of the tlp formation which lacks blood vessels. However, to finally confirm this hypothesis appropriate investigations of the tlp formation itself would be necessary, whereas it may be difficult to hit this short florid phase in the synovial tissue of RA patients.

Comparison tumour-like proliferation – malignant tumour

The term "tumour-like proliferation" (tlp) raises the question in how far these synovial cell formations compare and contrast with a malignant tumour. The differences are as following:

- Most malignant tumours (MT) grow slowly and its growth is coordinated with the accompanying vascularisation. The MT accordingly has an adequate blood supply.
  - In contrast, the tlp tissue develops so rapidly that a vasculature has insufficient time to develop.
- Most MT have a long life-span, due to an adequate blood supply.
  - In contrast, the tlp tissue is fated to die soon as, on the one hand, the highly active cell masses are avascular and, on the other hand, the multi-layered, densely packed cell mass in the joint space has insufficient oxygen.
- An essential difference lies in the way in which the cell mass penetrates into normal tissue.

An invasion of MT cells into the extracellular matrix faces a dense meshwork of collagen fibres, embedded in aggrecan and glycoprotein gel. This sealed architecture forms a barrier that can only be breached with matrix degrading enzymes. According to the studies of Fidler et al. (1978), Pauli et al. (1983), Weiss and Ward (1983), and Woolley (1984), membrane associated factors of MT cells induce the synthesis and release of matrix degrading enzymes in the surrounding mesenchymal cells. Collagenolysis occurs secondary to a physical alteration of the matrix due to an accumulation of glycosaminoglycans and is accompanied by an increase in water content (Knudson et al. 1990). Cathepsin B plays a particular role in this regard and is synthesized and released by stimulated host cells under the influence of MT cells and activates collagenase (Graf et al. 1981; Trabandt et al. 1991). Sloane et al. (1981) have demonstrated a synthesis of cathepsin B in carcinoma metastases. In this manner, a pathway is cleared before the invasion of proliferative MT cells.

Matrix degrading enzymes

In contrast, the invasive process of tlp masses takes an entirely different course: The attacking synovial masses themselves dispose of a sufficient proteolytic potential to degradatively penetrate into the cartilaginous and osseous matrix. Studies of the work group of Harris and Werb offer a convincing explanation for this: As early as in 1969, Harris and colleagues could prove collagenase secretion in synovial cultures of patients suffering from various joint diseases. In 1974, Werb and Burleigh detected a specific collagenase in monolayer cultures of rabbit fibroblasts. In 1970 already, Harris stresses the significance of synovial collagenase with regard to the pathogenesis of RA (Harris et al. 1970).

In 1990, Trabandt et al. made an important discovery. They found in patients with RA a high expression of cathepsin L in the tlp cells at the invasive front of the articular cartilage.

Already in early stages of RA, but also in other arthritides, an expression of mRNA is provable in the lining cells as well as in the synovial stroma (Cunnane et al. 1997). These findings argue for the early presence of proteases under the influence of unspecific inflammatory triggers of different genesis.

If, however, secretion of proteolytic enzymes is indeed a quantitatively different but non-specific function of the synovial cells, then the important question arises, why a synoviogenous destruction of joint tissue is only observed in RA. This can be answered as follows: Proteolytic enzymes can only be effective if in close contact with the substrate, namely cartilage and bone. If this is not the case, they will be paralyzed by the inhibitory potential of the synovial fluid (see p. 84).

In RA, the condition for a destructive effect of degradative synoviogenous enzymes is fulfilled. Assumption is, however, the aggressive encroachment of synovial tlp masses onto cartilage and bone; hereby the interference of inhibitors is eliminated! Moreover, it can be assumed that the highly actively secreting tlp cells, in contrast to the regular synovial cells, have a much higher potential for enzyme production.

The effect of these enzymes that initially degrade aggrecans and then the collagen fibre network can be seen in Figs. 3.24 and 3.25.

End stage of joint process

The chronic relapsing and remitting process of joint destruction in RA comes to a halt when the fight for years has so destroyed the synovial tissue as well as its target tissues, i.e. articular carti-

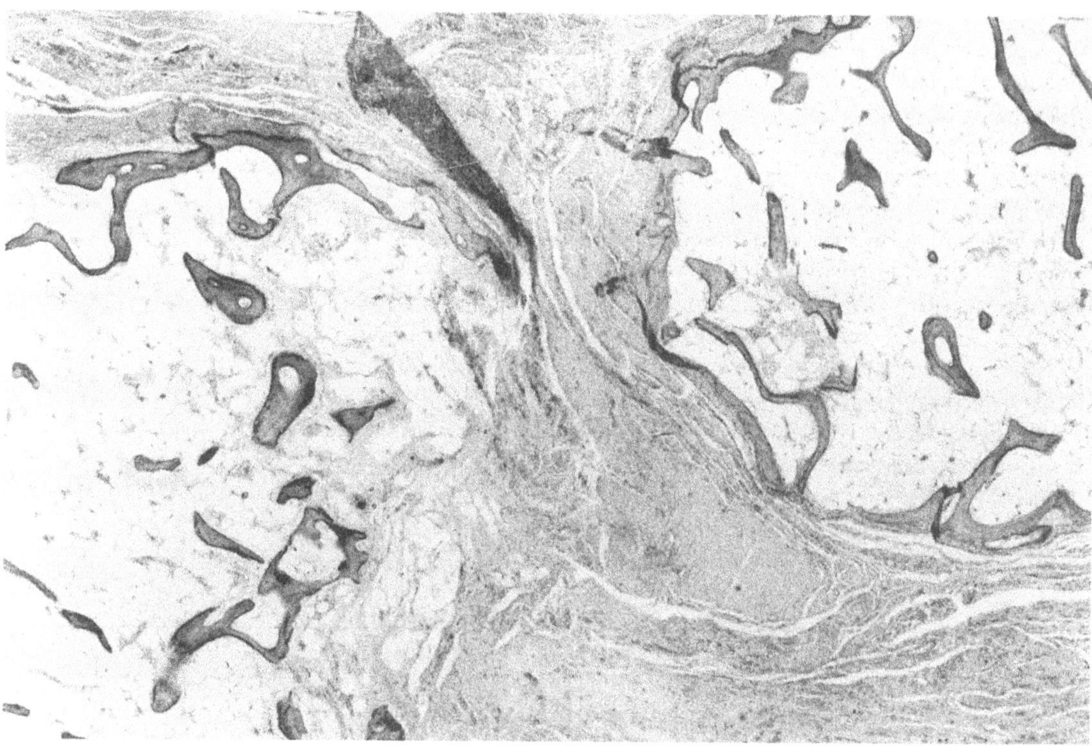

Fig. 3.43
Rheumatoid arthritis

Metatarsophalangeal joint. Fibrous ankylosis

lage and adjoining bone, that the structural basis for the exudative-inflammatory as well as the proliferative-destructive processes has disappeared.

The morphological picture of a burnt out joint gives an indication of the character and of the immense destructive potential of the RA process. Often there are only islands of articular cartilage remaining. If bone is predominantly affected by the invasive process, the articular surface may remain intact (see p. 96).

However, the original form is lost, firstly through loss of the underlying bone structure and secondly due to irregular loading of the cartilage leading to structural disturbances in the joint surface (see Fig. 3.39).

Fibrous ankylosis

Disappearance of the articular space and coalescing of both with scar tissue covered articular surfaces are not seldomly observed as result of lack of movement. In this fibrous ankylosis, the remnants of the articular structures lie, incorporated in the fibrous scar tissue in general, without any reaction (Fig. 3.43). This fibrous scar tissue in general has no tendency for ossification. An osseous bridging between the destroyed joint elements is characteristic for PSA and other diseases of the group of SSA (see p. 189).

Traces of penetration

Particularly noticeable is the destruction of adjoining bone: the scar tissue-filled tracks of previous episodes of synoviogenous invasion can be observed. Sites of penetration are sealed off from the remaining marrow space by irregular new bone formation. Occasionally evidence of osteoblastic activity may be seen.

Cysts containing debris

When the cartilage surface as well as the subchondral bone lamellae have been invaded, cystic lesions may be found in the

marrow space, which are either filled with scar tissue or else may contain fibrin as well as cartilage and bone fragments.
Rarely, occasional osteoclasts may be seen amongst the bone remnants. Further away from the joint, the bony trabeculae are thinned. In the region of the joint, the marrow space is fibrosed and often contains small collections of lymphocytes.

Secondary osteoarthrosis

As long as the articular cartilage is not destroyed and replaced by pannus scar, the surface demonstrates fissures and evidence of abrasion, whereas osteophytes in the form of secondary osteoarthrosis deform the joint rim. In cases where the cartilage is replaced by pannus scar, it is not uncommon to observe true villous synovial vegetations, which have developed from the scar tissue (see p. 103).
Concurrent with destruction of the joint surface, the synovial tissue also loses its original structure.

Fibrosis of the villous stroma

At first there follows fibrosis of the villous stroma with flattening or loss of the lining cells. The remaining portions of synovial tissue become increasing fibrotic. The number of local fibroblasts progressively diminishes and finally also the blood vessels disappear.

Hyalinisation of collagenous tissue

The loss of blood supply leads to necrosis of the remaining fibroblasts and to hyalinisation of the collagenous tissue.
The degenerated, previously plastic synovial tissue has now become transformed into a stiff scar tissue. This gets trapped between the rough and incongruent joint surfaces and becomes increasingly torn and frayed. It is understandable that such a denatured and destroyed synovial membrane is no longer in the position to perform sufficient nutritive functions for the remaining cartilage and at the same time is a favourable site for the settlement of bacteria ("bacterial superinfection"; see p. 386).

Secondary osteoporosis

Progressive osteoporosis and loss of joint function give rise to an increasing fracture risk for RA patients. In a retrospective study of 85 RA patients, Fitzek et al. (1989) documented 107 fractures of the peripheral skeleton. Forty-four traumatic fractures in 31 patients contrasted with 63 pathological fractures in 54 patients. Steroid therapy also played a role.

3.8 Cervical Vertebral Column

Axial manifestation of RA

In the context of RA, Schilling (1984) terms the cervical vertebral column the "fifth extremity". Neck pain, which occurs in about half of the patients with RA, is the most frequent manifestation of cervical spine involvement, although half of these patients have normal cervical spine radiographs (Hardin and Halla 1993). Indeed, the cervical vertebral column shows a predilection for various rheumatic (arthritic) diseases. Apart from degenerative processes like osteochondrosis, spondylosis, spondylarthrosis, oncovertebral arthrosis, facet arthrosis, and spondylosis hyperostotica, the cervical vertebral column is affected in AS (see p. 194) and in adult as well as in juvenile RA (see p. 174). Thereby, changes take place in the apophyseal, atlanto-axial, and discovertebral joints as well as in the adjacent structures such as the spinous processes of the vertebrae (Fig. 3.44).

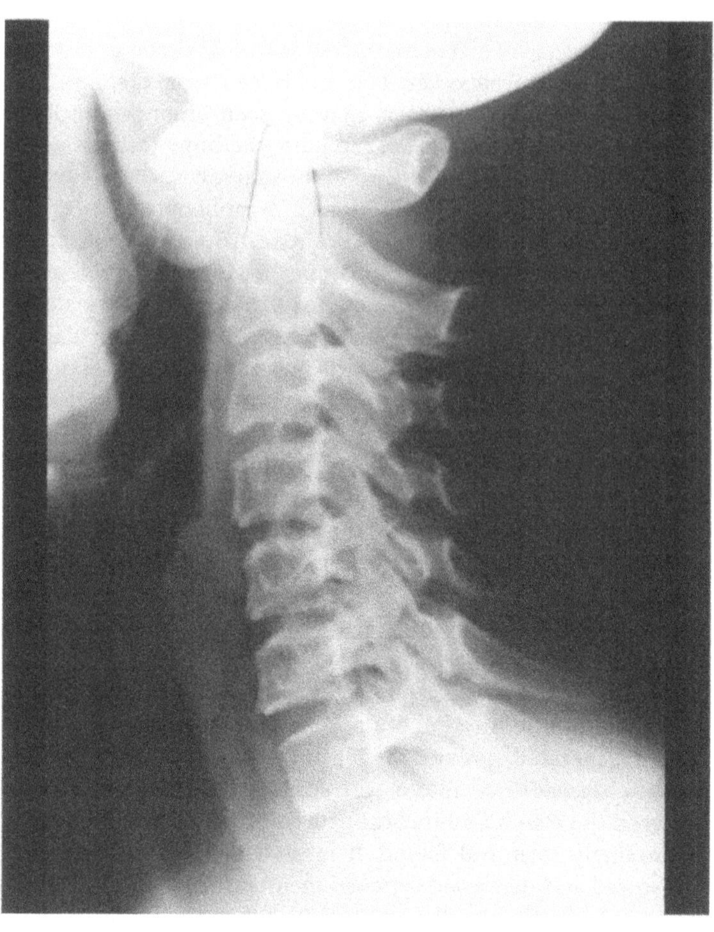

Fig. 3.44
Rheumatoid arthritis

52-year-old woman, RA for 18 years. Severe fixed atlanto-axial dislocation. Atlanto-odontoid distance 12 mm (*contours marked*). Spondylodiscitis at the front of the lower margin of the vertebral bodies C3 and C4. Intervertebral arthritis C 4/5 and C 5/6 (*unsharp contours*). (X-ray, M. Schacherl)

In adult RA, various mechanisms may contribute in a joint effort to the destruction of the cervical vertebral column which is a threat to function and life:

Spondylodiscitis

1. Discitis (non-reactive destruction of the intervertebral disk)
2. Spondylodiscitis
3. Destructive intervertebral arthritis with subsequent dislocation
4. Atlanto-axial dislocation
5. Osteolysis of the odontoid process
6. Osteolysis of the spinous process C7

The final stage of rheumatoid destruction of the cervical vertebral column thus results from a combination of inflammatory, mechanical, and osteolytical processes. The apophyseal, atlanto-axial, and discovertebral joints are the sites where inflammatory processes are triggered. In contrast to PSA where similar changes may take place, in RA the destructive and destabilizing aspect is predominant.

Bony erosions

Bony erosions predominate in apophyseal joints, the anterior and posterior aspect of the odontoid process, and the vertebral body

end-plate regions. Radiological findings of disk space loss and vertebral body erosions in the absence of osteophytosis suggest the diagnosis of RA in the vertebral column.
Forward subluxation of the atlas with respect to the axis is a common finding. Subaxial subluxations are characteristic and the resulting radiograph of the cervical vertebral column is termed the "step-ladder" appearance.
A serious complication in seropositive RA patients with atlanto-axial subluxation is spinal cord compression.

3.9 Cricoarytenoid Joints

In the context of the general affection of joints in RA, in most cases the cricoarytenoid joints are not spared. In 1880, Mackenzie described for the first time their involvement in patients suffering from RA.
Since, however, their clinical manifestation is not a characteristical sign, they are in general overlooked or misinterpreted. Thus, dyspnoea on exertion and inspiratory stridor in chronic cricoarytenoid arthritis are often interpreted as psychoneurosis or asthma (Leicht et al. 1987). The involvement of the larynx in patients with RA has been revealed during autopsy in 45%–86% (Bolten 1991). The histological changes show no difference in quality from those changes observed in the remaining diarthrodial joints with regard to lympho-plasma cellular infiltrates, proliferation of the synovial villi, and synovial destruction of the articular surface. The process can burn out in the form of a fibrous ankylosis of the cricoarytenoid joints. Endarteritis with amyloidosis was described by Wolman and coworkers in 1965. Ankylosis is supported by a long-lasting recurrence paresis. Furthermore, the cricoarytenoid arthritis may become complicated by bacterial superinfections (see p. 395; Woldorf et al. 1971; Jurik et al. 1985) and thus trigger a life-threatening obstruction of the respiratory tract which then requires an endotracheal intubation.

3.10 Extra-Articular Manifestations of RA ("Rheumatoid Disease")

There are two mechanisms imprinting the extra-articular manifestations of "rheumatoid disease": on the one hand, unspecific inflammatory processes, characterized by exudation and proliferation, on the other hand, primary necrotizing processes, specific for RA. Both mechanisms can take place at the same organs. Primary necrotizing processes show a preference for collagen type I structures.
Although "rheumatoid arthritis" owes its name to the prominent articular effects, the term hides the multidimensional nature of the disease. Involvement of the tendon sheaths, tendons, bursae, joint capsule, lungs, pleura, peritoneum, pericardium, myocardium, blood vessels, and sclera may all contribute to the full clinical picture. On occasions the joint process may be a minor consideration, overshadowed by life-threatening systemic features.

Considering the cardiac involvement in RA, Lebowitz in 1963 proposed the term "rheumatoid disease" in this context.
In 1973, Gordon and colleagues demonstrated the contribution of extra-articular manifestations to the clinical features of 127 patients with definite RA. Such features were found in 76% of patients and included subcutaneous nodules (53%), lung fibrosis (20%), digital vasculitis (15%), skin ulcers (15%), lymphadenopathy (12%), non-compressive neuropathy (10%), splenomegaly (9%), episcleritis (9%), and pericarditis (2%). It should be emphasized, however, that clinical parameters reflect gross changes only: the exact extent of extra-articular involvement in RA could only be determined by autopsy.
However, there is a clear preference of seropositive patients with RA to develop extra-articular manifestations.

3.10.1 Unspecific Exudative-Inflammatory Processes

The involvement of structures outside the joint is dependent on the particular tissue involved and occurs in three different forms:
1. In common with joints, tendon sheaths possess synovium and the disease process is correspondingly similar.
2. Pericardium, pleura, and peritoneum are covered by a serosal membrane, which can participate in exudative/inflammatory reactions.
3. In contrast to the surface structures in 1 and 2, deeper connective tissue containing collagen type I may be involved in a primary necrotizing process ("rheumatoid nodules") which is specific for RA.

Tendon sheaths

The process that occurs in tendon sheaths is analogous to that within the joint. In both instances, acute synovitis is characterized by discrete fibrin polymerisation on the synovial surface and proliferation of the lining cell layer. Multiple small villi are a frequent finding and they may be more elongated than in joints.
Lymphocytes, plasma cells, and occasional lymph follicles with germal centres can be seen in the synovial stroma, especially in the villi. Stromal proliferation can become marked in the synovial membrane of the tendon sheath, with the appearance of tlp. However, in contrast to the situation in the joint, it is extremely rare for invasion of the tendon to occur.
The uncharacteristic inflammatory process can cause the appearance of blood vessels between the fibre bundles of the tendon, associated with small groups of lymphocytes.
A consequence of tenosynovitis frequently associated with RA is the carpal tunnel syndrome (CTS; see p. 427).
Generally in RA, the pericardium, pleura, and peritoneum (see p. 110) behave in a similar fashion as might be expected from their similar structure.
Exudative inflammatory changes often occur, although generally asymptomatic and documented only at autopsy.

Pericardium

Exudative inflammations often occur in leaving scars or resulting in a loose mobile bridge of connective tissue between visceral and parietal pericardium. In contrast to the tuberculous pericarditis,

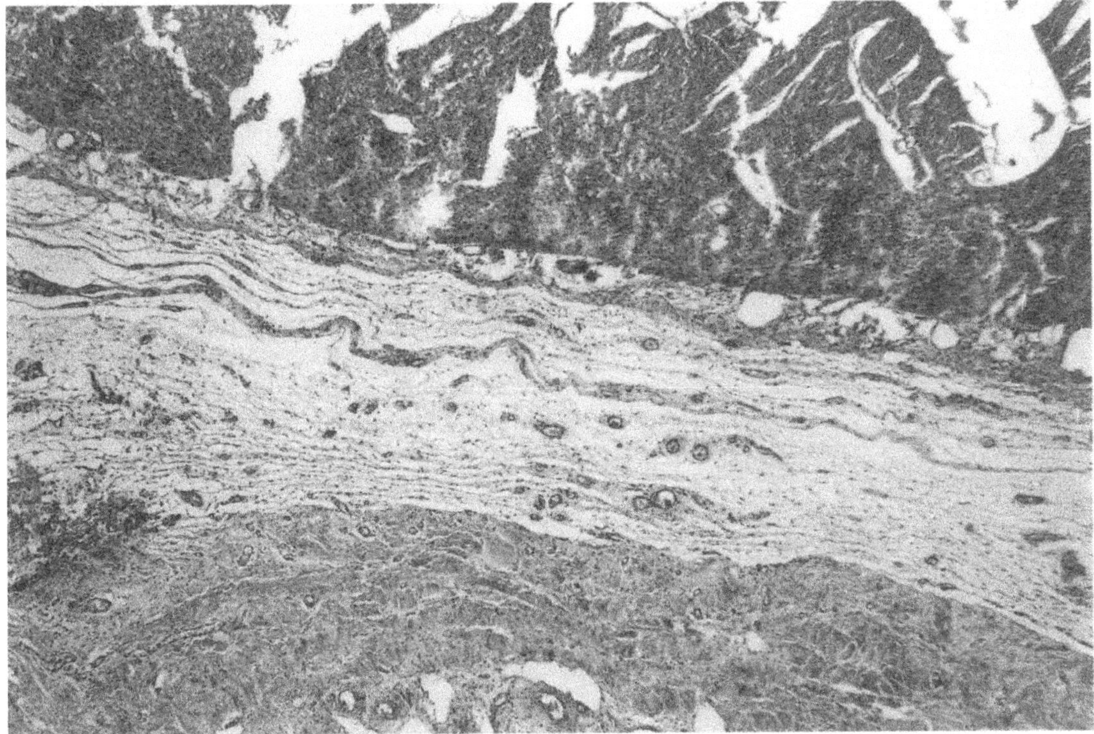

Loose bridge of connective tissue between epicardium and pericardium following pericarditis

Fig. 3.45
Rheumatoid arthritis

these pericardial adhesions never calcify and are clinically insignificant, because here a loose displaceable layer develops between both surfaces in the course of time. The diagnosis is usually documented only by the pathologist (Fig. 3.45).

Pleura

In the context of RA exudative inflammatory processes on the pleural surface can frequently be observed, in general occurring discreetly and not assuming clinical significance. They may leave loose fibrous adhesions, which will be detected only by a post mortem examination (approx. 50% of RA patients; Medsger 1986). This is only of little, if any functional importance especially since here, too, in the course of time a loose displaceable layer develops in the region of the adhesions.

Peritoneum

Basically, the peritoneum can also, like any serous membrane, turn unhealthy during an RA polyserositis, with fibrin exudation, fibrosation, and adhesion of the peritoneal surfaces. In contrast to pericardium and pleura, peritoneal involvement recedes into the background. (Exact observations, however, allowing a quantitative evaluation do not exist.)

3.10.2 Specific Processes: Rheumatoid Necroses ("Rheumatoid Nodules")

While in RA the inflammatory and destructive processes at joints and tendon sheaths are in the centre of interest, additional primary necrotizing processes can occur in the depth of collagenous tissue structures in patients with seropositive RA.

3.10.2.1 Localization of Rheumatoid Necroses

The fact that in RA necrotic processes are generally only observed in form of "skin nodules" ("key fossil" of RA) has led to an underestimate of their importance for the patient. According to the site of involvement, nodules can simply be a cosmetic problem or they may give rise to more serious, functional problems by destruction of a tendon for example. When the heart or blood vessels are affected, their occurrence may be life-threatening.
The fact that we saw in material gained from forefoot surgery in seropositive RA patients in 64% clinically not suspected RA-necroses in the subcutaneous tissue of the plantar surface (see p. 116), gives the idea that there is a generalized clinically latent tendency for necrotizing processes in these patients.

Skin

In the skin, the rheumatoid nodule is primarily found at sites subject to repeated minor trauma, such as the elbow, fingers or heel. Generally, the nodule is situated within thickened subcutaneous connective tissue, in most cases in the neighbourhood of a bony substratum (Figs. 3.46–3.49).
It is only rarely that rheumatoid nodules are found in the cutis itself. The clinically defined rheumatoid nodule in fact often consists of several necrotic centres which are surrounded by a single fibrous capsule.
According to our experiences, "rheumatoid nodules" are mixed up very often with the granuloma anulare above all in juvenile patients (see p. 124).

Joint capsule

Nodules are also relatively common in the joint capsules. They almost invariably lie in the stratum fibrosum and only very rarely in the synovial membrane itself. In this case, they erode through to the synovial surface. The resulting picture may be confused with fibrin deposition in which the palisade can resemble a rather cylindrical lining cell layer (Fig. 3.50).

Tendons

Although the inflammatory process of tenosynovitis may spread to the tendon by way of the blood vessels, generally the tendons are left intact. On the other hand, however, nodules occurring in the tendon can be very destructive and lead to tendon rupture (Fig. 3.51). In a 68-year-old patient with seropositive RA, we have seen destruction of the palmaris longus tendon over a 1.5 cm area, caused by more than 30 closely packed, early but prominent necrotic nodules.

Lung and pleura

The collagenous scaffold of the lung may be involved in the necrotizing process. Nodules are predominantly lying in the region of the pleura or in an interlobar fissure (see p. 148).

Pericardium

Rheumatoid nodules may also occur in the pericardium. It is a moot point, whether previous pericardial adhesions are a precondition for their formation (see p. 136).
Macroscopically, the nodules situated above the visceral pericard surface show great similarity to tuberculous foci (see p. 119).

Myocardium

This necrotic process can have dramatic consequences when the fibrous skeleton of the heart or pre-existing scar tissue are involved, which mainly consist of collagen type I. Nodules may establish themselves in the neighbourhood of a heart valve and may cause valvular insufficiency (see p. 137).

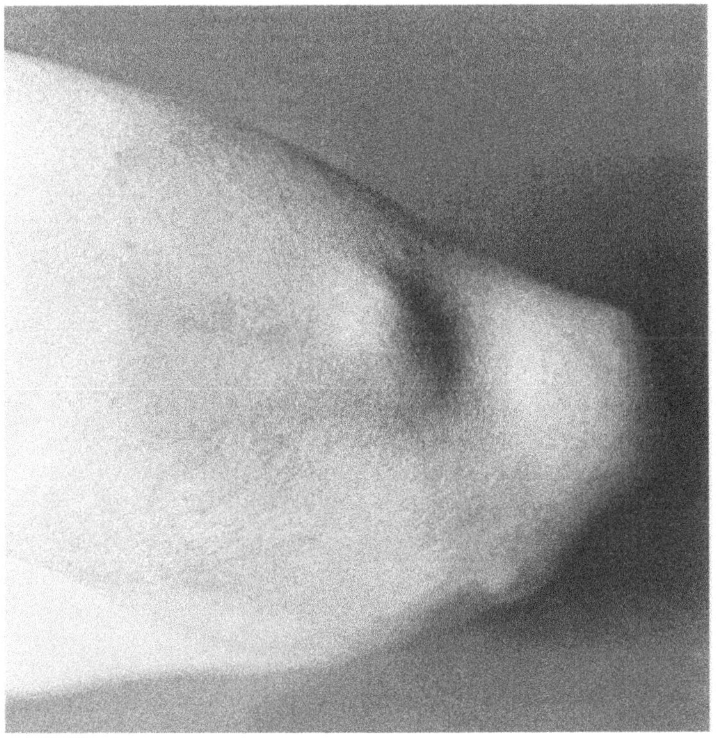

"Nodular rheumatism" overlying the ulna. There is also swelling of the olecranon bursa

Fig. 3.46

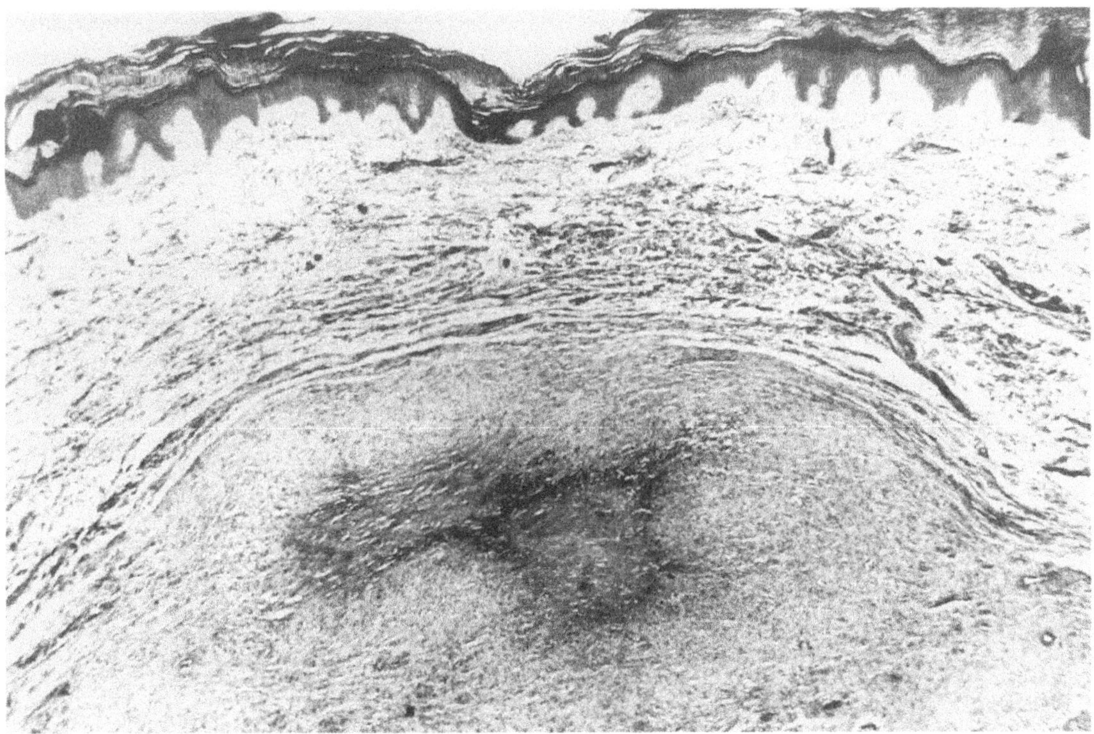

Subcutaneous rheumatoid nodule close to the dermis

Fig. 3.47
Rheumatoid arthritis

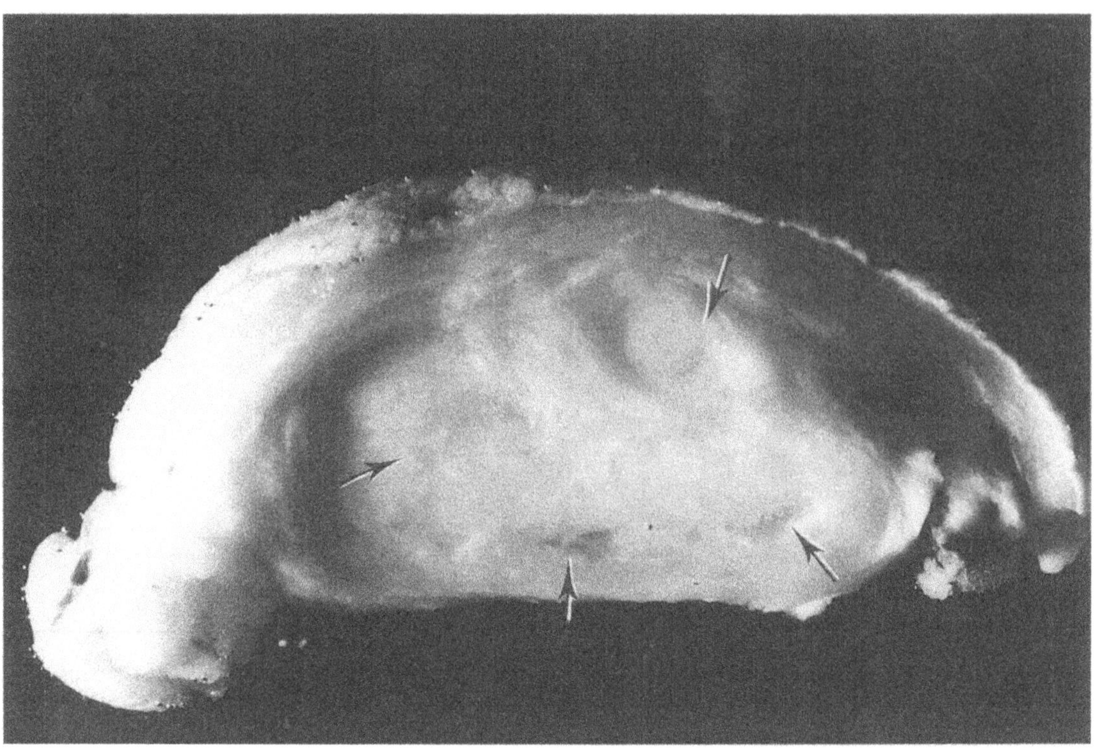

Fig. 3.48
Rheumatoid arthritis

Cut surface of a subcutaneous rheumatoid nodule with several centres of necrosis (*arrows*)

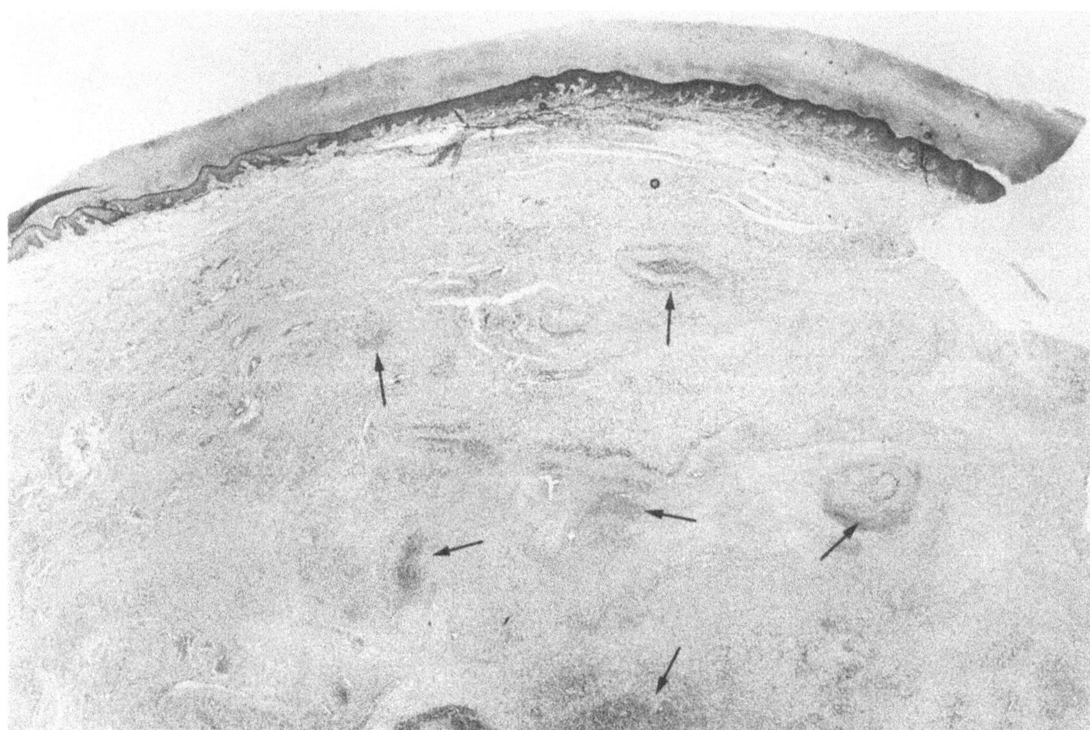

Fig. 3.49
Rheumatoid arthritis

Subcutaneous rheumatoid nodule with several central necroses (*arrows*). The vicinity is scar-like thickened

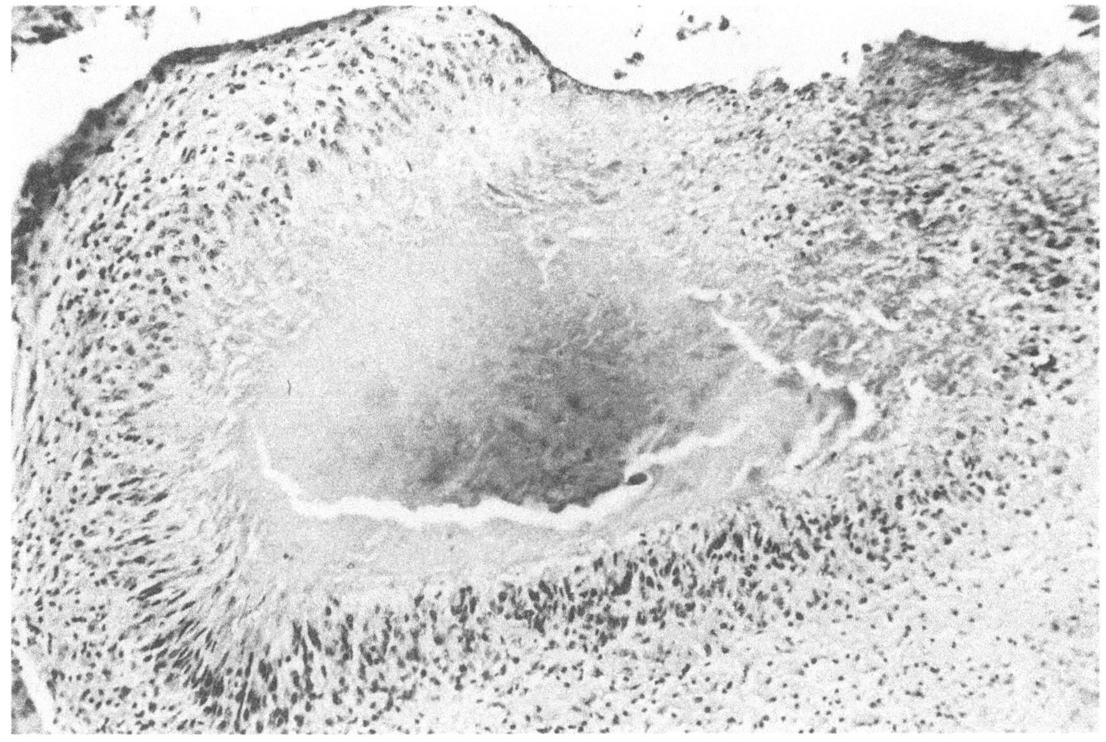

Rheumatoid necrotic nodule in a synovial villus. The necrosis has reached the eroded surface

Fig. 3.50
Rheumatoid arthritis

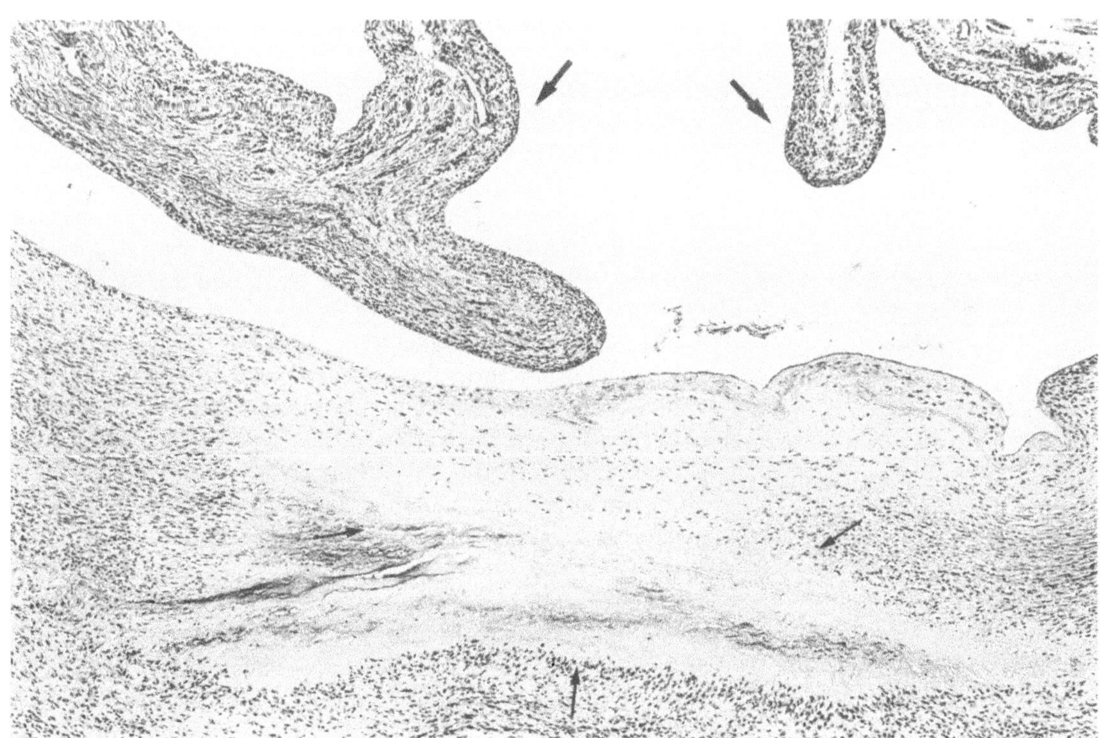

Rheumatoid necrosis in a tendon (*arrows below*). *Arrows above*, synovial villi from the tendon sheath

Fig. 3.51
Rheumatoid arthritis

The collagenous connective tissue of vessels situated in the depths of the heart muscle is itself seldomly subject to RA-necroses. Hereby, the neighbouring myocardial fibres perish. Clinically it is possible for such a process to be confused with ischaemic cardiac infarction and, after multiple occurrences or involvement of the conducting system, it may be fatal (Cruickshank 1954; Fassbender 1963, 1975; Ahern et al. 1983; see p. 143).

Sclera

Apart from inflammatory eye disease, which frequently accompanies RA, rheumatoid nodules may occur in the dense collagenous tissue of the sclera. The dramatic consequences of this necrotic scleritis are clear from its synonym "scleromalacia perforans" or "necrotisans", which often leads to loss of the eye (see p. 151). The histological picture of these eye processes corresponds to the well-known pattern: central necroses with surrounding cell palisade. Inflammatory infiltrates can encroach from a neighbouring episcleritis on the necrotizing process and can intersperse the marginal palisade with neutrophils and lymphocytes.

Blood vessels

Primary necrotizing processes may also occur in the wall of arteries and veins. The necrosis may be confined to a single segment of the vascular wall or at the other extreme, the whole vessel may be involved.

The vascular wall necrosis in RA is also confined by a sequestrum shaped cell palisade. If necrosis affects the full circumference, fibroblasts may lie radially arranged in form of a ciliary crown. This picture corresponds to the classical model of the rheumatoid necrosis (see p. 135).

Bursa

The fibrotic capsule of a bursa is a typical site for nodule formation.

Predisposing factors include the thick layer of collagen type I as well as the mechanical trauma which is both typical for the localization of bursae and also for rheumatoid nodules.

Plantar surface

The highest frequency of RA-necroses we found in the subcutaneous tissue of the plantar surfaces of patients with seropositive RA. In the thickened skin of the sole, which was removed on occasion of a Clayton operation, we found in 221 patients 122 times (64%) at least one, but mostly, however, several typical RA-necroses ("RA-nodules"). In most of the patients, such nodules were not noticeable and also the nodules on the plantar surface were clinically latent. The decisive role of mechanical irritation for the formation of RA-necroses in seropositve patients is confirmed by this localization: as the mechanical irritation under pressure of bodily weight is greatest in bones of the metatarsophalangeal joint, RA-necroses are to be expected here first.

The unexpected high frequency of RA-necroses in the plantar region allows us also to draw conclusions to the tendency of a general occurrence of necrotizing processes in seropositive RA patients. One goes surely not wrong if one accounts the primary necrotization as the third pathogenetic component, besides inflammatory and destructive processes, in the overall picture of the disease even in patients without visible cutaneous nodules.

3.10.2.2 Development of Rheumatoid Necroses

We have been able to document the following phases in the development of a rheumatoid nodule:

Phase I

Single collagen fibrils and fibres swell and become eosinophilic. This eosinophilic fibrinoid material has been regarded by some authors as altered local collagen or ground substance, by others as deposited extrinsic material such as fibrin, serum proteins, or nucleoprotein (Movat and Moore 1957). We as well as Sokoloff and coworkers (1953) identified this fibrinoid material in the early nodule as fibrin. The neighbouring fibroblasts die and become indistinct. Connective tissue cells in the region show a mobilization with irregular proliferation (Figs. 3.52, 3.53).

The bordering living tissue contrasts sharply with the necrotic centre, and a cell palisade starts to form.

In this first phase, many small nodules may converge to form a single rheumatoid nodule. It should be emphasized that no lymphocytes, plasma cells, neutrophils, macrophages, or new vessels are discernible in the generation of the nodule. The necrosis of tissue occurs without a reactive inflammatory response.

Phase II

The necrotic centre develops its ultimate size and form. Cellular recruitment is marked with the formation of a complete palisade (Fig. 3.54).

The necrosis is homogeneous on light-microscopy. The completed palisade comprises large, elongated cells with plentiful cytoplasm and spindle-shaped to oval nuclei, radially arranged around the necrotic centre. The sequester-like boundary between necrotic centre and cellular surround is impressively sharp. One is under the impression that the palisade cells touch with their "feet" the necrotic core. The necrosis and palisade become on the outside encased in a fibrous capsule. Perivascular infiltration by lymphocytes is rare. Single neutrophils may invade. C5a in the necrotic centre explains their attendance.

Phase III (After Months to Years)

Through the accumulation of calcium salts, the necrotic centre may become mildly basophilic and over the course of time disintegrates, or more rarely with surface contact, liquifies (Fig. 3.55). At this stage, the necrotic centre may contain occasional neutrophils. The palisade has faded and has been partially or completely replaced by fibroblasts and groups of macrophages. The sequestered, walled off necrosis may persist in this manner for years surrounded by a thick, fibrous capsule sparsely populated with cells. It is only after many years that secondary fibrosis of the degenerated necrosis can occur – the initial shape, although faint, remains recognizable and bears witness to the nature of the original process (Fig. 3.56).

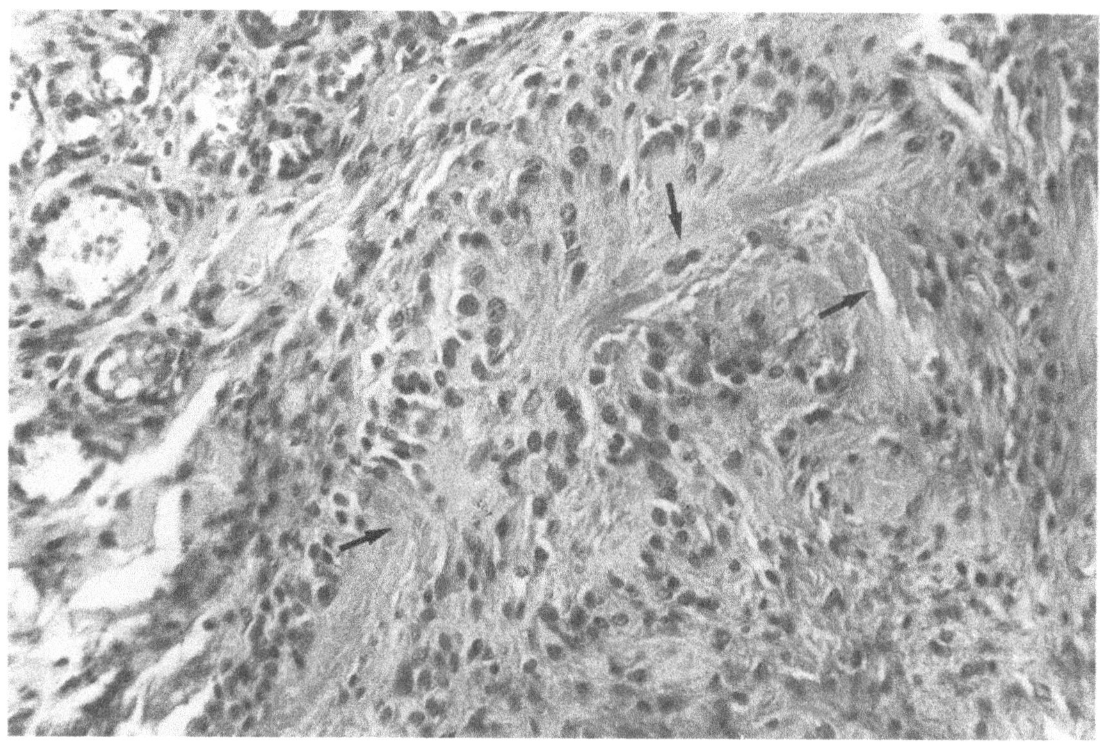

Fig. 3.52
Rheumatoid arthritis

Starting rheumatoid necrosis (*arrows*) of single collagen fibre bundles in a tendon with a well-formed palisade (Necrosis Phase I)

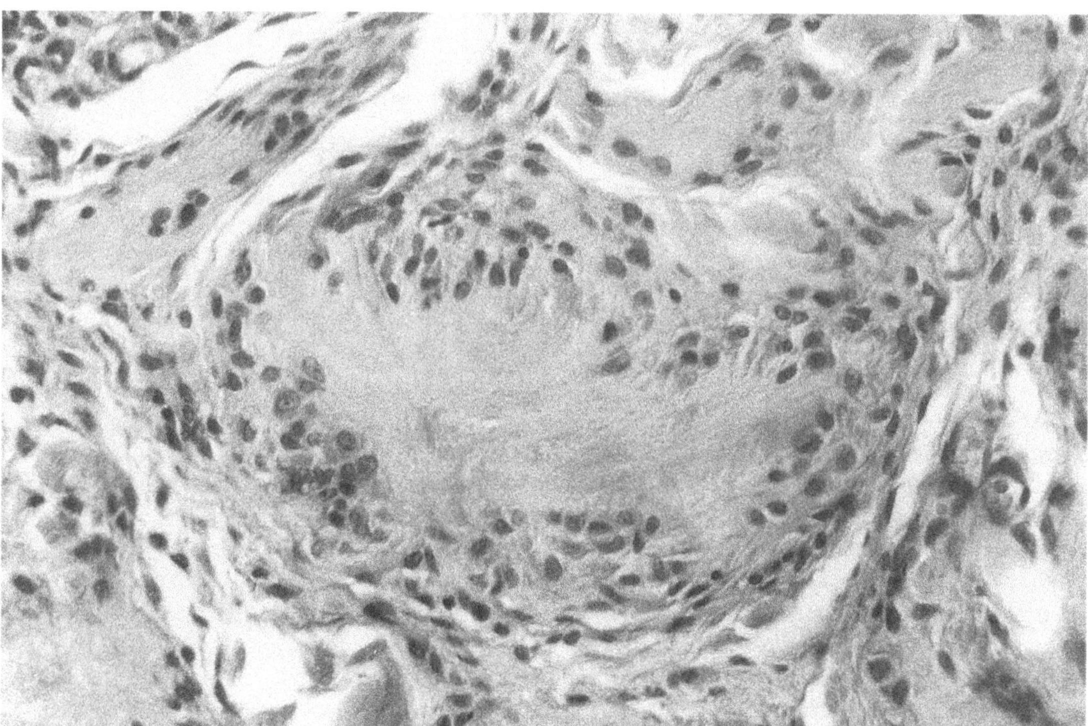

Fig. 3.53
Rheumatoid arthritis

Early rheumatoid necrosis of individual collagen fibre bundles in a tendon showing pronounced reaction by connective tissue cells (Necrosis Phase I)

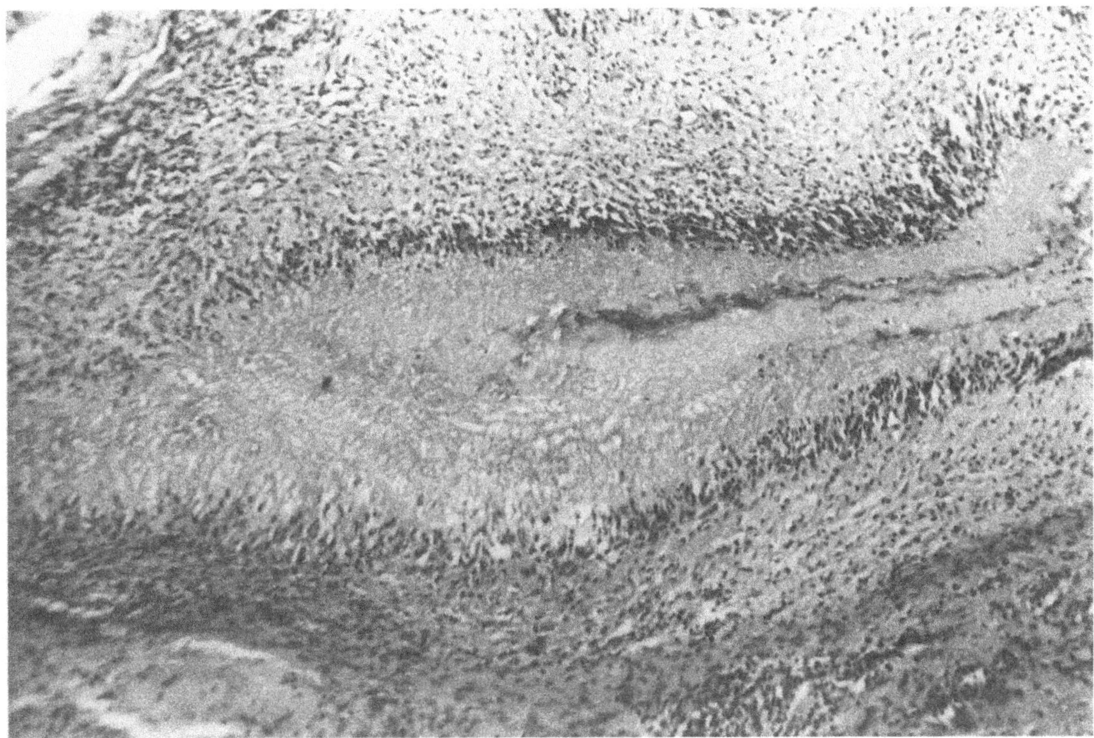

Rheumatoid necrosis (Phase II) in the subcutaneous tissue of the plantar surface

Fig. 3.54
Rheumatoid arthritis

In many respects, the rheumatoid nodule resembles a tuberculous nodule. The central necrosis is not organized but is encapsulated: in both cases, the necrotic centre is treated like a sequestration and isolated from the surrounding tissue.

3.10.2.3 Pathogenetic Hypotheses of Rheumatoid Necroses

In the field of general morphology, the rheumatoid nodule is considered to be an uncommon phenomenon. Its development is outlined in various hypotheses. One hypothesis claims a vascular occlusion to be the underlying process. If this were the case, neutrophils, macrophages, fibroblasts, and angioblasts immediately would infiltrate the necrotic area, absorb the disintegrated tissue and build up granulation tissue, as is the case in any infarction, but this never has been observed in rheumatoid nodules.
The fact that the necrotic centre is surrounded by a dense palisade of connective tissue cells which never penetrate the boundary line into the necrotic area as well as the configuration of the rheumatoid nodule do not support this hypothesis.
Another hypothesis, which claims the development of rheumatoid necroses is caused by neutrophils, is not valid since in the early developmental phases of the rheumatoid nodule no neutrophils are found. Furthermore, the tissue destruction due to neutrophils would result in the formation of an abscess instead of an acellular destruction of collagen fibres.

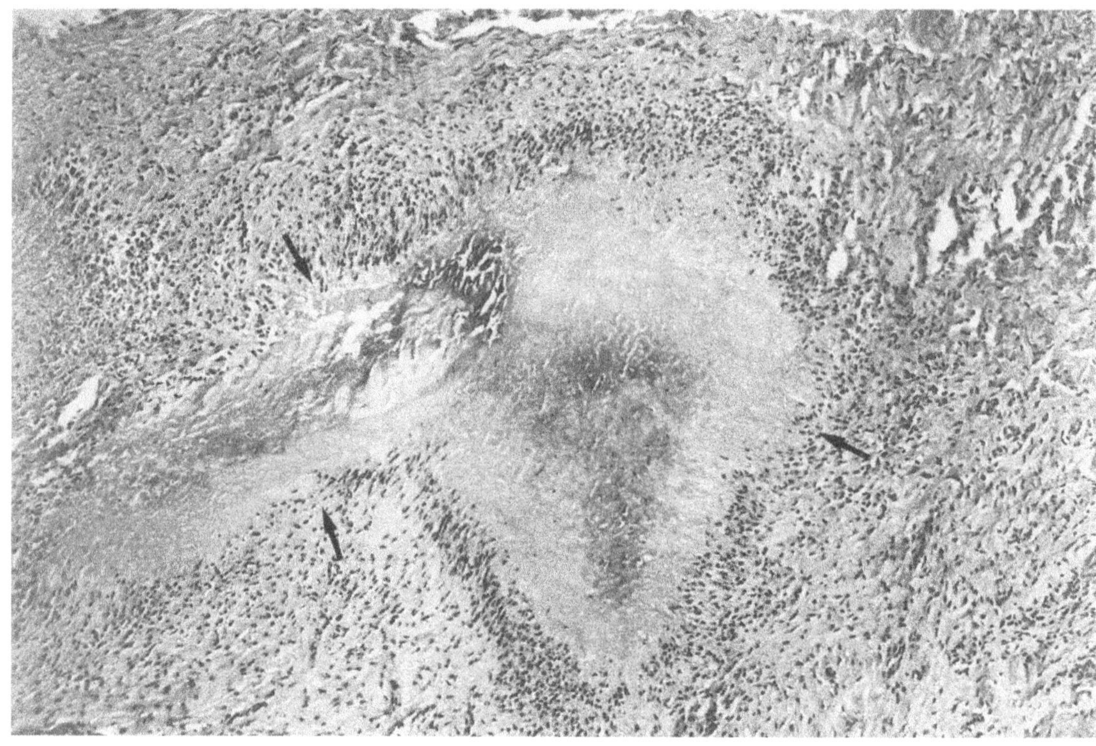

Fig. 3.55
Rheumatoid arthritis

Older rheumatoid necrosis surrounded by a fibrous capsule. Deposition of calcium salts in the centre. The palisade has faded and is partly replaced by fibroblasts and macrophages (*arrows*) Necrosis Phase III)

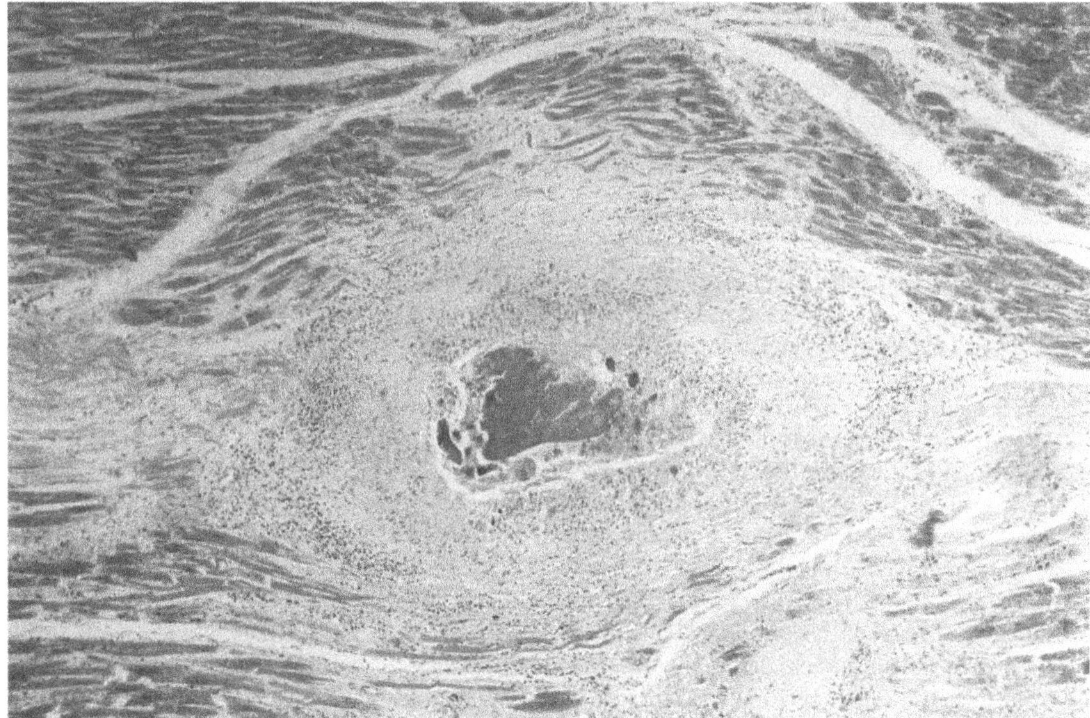

Fig. 3.56
Rheumatoid arthritis

An old scarring rheumatoid necrotic focus in the myocardium. Centrally, there are calcified muscle remnants surrounded by the remainder of a palisade showing extensive scarring (Necrosis Phase III)

The presence of immunoglobulin and HLA-DR (Hedfors et al. 1983) within the rheumatoid nodules does not offer an explanation for the devitalisation of the connective tissue without corresponding cell involvement.

Role of rheumatoid factors

Nevertheless, humoral-immunological components must take part in the development of rheumatoid necroses, since on principle they are linked to the presence of IgM rheumatoid factor, demonstrated by conventional methods (Waaler-Rose test, latex fixation test; see p. 58).

Another pathogenetic component is seen in minor tissue lesions predominantly found at mechanically exposed areas (e.g. elbows, ankles, balls of the foot).

Mechanically induced irritation facilitates the influx of serum containing rheumatoid factors into the tissue. Nevertheless, this hypothesis lacks the binding link between the role of rheumatoid factors, on the one hand, and the activation of procollagenase, on the other.

Role of collagenases

According to our observations, a high-grade proliferation of local fibroblasts precedes the formation of a RA-necrosis (Fig. 3.57). Thus, dense cell formations, which remind of the tlp in the synovial tissue, are created. The cells show relatively large, light vesicular nuclei. Mitoses are to be found, but rarely. At first, tiny gaps appear in this "lawn" of cells. Later, these develop into narrow or round foci of necrosis that grow and may blend into one with adjacent foci. The young necroses are encompassed by a "lawn" of proliferated fibroblasts, into which also macrophages immigrate. After a short period of time, they differentiate into the characteristic palisade that consists of radially arranged, long, narrow cells with large nuclei (Fig. 3.58). The palisade separates the necrotic centre from its surroundings. Over time, the surrounding fibroblastic cellular elements fade away. A capsule consisting of collagen fibres takes their place, it may exist for months or even years. The augmentation of fibres leads to an increase in the capsule's density in the course of time. We risk the hypothesis that collagenases released during the break-down of the compact fibroblasts, which contain procollagenase, initiate the necrosis. Harris (1972) demonstrated that culture supernatants of nodule tissue contained collagenase and a neutral protease. Also in the experiments by Ziff and coworkers (1953), in which the necrotic centres of nodules were extracted and the residual tissue examined histologically, a connective tissue framework remained following extraction. The extracted material was free of collagenous protein, which indicates that the central necrosis of the RA-nodule is the work of degrading enzymes. As long as they are fresh, remnants of this cell proliferation are noticeable surrounding them (Fig. 3.59). Later, the vicinity becomes increasingly necrotic. Only the radially arranged palisade of large, narrow cells continues to exist over several months.

Elements of cell palisade

For years, the elements surrounding the rheumatoid necrosis have aroused particular attention. Parallels exist between the palisade cells in the necrosis and the cells constituting the synovial membrane. Both contain TNF-α, IL-1β, and identical cell adhesion molecules (Wikaningrum et al. 1998). The question whether palisade cells are macrophages or fibroblasts is mainly decided in

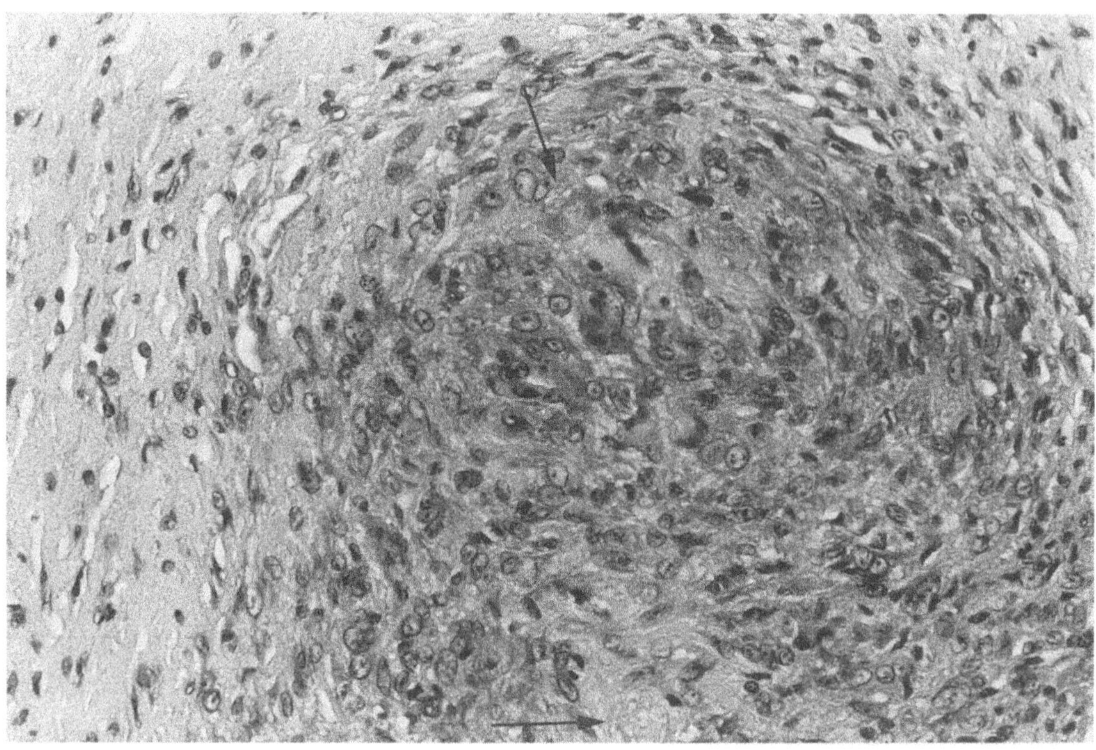

Fig. 3.57
Rheumatoid arthritis

Birth of an RA-necrosis in the region of high-grade proliferation of synovial fibroblasts. *Arrows*, cell gaps with tiny necroses

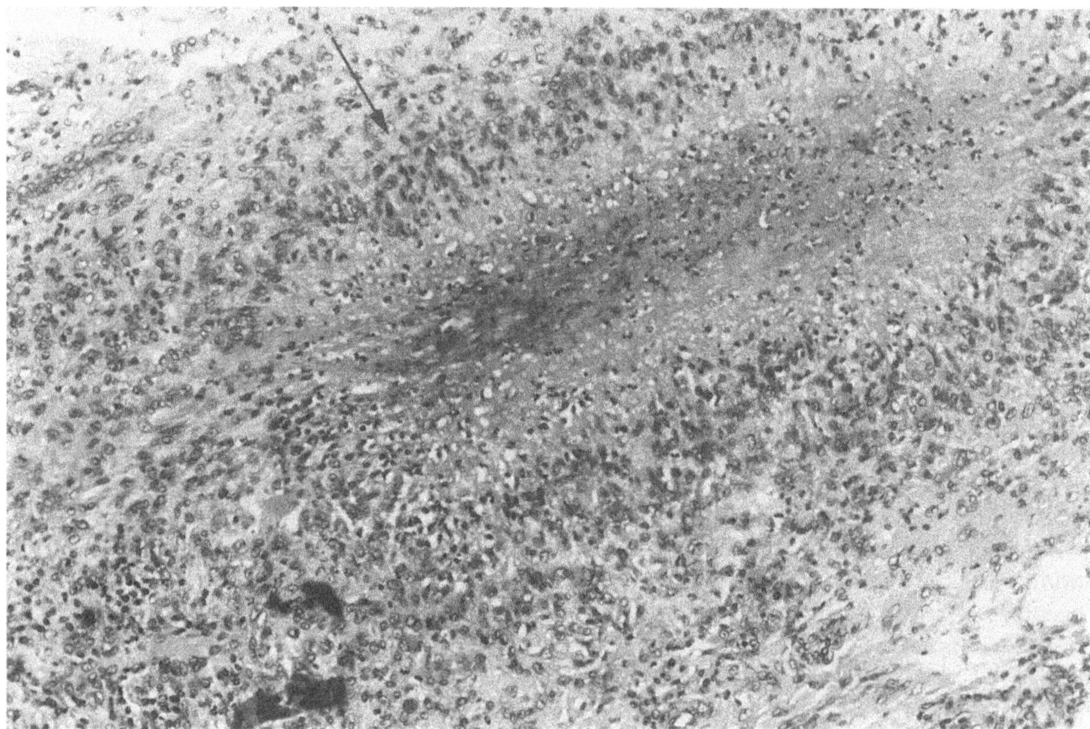

Fig. 3.58
Rheumatoid arthritis

Early RA-necrosis. At the margin of the necrosis, a beginning cell palisade (*arrow*) is recruited from the "lawn" of proliferated fibroblasts and some macrophages

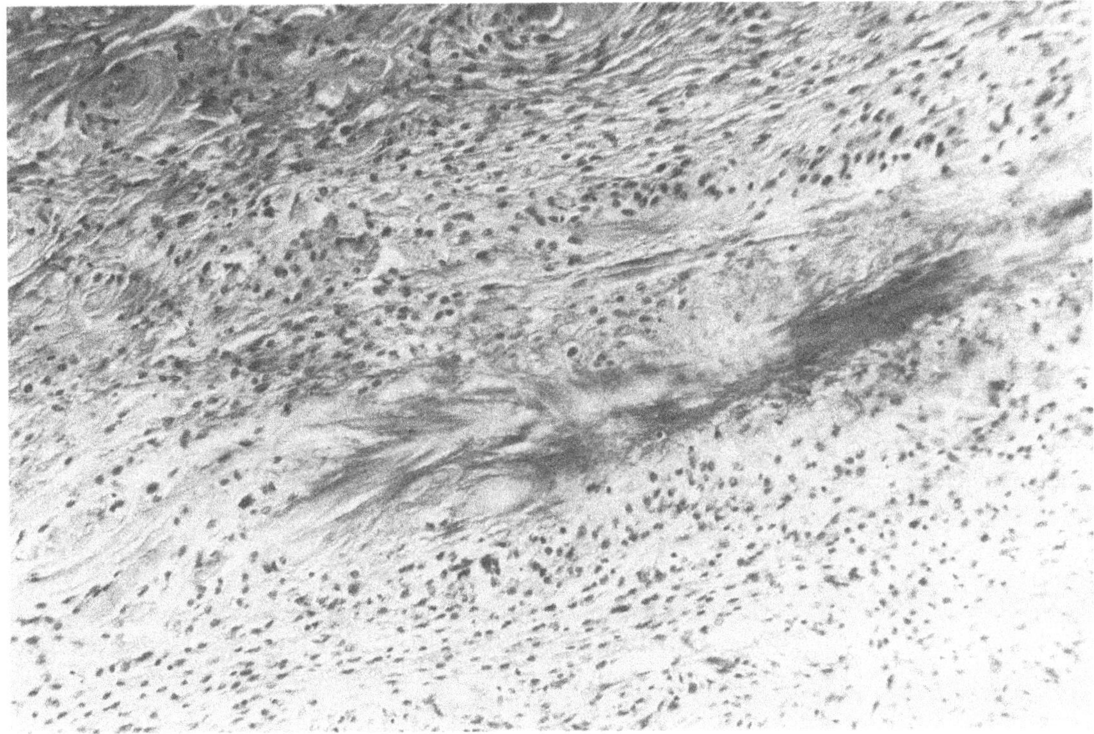

Rheumatoid nodule showing individual collagen bundles with surrounding palisade in the subcutaneous layer

Fig. 3.59
Rheumatoid arthritis

favour of macrophages. According to the studies performed by Hedfors et al. (1983), staining for HLA-DR and OKM1 indicates that the cells within the palisades are macrophage-like cells. Their marked proliferative activity is evident from their OKT9 reactivity. Edwards and coworkers (1993) consider the palisading cells to be a combination of macrophages and fibroblasts; the latter, however, show no signs of synoviocyte differentiation. The discrepancies between the different understandings might be due to different developmental phases of the nodules examined. According to our observations, fibroblasts prevail in the later stages of development. Electron-microscopic studies by Cochrane et al. (1964) of the necrotic centre have demonstrated collagen and reticulin fibres, fibrinoid material, cellular organelles, and fat globules in the necrotic debris.

Electron-microscopic studies

The fact that rheumatoid necroses never occur in rheumatoid-factor-positive individuals who are not suffering from RA, may be explained by the studies of Natvig and colleagues (1988). They found differences between the rheumatoid factors of patients with RA and those of healthy seropositive individuals. The latter virtually all show rheumatoid factor antibodies of the IgM type, whereas in patients with RA both IgM and IgG antibodies are found. It is quite likely that only the IgG rheumatoid factors are of pathogenetic nature while the IgM rheumatoid factors appear to escape into the blood circulation where they probably do not cause much harm.

3.10.2.4 Differential Diagnosis Between Rheumatoid Necroses and Other Forms of Necroses

Although the fully developed nodule with its characteristic features is specific for RA, there is a second phenomenon which could be very similar and in our experience is frequently mistaken for the rheumatoid nodule, namely, granuloma anulare. In contrast to the former, granuloma anulare is only found in the skin and generally in the dermis. Owing to the extreme similarity of both conditions, diagnosis can be very difficult especially as RA-necrosis is rarely found in the cutis and the granuloma anulare can be subcutaneous.

Despite possibilities of confusion, we have been able to find some features helpful in their differential diagnosis:

Rheumatoid necrosis

- ▸ Rheumatoid necrosis
  1. Clinical features: occurrence only in seropositive RA patients.
  2. Site: generally subcutaneous.
  3. Form: usually round to oval, may also be branched.
  4. Tendency for deposition of calcium salts and degeneration.
  5. Complete palisade of regular, elongated fibroblasts.
  6. Surrounding fibrous capsule.
  7. Occurrence at mechanically exposed sites.

Granuloma anulare

- ▸ Granuloma anulare
  1. Clinically and serologically unassociated with articular or other systemic disease. No rheumatoid factors!
  2. Site: generally in the skin (Fig. 3.60).
  3. Form: predominantly elongated with irregular collagen fibre bundles which extend often like a swallow-tail into the neighbouring tissue (Figs. 3.61, 3.62).
  4. No tendency of the necrosis to degenerate.
  5. No complete palisade with ordered fibroblasts. Usually, the necrosis is surrounded by an irregular array of cells consisting of macrophages and connective tissue cells.
  6. Generally, no surrounding capsule. In the immediate vicinity, lymphocytes may be found around small blood vessels.
  7. No dependency on mechanical expositions (Figs. 3.63, 3.64).

"Pseudorheumatoid nodule" ("Type X")

Apart from these two skin conditions which can be distinguished by their characteristic features, a third type of necrosis rarely may be observed, which does not fall into either group. Since the clinical and serological features of RA are lacking, there is a tendency to include this entity under the label of granuloma anulare or to use the term "pseudorheumatoid nodule" (Mesara et al. 1966; Williams et al. 1977; Cohen 1983). Not only do we consider the term "pseudorheumatoid nodule" to be of little use, we feel that it invites confusion as a non-existent connection with RA or other rheumatic condition is suggested. For this reason, we have called this form of necrosis "Type X", in order to distinguish it from granuloma anulare, on the one hand, and to avoid the suggestion of any serological connection, on the other. The term "Type X" simply represents a convenient peg, until the pathogenetic processes are understood or a more suitable term is found.

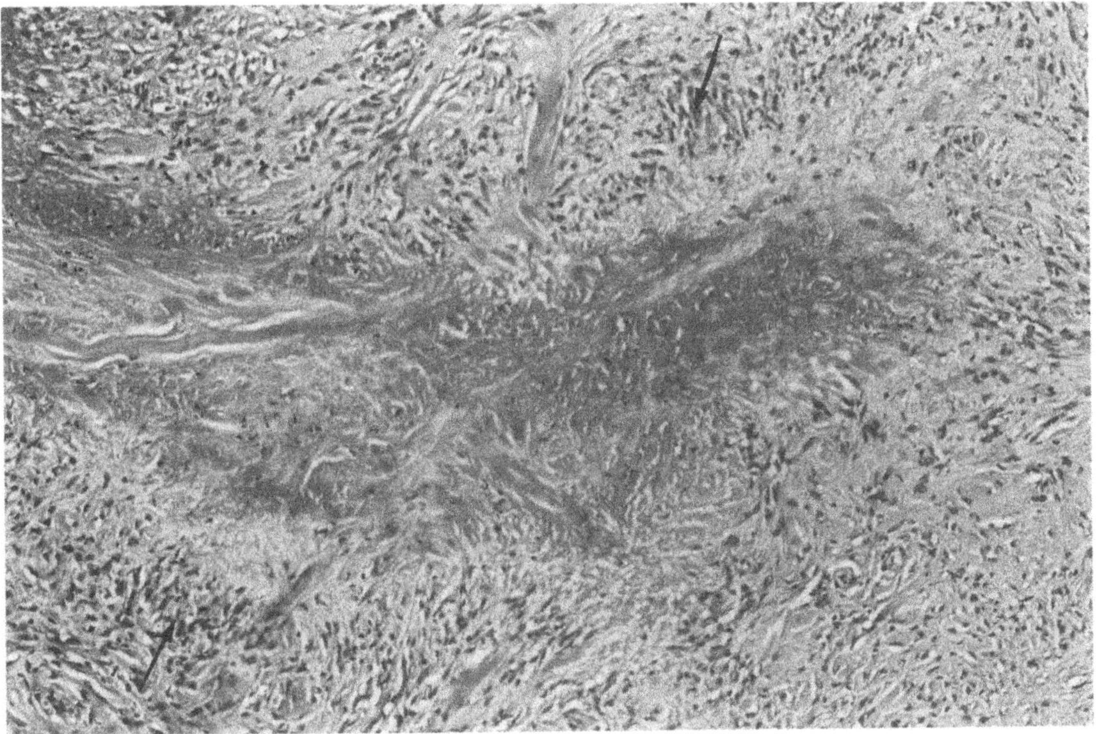

Fig. 3.60
Granuloma anulare

In the necrotic centre, the collagen fibres are partly preserved, radiating into the vicinity. Only in some parts a disarranged palisade of mixed cells (*arrows*)

- "Pseudorheumatoid nodule" ("Type X")
  1. No clinical evidence of RA or other rheumatic disease. Rheumatoid factors are absent.
  2. Site: both in the skin and subcutaneous tissues.
  3. Form: the necrosis is large and round to oval in shape.
  4. The necrosis is more prominent than it is the case in granuloma anulare.
  5. The palisade comprises radially situated fibroblasts, with staggered macrophages.
  6. No fibrous capsule.

Of the three types, rheumatoid nodules can be clearly distinguished by the presence of rheumatoid factors acting in this case as a marker.

Skin nodules in RF and JCA

Skin nodules also occur in RF (see p. 50) and in juvenile chronic artheritis (JCA) (see p. 174). The histological picture is similar for both, but is distinct from the rheumatoid nodule in RA. In RF and JCA, the centre consists of a banded, fibrinoid necrosis. The primary necrosis of collagen bundles that is a feature of RA or granuloma anulare is absent. Instead of a palisade of fibroblasts, an irregular collection of macrophages, lymphocytes, and neutrophils can be seen. The collagenous fibrous capsule which is a feature of RA does not form.
However, there is one exception, namely, the necrotizing processes found in the seropositive poly-articular form of JCA which are indistinguishable from the rheumatoid nodules seen in adult RA.

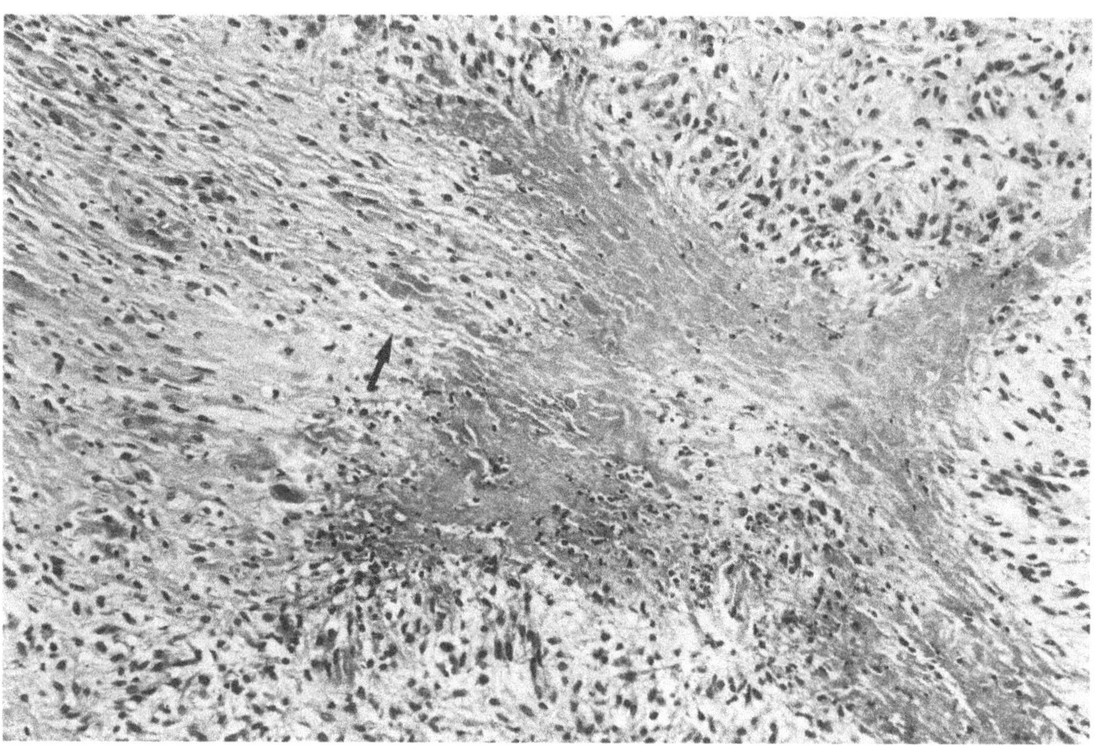

Fig. 3.61
Granuloma anulare

Typical swallow-tail formation. The necrotic centre is only in parts surrounded by a palisade of mixed cells *(arrow)*. Collagen fibres are radiating into the vicinity

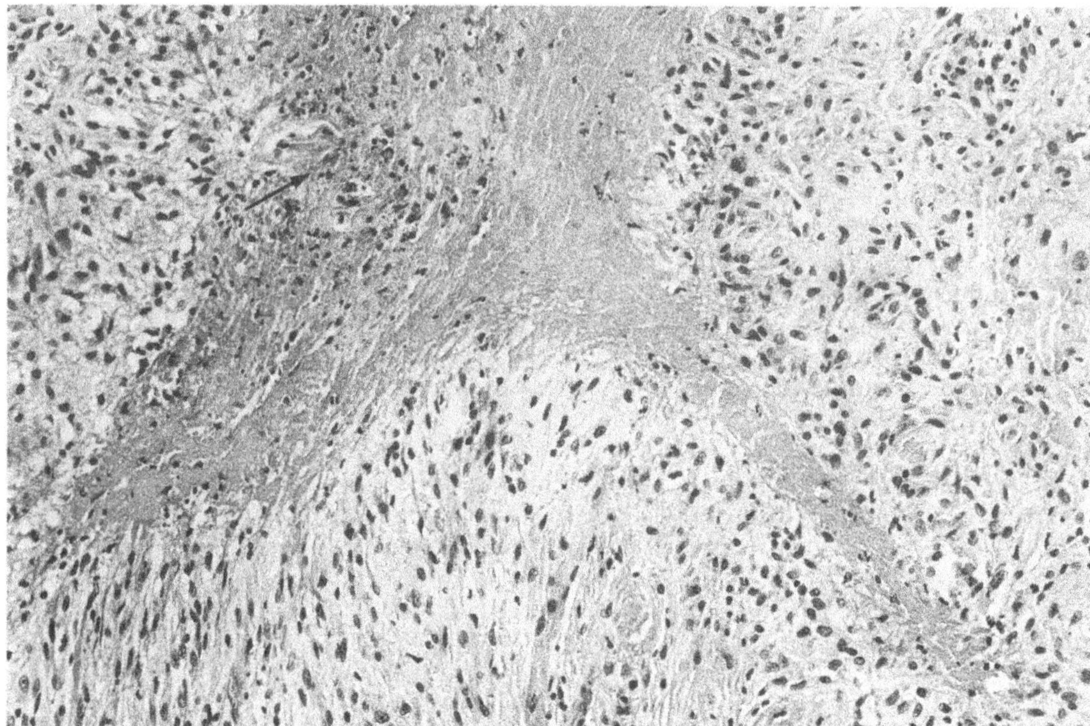

Fig. 3.62
Granuloma anulare

Typical swallow-tail. Necrotic collagen fibres, surrounded by staggered macrophages and fibroblasts, in between few lymphocytes. In the necrosis some immigrated neutrophils

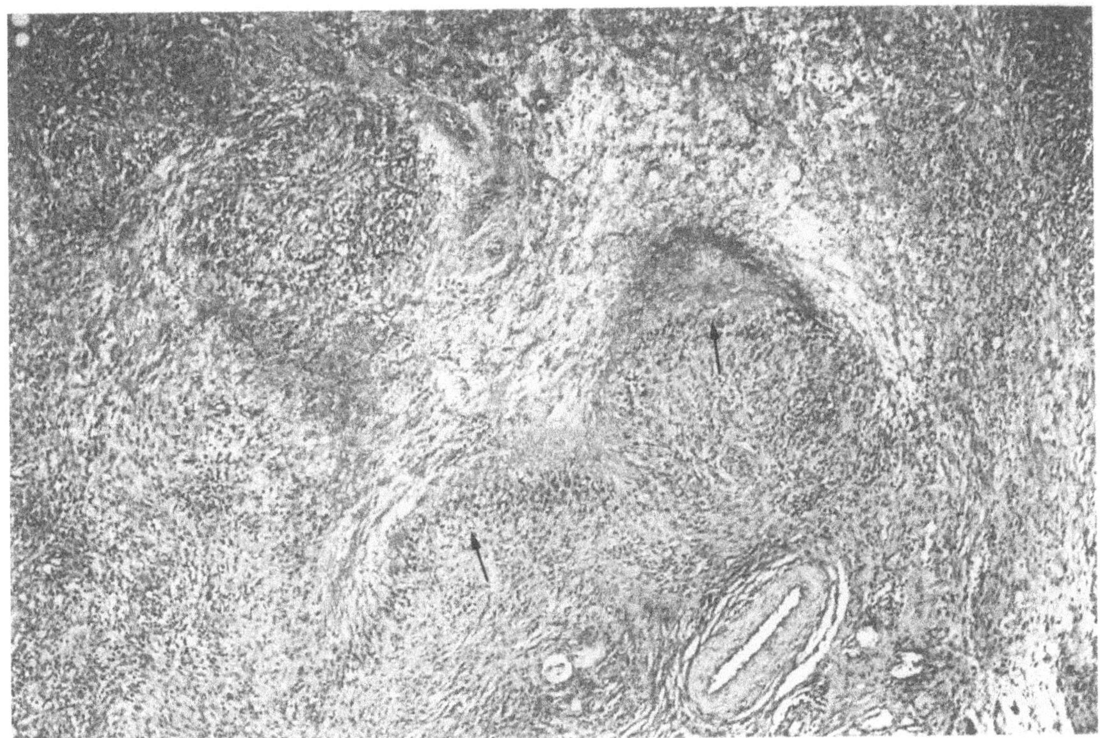

Swallow-tailed necrotic area. In the lower part, not fully developed cell palisade (*arrows*). The other regions are surrounded by partly staggered macrophages. In the vicinity, newly formed blood vessels surrounded by lymphocytes

Fig. 3.63
Granuloma anulare

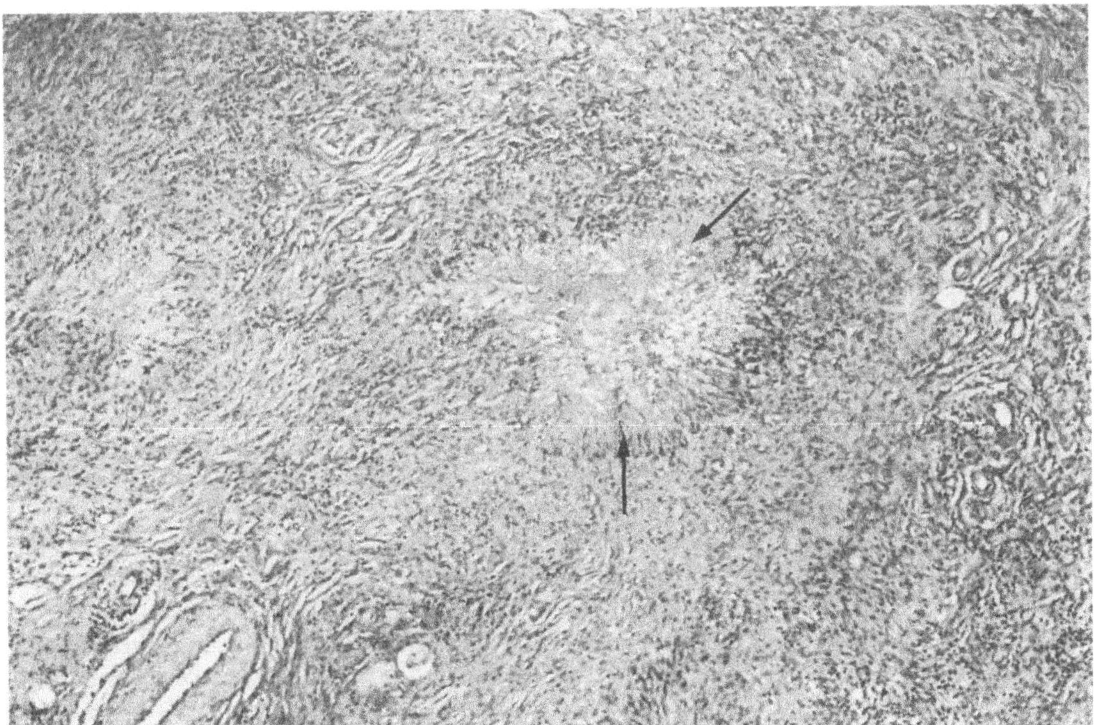

Not fully developed cell palisade (*arrows*). The other regions are surrounded by macrophages. In the vicinity, newly formed blood vessels and lymphocytes

Fig. 3.64
Granuloma anulare

3.11 Visceral Manifestations of Inflammatory and Necrotizing Processes in RA and Their Nosological Importance

With the affection of visceral tissues (blood vessels, heart, lung, eye) RA no longer can be considered to be merely a joint disease but a systemic "rheumatoid disease" and thus steps into a new, significant clinical dimension. At this point, patients generally are in an advanced stage of the primary disease and show high titres of rheumatoid factors.

In RA, a disease in fact dominated by inflammatory mechanisms, the vascular system is involved from the onset of the disease. In the context of the local inflammatory process, capillaries, arterioles, and venules undergo endothelial changes which at that early point of time not yet justify the term vasculitis.

3.11.1 RA-Vasculitis

In the context of rheumatoid vasculitis, arteries, predominantly small and seldom of medium size, and, more rarely, veins may be affected, whereby the arterial disease prevails the clinical symptoms. To determine the actual dimension of the vasculitis process in RA, systematic post mortem investigations of the entire vascular system are required.

Localization of RA-vasculitis

The clinical profile of RA is mainly characterized by the involvement of vessels in the following manner:

1. Distal arteritis can result in gangrene of fingers and toes.
2. Arteritis involving adjacent nerves can initiate peripheral neuropathies.
3. Arteritis in the heart, lung, colon, kidney, and pancreas can result in tissue infarction.

The morphological picture of vasculitis in RA is variable and with intensification of the process increases its characteristic aspects sometimes reaching specificity. Since damaging factors (e.g. antibodies, immune complexes) initially come into contact with the endothelial tube, pathological changes can be demonstrated at the endothelium which we described as "progressive transformation" (Simmling-Annefeld and Fassbender 1979). Already on light-microscopic examinations of semi-thin sections, capillaries, arterioles, and venules of the synovial membrane in RA reveal swelling of the endothelial cells, which project button-like into the lumen (Figs. 3.65–3.67).

In RA, arteries and veins can also be submitted to inflammatory processes which are characterized by proliferation of the intima and infiltration of the vascular wall by neutrophils.

These processes, however, are non-specific and ubiquitous. This statement is still valid, even when, under the influence of neutrophil enzymes, the media disintegrates. Thus, in RA a necrotizing arteritis of this origin may occur, but without being characteristic or of diagnostic value.

Medial necroses

Medial necroses, however, surrounded by proliferated intimal and adventitial cells, are a characteristic feature of RA. These me-

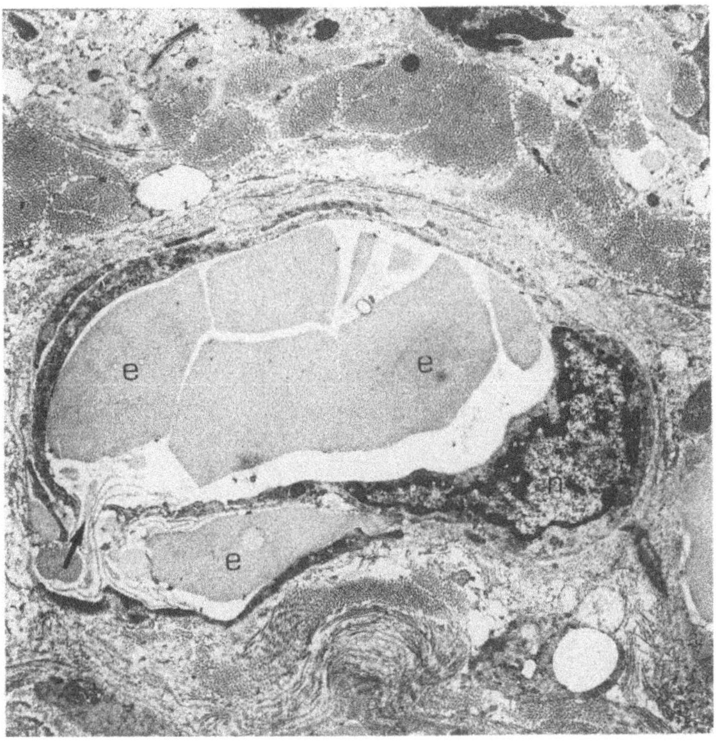

Venule within the synovial tissue. Plasma exudation between the extensions of two endothelial cells (*arrow*). *N*, endothelial cell nucleus; *E*, erythrocyte. (Electron micrograph)

Fig. 3.65
Rheumatoid arthritis

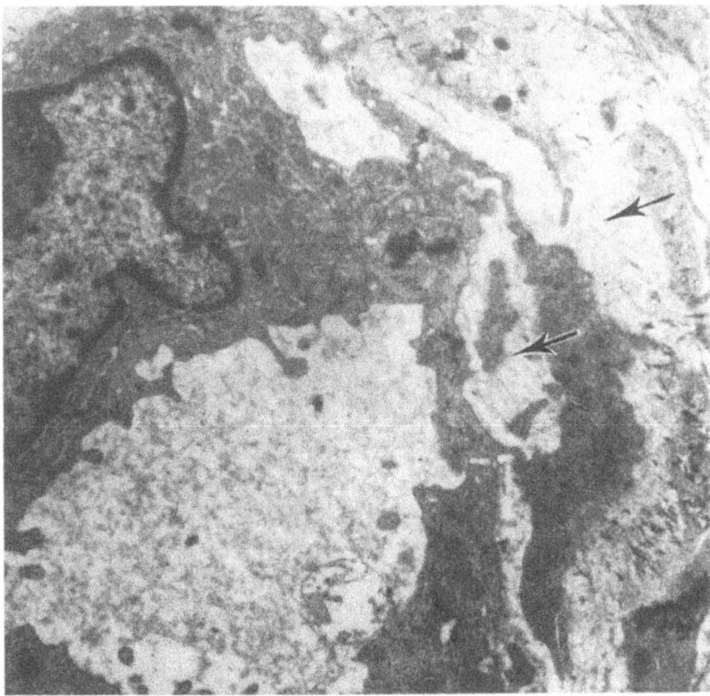

Venule in the synovium. The endothelial cell resembles a fibroblast with extensive endoplasmic reticulum and many mitochondria. There is a fissure between the projections of two endothelial cells with plasm exudation (*arrows*). (Electron micrograph; Bierther and Wegner 1971)

Fig. 3.66
Rheumatoid arthritis

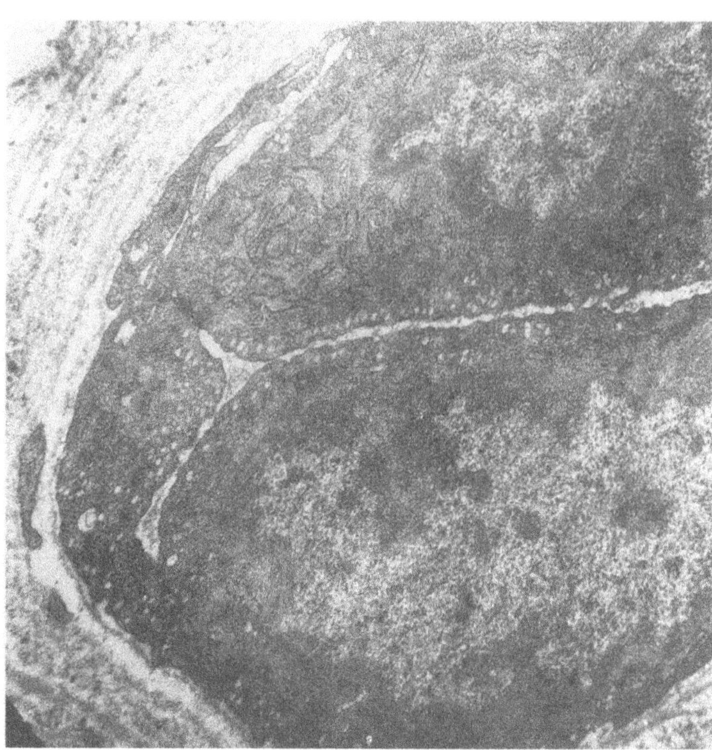

Fig. 3.67
Synovial capillary

Endothelial cells on either side of the slit-like lumen show nuclei. Prominent rough endoplasmic reticulum. *Left*, multi-layered basement membrane. (Electron micrograph; Bierther and Wegner 1971)

dial necroses may affect one segment only or the full circumference of the vascular wall. In the beginning, the proliferating adventitial connective tissue cells are arranged in a disordered way, but with further formation on the necrosis they become radially oriented and subsequently form a palisade consisting of long cells with oval nuclei rich in chromatin. If the vessel has become necrotic in its full circumference, the radially oriented connective tissue cells seem to "stand with their feet" on the necrotic vascular tube, a picture that shows resemblance with a monstrance. It is noteworthy that none of these cells invade the necrosis, rather, the boundary line between the vital cell palisade and the necrotic vascular tube is highly demarcated like a sequester. While neutrophils are found in the intima and occasionally also in the adventitia, the necrotizing process of the media in RA progresses without involvement of neutrophils, lymphocytes or macrophages. According to our observations, this phenomenon – focal necrosis without cell content, surrounded by a dense, radially oriented connective tissue cell palisade – is the equivalent to the rheumatoid nodule and thus is specific for the seropositive RA (see p. 117). In rheumatoid vasculitis, we never observed aneurysm, as is the case in panarteritis nodosa.

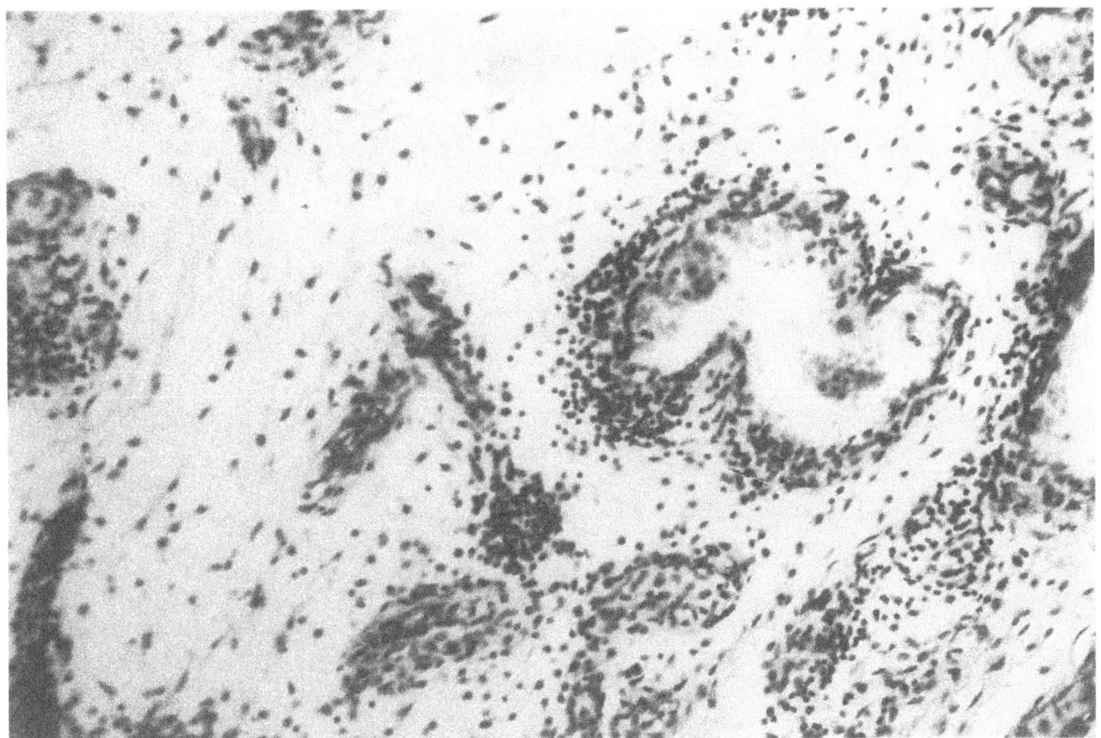

Lymphocyte infiltrates surround small vessels in the synovial membrane

Fig. 3.68
Rheumatoid arthritis

We classify vascular processes in RA into three categories:

1. Not characteristic for RA:
   - Perivascular lymphocytic infiltration (Fig. 3.68).
   - Perivascular neutrophil infiltration with involvement of the vascular wall.
   - Proliferation of the intima with and without infiltration of the media by neutrophils.
2. Characteristic for RA:
   - Medial necroses with cell proliferation of intima and adventitia, possibly mixed with neutrophils (Figs. 3.69, 3.70).
3. Specific for RA:
   - Segmental or complete medial necroses without cell content surrounded by a radially oriented palisade of connective tissue cells (Figs. 3.71–3.77).

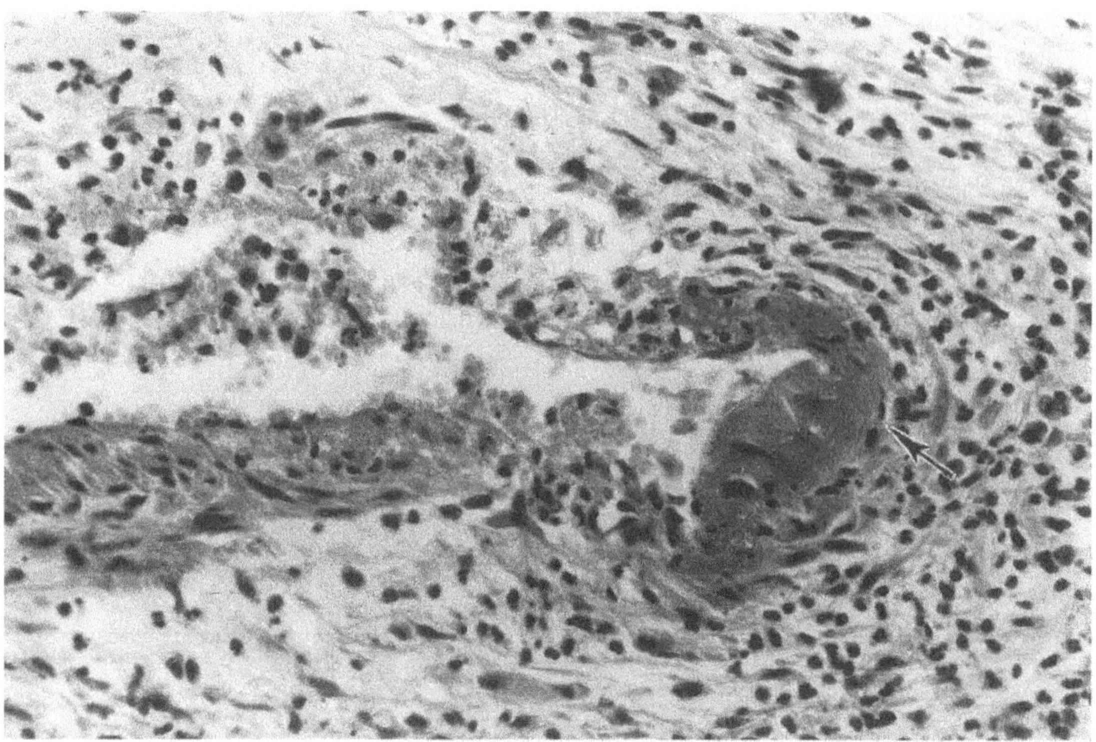

Fig. 3.69
Rheumatoid arthritis

Small artery in skeletal muscle. To the left, there is polymorph infiltration of the media, with necrosis at the right side (*arrow*)

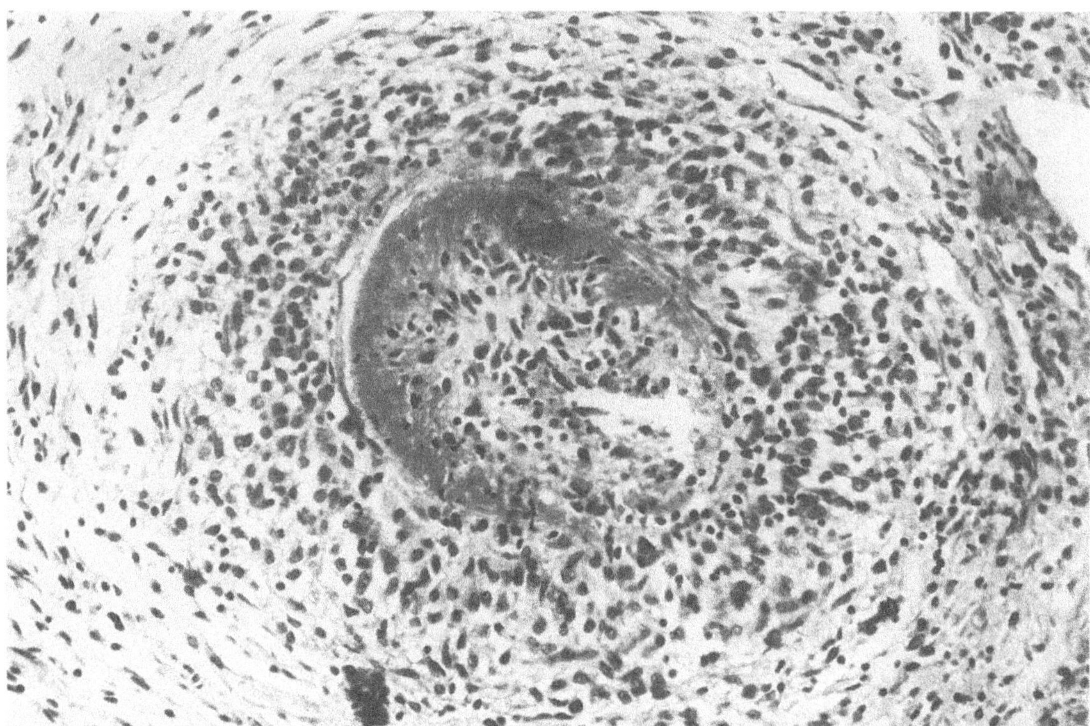

Fig. 3.70
Rheumatoid arthritis

Crescent-shaped medial necrosis with reactive proliferation of adjacent intima and adventitia of a small adrenal vessel

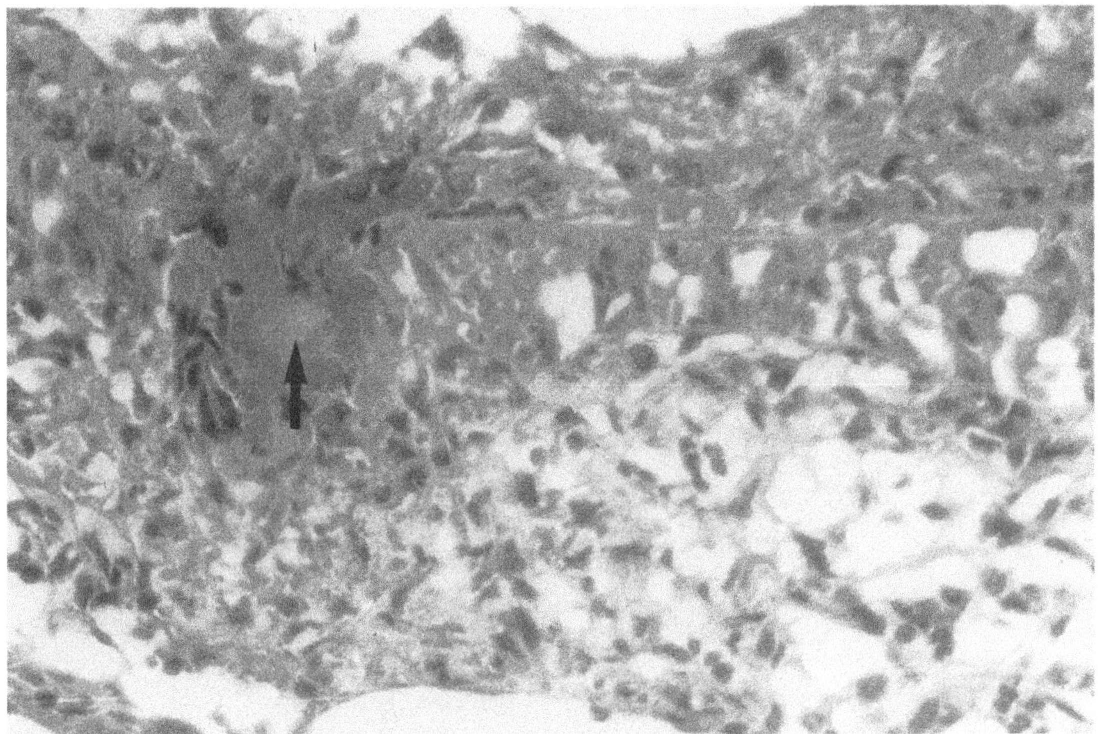

Total necrosis of a small branch of an artery also showing extensive medial necrosis (*arrow*)

Fig. 3.71
Rheumatoid arthritis

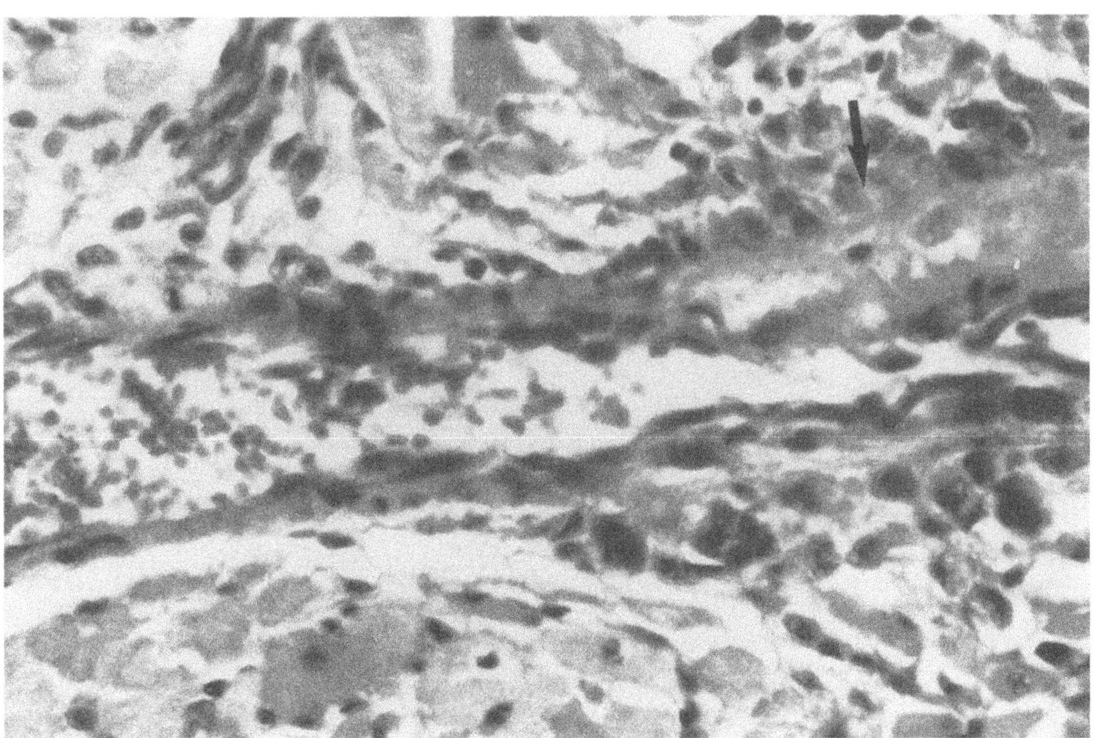

Artery of cardiac muscle with normal media on the left and necrosis on the right. Palisade formation at right top (*arrow*)

Fig. 3.72
Rheumatoid arthritis

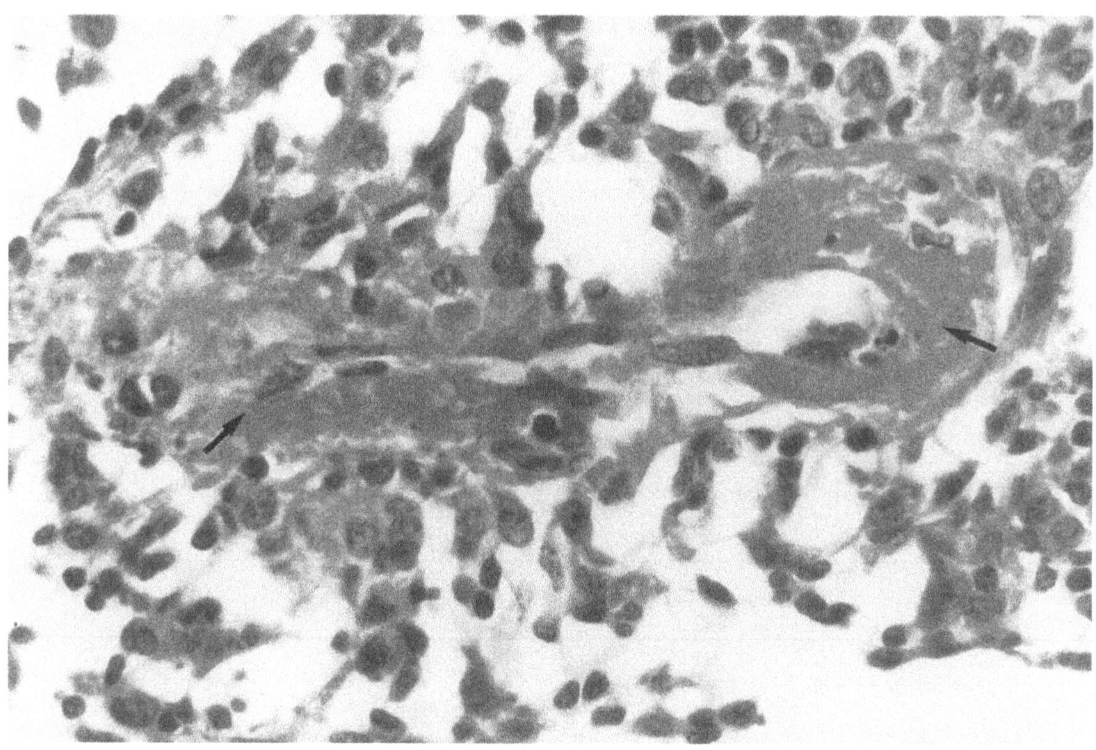

Fig. 3.73
Rheumatoid arthritis

Fresh necrosis of a small renal artery. Above and to the right, there is a formed palisade (*arrows*)

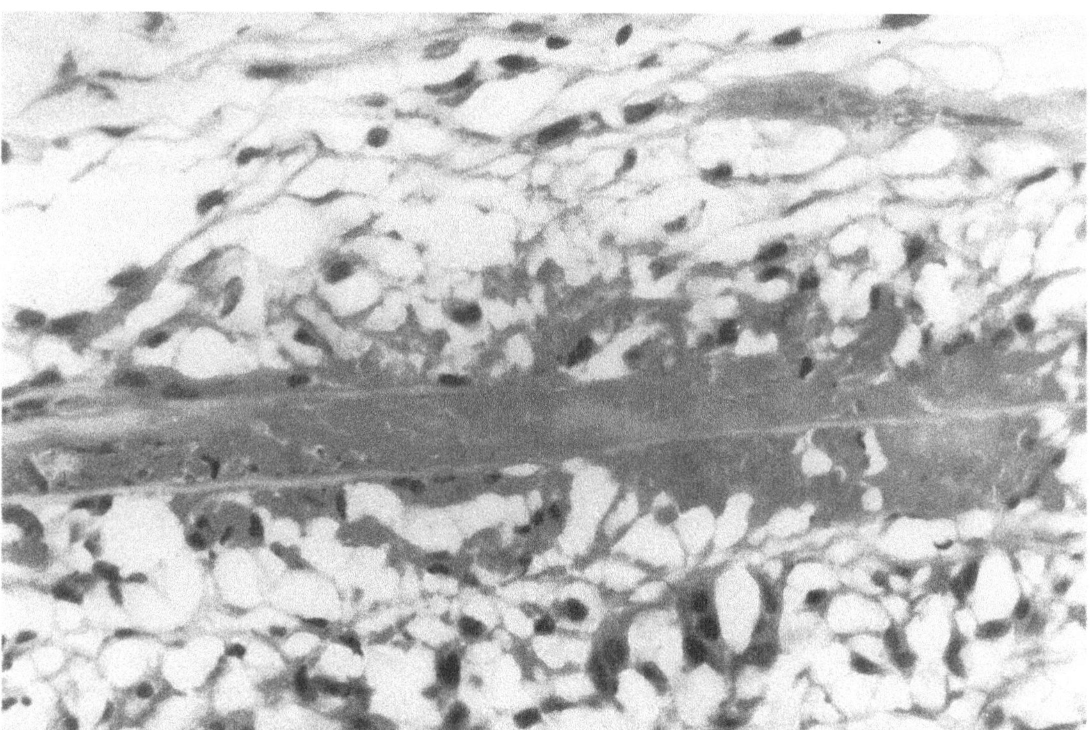

Fig. 3.74
Rheumatoid arthritis

Fresh necrosis affecting the internal elastic lamina of a medium-sized artery. Early proliferation of surrounding connective tissue cells with a suggestion of a radial arrangement

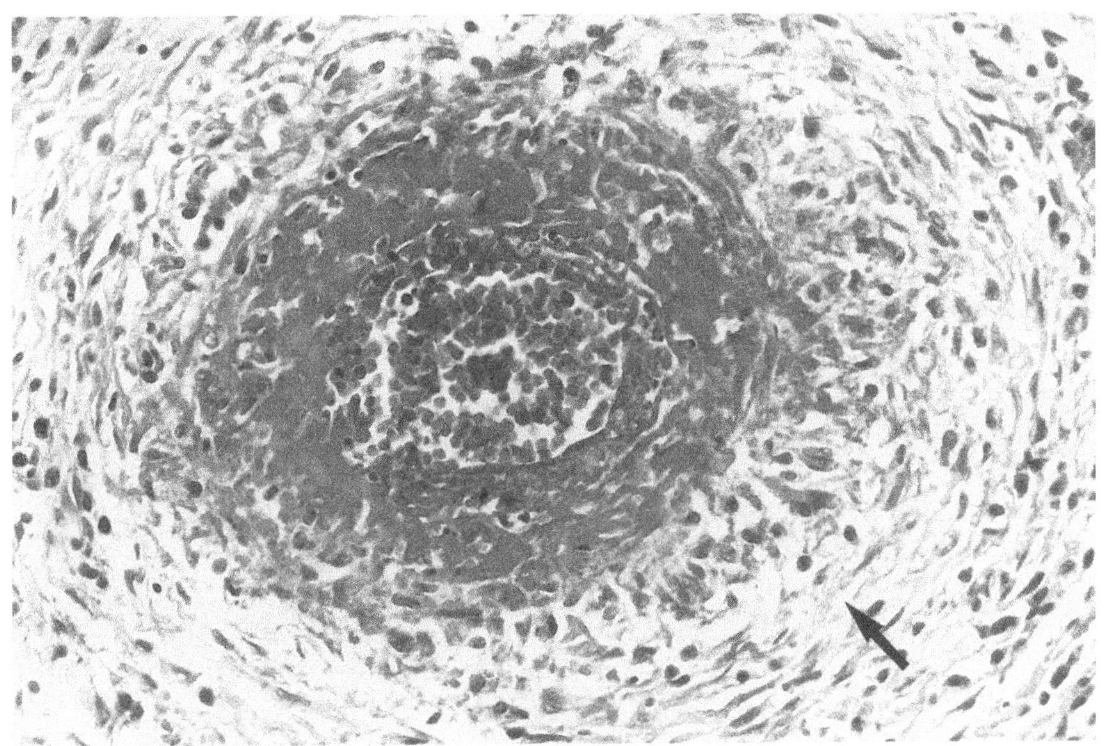

Total necrosis of a renal artery with preservation of lumen. There is a well-formed cellular palisade (*arrow*)

Fig. 3.75
Rheumatoid arthritis

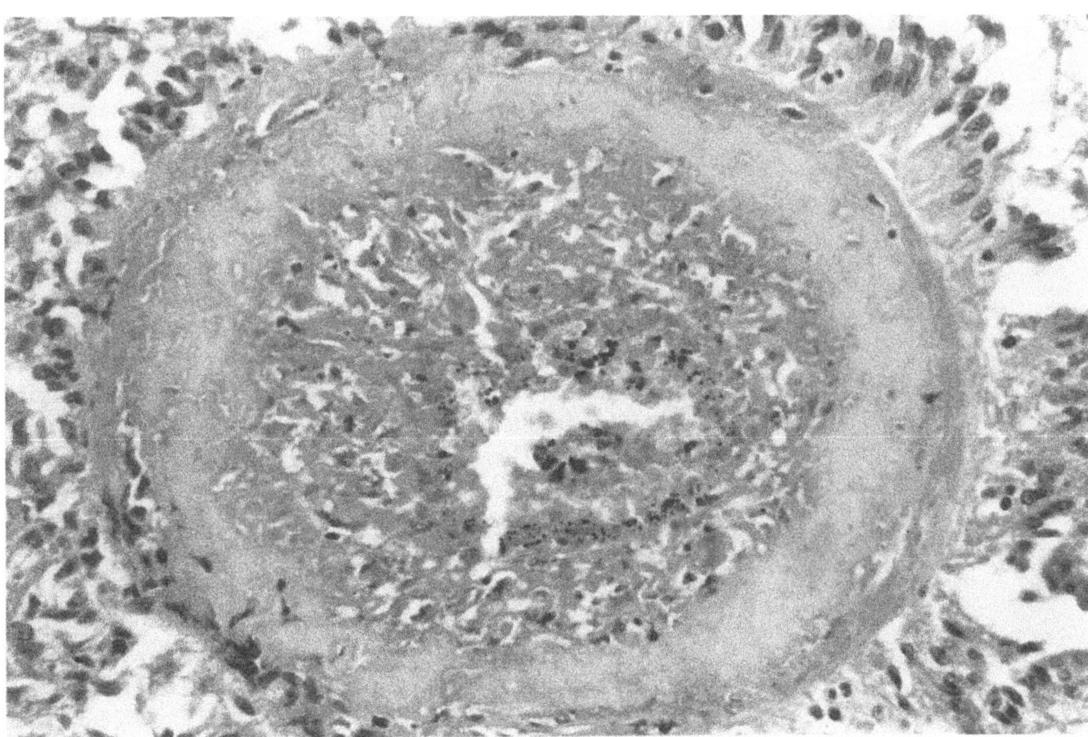

Total necrosis of all layers of a renal interlobular artery. A palisade is clearly recognizable, with proliferation of connective tissue cells

Fig. 3.76
Rheumatoid arthritis

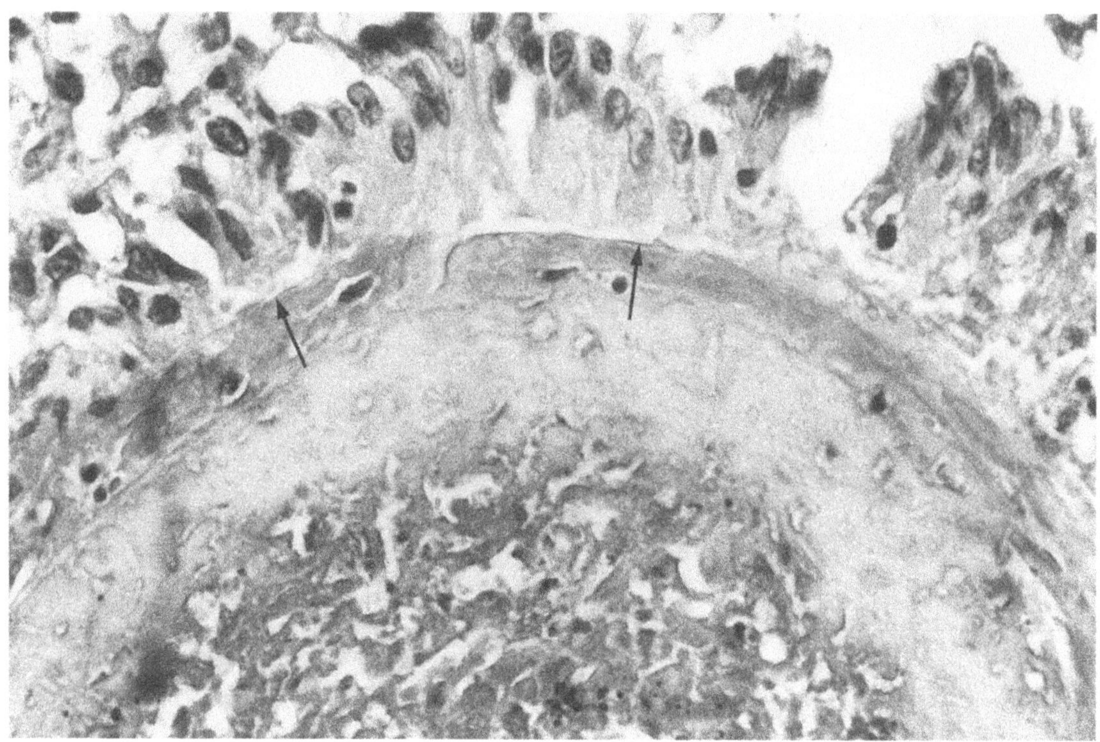

Fig. 3.77
Rheumatoid arthritis

Segment from Fig. 3.76. Sharp demarcation between life and death: between necrotic arterial tissue and highly proliferated cell palisade (*arrows*)

3.11.2 Heart

The disease of the heart which is triggered by the mechanisms of RA impressively shows how little the designation RA describes the real character of the disease and its clinical profile. Indeed, the joints and the tendon sheaths are the main sites of manifestation in RA, in contrast to RF, a disease which "only licks the joints, but bites the heart" (Lasègue 1864; see p. 10) but in the course of RA, all layers of the heart (pericardium, myocardium, and rarely also endocardium) can also be affected. Thereby, completely different specific and unspecific processes can manifest themselves in the different structures and can, under certain circumstances, lead to a fatal combination.

Pericardium

Pericarditis and its residual scarring may be quite frequently observed in RA. Quoted incidence varies between 20% and 50% (Baggenstoss and Rosenberg 1941: 5 out of 25 rheumatoid autopsies; Young and Schwedel 1944: 19 out of 38; Egelius et al. 1955: 7 out of 13; Sokoloff 1964: around 40%). Our own data from autopsies of nine children with a juvenile form of RA showed features of healed pericarditis in seven cases (Fassbender 1967a).
The differentiation from the pericarditis of RF is mainly one of degree: the rheumatoid inflammatory process is in general not acute and severe, but more chronic than that of RF. The fibrinous exudate is smaller in amount and becomes organized without leaving fibrinous masses and calcification does not ensue. Fibrous pericarditis and its obstructive sequelae are not associated with RA.

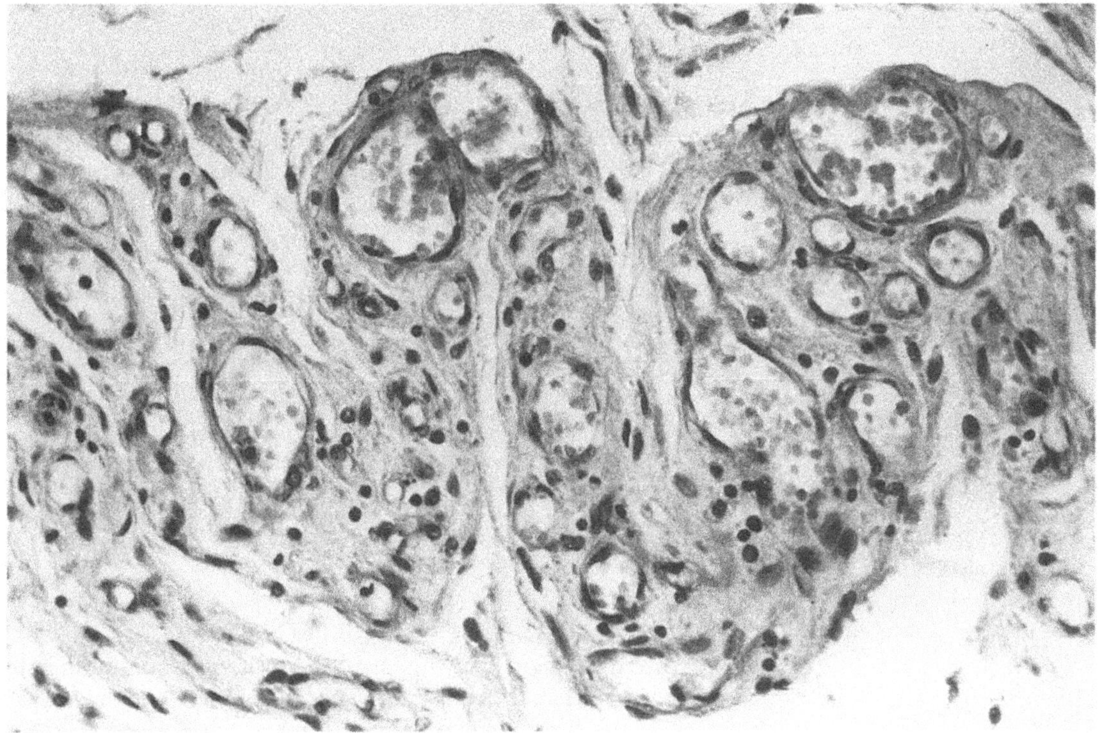

Prominent formation of new vessels in a pericardial scar

Fig. 3.78
Rheumatoid arthritis

Organization of the inflammatory exudate is affected by cardiac movements. This results in a loose mobile bridge of connective tissue between visceral and parietal pericardium. Fat cells appear in this loose scar tissue which furthers its mobility. Newly formed blood vessels follow a circuitous path which similarly allows for movement (Fig. 3.78).
In summary, rheumatoid pericarditis is a process of low-grade intensity. The connective tissue resulting from organization of the inflammatory tissue has the structure of a mobile layer, thus not interfering with normal cardiac action. It is, therefore, not surprising that the pericarditis of RA and the consequential scarring are usually not noted clinically and the diagnosis is usually made by the pathologist.
This macroscopically indifferent picture of scar tissue is accompanied by variable microscopic appearances. The tissue contains foci of diffusely arranged lymphocytes and plasma cells. There is an occasional neutrophil and freshly deposited fibrin may occur in the vicinity of new capillaries and venules. Some infiltrating cells are found in the subepicardial adipose tissue. At the surface, the lining cells are swollen so that they resemble a palisade. Occasionally, the loose scar tissue contains small remnants of serosal elements with large mesothelial cells which may form several layers and contain large nuclei. This resembles the findings in the pericarditis of RF (see p. 35).
Besides these unspecific, subacute, chronically progressing fibrinous exudative processes, a necrotic process which is specific for RA can establish itself in the collagenous tissue of the peri-

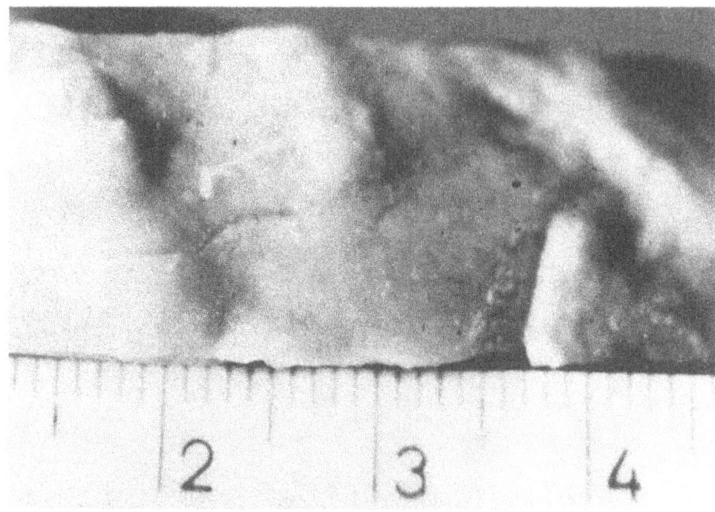

Fig. 3.79
Rheumatoid arthritis

Rheumatoid necroses in the pericardium

cardium in patients who are seropositive. Nodules thereby appear which arch against the epicardium. These nodules are yellow at the cut surface and reminiscent of tuberculous caseation foci (Figs. 3.79–3.81). The nodules can ulcerate and discharge their necrotic material into the pericardium and, thus, give rise to the clinical picture of acute pericarditis. Interesting in this respect is the transformation of the fibroblasts (the mesothelial lining cell layer has already disappeared at this stage): a dense formation of large cylindrical cells can be observed, which correspond to the type of cell palisade of RA-necrosis ("rheumatoid nodule"), but also have a significant similarity to the highly proliferating lining cells of the synovial stroma. The behaviour of the pericardium is thus identical to that of the cellular transformation which can occur at the pleural surface in seropositive patients. It is obvious therefore to view the palisade-like proliferation of the mesenchymal cells as a characteristic of seropositive RA.

Myocardium

Also in the myocardium, processes can occur which are unspecific as well as specific for RA.

Non-specific myocarditis

The myocardium may be variously affected in the course of RA. A non-specific interstitial myocarditis is found quite frequently. Collections of lymphocytes, plasma cells, and histiocytes sometimes occur in the vicinity of small vessels. The left ventricle, near the mitral ring, is affected with much greater frequency than the right ventricle. Interstitial myocarditis is occasionally accompanied by foci of muscle necrosis. This may be of sufficient prominence to resemble Fiedler's myocarditis (Sokoloff 1964). Our own observations in two cases of Still's disease showed small areas of myofibril necrosis, surrounded by small numbers of diffusely situated histiocytes, a few lymphocytes, and an occasional eosinophil. These two children died from cardiac failure (Fassbender 1967a; Figs. 3.82–3.84).

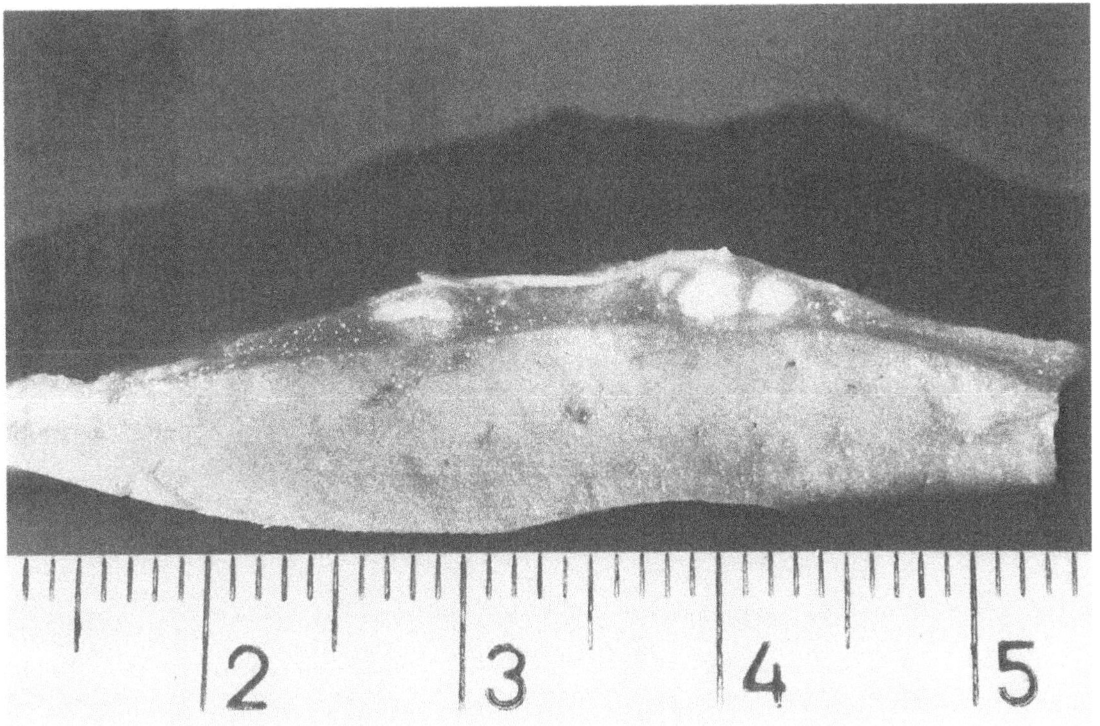

Section of rheumatoid necroses in the pericardium (see Fig. 3.79)

Fig. 3.80
Rheumatoid arthritis

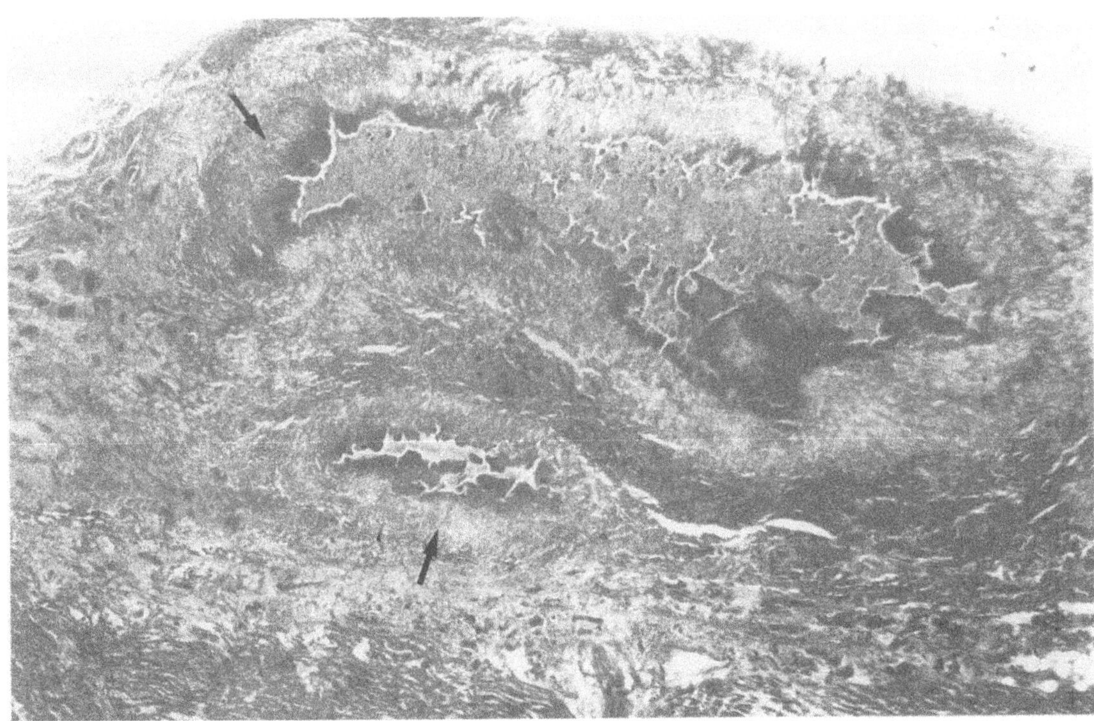

Large (*upper*) and small (*lower*) rheumatoid necrotic centres (*arrows*) stretching the epicardium outwards. Some calcification has occurred

Fig. 3.81
Rheumatoid arthritis

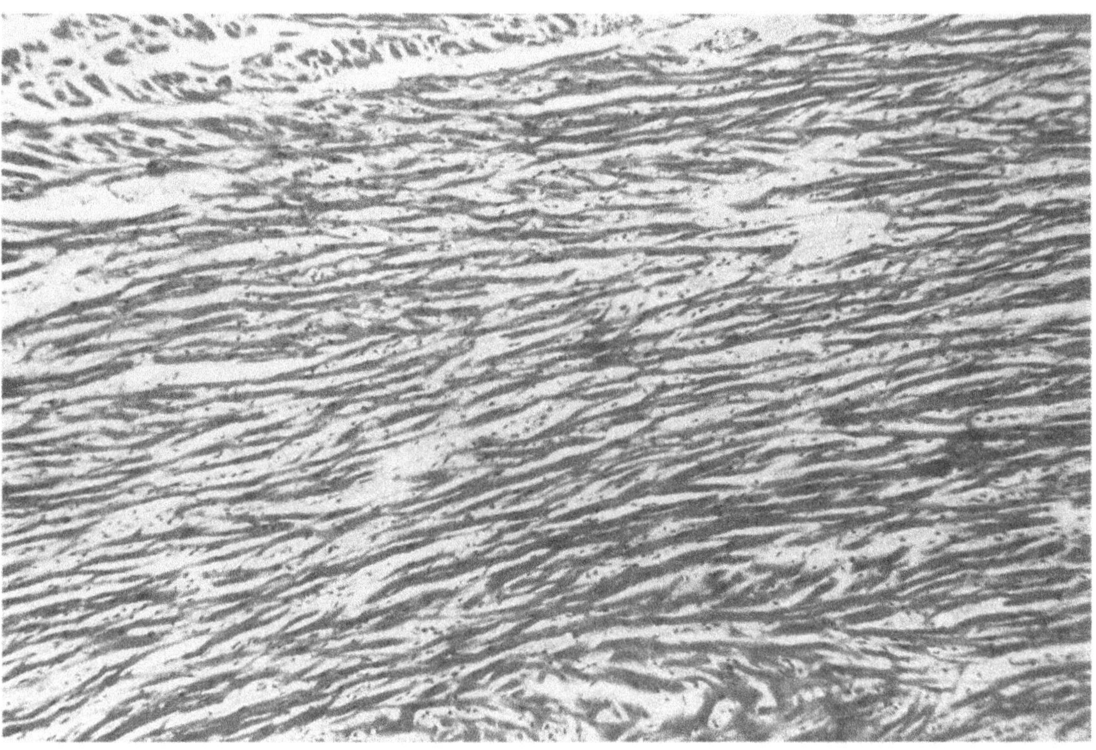

Fig. 3.82
Rheumatoid arthritis

Diffuse myocarditis with atrophy of muscle fibres and interstitial oedema

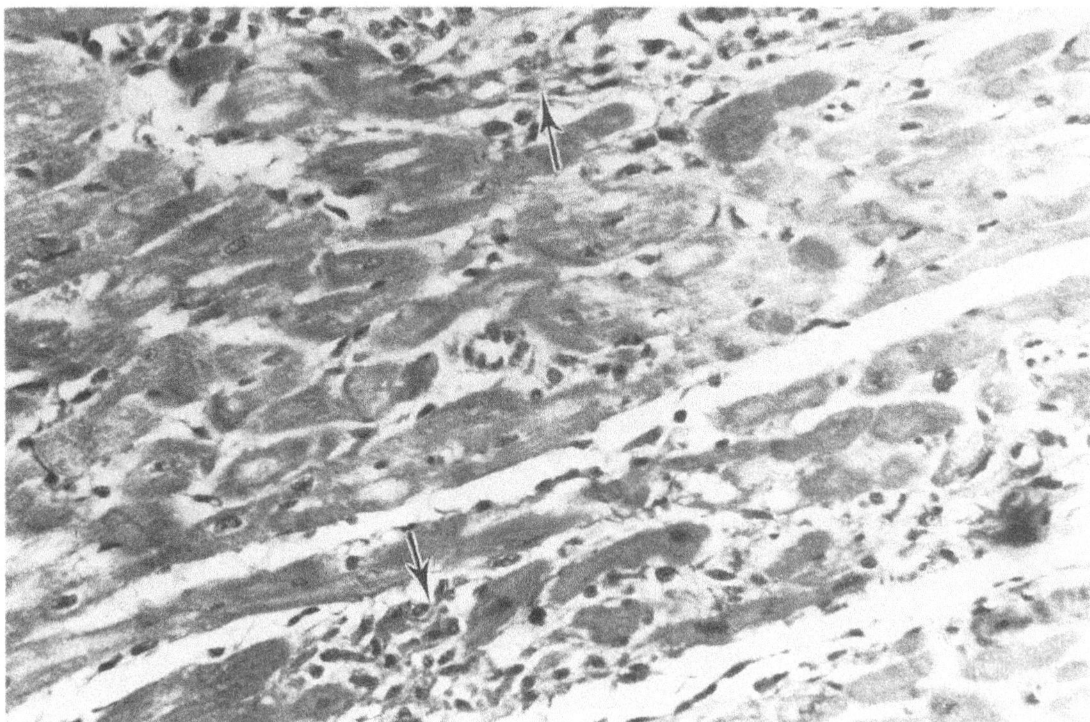

Fig. 3.83
Rheumatoid arthritis

A focus of myocarditis with local muscle fibre necrosis (*arrows*) and early reaction by connective tissue cells

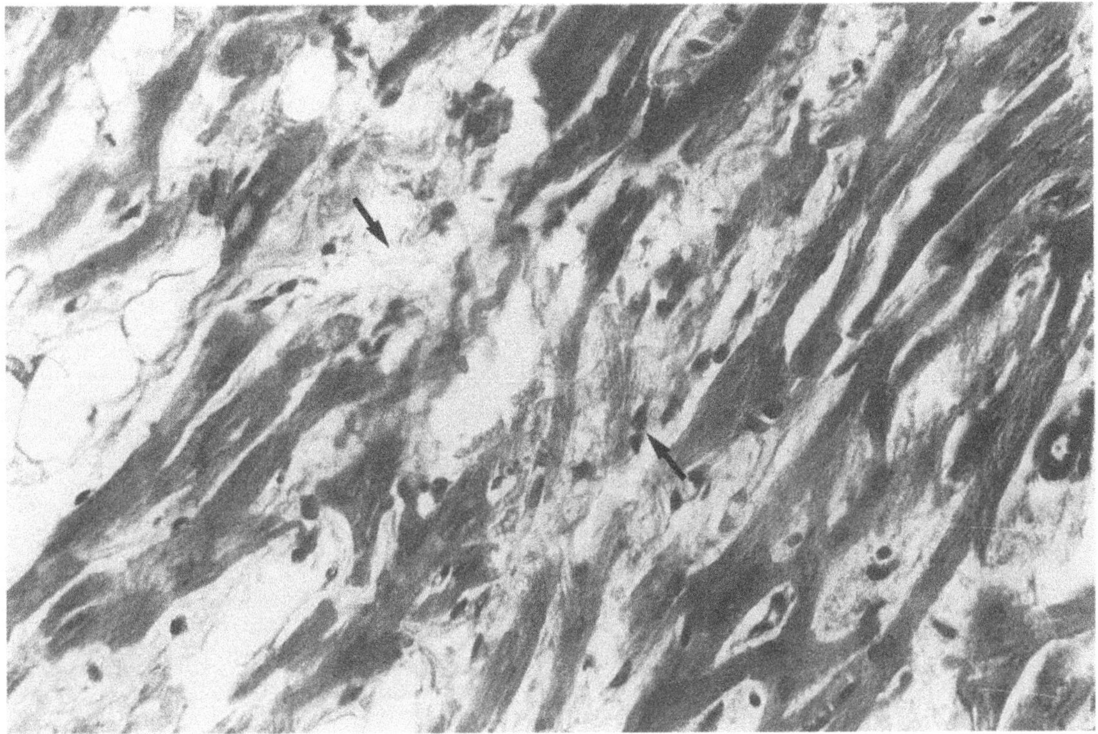

Diffuse myocarditis, necrosis of muscle fibres (*arrows*), and interstitial oedema

Fig. 3.84
Rheumatoid arthritis

Specific myocarditis

The myocardium may, however, also be affected by typical necrotic rheumatoid nodules, analogous to those of the subcutaneous tissue, joint capsule, tendon or lung etc. (see p. 12). These necroses are very much larger than Aschoff bodies. With ageing, the lesions change from a white to a yellow discolouration. The myocardial nodular necrotic foci were first described by Baggenstoss and Rosenberg (1941). They occur in the epicardium, the myocardium, and in the valve rings, which may give rise to valve incompetence. Their frequency is not known with certainty, the reported incidence in RA ranging from 2 out of 19, 7 out of 36, 5 out of 100, to 10 out of 43 in variously reported autopsied cases (Sokoloff 1964). The myocardial necrotic nodules occur more frequently in the left ventricle than in other cardiac chambers. They do not have a distribution which would suggest confinement to areas supplied by particular coronary vessels or their branches (Figs. 3.85, 3.86).
The necrotic zones may, according to the duration of the process, show the remains of myocardial fibres, which can undergo calcification. With time, the necrotic focus may become replaced by acellular collagenous scar tissue. Organization and scarring, however, only, if at all, take place after a period of months or years, in contrast to the speed with which this evolution occurs after a cardiac infarct.
The typical morphological appearances of the rheumatoid nodule, in the shape of the cell palisade, differs with age of the lesion: whereas the early lesion shows islands of circumferential cell ag-

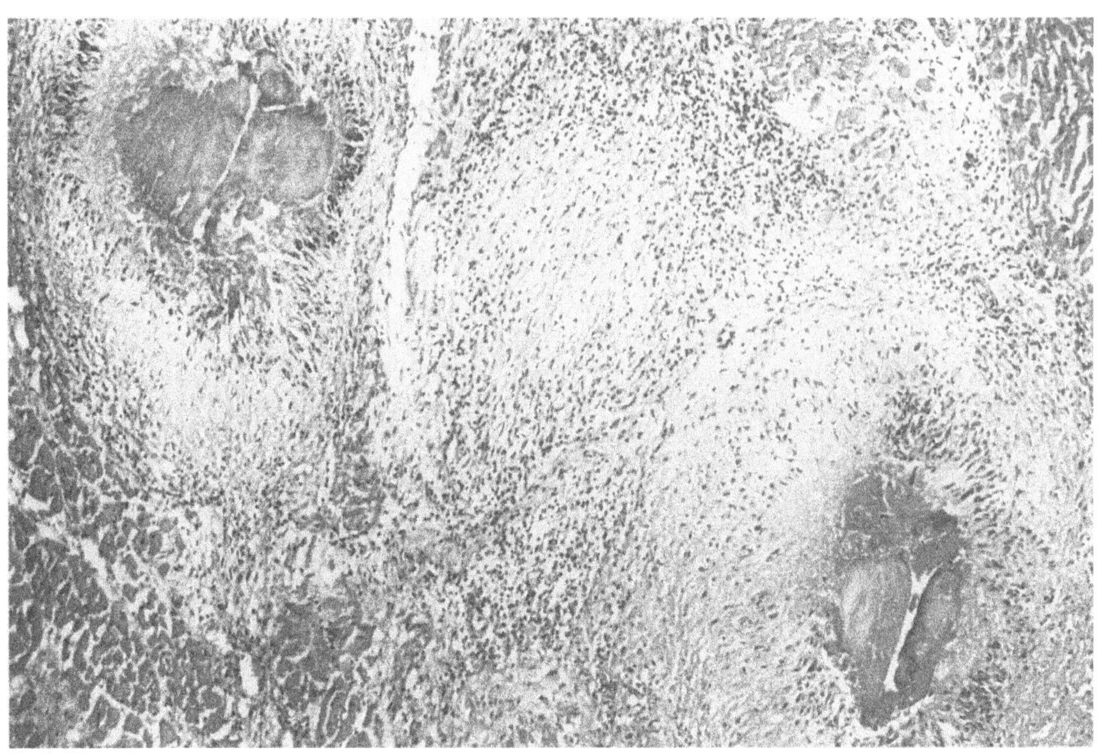

Fig. 3.85
Rheumatoid arthritis

Two rheumatoid necrotic foci in the myocardium. There are necrotic muscle fibres in the centre with surrounding palisade and fibrosis

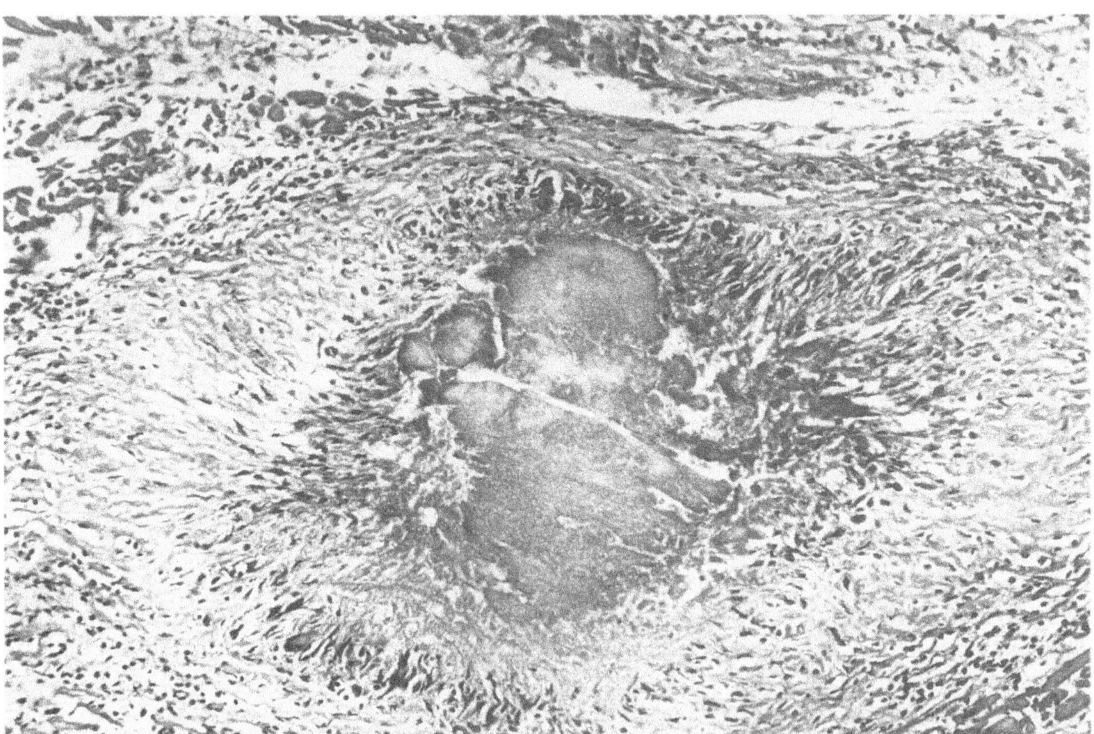

Fig. 3.86
Rheumatoid arthritis

A more advanced rheumatoid necrotic focus in the myocardium. The central area consists of necrotic secondary calcified muscle fibres; the palisade is beginning to disappear in places. The area is surrounded by scar tissue

gregation, the fully developed palisade of connective tissue cells develops later and consists of fibroblasts and histiocytes. These cells show a weakly eosinophilic cytoplasm and an oval nucleus, rich in chromatin. The palisade forms a sharp division between necrosis and intact myofibres. As with such nodules in other anatomical situations, invasion of the necrotic area by fibroblasts or angioblasts is not apparent. The palisade disappears with time, leaving a spherical scar (Figs. 3.87, 3.88). It is much larger than the scar of the Aschoff node, and shape and size allow for differentiation from the scar left by an infarct.

Clinically and electron-cardiographically, it is possible for a myocardial necrotic nodule to be confused with cardiac infarction.

The appearance of necroses in the myocardium is not per se plausible. On the one hand, all known RA-necroses ("rheumatoid nodules") develop in collagenous tissue of type I, on the other hand, we are unaware of any necroses in skeletal muscle tissue. Also, the latest statement of Bely and Apathy (1991a) on the vascular genesis of the RA-necroses, i.e. their appearance based on an infarction, does not offer an explanation since the RA-necrosis has no similarity to an infarction, neither with respect to its development, form, and structure nor to its cell content. In particular, infarcted tissue rapidly becomes organized by granulation tissue and is surrounded by a wall of neutrophils (see p. 119). All this is not valid for the RA-necroses, neither in the myocardium nor at other locations. The necrotic centre does not become organized but is walled off like a sequester from the healthy tissue by a cell palisade and later by a collagenous capsule.

Since the myocardial necrosis is a morphological analogy of all the other RA-necroses, an identical mode of development must also be assumed (see p. 117). Hereby the collagenous interstitium is primarily degraded and the muscle cells are secondarily drawn into this destruction.

Endocardium

Although endocarditis in the narrower sense does not fit into the mosaic of RA-disease, the heart valves in seropositive patients can be affected by the necrotizing process in the collagenous framework of the valve ring, their function thus becoming diminished (Fig. 3.89). Sokoloff (1964) reported the following order of heart valve involvement: mitral, aortic, tricuspid, and pulmonic. In 12 RA patients with heart involvement, Bely and Apathy (1991a) found 4 cases of rheumatoid nodules in the valve region.

Coronary arteries and their branches

In the course of general vasculitis in RA (see p. 128), Bely and Apathy (1991a) found generalized vasculitis in 19 out of 100 RA patients, the coronary vessels were affected in 12 cases. The main branches were also diseased in 6 cases, whereas the arteritical processes occurred, in agreement with the observations of Sokoloff (1963), mainly in the small arteries of the myocardium. The histological picture of the arteritides, also at other locations, is influenced by the primary extent of the lesion, the duration of the process, and probably also by the influence of antiphlogistic and cytostatic agents.

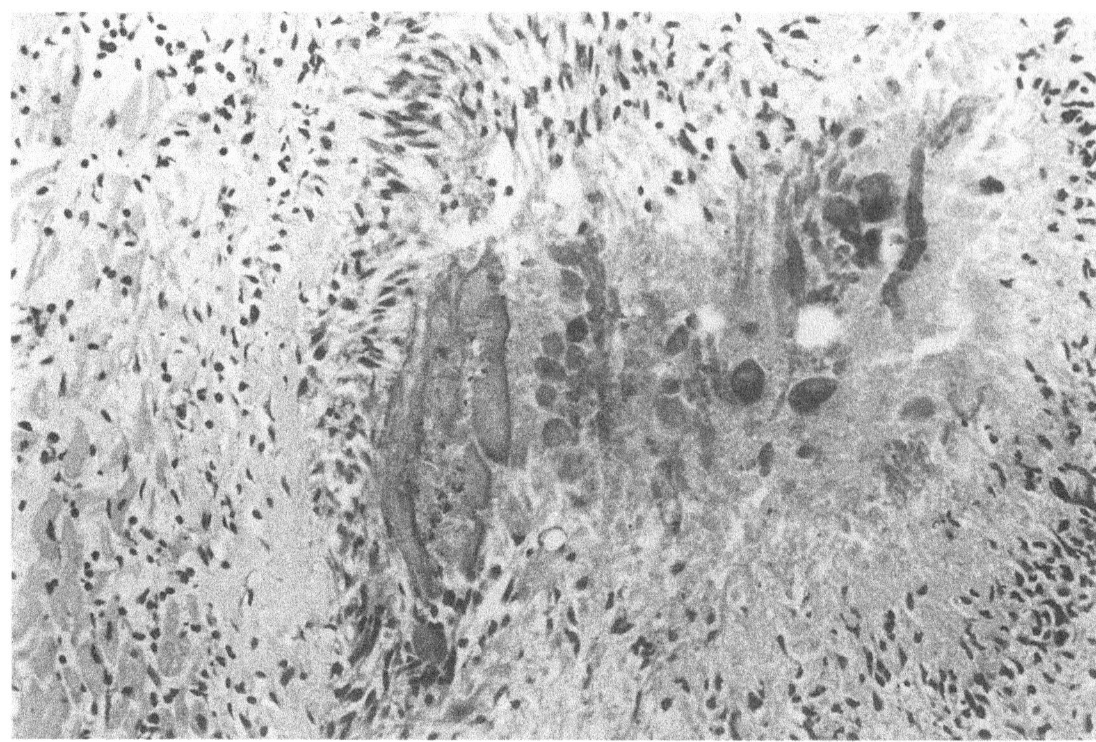

Fig. 3.87
Rheumatoid arthritis

Rheumatoid necrosis in the myocardium. Centrally, there are individual necrotic calcified muscle fibres but the palisade is waning

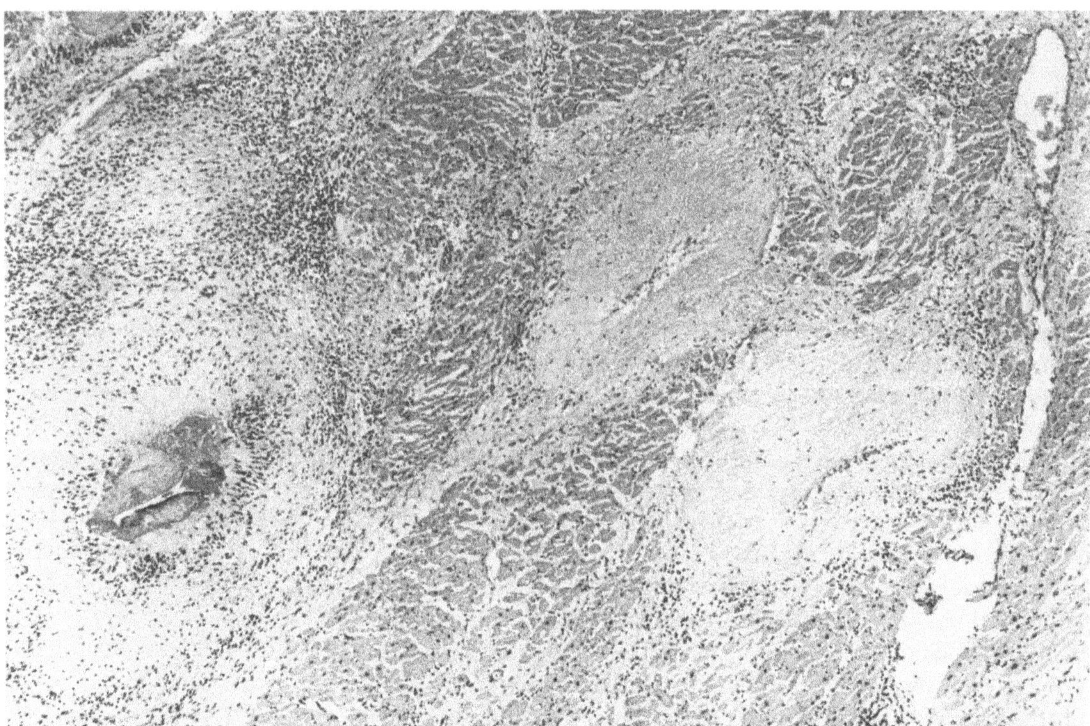

Fig. 3.88
Rheumatoid arthritis

The rheumatoid necrosis on the *left* shows centrally necrotic muscle fibres and part of a palisade. On the *right,* there are two entirely scarred foci

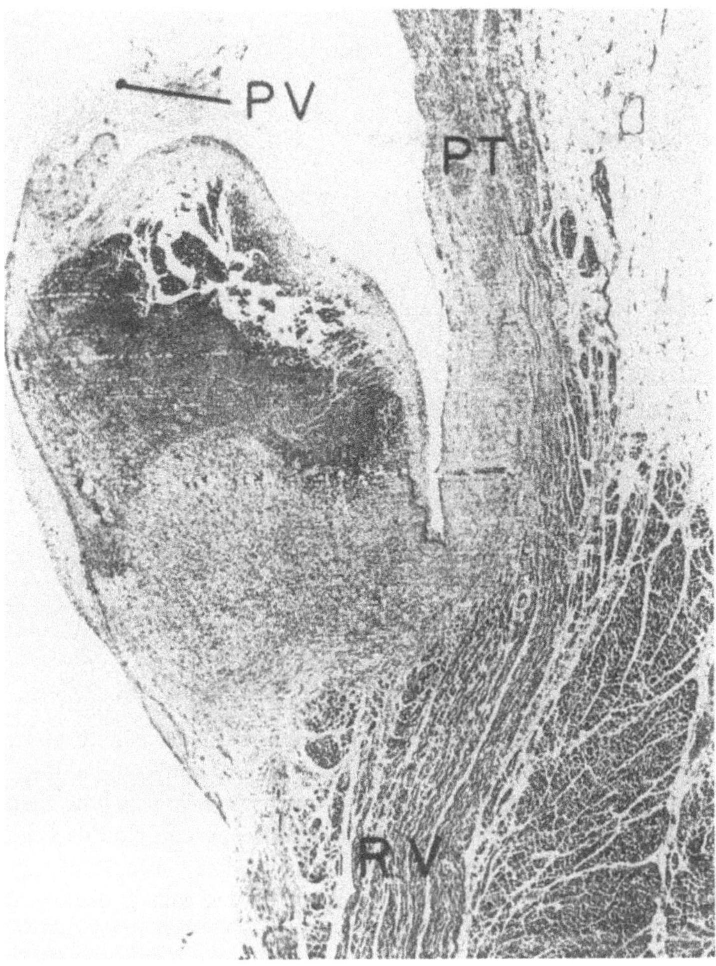

Fig. 3.89
Rheumatoid arthritis

Rheumatoid necrosis in subendocardial tissue reaching into the neighbouring valve. *PV*, pulmonary valve; *RV*, right ventricle; *PT*, truncus pulmonaris. (Roberts 1968)

The primary lesion of the sub-epicardial and intra-myocardial arteritis corresponds to the general basic pattern of RA-vasculitis (see p. 128).
Characteristic is the more or less pronounced fibrinoid necrosis of the media, which affects the intima and adventitia and, by secondary thrombosis, can occlude the vessel. Whereas RA-necroses themselves destroy only relatively small muscle foci, the arteritical vascular occlusion can, under certain circumstances, lead to widespread infarctions, which can even lead to death.

Amyloid deposits in the heart

In RA and systemic JCA (Morbus Still), the deposition of amyloid in the heart, in general, does not affect the cardial function and remains clinically unnoticed. At autopsy we found in RA as well as in JCA pavement-like deposits of varying extent in the endocardial ventricles of the right atrium (Fig. 3.90). Also we saw amyloid deposits in the sarcolemma tubules, with entwining around the muscle fibres. Most frequently, we found deposition of amyloid plaques in the media and adventitia of cardiac veins, less often in myocardial arteries.

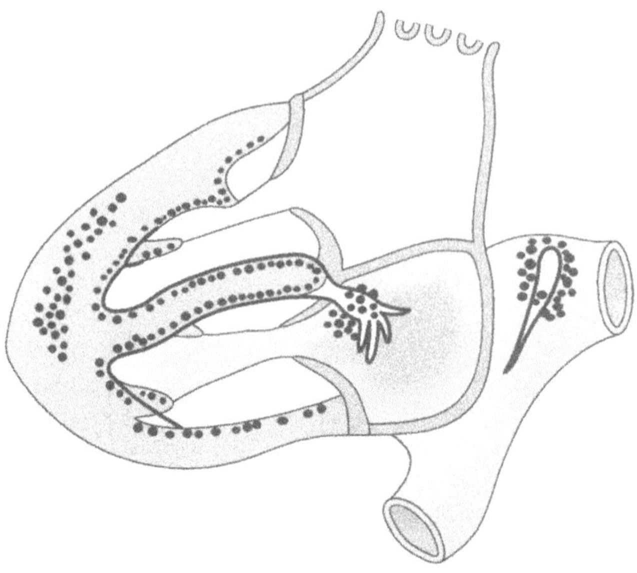

Fig. 3.90
Still's disease

Localization of amyloid in the hearts of nine children

The vascular lumen, however, always remained clear. In some cases, also the heart valves contained bands of amyloid (Fassbender 1967b). At autopsy of children with systemic JCA who died whilst seemingly healthy, we observed that heart amyloidosis can have dramatic consequences. Here we found as the cause of sudden death massive deposits of amyloid in the muscle plexus of sinus nodules, of artero-ventricular nodules, and the Purkinje fibres (Fassbender 1967b; Figs. 3.91, 3.92). We thus believe that amyloidosis of the heart remains clinically latent as long as it does not lead to the entwining of larger myocardial sections or affects the conduction system. While the appearance of a secondary amyloidosis (AA-amyloidosis; see p. 155) in RA is estimated with the aid of rectal or gingival biopsies to be about 5% (Arapakis and Tribe 1963), the post mortem examinations revealed a frequency of 26% (Calkins and Cohen 1960). At autopsy of 100 RA patients, Bely and Apathy (1991a) found in 24 cases a secondary amyloidosis (AA-amyloidosis). We regard as remarkable that in 23 of these 24 patients, amyloidosis of the heart was also observed which actually corresponds to a primary AL-type amyloidosis. This finding leads to the conclusion that in RA patients with certified amyloidosis, amyloid deposits in the heart must also be taken into consideration.

3.11.3 Lung and Pleura

Besides the heart, only the lung and pleura can be addressed as a site for a proper "organ manifestation" of RA. Contrary to earlier opinion, the lung and pleura are relatively frequently involved in RA. This is more often the case in seropositive than in seronegative patients. Either the pleura or the pulmonary parenchyma may be affected, the lesion being of an inflammatory or necrotizing nature.

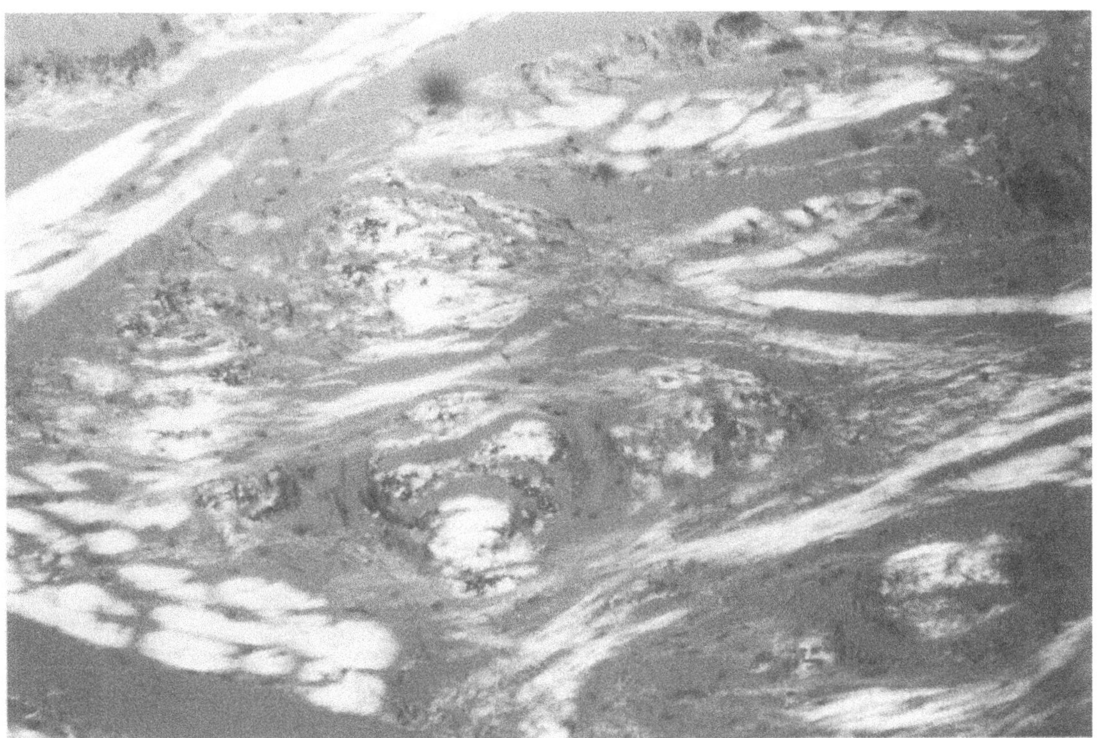

A photograph taken with polarized light of amyloid in the conducting system of a 16-year-old child

Fig. 3.91
Still's disease

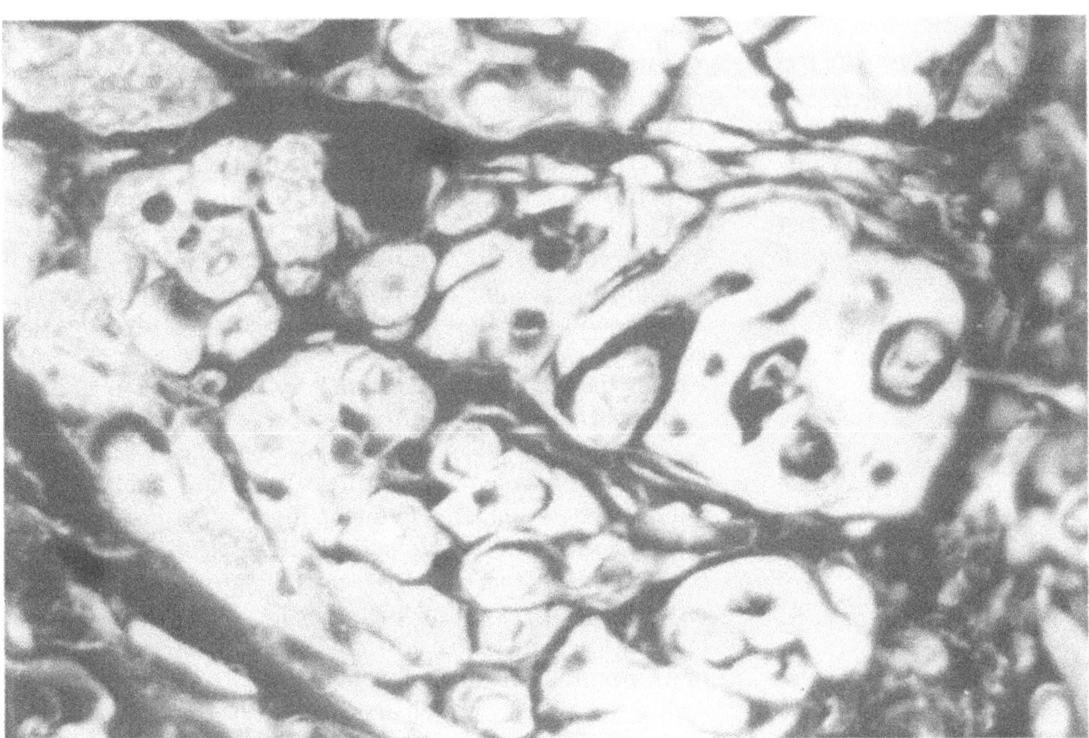

Photo by polarized light of amyloid surrounding fibres in the myocardium of the right ventricle of a 7-year-old child

Fig. 3.92
Still's disease

Table 3.5. Lung processes found in autopsy of 100 patients with classical rheumatoid arthritis (Bely and Apathy 1991b)

	Male	Female	Total
Vascular lesions (necrotizing vasculitis)	4	11	15
Rheumatoid nodule	0	3	3
Interstitial pneumonia	18	38	56
Rheumatoid pneumonia	1	4	5
Rheumatoid pleuritis	12	18	30
Bronchiolitis obliterans	0	1	1
Special forms Caplan's syndrome	0	0	0
Special complications Amyloidosis	5	19	24
Non-specific complications Airway infections	16	29	45

The evaluation of the prevalence of lung involvement in RA depends on the chosen investigation methods. According to Bely and Apathy (1991b), 1.6% of lung involvements are revealed radiologically, 40% spirometrically, and 56% by autopsy.
At autopsy of 100 patients with classical RA, the authors found different lung processes (Table 3.5).
We would like to divide the most significant forms of lung and pleural involvement in RA into unspecific and specific processes.

Unspecific fibrinous pleuritis

The effusion in unspecific fibrinous pleuritis is rarely so strong that it appears clinically. The fibrin is eventually organized, leaving fibrous adhesions of variable extent. This is only of little, if any, functional importance. Evidence for pleural involvement is usually only obtained at autopsy, when it is found with considerable frequency.

Pleural necroses

Besides these unspecific inflammatory reactions of the serosal pleural surfaces, specific RA-necroses (see p. 112) can establish themselves in the collagen framework of the pleura in seropositive RA. The nodule on the pleural surface does not acquire its full distinction compared to that in the depth of the tissue. The central necrotic tissue can spread in the pleural space where instead of the flat mesothelial pleural lining cell layer, a radially directed superficial cell palisade develops which is mixed with multinuclear giant cells, equivalent to the concentric cell palisade of RA-necrosis ("rheumatoid nodule"; Fig. 3.93). The collapse of such a nodule into the pleural region can trigger a clinically relevant exudative pleuritis.

RA-necroses in the lung

RA-necroses ("rheumatoid nodules") in the lung correspond in their form and construction to the typical pattern (see p. 117). These nodules are mainly located in the vicinity to the pleura or

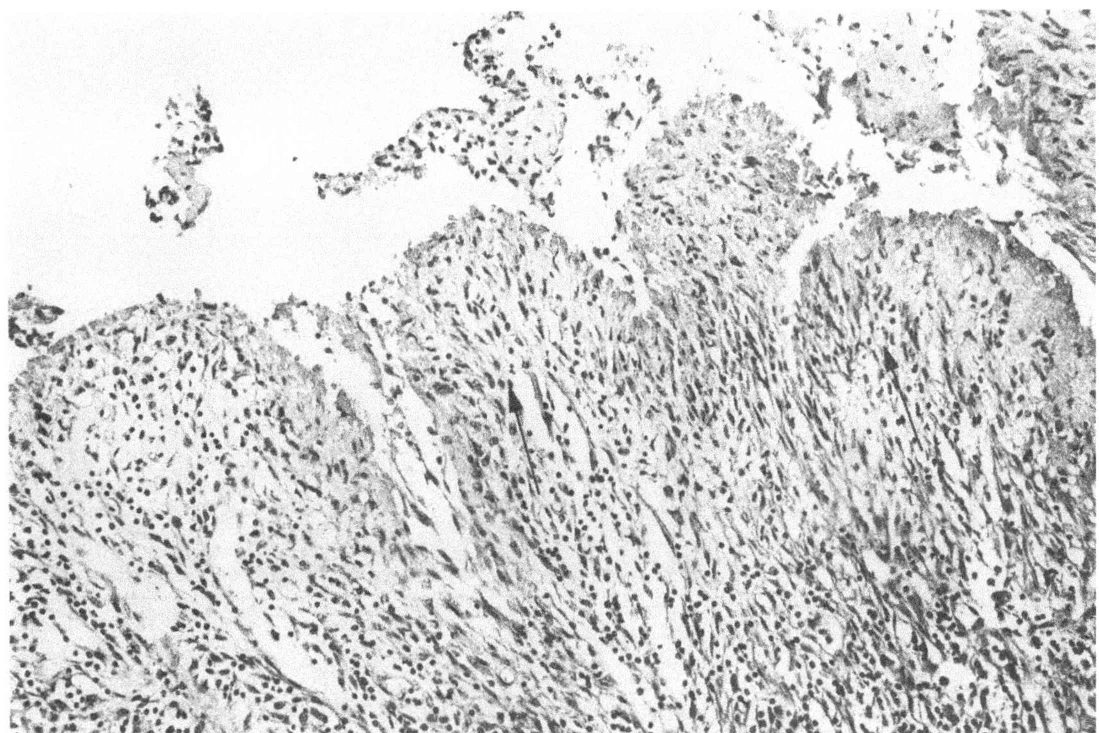

Spread rheumatoid necrosis on the surface of the pleura. The decaying necrotic material is surrounded by a palisade-like proliferation of connective tissue cells. In the depth, scattered lymphocytic infiltration. (Biopsy, 28-year-old woman)

Fig. 3.93
Rheumatoid arthritis

in the region of the interlobular spaces. Their diameter is rarely greater than 2 cm. Whereas single nodules are clinically insignificant, the conflux of several necrotic foci can lead to an atelectasis of larger areas of the lungs. The collapse of such a nodule into the pleural space can trigger a pleuritis (see above) and, under certain conditions, a pneumothorax. These lung foci can be detectable for years by X-ray. The necrotic centre can, however, soften and liquefy. Since the radiological detection of such nodules has to be distinguished diagnostically from tumour metastases or tuberculomata, the diagnosis can be certified by the existence of rheumatoid factors and also, if necessary, by biopsy.

Caplan's syndrome

In 1953, Caplan described the simultaneous occurrence of lung nodules and RA in coal miners. Compared with a group of 14,000 miners with no joint disease, those with RA were 60% more likely to suffer from pneumoconiosis, characterized by appearance of lung nodules. These nodules are sharply outlined on the radiograph, have an average diameter of 0.5–5 cm and lie in the periphery of both lungs (Figs. 3.94, 3.95). The histological structure of these nodules closely resembles the rheumatoid nodules. In the surrounding tissues, carbon is stored in the macrophages. Tests for rheumatoid factors are generally positive in Caplan's syndrome. These lung nodules may cavitate and create a bronchopleural fistula.

Interstitial pneumonitis

Interstitial pneumonitis is a lung disease which occurs in the form of inflammatory foci in the region of the interstitium. The

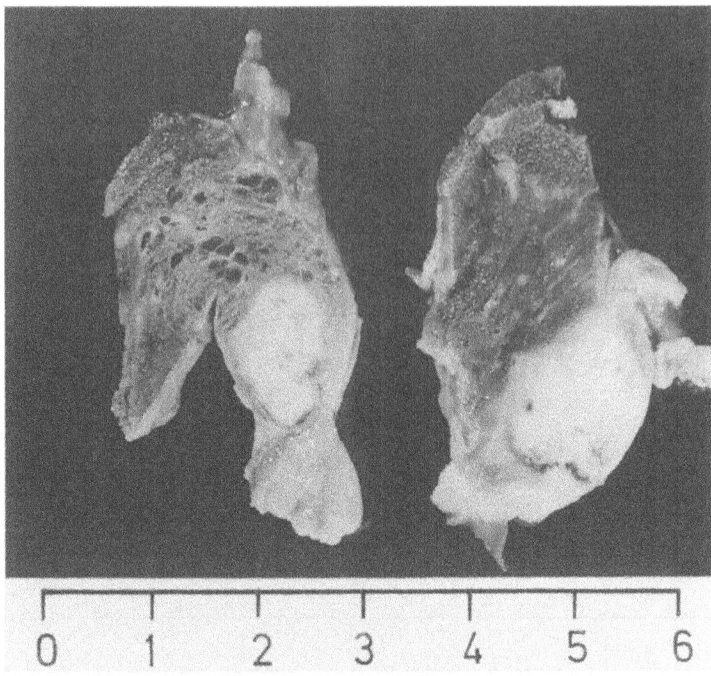

Fig. 3.94 Caplan's syndrome Cut surfaces of two pulmonary nodules. (Castleman 1967)

framework of the lung is oedematously loosely structured. The blood vessels are hyperaemic. Neutrophils are found occasionally. The alveoli contain a protein-rich exudate. Later stages are characterized by lympho-plasmacytic infiltrates and proliferating fibroblasts.

Interstitial fibrosis

Thus the progression towards interstitial fibrosis is facilitated, in which the whole interstitium is included. In the X-ray picture, this process appears as a diffuse reticulonodular network whereby "honeycomb"-like structures can appear (Dixon and Ball 1957). Morphologically, a diffuse collagenization of the lung framework occurs, dispersed by a mononuclear cell infiltration. Interstitial fibrosis can lead to respiratory insufficiency, pulmonary hypertension, and heart failure.

Arteritis

Bely and Apathy (1991b) found 15 cases of arteritis in the lung amongst 100 autopsies of RA patients. All types of RA-vasculitis (see p. 128) can thus be present in this way. The characteristic, necrotic form of rheumatoid arteritis is linked to the presence of rheumatoid factors.

Amyloidosis

In 24 out of 100 RA patients, Bely and Apathy (1991b) found amyloid deposits in the lung in the course of a general secondary (AA-) amyloidosis. The amyloid thereby deposits itself preferentially in the wall of the arterioles and arteries. Later, deposits also occur in the alveolar septa. The clinical significance of this amyloid localization is not unequivocally proven, although the widened alveolar septa can react to the amyloid by fibrosis.

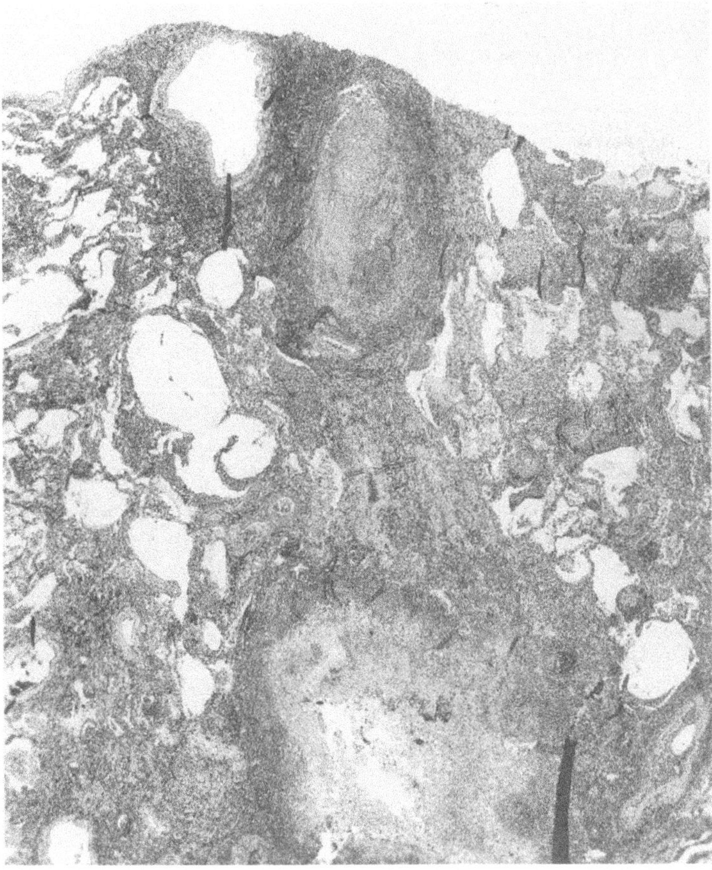

Small nodule in the pulmonary interstitium. (Castleman 1967)

Fig. 3.95
Caplan's syndrome

3.11.4 Eye

The importance of rheumatoid factors for the generalization of RA ("RA-disease") is demonstrated by the fact, amongst others, that in about 10% of seropositive RA patients the eyes are also affected (Epstein 1986). Bilateral keratoconjunctivitis is most frequent. The causes are atrophy and cirrhotic changes in the lacrymal glands. The reduced lacrymal secretion is accompanied by an increased viscosity. With additional dryness of the mouth and oropharynx it becomes a question of Sicca syndrome (see p. 163).
Less frequent, but more dramatic are the diseases of the sclera in which two basically different processes can be distinguished:
1. A superficial episcleritis
2. Scleritis proper

Episcleritis may arise from a variety of causes and only has an ill-defined relationship to RA. There is dilatation of the superficial conjunctival and episcleral vessels. Scleritis, however, is marked by various pathological changes. These may be of an inflammatory nature and consist of oedema and perivascular infiltration by lymphocytes, plasma cells, and neutrophils. The pathogenesis of "granulomatous scleritis" is more difficult to interpret. There

"Granulomatous scleritis"

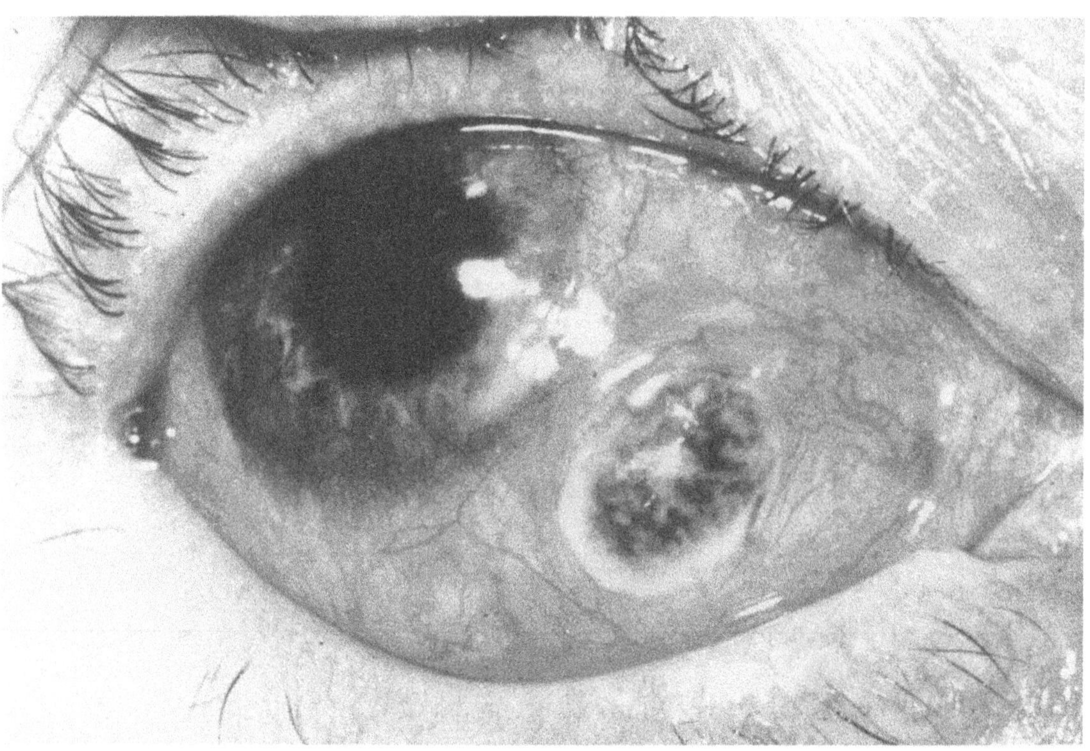

Fig. 3.96
Rheumatoid arthritis

Rheumatoid necrosis in the eye: scleromalacia. (Witmer 1970)

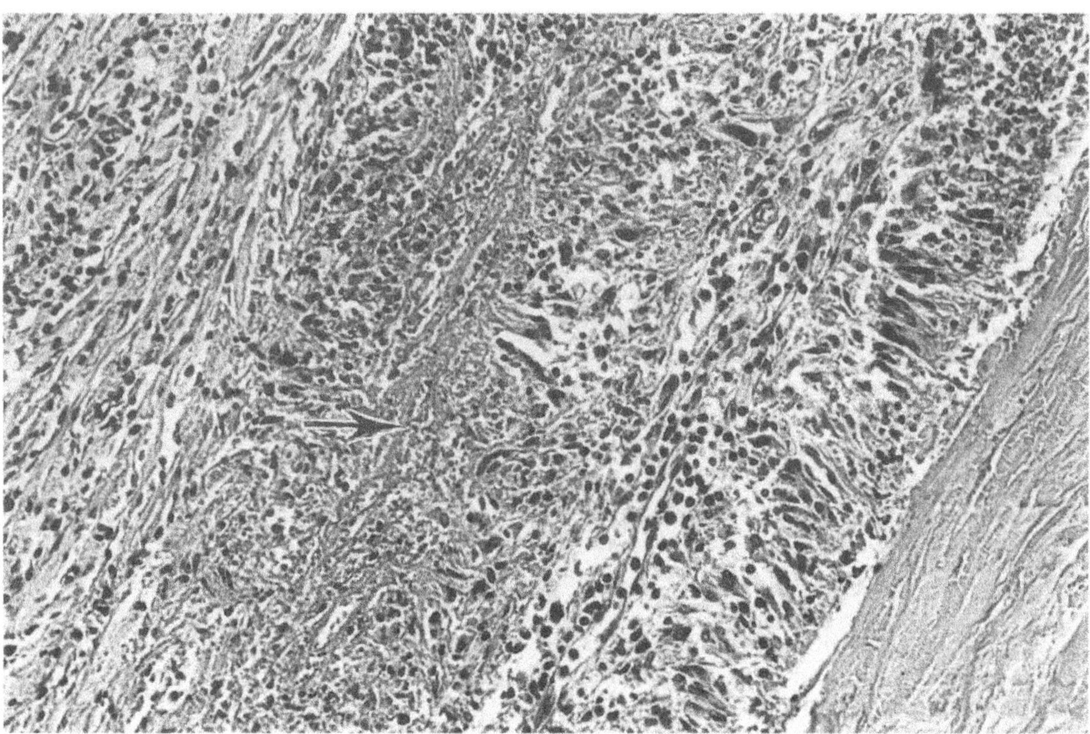

Fig. 3.97
Rheumatoid arthritis

Rheumatoid necrosis in the eye: perforating scleromalacia (granulomatous scleritis). Central necrosis (*arrow*) with typical cellular palisade in the sclera. (Lüders and Klemens 1963)

are papers reporting multiple "granulomata" with necrosis (Remky 1972). Such necrotic foci were reported to be surrounded by lymphocytes, histiocytes, and new capillaries. Gärtner (1959) described a homogeneous appearance of vascular walls with proliferation of histiocytes and multi-nucleated cells. The centre of these granulomata is a necrotic focus. These determine the ocular involvement and have been variously named "scleromalacia perforans" or "scleritis nodularis necroticans" (Franceschetti and Bischler 1950; Gärtner 1959; Figs. 3.96, 3.97). These are terms covering the same process, which, although the features are variable, may lead to destruction of an eye.

The disease processes of the sclera are explicable in terms of its anatomical structure. The loose episcleral tissue is particularly vascular, and it is here that inflammation occurs. On the other hand, the sclera proper is a dense structure of collagen (type I and III) and very avascular which does not readily allow for inflammation to occur. However, as in other collagenous structures, rheumatoid necrotic foci may be found. These are surrounded by a palisade of fibroblasts in the fashion typical of the rheumatoid nodule. This would seem to be the basis of "scleromalacia perforans" and "scleritis nodularis necroticans" and the inflammatory features at the periphery are features secondary to this. This view tallies with the fact that granulomata of the sclera occur in seropositive patients who also have rheumatoid nodules in other sites.

Anterior uveitis

Anterior uveitis is diagnosed in about 5% of cases of juvenile RA. This is clearly an inflammatory process unrelated to serum rheumatoid factor. Complications are the formation of posterior synechiae which become attached to the anterior surface of the lens, early cataract formation and association with superficial bands of calcification of the cornea. This complex forms a serious complication of the juvenile form of the disease and can lead to blindness.

3.11.5 Lymph Nodes

In a disease such as RA which is to such an extent dominated by immunological mechanisms, involvement of the lymphatic system is, in principle, to be expected. Lymph node swellings are observed in about 50%–75% of RA patients (Robertson et al. 1968) whereby particularly the draining lymph nodes of the extremities in the axillary and inguinal regions are affected. The prevalence is higher in male patients and lymphadenopathy is more common in seropositive patients.

Lennert (1961) found that individual nodes had diameters of up to 5 cm. Consistency is usually rather firm; the cut surface is light grey with occasional pink areas. The histological appearance shows characteristic features:

1. Secondary follicles are usually present which may be so impressive in number and in size that Brill-Symmers disease is simulated. These follicles contain plasma cells and germinoblasts, i.e. mostly small cells. The process is clarified as follicular lymphatic hyperplasia (Fig. 3.98).

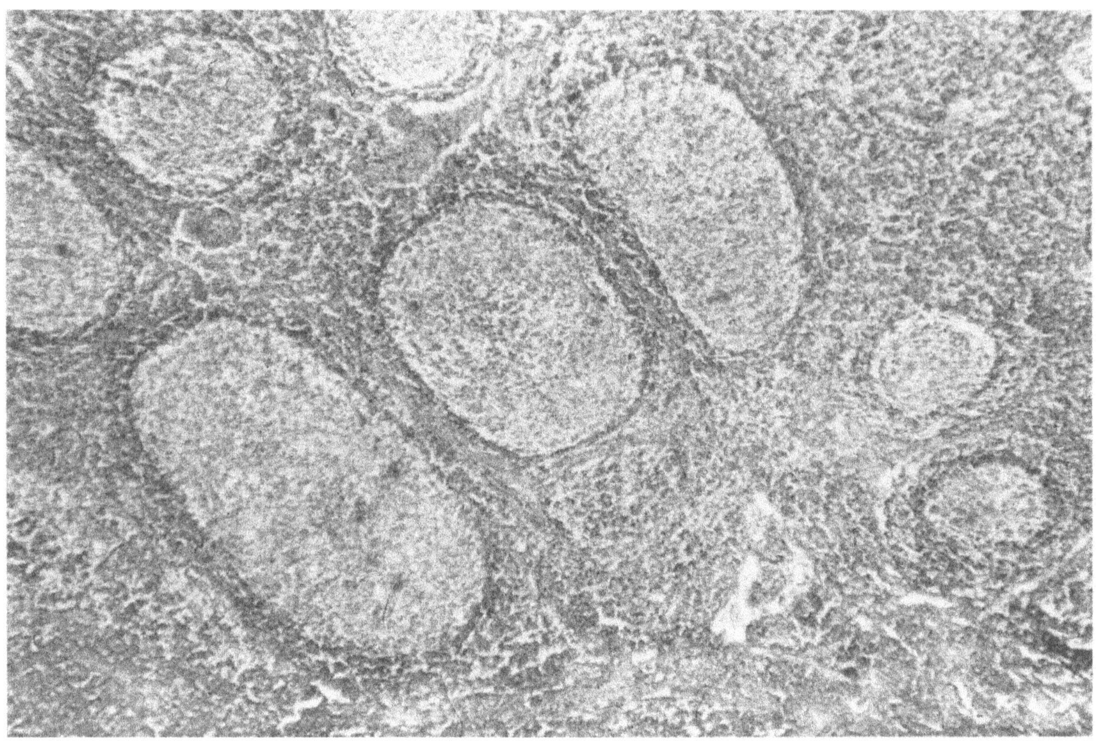

Fig. 3.98
Rheumatoid arthritis

Marked follicular hyperplasia; sinus catarrh (axillary node). (Lennert 1961)

2. The sinuses are very prominent with swollen endothelial cells and are filled with a large number of neutrophils (Lennert 1961).
3. The medulla shows hyperplasia of lymphocytes and plasma cells.
4. Lennert considered PAS-positive granules in sinus cells to be indicative of RA. None of these features is specific for RA except the expression of an enhanced immune response during the course of the disease (1961).

Lymphoma

The cytological uniformity helps to distinguish it from a malignant lymphoma. Cytological studies of lymph node aspirate may reveal active centriblast cells without malignant features (Symmons et al. 1985). Their presence correlates with markers of T cell activation in the peripheral blood. In summary, one can conclude that significant lymphadenopathy in RA correlates with disease severity, duration, and male sex. It is also associated with depressed lymphocyte reactivity and alteration of CD4:CD8 subset ratios, abnormalities similar to those seen in Felty's syndrome (Symmons et al. 1987). The question arises as to what extent these changes dispose for the increased occurrence of lymphoma which was observed in male RA patients.

3.11.6 Felty's Syndrome

In 1924, Felty described five patients with deforming arthritis, splenomegaly, and leukopenia. This triad, which was extended to include lymphadenopathy, anaemia, and thrombocytaemia, gained nosological autonomy as Felty's syndrome. The full symptomatic feature occurs only in seropositive patients with long-standing and severe articular disease. Frequently, vascular lesions are also observed, underlining the relationship to systemic rheumatoid disease. Further characteristic features of Felty's syndrome are hyperpigmentation and chronic leg ulcers on the lower extremities, both of which are common in RA patients with rheumatoid vasculitis, but are also seen in RA patients without any overt evidence of vasculitis. Therefore, it is reasonable to regard Felty's syndrome as an extreme, malign variant of RA.

3.11.7 Systemic Amyloidosis in RA

With amyloidosis we are dealing with the deposition of insoluble proteinaceous material in the extracellular matrix of several organs. Amyloid is an amorphous, eosinophilic, glassy, hyalin substance. The involved organs develop a rubbery, firm consistency and a waxy, pink or grey appearance.

Histological identification

By standard histological methods, amyloid appears as a homogeneous eosinophil substance. Van Gieson allows for some differentiation, collagen being deep-red, while amyloid is yellowish-orange.

Physically, Congo red is bound to the glycoprotein moiety of amyloid. However, elastic fibres and other structures of small blood vessels may also stain with Congo red and thus amyloid may be simulated. The PAS reaction of the material is positive and it is stained metachromatically by methyl violet. By polarization, the behaviour of the amyloid is positively bifringent and by staining with Congo red the amyloid itself shows an intensive green dichroism.

All types of human amyloid consist of non-branching rigid fibrils with approximately 100 Å in diameter. The individual filament has a diameter of about 70 Å and tends to aggregate laterally. Each filament has subunit protofibrils of 30–35 Å in diameter. The X-ray diffraction picture of the isolated amyloid fibrils is that of a cross-β pattern. The pleated sheet of Pauling and Corey indicates that the polypeptide chain runs transversely to the fibril axis of the specimen (Cohen and Skinner 1986).

Table 3.6 shows the types of amyloid and amyloidosis which can be distinguished at present.

Missmahl (1965) subdivided amyloid according to its structural association into a peri-reticular and a peri-collagenous variety. In RA, association is usually with reticulin fibres. However, in the cases of cardiac involvement (see p. 146) the peri-collagenous type was found.

According to hitherto observations, the development of amyloidosis in RA occurs only after a long course of illness, in no case less than 2 years, and may sometimes lead to life-threatening

Table 3.6. The 1990 guidelines for nomenclature and classification of amyloid and amyloidosis (Cohen 1991)

Amyloid protein	Protein precursor	Protein type of variant	Clinical
AA	apoSAA		Reactive (secondary) Familial Mediterranean fever Familial amyloid nephropathy with urticaria and deafness (Muckle-Wells syndrome)
AL	Kappa, lambda (e.g. k III)	Ak, A (e.g. A k III)	Idiopathic (primary), myeloma or macro-globulinemia-associated
AH	IgG 1 (γ1)	Aγ1	
ATTR	Transthyretin	e.g. Met 30	Familial amyloid poly-neuropathy (Portuguese)
		e.g. Met 111	Familial amyloid cardiomyopathy (Danish)
		TTR or Ile 122	Systemic senile amyloidosis
AApoAI	apoA1	Arg 26	Familial amyloid poly-neuropathy (Iowa)
AGel	Gelsolin	Asn 187 (15)[a]	Familial amyloidosis (Finnish)
ACys	Cystatin C	Gln 68	Hereditary cerebral haemorrhage with amyloidosis (Icelandic)
AB	B protein precursor (e.g. BPP_{695}[b])	Gln 618 (22)	Alzheimer's disease Down's syndrome Hereditary cerebral haemorrhage amyloidosis (Dutch)
AB_2M	B2-microglobulin		Associated with chronic dialysis
AScr	Scrapie protein, precursor 33-35 cellular form[c]	Scrapie protein27-30	Creutzfeldt-Jakob disease, etc.
		e.g. Leu 102	Gerstmann-Straussler-Scheinker syndrome
ACal	(Pro)calcitonin	(Pro)calcitonin	Medullary carcinoma of thyroid
AANF	Atrial natriuretic factor		Isolated atrial amyloid
AIAPP	Islet amyloid polypeptide		Islets of Langerhans Diabetes type II, insulinoma

AA, amyloid A protein; *SAA*, serum amyloid A protein; *apo*, apolipoprotein; *L*, immunoglobulin light chain; *H*, immunoglobulin heavy chain. Non-fibrillar proteins, e.g. protein AP (amyloid P-component), excluded.

[a] Amino acid positions in the mature precursor protein; the position in the amyloid fibril protein is given in parentheses. [b] Number of amino acid residues. [c] Molecular mass (kDa).

From Natvig JB, Førre O, Husby G et al. (eds) (1990) Amyloid amyloidosis; Kluwer Academic Publishers, Dordrecht (modified and reprinted with permission).

complications. This refers to the secondary or reactive type of the AA-amyloid.

Incidence of secondary AA-amyloidosis

The actual incidence of secondary AA-amyloidosis in RA is difficult to determine. Estimates of frequency vary, depending on whether they are based on clinical symptoms or bioptic or autoptic findings. From post mortem series, the approximate frequency of amyloidosis in RA ranges from 26% (Calkins and Cohen 1960) to 24% (Bely 1990), other investigators assume an overall incidence of amyloid in RA between 5% and 15% (Missen and Taylor 1956; Husby 1985; Mutru et al. 1985). Rectal biopsies in 115 consecutive RA patients with long-standing disease showed an ante mortem amyloidosis prevalence of 5.2% (Arapakis and Tribe 1963). While reviewing the divergent results, it is important to take into account the varying age, duration, serological behaviour, and severeness of the illness among the under "RA" classified patients.

Renal involvement

Renal involvement is the most significant clinical feature of AA-amyloidosis in RA. This may manifest itself as low-grade albuminuria or as in the case of about a fourth of these patients as severe nephrosis or renal insufficiency with widespread destruction of nephrons. This latter event, which is the major contribution to the mortality caused by amyloidosis secondary to RA, may not be associated with hypertension. By autopsy, Bely (1990) found in 21 out of 24 RA patients with secondary generalized AA-amyloidosis renal amyloid. In the kidney, amyloid deposition occurs in the basement membrane of small arteries and glomerular capillaries. Electron-microscopically, amyloid is closely related to the mesangial cells and to the glomerular endothelium. Amyloid extends to replace the glomerulus, resulting in a homogeneous, eosinophil body. The basement membrane of tubules is also affected. Needle biopsy is particularly suitable for diagnosis, since glomerular involvement is widespread throughout the kidney.

Liver

Hepatic AA-amyloid is deposited in the reticular network between parenchymal cells and Kupffer cells. Adjacent parenchyma may atrophy, the size of the liver increases. Macroscopically, the lobular pattern is accentuated. Thin slices may take an transparent appearance in extensive amyloidosis. Nevertheless, hepatic function is sufficiently preserved so as not to endanger life.

Spleen

In the spleen, AA-amyloid is similarly deposited around the reticular stroma. The involvement of splenic follicles gives rise to an appearance termed "sago" spleen. If, however, a diffuse involvement occurs in the red pulp, the cut surface becomes bright-red and shiny and a thinly cut slice is sometimes transparent. (This has been termed "ham" spleen in the German literature.) Asymptomatic splenomegaly, which may be massive, occurs.

Adrenal gland

AA-amyloid may cause an increase in adrenal size. The macroscopically greyish-white material is deposited around the reticular stroma and may affect all three anatomical zones, depending on the extent of amyloidosis. This may, as in the case of the liver, cause necrosis of parenchymal cells without apparent clinical impairment of adrenal function.

Amyloidosis of the liver [according to Bely (1990) in 77.3% of deceased RA patients with secondary generalized AA-amyloidosis], spleen (86.7%) or adrenal gland (85%), however, is frequent but of no or only slight clinical significance.

Gastrointestinal tract

The frequent involvement of the rectal mucosa in RA by AA-amyloid offers a ready approach for biopsy which carries only a minimal risk and a very good chance of correct diagnosis. In post mortem series, Missmahl (1972) found the rectal mucosa to be involved in 80% of cases of generalized AA-amyloidosis, Bely in 100%.

Lung

In the lung, AA-amyloid is able to deposit in the wall of arterioles, arteries, more seldom also in the alveolar septa (see p. 150).

Joints

While in the course of a secondary AA-amyloidosis in RA the deposition of amyloid in the joint itself plays no role, AL-amyloid can be deposited in the articular cartilage in patients with multiple myeloma and thus can destroy it (Uehlinger 1973).

Heart

In the course of a generalized secondary AA-amyloidosis in RA, amongst the characteristic peri-reticular deposits in the kidney, the adrenal gland, the liver, the spleen as well as in the gastrointestinal tract, also peri-collagenous deposits in the heart can occur, as they are reserved for the type of an AL-amyloidosis (see p. 145).

3.11.8 Late Onset RA

In about 4/5 of the cases, RA begins lingeringly between the ages of 25 and 50, whereby females are afflicted three times more often than males. In the remaining 1/5 of the cases, the disease starts only after the 60th year of life, and males and females are almost equally often affected. This late onset RA is characterized by its acute onset with asymmetrical attack, particularly also of the large joints.

The prognostic evaluation of this RA type is different. Dequeker and coworkers (1966) as well as Kaiser (1969, 1989), amongst others, point out the unfavourable progress of RA starting at this age. Our morphological observations of joint tissues of patients with late onset RA are also indicative of its highly destructive nature. These findings have been opposed by other authors who judge the prognosis of this late onset RA as rather positive (Forestier and Charmant 1950; Francon 1957; Corrigan et al. 1974). In the course of an evaluation of 133 elderly-onset RA patients (onset 60 years of age or later), Shiozawa and coworkers (1997) found a better joint prognosis compared with that for patients with earlier onset of RA.

A key to solve this apparent contradiction is given by Healey (1986) and Caroit and coworkers (1987) by dividing the late onset RA into three groups with different clinical symptoms and prognoses. Thereby, about 65% of the cases belong to the classical form of late onset RA which attacks particularly also the large joints and which is characterized by a fast, progressing joint destruction. Rheumatoid factors are detectable in most of the patients.

This is opposed by two other forms of late onset RA with benign progress. A type to which about 10% of the cases belong occurs together with Sicca syndrome (see p. 161) and shows a persistent

synovitis of the hand and MCP joints which, however, progresses without joint destruction although most of the patients are seropositive.
A further late onset type of RA occurs only after the 70th year and accounts for about 25% of the cases. The male-to-female ratio is 4:3. Characteristic is the often acute onset with a pronounced symmetrical myalgic syndrome in the shoulder region. Further characteristics are a high inflammatory activity as well as the attack of large and small joints. Most of the time, rheumatoid factors are not detectable. Since this type of late onset RA is mostly myalgic, confusion with polymyalgia rheumatica (see p. 276) is likely at the onset.
From the standpoint of the pathologist, significant doubts arise as to whether these two special forms which progress without joint destruction justify the term late onset "RA". On the other hand, no doubt exists that the first, the malignant group, belongs to the RA which is characterized not only by the presence of rheumatoid factors, but also by the joint destruction which is typical of RA.

3.11.9 Mortality

To what extent RA can be considered as cause of death may only be determined with more autopsy series. However, investigations of this kind are rare, which is understandable when one takes into account the chronic character of this disease, which tends to burn out with increasing age. Usually, those patients die at home and therefore no post mortem examination takes place.
A series of extensive follow-up studies endeavoured to estimate the risk of death for RA patients (Gordon et al. 1973; Mutru et al. 1985; Mitchell et al. 1986; Symmons 1988). The different authors agreed consistently on the basis of their observations, that RA, when commencing after the 40th year of age, shortens life expectancy of patients by up to 50%, in contrast to control groups. According to observations of Gordon et al. (1973), the death rate (over a period of 5 years) in patients with RA who have extra-articular manifestations is twice as high as in patients with exclusively articular affection.
With regard to the studies at hand, there are principally three distinct processes responsible for the fatal course of the disease:
- Specific complications of RA
- Non-specific complications of a chronic disease
- Complications conditioned through therapy

The first group includes:
- Amyloidosis: secondary generalized amyloidosis may result in fatal renal insufficiency.
- Atlanto-axial dislocation: may result in tetraplegia and fatal respiratory paralysis.
- Rheumatoid necroses ("rheumatoid nodules"): may be of considerable clinical significance and of possibly fatal outcome if the necrotizing processes take place in the lung, myocardium, heart valve, and blood vessels (see p. 112), espe-

cially the coronary vessels, above all, if the conduction system is affected.

- Rheumatoid lung affection: involvement of the lung in form of interstitial fibrosis jeopardizes the patient's life (see p. 150).

The second group includes:

- Non-specific systemic infections: all statistics on the cause of death in RA patients blame those infections to be the primary cause, e.g. bronchopneumonia, pyelonephritis.
- Sepsis, initiated from the affected joints (see p. 385) or bacterial-purulent superinfection (see p. 395).

The third group includes:

- Predominantly fatal haemorrhages of gastric ulcers following applications of steroidal and non-steroidal antiphlogistic agents. The increased susceptibility for infections which may lead to sepsis can be attributed to the antiphlogistic drugs, especially also the immune suppressive therapy.
- Though the therapy with gold is being accompanied by severe side effects, fatal outcome is rare. Aplasia of the bone marrow occurs in less than 0.5% following application of gold (McCarty et al. 1962b). In such cases, pancytopenia progresses with severe infections and haemorrhages and is fatal in 60%. In rare cases, gold therapy can cause enterocolitis which may be fatal in approximately 50% (Stein and Urowitz 1976; Fam et al. 1980).

In a prospective study over a time period of 10 years, Kellgren and O'Brien (1962) found a mortality rate of 27% in seropositive RA patients, in contrast to 15% in RA patients without detectable rheumatoid factors. The worse prognosis for seropositive patients is plausible, as the development of necrotizing processes, amongst them necrotizing vasculitides, is elementarily bound to the presence of rheumatoid factors.
From the pathological-anatomical point of view, the final clarification of the pathomechanisms leading to death in RA remains unanswered as long as access to results based on a large number of autopsies is limited.

4 Sjögren's Syndrome

4.1 Definition

Sjögren's syndrome (SS) is a chronic inflammatory disease characterized by diminished lacrimal and salivary gland secretion (the sicca complex) resulting in keratoconjunctivitis sicca and xerostomia (Talal et al. 1987). The glandular insufficiency is secondary to lymphocytic and plasma cell infiltrations. The term autoimmune exocrinopathy has been introduced for SS (Strand and Talal 1980). Both a primary and a secondary form of this disease are recognized. Approximately 25% of patients with an associated rheumatoid arthritis (RA) are considered to have secondary SS; a small percentage may have another associated connective tissue disease. Primary SS is diagnosed in the absence of another connective tissue disease.

Sicca complex

Secondary SS

Primary SS

SS is particularly important among the autoimmune diseases for two reasons. First, perhaps 2 to 3 million individuals are affected in the United States. Second, in SS, a benign autoimmune process can terminate in a malignant lymphoid disorder. The disease offers potential insight into the mechanisms whereby immunological dysregulation may predispose a person to a malignant transformation of B cells already involved in an autoimmune process (Talal 1993).

4.2 History

Mikulicz's disease

In 1892, Mikulicz (1937–1938) reported a man with bilateral parotid and lacrimal gland enlargement associated with massive round cell infiltration. In 1925, Gougerot described three patients with salivary and mucous gland atrophy and insufficiency progressing to dryness. Two years later (1927), Houwer emphasized the association of filamentary keratitis, the major ocular manifestation of the syndrome, with chronic arthritis. In 1933, Henrik Sjögren reported detailed clinical and histological findings in 19 women with xerostomia and keratoconjunctivitis sicca, of whom 13 had chronic arthritis. In 1953, Morgan and Castleman concluded that SS and Mikulicz's disease were the same entity.

Ocular manifestation

4.3 Etiology

Multifactorial origin

Autoimmune disorders have a multifactorial origin with elements of:

Genetic and immunological control

1. Genetic control related to the activity of specific immune response genes.
2. Immunological control exerted by regulatory T-dependent lymphocytes (suppressor and helper T cells).
3. Possible viral influences, although such influences are not yet clearly established.
4. Sex hormone modulation of immune regulation in which estrogens enhance and androgens suppress autoimmunity (Ansar et al. 1985).

HLA-B8 and HLA-DR3

SS is one of several autoimmune diseases associated with the histocompatibility antigens HLA-B8 and HLA-DR3, which is an indication of the genetic predisposition. Primary SS in males is associated with HLA-DRw52 but not with HLA-B8 or HLA-DR3 (Molina et al. 1986).

Animal models

Several spontaneously autoimmune mouse strains, particularly the MRL mice, have features of SS. Transgenic mice containing the HTLV-1 tax gene develop salivary gland lesions resembling SS.

4.4 Epidemiology

As in most autoimmune diseases, there is a predilection for middle-aged and elderly females. Primary SS in men is an uncommon condition (Anaya et al. 1995). Definite sicca syndrome was found in 3.5% of females and 2.8% of males over the age of 80 years. There was no association between the prevalence of autoantibodies and keratoconjunctivitis sicca or xerostomia in these individuals, suggesting that senile atrophy of the secretory apparatus rather than immunological injury was the underlying etioloy. In the United Kingdom, the incidence of keratoconjunctivitis sicca in RA patients is 11%, whereas xerostomia occurs in only 1% of these patients (Whaley and Alspaugh 1985). High incidences of salivary gland abnormalities are found in patients with systemic lupus erythematosus (SLE; Alarcón-Segovia et al. 1974a) and scleroderma (Alarcón-Segovia et al. 1974b; Cipoletti et al. 1977).

An exact prevalence of SS is unknown but it is probably the most common connective tissue disease after RA. One can reasonably predict a prevalence of 0.5% (Talal 1986). In post mortem examinations of RA patients, lymphocytic infiltration of the submandibular glands were found in all of these patients (Waterhouse and Doniach 1966). In many cases, these pathological alterations had not manifested clinically. It may be assumed that regarding the prevalence of salivary gland disease only an approximate estimation can be made.

4.5 Clinical Manifestations

More than 90% of patients are women; the mean age is 50 years. The disease occurs in all races and in children (Chudwin et al. 1981). The two most common presentations are:

Sicca syndrome and RA

1. The insidious and slowly progressive development of the sicca complex in a patient with chronic RA.

Oral and ocular complications

2. The more rapid development of a severe oral and ocular dryness, often accompanied by episodic parotitis, in an otherwise well patient.

About 50% of patients with keratoconjunctivitis sicca have additional features of SS. The most common ocular complaint is a sensation, described as "gritty" or "sandy", of a foreign body in the eye. Ocular complications include corneal ulceration or vascularisation, followed rarely by perforation.

Salivary gland insufficiency

Dryness may also involve the nose, the posterior pharynx, the esophagus, the larynx, and the tracheobronchial tree and may lead to epistaxis, hoarseness, recurrent otitis media, bronchitis, or pneumonia. Half these patients have parotid gland enlargement, often recurrent and symmetric.

Arteritis

The arteritis of SS resembles classic RA in its clinical, pathologic, and roentgenographic features. Keratoconjunctivitis sicca develops in about 10%–15% of patients with RA. Arthralgias and morning stiffness without joint deformity may occur in patients with the sicca complex.

Visceral complications

Fourty percent of patients show an interstitial nephritis. Splenomegaly and leukopenia, suggestive of Felty's syndrome and vasculitis with leg ulcers and peripheral neuropathy, may appear even in the absence of RA.

Raynaud's phenomenon

Raynaud's phenomenon occurs in 20% of the patients (Talal 1993). A variety of pulmonary disorders may be present (Fairfax et al. 1981; Segal et al. 1981; Constantopoulos et al. 1985; Vitali et al. 1985). Peripheral or cranial neuropathy may cause symptoms of dysesthesia or paraesthesia. Facial pain and numbness can accompany trigeminal neuropathy. Chronic thyroiditis of the Hashimoto type is present in 5% of patients. SS is found in 52% of patients with primary biliary cirrhosis and in 35% of patients with active chronic hepatitis (Talal 1993).

Moreover, the skin, pancreas, and glands of the vaginal tract, but in general all organs may also be involved in the course of SS.

Laboratory findings

Rheumatoid factors in patients with SS are positive in approximately 70%. Antinuclear antibodies (ANA; up to 85%) and characteristic, but unspecific autoantibodies against ribonucleoproteins (up to 65%) Ro/SSA (anti-Ro) and La/SSB (anti-La) are produced (Pease et al. 1989; Venables et al. 1989; Anaya et al. 1995; Youinou 1995; Tengnér et al. 1998).

4.6 Pathology and Pathogenesis

The term "benign lymphoepithelial lesion" mainly refers to the morphological picture of the salivary glands. SS, however, is also characterized by lymphocytic and plasma cell infiltrations of lacrimal glands and exocrine glands in the respiratory tract, gas-

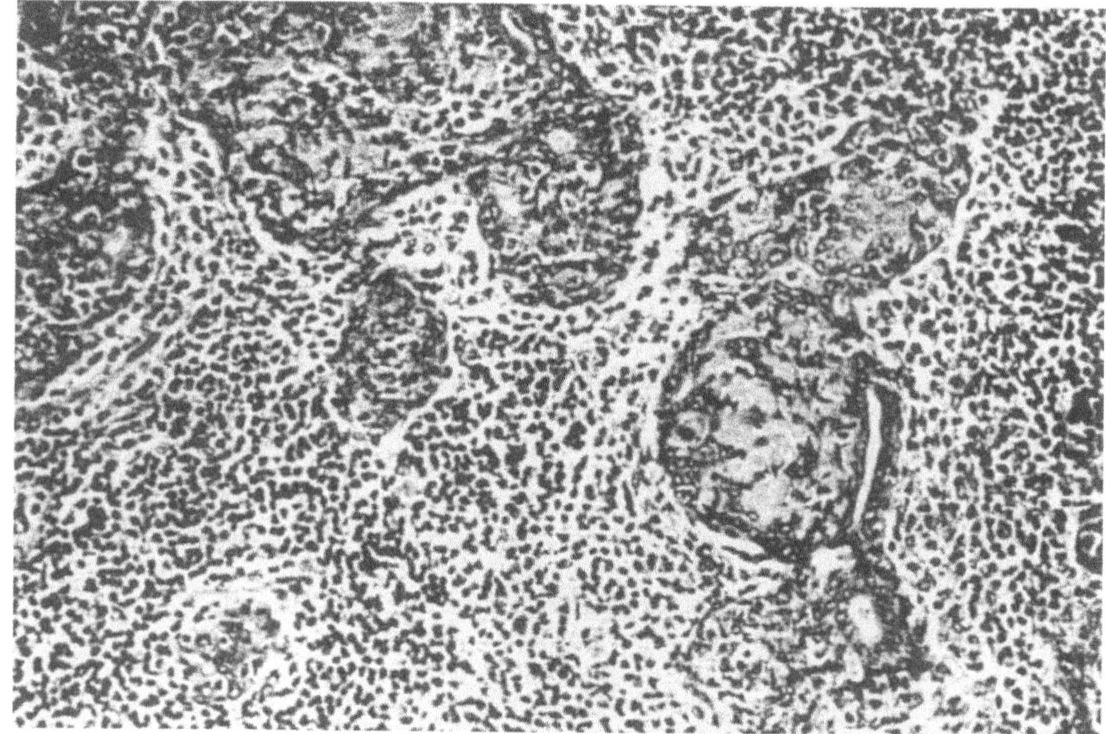

Fig. 4.1
Sjögren's syndrome

Chronic myo-epithelial parotitis. Dense lymphocytic infiltration of parotid tissue with inclusion of islands of myo-epithelial cells (female patient aged 48 years). (Seifert 1971)

trointestinal tract, vagina, pancreas, and kidney. Parotid and submaxillary but also the minor (gingival, labial, and palatine) glands are affected.

Myo-epithelial sialoadenitis

Knowledge of the histopathology of the glands was derived from autopsy and biopsy material. Seifert (1966) coined the term myo-epithelial sialoadenitis. This was designed to include the alteration of the parenchyma with atrophy of secretory elements, distension and other duct changes, lymphoid and plasma cell infiltration, and finally fibrosis of the parenchyma.

Systemic disease

These pathological features are seen in the salivary as well as the lacrimal glands but tend to be most marked in the parotid. Involvement of the pancreas, the mucous and serous gastric glands, and the secretory glands of the bronchi and genital tract has also been noted. The fact that also mucal glands of trachea and bronchus as well as lung, kidney, and skeletal muscles can be affected by lymphoid infiltrates, points to the systemic character.

Myo-epithelial crescents

Obstruction of salivary ducts

Considerable importance has been ascribed to the occurrence of myo-epithelial crescents. They arise from the proliferation of duct epithelial cells with spherical nuclei and from the myo-epithelium which has elongated darkly staining nuclei. These formations cause narrowing and even obstruction of small to medium-sized salivary ducts (Figs. 4.1–4.3). With time, these crescents may undergo regression with hyalinisation and collagen formation in the region of basement membranes.

Atrophy of glandular parenchyma

The lumina of salivary ducts may contain remnants of PAS-positive material as remains of desiccated secretion. The secretory

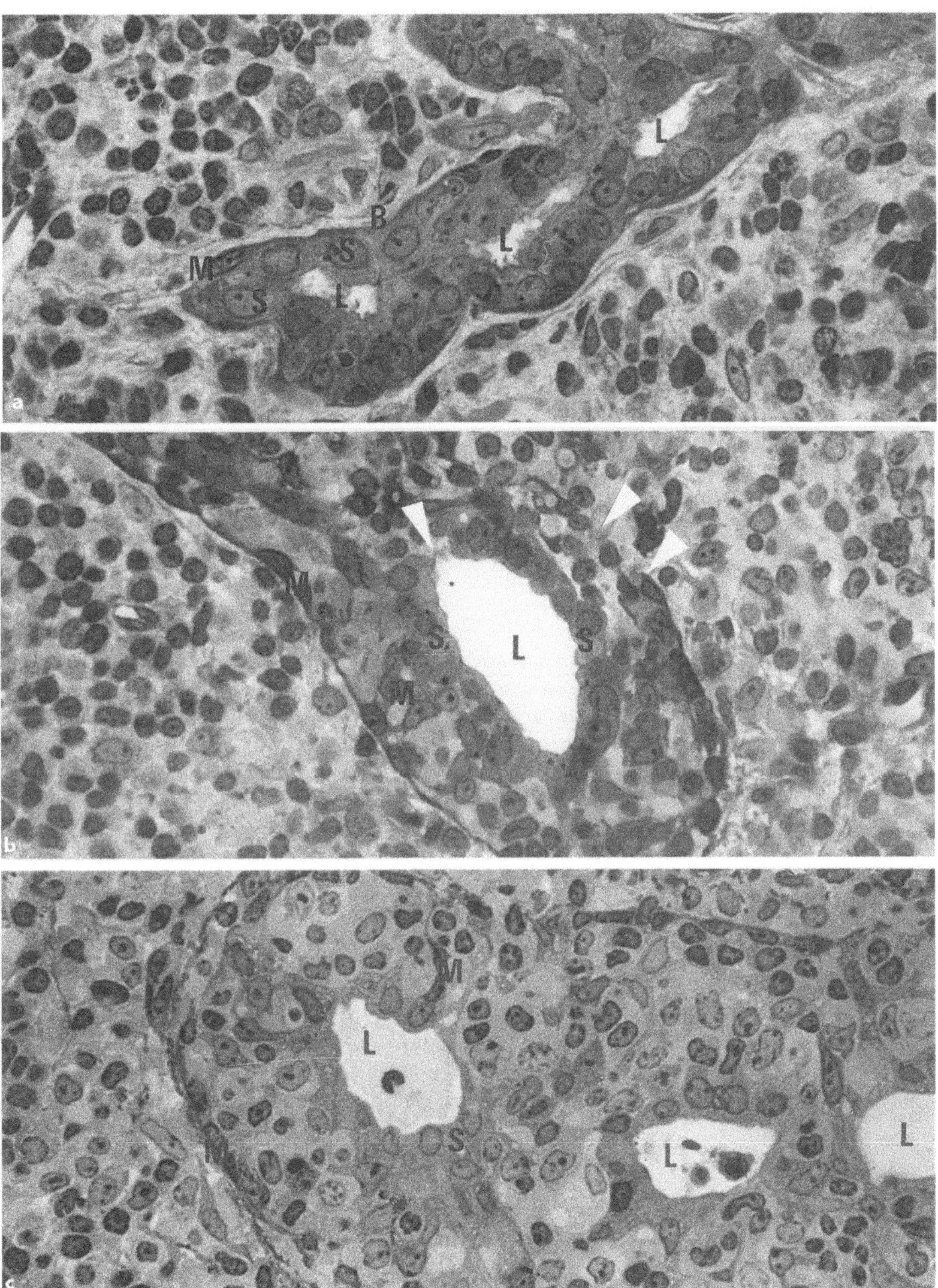

Myo-epithelial sialoadenitis. **a** Duct showing typical structure (*L*, lumen; *S*, epithelium; *M*, myo-epithelium; *B*, basement membrane). Interstitial lymphocyte infiltration. **b** Myo-epithelial island: distended lumen (*L*) with incomplete surrounding epithelium (*arrow*). *M*, myo-epithelial proliferation. Circumscribed dissolution of basement membrane with early lymphocyte infiltration (*twin arrows*). *S*, epithelium. **c** Myo-epithelial island with increased lymphocyte infiltration (semi-thin sections). (Donath and Seifert 1972)

Fig. 4.2a–c
Sjögren's syndrome

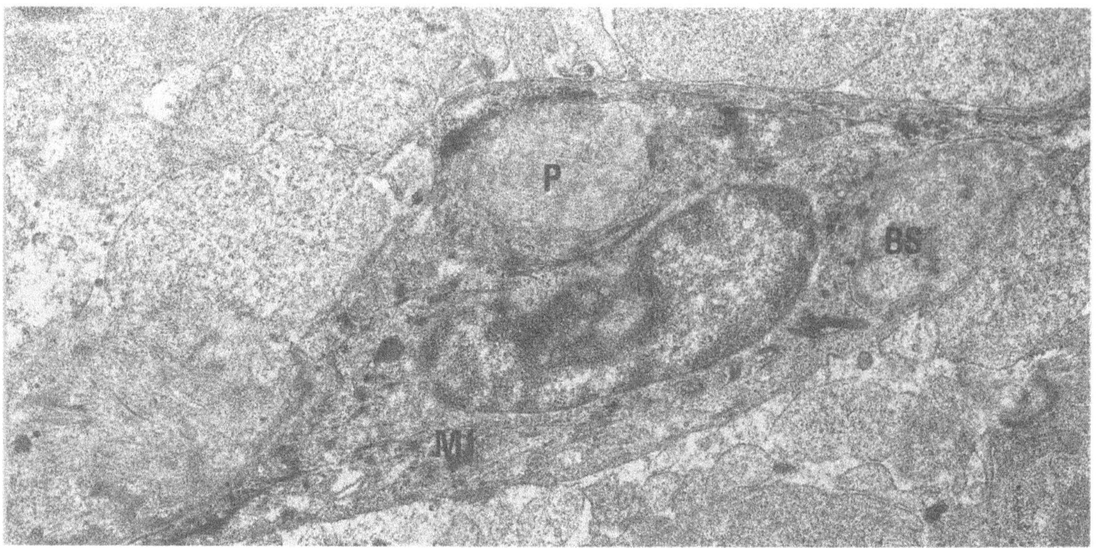

Fig. 4.3
Sjögren's syndrome

Myo-epithelial sialoadenitis. Myo-epithelial cell with intracytoplasmic, membrane-limited, basement membrane-like substances (*BS*), partly tropo-collagen (*P*), myofilaments (*Mf*). (Electron micrograph, 1:9,000; Donath and Seifert 1972)

acini may atrophy to such an extent that a salivary gland may give the appearance of a tumour consisting only of lymphocytic infiltrates and myo-epithelial crescents. It is difficult to envisage any pathogenic connection between SS and RA. The morphological appearance can only be regarded as inflammatory within the widest limits of the term. Definite exudative and proliferative features are absent.

T lymphocyte infiltration

HLA-DR-positive epithelial cells

The question whether the destruction of gland parenchyma precedes or follows the lymphocytic infiltration is answered by the studies of Lindahl et al. (1985) and Fox et al. (1986). It could be shown that numerous glandular epithelial cells in the salivary glands are HLA-DR-positive. The HLA-DR-positive epithelial cells are in close proximity surrounded by lymphocytic infiltrates in which activated CD4+ T-helper cells are the most prominent population represented (Adamson et al. 1983; Lindahl et al. 1985; Kong et al. 1997). It appears that the early lymphocytic infiltrations, which are predominantly periductal and give rise to minimal ductal damage, consist of immunoglobulin-bearing B lymphocytes whereas acinar destruction is associated with increasing T lymphocyte infiltration. The predominant T lymphocyte subset in the salivary gland infiltrates is CD4+ (i.e. of the helper-inducer population; Fox et al. 1982). It is uncertain if the tissue damage is due to antibody-dependent cell mediated lymphocytotoxicity or to cytotoxic antibodies. In early stages of the disease, one can find scattered lymphoid cell infiltrations around small intralobular ducts. In proportion to the extent of this infiltration, the acinar atrophy is varying. In rare cases, lymph follicles containing germinal centres may develop. There is a risk for malignant transformation of these primarily benign alterations. The T lymphocyte infiltration represents the early phase of SS in which a cell mediated immune response gives rise to the initial

Cytotoxic mechanisms

parenchymal damage while the later augmentation of B lymphocytes and plasma cells causes an increase in tissue damage by antibody-dependent lymphocytotoxicity or the production of lymphocytotoxic antibodies (Whaley and Alspaugh 1985). In the salivary glands of patients with SS, B and T lymphocytes as well as elevated levels of IgA and IgM rheumatoid factor are also found. These are in part synthesized locally but mainly serum derived (Dunne et al. 1979).

IgA and IgM rheumatoid factor

"Pseudolymphoma"

Occasionally, lymphocytic infiltration of the salivary glands can be so pleomorphic and invasive that it is difficult to differentiate from a malignant neoplastic process. The lymphatic infiltration of the exocrine organs in SS is generally mild, however, it can occasionally become very intensive. From an originally stable process a so-called pseudolymphoma can develop in lungs, kidneys, and salivary glands. Sometimes the lymphoproliferation can also become generalized to produce lymphadenopathy, lung infiltration, fever, and loss of weight reminiscent of a malignant lymphoma (Talal and Bunim 1964).

Generalized lymphoproliferation

Histologically, two types of pseudolymphoma can be differentiated, one consisting of plasmacyte infiltrations and another of small and large lymphocytes or plasma cells and large reticulocytes. The damage to normal lymphatic structure and capsule infiltration can make the differentiation between benign and malignant lymphoproliferation more difficult. The danger that from an initially benign lymphoproliferation a malignant lymphoreticular neoplasm develops is considerably increased in patients with SS (Zufferey et al. 1995; Kruize et al. 1996).

Malignant degeneration

Malignant lymphomas can develop in certain cases from pseud olymphomas after many years. Patients with SS have an increased risk for development of malignant lymphoma (Zufferey et al. 1995; Kruize et al. 1996). A report from the US National Institutes of Health (NIH) suggests that the risk rate for developing non-Hodgkin's lymphoma in SS is 44 times higher than normal (Kassan et al. 1977). This accords with the continuous transition of an autoaggressive inflammation to a malignoma.

Autoimmune phenomena

SS belongs to the autoimmune diseases which are associated with histocompatibility to antigens HLA-B8 and HLA-DR3. The class II MHC antigens predispose to the development of autoimmune diseases. Also the evidence of characteristic autoantibodies Ro/SSA and La/SSB, and ANAs stands for it (Youinou 1995). A particular number of patients tend to have immunological reactions against viruses or viral-altered host antigens. SS can be therefore an autoimmunological precursor syndrome of RA or other defined collagen diseases. Rheumatoid factors are present in approximately 3/4 of SS patients. The spectrum of antinuclear antibodies in SS merges with those seen in SLE. Also an antibody specific for salivary duct epithelium has been observed by indirect immunofluorescence in 50% of SS patients (Talal 1986; Bodeutsch et al. 1992).

"Primary SS"

Drosos and colleagues (1988) described a primary SS which appeared independent of systemic disease. They found in 80% of lip biopsies which had been volunteered by 62 sympton-free older people histological changes of varying definition which corresponded to those of SS. It is notable that these changes were only found in women.

5 Juvenile Chronic Arthritis*

5.1 Definition

The term "juvenile chronic arthritis" (JCA) does not define a nosological entity. It represents today more an overall conception comprising different disease entities differentiated according to the initial constitutional condition of the patient, the pathogenesis, the onset of the illness, the pattern, and the character of the disease process.

5.2 History

In 1864, Cornil described for the first time the case of a 29-year-old female whose progressive arthritis had started at 12 years of age. In 1890, Diamantberger reported more than 38 children with rheumatoid arthritis (RA). However, it was only the masterly description by Still (1897) of a "form of chronic joint disease in children" which established the unique position of JCA as an independent disease. Still described 12 children with a polyarthritis distinguishable from RA and 6 children in whom there was no difference from the adult form of RA. The first group had a generalized lymphadenopathy and splenomegaly, and frequently pericarditis, involvement of the cervical spine with episodes of fever, and retardation of growth.

5.3 Epidemiology

It is difficult to estimate the exact frequency of JCA as the oligoarticular forms in particular are often unrecognized. JCA occurs in every climatic zone and all races. Bywaters (1968), in his studies of the town and country districts of Berkshire (UK), calculated an incidence of 6 per 10,000 school children. The prevalence of JCA in USA is estimated to be about 0.16–0.43 per 1,000 children (Cassidy and Nelson 1988; Gewanter and Baum 1989).

Synonym: juvenile rheumatoid arthritis

5.4 Diagnostic Criteria

The criteria for the classification of JCA revised in 1989 by the American College of Rheumatology (Cassidy et al. 1989) are:

1. Age of onset: less than 16 years.
2. Arthritis in one or more joints defined as swelling or effusion, or the presence of two or more of the following signs: limitation of range of motion, tenderness or pain on motion, or increased heat.
3. Duration of disease: longer than 6 weeks.
4. Type of disease onset during the first 6 months classified as:
   - Polyarthritis: five or more joints.
   - Pauciarticular disease (oligoarthritis): four or fewer joints.
   - Systemic disease: arthritis with intermittent fever.
5. Exclusion of other forms of juvenile arthritis.

According to our present state of knowledge, five groups of JCA can be distinguished (Table 5.1), but probably an extension of this nosological classification can be expected in the future.

5.5 Clinical Features

The general clinical picture shows in the five groups clear differences which demonstrate the unique character of the respective forms of JCA.

In contrast to adult RA, in general, JCA in all age groups is characterized by the primary involvement of the large joints of the lower extremities, predominantly knee and foot joints. Sometimes the hand and elbow joints are also involved; and occasionally also the small joints of the hand and foot, too.

Systemic JCA (Still's disease)

Group 1

Systemic JCA, starting in early childhood, is characterized by fever, exanthema, hepatosplenomegaly, polyserositis, and leucocytosis. The patients in early childhood are particularly endangered by infection. The risk of amyloidosis is approximately 15%. The joint involvement is 60% polyarticular and 40% oligoarticular and the large and small joints can be affected symmetrically. Joint destruction in cases with a polyarticular onset is considerably greater than in those with an oligoarticular onset.

Polyarticular seronegative JCA

Group 2

Polyarticular seronegative JCA, which occurs approximately 70% in young females of all age groups may be preceded by mild general symptoms. The pattern of joint involvement corresponds to that of the seropositive form, except that the distal interphalangeal joints can be affected. The progress is, however, substantially more favourable than in the seropositive form and the disease process of the joints can come to a standstill.

Polyarticular seropositive JCA

Group 3

In polyarticular seropositive JCA which affects mainly females of school age, the systemic symptoms may be mild. Rheumatoid

Table 5.1. Five sub-groups of JCA according to Schaller (1977)

	Group 1	Group 2	Group 3	Group 4	Group 5
Disease	Systemic JCA (Still's disease)	Polyarticular RF negative JCA	Polyarticular RF positive JCA	Oligoarticular JCA - type I	Oligoarticular JCA - type II
% JCA-patients	20	25	10	30	15
Proportion of sex	m=f	70% f	80% f	80% f	90% m
Disease onset	Early childhood	Entire childhood	Late childhood school age	Early childhood infancy	Late childhood school age
Joint involvement	Large + small joints, (poly-, oligoart.) symmetric	Large + small joints, symmetric	Large + small joints, symmetric	Single joints, asymmetric	Large + small joints, asymmetric
Cervical spine	65%	Frequently	Frequently	Rarely	Rarely
Sacroiliitis	Very rarely	None	Rarely	None	Generally
Iridocyclitis	None	Rarely	None	50% chronic	20% acute
Visceral involvement	Spleen, liver, heart, lymphocytes	None	None	None	None
Amyloidosis	Approx. 15%	Rarely	Rarely	Rarely	Rarely
Fever	Approx. 97%	None	None	None	None
Rheumatoid factor	Negative	Negative	100%	Negative	Negative
Antinuclear antibodies	Negative	20%	50–75%	60–80%	Negative
HLA typing	?	?	DR 4	DR 5, DR 8	B 27
Prognosis	Severe arthritis in 25%	Severe arthritis in 10–15%	Severe arthritis in more than 50%	Eye lesion in 10–30%	Subsequent spondylo-arthropathy

factors are demonstrated in 100% of cases and an association exists with HLA-DR4. As in adult RA, large and small joints of the upper and lower extremities are affected symmetrically (with the exception of the distal interphalangeal joints). Infrequently, the sacroiliac joint is involved. Joint destruction progresses as severely as in adult RA.

Group 4

Oligoarticular JCA (type I)

In oligoarticular JCA (type I), generalized symptoms are rare but the primary danger is of a chronic iridocyclitis in 50% of patients. There is a high risk of defective healing or blindness.

There is an association with HLA-DR5 and HLA-DR8. The joint disease in this oligoarticular form of JCA which starts in early childhood and affects predominantly young females progresses particularly mildly. Joint involvement is asymmetric and limited to single, usually large joints (knee). Joint destruction may be totally absent and the process can completely resolve with appropriate therapy.

Oligoarticular JCA (type II)

Group 5

Oligoarticular JCA (type II) is characterized by the facts that 90% of the almost exclusively young male patients are HLA-B27 positive, and that it can develop into the clinical picture of juvenile ankylosing spondylitis (AS; see p. 188). Thus, there is a possible progression to the group of diseases of the seronegative spondarthritides (SSA). In 20–30% of patients, an acute iridocyclitis occurs. The joint involvement is asymmetric and both large and small joints can be affected. It is pathognomonic that there is a progressive bilateral involvement of the iliosacral joint over a long time. Often the hip and the metatarsophalangeal joint of the big toe are also affected. The X-ray picture frequently shows bony spur growths of the calcaneus (enthesopathy; see p. 182). The involvement of the lumbar vertebrae (more rarely the cervical vertebrae) completes the clinical picture of a juvenile spondylitis.

5.6 Pathology

We owe to Bywaters the first comprehensive documentation of 32 post-mortem investigations made in Taplow (UK) between 1974 and 1976 (1977). His findings agree with those which we have collected in 21 children aged between 2.5 to 16 years who had died of JCA in the period of 1959 to 1978 in the Children's Rheumatism Clinic in Garmisch-Partenkirchen (Germany). These concerned, except one seropositive polyarticular case, children of the systemic Still group. Basically, it can be said that qualitatively morphological changes in these cases do not differ essentially from those in adult RA.

Joint disease process

Bywaters (1976) emphasized the similarity of the synovial disease process in JCA and adult RA. These observations are, however, difficult to reconcile with the essentially milder clinical course of oligoarticular forms of JCA. Cassidy (1985) observed in X-ray investigations of children with JCA that marginal erosions and narrowing of the cartilaginous space did not occur before 2 years of active disease even in the child with polyarthritis. In some children with oligoarticular affection, he found no erosions even after one or two decades of constant effusions.

In our post-mortem reports of 21 children with JCA, we found, in accordance with the X-ray observations of Cassidy, severe joint destruction only in patients with systemic JCA (group 1) who had been confined to bed for a long period. An extreme case was that of a 14-year-old boy with polyarticular systemic JCA (Still's disease) who had remained for years in bed untreated and died of myocarditis. We found a total ankylosis of all the large joints of the upper and lower extremities and of the joints of the jaw.

Retrospectively it is not to be excluded that it concerned a juvenile AS. In one case of a 14-year-old girl who had a seropositive polyarticular JCA (group 3) of early onset and died of renal amyloidosis, the joint destruction was histologically of the adult RA type. In addition, we found arterial necrosis (see Fig. 3.75) which we have otherwise only seen in patients with seropositive adult RA. In the remaining cases, the joint capsule was thickened and the synovial membrane hyperplastic, joint cartilage and subchondral bone, on the other hand, were fully or largely intact. The cause of death was myocarditis or renal infection.

It could be expected that the key information about the disease process of the joint would be provided by the state of the synovial tissue. However, it must be recognized that the changes in the synovial tissue caused by local and systemic inflammatory diseases are never stationary; individual histological findings are momentary records which are solely evidence of the condition of the synovial tissue at a specific point in time. Nevertheless, in a great number of synovial biopsies, taking into account individual variations, certain differences are found compared with the synovial changes in adult RA.

Synovial tissue

In the Zentrum für Rheuma-Pathologie (Mainz, Germany) up to December 1999, 511 synovial biopsies of JCA patients were examined. The JCA tissue shows the following similarities to adult RA: the synovial tissue is hyperplastic. There is a moderate new villous formation formation of medium length and breadth. Discrete fibrin remnants can lie on the villi surface. The lining cells are in general cubic or tall cylindrical. The synovial stroma is loosely fibrosed and contains predominantly focal layered lymphocytes as well as a scattered distribution of plasma cells. Neutrophils are neither associated with synovitis of adult RA nor with JCA, as Bywaters and Ansell reported as early as 1965.

The synovial changes in JCA can be distinguished from those of adult RA by the following factors: the synovial hyperplasia is in general less than in RA. The synovial stroma cells can proliferate to a high degree only in seropositive polyarticular adult JCA (group 3), but not in the oligoarticular forms (groups 4 and 5); we have never seen this kind of excessive proliferation as in RA. Focal lymphocyte infiltrates are more consistently found in JCA than in RA. True lymph follicles with germ centres are in both extremely rare. Plasma cells are found more frequently in JCA than in RA. In agreement with Bywaters (1970), we have never seen rheumatoid necroses except in one case with seropositive adult JCA (group 3). They are, however, basically possible in seropositive polyarticular JCA (group 3). The absence of aggressive synovial cell proliferation in the oligoarticular forms (groups 4 and 5) is an explanation for the mild course of the disease as well as for the non-appearance of joint destruction.

Sacroiliac joint

A bilateral symmetrical sacroiliitis is pathognomonic for the HLA-B27 associated oligoarticular JCA (group 5), 90% of which occur in boys. In polyarticular seropositive JCA (group 3), sacroiliitis is rare. The observations of Bywaters (1968) are unusual, that in the sacroiliac joints of some of the children who had died of systemic JCA (Still's disease) he found breaks in the surface of the joint which were filled with granulation tissue. These discrete changes were thus clearly distinct from the early changes of HLA-B27 associated oligoarticular JCA (group 5) which is characterized by wide-spread inflammatory destruction of cartilage more marked on the iliac side and destruction of underlying bone. The onset and development of sacroiliac disease can only be judged by X-ray investigations, as occasional pathological-anatomical findings, particularly the early stages, do not provide an adequate basis. Schilling and coworkers (1963) believe that the iliosacral joint is capable of reconstruction at the earliest in the 10th year of age. The changes are nearly symmetrical, and in addition there is a radiological variegated picture which consists of the following phenomena: apparent widening of the joint space, curved marginal resorption, small cystic resorption bodies, bony thickening (sclerosis), and synostoses.

Cervical spine

In 25% of cases of adult RA, the cervical spine is affected in the form of cervical arthritis, which rarely ankyloses (see p. 107), whereas in two-thirds of children with systemic JCA (Still's disease) and less frequently in both polyarticular forms of JCA (seropositive and seronegative), a cervical arthritis occurs with an ankylosing tendency which can appear at an early stage of the disease. By contrast, in both of the oligoarticular forms of JCA involvement of the cervical vertebrae is rare.

Schilling et al. (1963) found in 18 adolescent patients with systemic JCA (Still's disease) and polyarticular joint involvement 13 instances of typical intervertebral joint synostoses with fusion of the upper and middle segment and hyperplasia of the corresponding discs and vertebral bodies. Mäkela and coworkers (1979) report a great number of afflicted children with inflammatory changes at the atlanto-axial joints (C1 and C2). Bywaters (1976) mentions a primary involvement of the apophyseal joints with ankylosis of C2–C3, lack of growth, and later a fusion of the vertebral bodies (Fig. 5.1). He maintains that due to the late development of the acquired uncovertebral joint space in childhood and the absence of disc degeneration, the cervical subluxation, characteristic of adult RA, is rare, occurring only at the atlanto-axial joint as a result of erosion of the dens and its attachments. Thus, fusion is common and subluxation is rare except at C1–C2. Bywaters (1976) made the observation that JCA patients may in later life develop subluxations in the region of the uncovertebral joint of the same type as in adult RA.

Skin nodules

Skin nodules are not infrequent in JCA. In patients with polyarticular seropositive JCA (group 3), which, however, constitute only approximately 10% of the five forms of JCA, they cannot be distinguished from the rheumatoid nodules of seropositive adult RA (see p. 124). In the other seronegative forms of JCA, these classical rheumatoid nodules never appear. The danger of a mistaken diagnosis lies in the fact that a granuloma anulare (see p. 125) can be exceedingly similar to a rheumatoid nodule, but in no way can a relationship be recognized to a rheumatic illness or to rheumatoid factors. In 20% of children with systemic JCA (Still's disease; Kölle 1970) and in 10% of the other seronegative JCA forms, skin nodules do in fact occur at mechanically exposed sites (Bywaters 1970). These are smaller, softer, and essentially more transient than the rheumatoid nodules of adult RA. Histo-

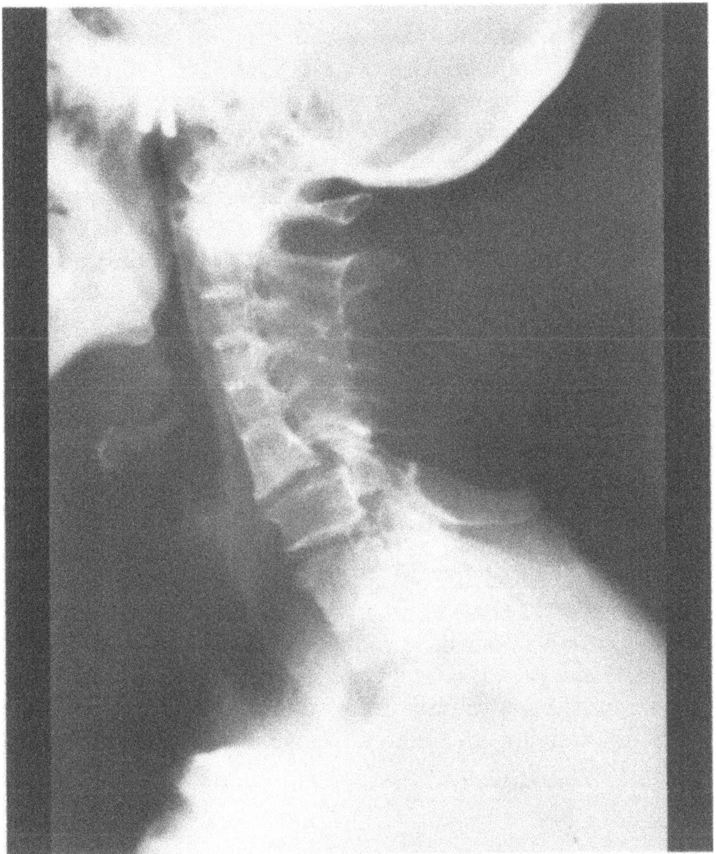

Cervical spondylitis following earlier Still's disease. Synostosis of intervertebral joints and hypoplasia of vertebral bodies and intervertebral discs from C3 to C7 (37-year-old female)

Fig. 5.1
Still's disease

logically, they are also fundamentally distinguished from the rheumatoid nodule: in place of central necrosis, there is a striped fibrinoid zone with layers of connective tissue cells and a few neutrophils, also there is not the continuous histiocyte palisade typical of the rheumatoid nodule. The changes are often not well defined and are subject to variation according to the age of the skin phenomena. Here again, it is apparent that no true rheumatoid nodules occur without the previous presence of rheumatoid factors!

Mortality

The mortality of JCA is simple to determine as death in childhood is an uncommon occurrence. In contrast, it is difficult to estimate RA as a cause of death in adults. At the present time, the mortality of JCA is approximately 10%, of which the majority of cases are Still's disease. In the autopsies of 21 children with JCA (see p. 172), we saw three cases of pyelonephritis as the cause of death.

Amyloidosis

The complication most dangerous for the life of the patient is amyloidosis (see p. 173). In contrast to adult RA, amyloidosis is a relatively frequent cause of death in JCA. Schnitzer and Ansell (1977) stated that about half of JCA patients with secondary AA-amyloidosis die within a period of 10 years from the establishment of the diagnosis. In statistics from Husby (1977), amyloidosis occurred in 5% of JCA children. Kölle (1975) found amyloidosis in 20% of children with systemic JCA (Still's disease). The variation in the frequency can be accounted for by the difference in diagnostic procedures. A greater accuracy is achieved by rectal mucous membrane or gingival biopsies. As systemic JCA (Still's disease) is associated with a particularly high amyloid frequency and simultaneously has the highest mortality, it is understandable that post-mortem cases of JCA record a high occurrence of amyloidosis. Amyloidosis was the cause of death in all six cases of Munthe (1972). We ourselves found in 10 of our 21 autopsies of children a secondary AA-amyloidosis with regular involvement of kidneys, adrenal glands, liver, and spleen. This is related to the duration of the illness in patients with systemic JCA (Still's disease) which is between 3.5 and 12 years. In addition, we also saw in six of these ten cases amyloid deposits in the heart, which strictly speaking classes them with the primary type of amyloidosis (see p. 158). In three cases, it was the cause of death. Schnitzer and Ansell (1977) reported a follow-up study from 1 to 28 years of 1272 patients who were classified as JCA although there occurred among them young patients with psoriatic arthritis (PSA) and AS. They found in 51 cases (4%) a secondary AA-amyloidosis. However, in a cohort of 243 of these patients who were followed for 15 years, an amyloidosis developed in 18 (7.4%) cases.

6 Seronegative Spondarthritides*

The discovery of common, clinical, radiological, and serological phenomena and, in particular, the common processes in the axial skeleton, as well as the familiar and genetic relationships has lead to the supposed concept "seronegative spondarthritides" (SSA). In 1976, Wright and Moll developed their concept of the

Concept of SSA

Synonyms: seronegative spondylarthropathies, seronegative spondylarthritides

SSA (today mostly known as "seronegative spondylarthritides" or "seronegative spondylarthropathies") for patients with seronegative polyarthritis associated with co-disease, in order to support the hypothesis that certain types of arthritis are closely interrelated. The most important feature is the fact that all members of the disease-group are seronegative for rheumatoid factors and that there is an association of each type of arthritis with ankylosing spondylitis (AS).

Prevalence of HLA-B27

In the 1960s, the serological analysis and recognition of human leucocyte antigens (HLA) assumed increasing importance and lead to the discovery that there is a relationship between HLA and rheumatic disorders. The increased prevalence of HLA-B27 in patients with seronegative spondylarthropathies has been known since 1973 (Brewerton et al. 1973; Schlosstein et al. 1973). In this context, Wright and Moll (1976) proposed, as a working hypothesis, to think of a large cluster of inherited immune responses, all frequently represented by the histocompatibility antigen HLA-B27 as a marker. Calin (1992) assumed that the phenotypic expression of the SSA presumably depends on an additional gene (or genes) which has not yet been ruled out and possibly further environmental triggers.

According to the criteria of the German Society of Rheumatology (Deutsche Gesellschaft für Rheumatologie 1999), the following diseases were added to the SSA-group:

Members of "SSA family"

1. Ankylosing spondylitis (AS)
2. Reactive arthritides (REAs; including Reiter's syndrome, RS)
3. Psoriatic arthritis (PSA)
4. Oligoarticular juvenile rheumatoid arthritis (JCA) type II
5. Ulcerative colitis (UC)
6. Crohn's disease (CD)
7. Whipple's disease (WD)

In how far WD is to be counted among the SSA is still being disputed.

Characteristic features of SSA

The SSA-group has, in the meantime, acquired a sharper profile which is characterized by the following features (Arnett 1986; Deutsche Gesellschaft für Rheumatologie 1999):

1. Oligo- or polyarthritis
2. Participation of the axial skeleton with sacroiliitis and/or spondylitis
3. Absence of serum rheumatoid factors
4. Lack of rheumatoid nodules
5. Frequent inflammatory involvement of tendon and fascial insertions (enthesopathy)
6. Onset predominantly in young adults and children
7. Strong familiar aggregation and intimate genetic association with HLA-B27
8. Tendency towards extra-articular manifestations including anterior uveitis (mostly in association with HLA-B27), conjunctivitis, aortitis, and skin lesions

Amor and coworkers (1990) extended this spectrum with the following further criteria:

9. Sausage-like toe or digit (dactylitis)

10. Non-gonococcal urethritis or cervicitis accompanying or within 1 month before onset of arthritis
11. Acute diarrhoea accompanying or within 1 month before onset of arthritis
12. Presence or history of psoriasis and/or balanitis and/or inflammatory bowel disease (IBD; ulcerative colitis, Crohn's disease)

Enthesopathy

Characteristic phenomena of the SSA include typical changes occurring at the transitional zone between tendons and bone.
In 1966, the Czechoslovakian rheumatologists Niepel and collaborators described changes that until today have been acquiring increasing importance in understanding the SSA. These changes were painful, radiologically defined bony appositions near the tendons radiating into the bone, in AS primarily in the region of the ischial tuberosities and the calcaneus. They described analogous processes in another 38 localisations within the skeleton. All these they considered to be "results of rheumatoid inflammations in tendinous and ligamentous insertions" and named them "enthesopathy".
In the interface between tendons and bone, the authors recognized the physiological weak point to be. The "enthesis" they defined under biomechanical aspects as follows: excessive strain and chronic over-exertion lead to ruptures of tendon fibres and to "enthesopathy", that may manifest in 38 points of tendon insertion in the skeletal system. The coherence between bone and cartilage is weakened in the process, the continuity of the cartilaginous zone is impaired, bone may become denuded, so that small portions of cartilage and bone are separated from each other by the pull of tendon fibres. "The damage induces repair, and with it the appearance of abundantly vascularized granulation tissue and the reconstruction in the bone and the cartilaginous zone" (Niepel and Sitaj 1979). Inflammation, oedema, and new bone formation result in the radiographically detectable manifestation of enthesopathy.
According to these authors, the structural weakness of the bond between tendon and bone also predisposes for the development of "enthesis spondylarthritica". While Niepel and his colleagues regarded enthesopathy merely as a structurally effected epiphenomenon in various disease entities, Schilling and Schacherl (1967) identified enthesopathy as a pathognomonic structural element of PSA and juvenile AS, that finds its manifestation in "ossifying tendostosis" and "capsulitis", and is radiographically visible as "protuberances" (Schacherl and Schilling 1967). In that way, enthesopathy advanced from a "phenomenon" to a still valid "symptom".
In 1971, Niepel's observations found their completion: Ball realized that enthesopathy was the general mechanism at the basis of the beginning and the further course not only of AS but also of all other members of the SSA-group.
Even if the importance of enthesopathy for the concept of SSA is undisputed today, the pioneer work of Niepel and Sitaj should not be forgotten. They were remarkably good observers.

Clinical manifestations

While the characteristic process of ossification develops slowly and may not be recognized for quite a long period of time, the clinical picture of SSA is characterized by asymmetrical arthritides, predominantly affecting joints in the lower extremities. In some patients, the symptoms may be transient and disappear completely, in others, they may reside. Some patients, especially those with AS and PSA, may develop the clinical picture of chronic arthritis.

Pathology

Although the pathological process amongst the various SSA differs in quantitative features, it is in many respects qualitatively analogous.

Bony metaplasia as general mechanism

The pathological picture of SSA is determined essentially by metaplastic processes in different structures. The tendency to bony metaplasia can be validated as a general mechanism for the SSA.

Our studies sustain the concept of Ball, already presented in 1971, based on his most painstaking investigations, stating that the ossification processes in all disease entities of SSA proceed according to the common principle of enthesopathy. There are two mechanisms involved in the enthesopathic process:

Two mechanisms of ossification

1. Desmal ossification which occurs at transitional zones between bone and collagen tissue. This form of ossification, which has also given this pathogenetic principle its name, is typical for enthesopathy. Bone and tendon or capsular tissue respectively are each made up of the same collagen type I.
2. Enchondral ossification, a very rare process in SSA, according to our observations and those of Ball, occurs only in the context of adjacent desmal ossification. It takes place in articular cartilage in patiens with PSA as well as in the nucleus pulposus, and in intervertebral articular cartilage in those with AS.

Bony metaplasia

The actual enthesopathic process is characterized by metaplasia of collagen fibres into fibrous bone. In contrast to Ball, we never observed inflammatory infiltrations or other signs indicating present or past inflammation in the site of bony metaplasia. The realization of this metaplastic tendency differs amongst the various SSA. The most pronounced is that in AS, less in PSA, RS, and the other REA, and least with IBD (CD, UC). Accordingly, the bony ankylosis characterizes the basic mechanism of the SSAs, the characteristics of which are:

Basic mechanism

1. A strict coherence with original bony structures.
2. A tendency of adjacent bones to fuse with each other.
3. The use of pre-existing fibre framework made up of collagen type I (enthesis) as a leading structure and the continuous incorporation into newly formed fibrous bone.
4. Ossification processes generally are multilocular and frequently take place synchronously.

In most cases, the histological changes of the synovial membrane of patients with different types of SSA allow a differentiation from synovial processes in rheumatoid arthritis (RA), osteoarthritis (OA) or bacterial synovitides.

Characteristics of synovial tissue

In 1975, we first discovered some characteristic features in the synovial membranes of patients with SSA. Since then, further studies on the synovial membranes of patients with PSA and those with incipient AS, as well as with other types of SSA have confirmed these observations (Espinoza et al. 1982; Fassbender and Fassbender 1992). The synovial membranes of patients with different forms of SSA exhibit the following characteristics:

1. The synovial villi are longer and smaller than in RA and OA.
2. Fibrosis is denser than in OA but not as compact as in RA synovitis.
3. The most impressive feature of SSA is the abundant development of numerous new small blood vessels at an early stage, especially in the periphery of the synovial villi. Blood vessels are tiny at first and lie closely beneath the lining cells.

Blood vessels

4. The lining cells proliferate considerably during the florid stage of the disease. The multi-staged layers of cuboidal to cylindrical cell elements form an impressing contrast to the fibrotic synovial stroma in which no synovial cell proliferation occurs. In the resting stage, the lining cells are flat and single-layered.
5. Fibrin exudation is very rare. If it occurs at all, only small amounts can be seen. Stronger fibrin exudations are signs of a bacterial superinfection (see p. 395).
6 Cell infiltration is not constant and it reflects the dynamics of the process. In active cases, lymphocytes and, in particular, plasma cells may in various combinations infiltrate the villi. In AS, however, plasma cells prevail which in extreme cases form a dense, lawn-like structure. Neutrophils do not participate in SSA synovitis. We never observed true lymph follicles. Depending on the systemic process, the cell infiltration can regress and with increasing fibrosis become sparser. Altogether, the lympho-plasmocytic cell infiltration is not characteristic, can appear in all forms of arthritis, and can be used for diagnosis in SSA only in combination with the other histopathological features, especially with the typical pattern of vascularisation. The morphological picture is characteristic for the different members of the SSA family. It is crucial, therefore, to perform a surgical biopsy at the earliest possible stage because, with further progress of the disease, some of the characteristic morphological features may disappear.

Cell infiltration

Low-grade smouldering process

The overall impression of the events in the synovial membrane in SSA is that of a low-grade smouldering process with only traces of short-lived active phases which leave behind fibrosis and an increased formation of villi. Lymphocytes and plasma cells are evidence of the systemic immunological process and not the expression of an actual inflammation. In patients with SSA, we have never seen proliferation of immature synovial stroma cells, such as it occurs in RA (tumour-like proliferation, tlp; see p. 75). This supports our observation that in the SSA-group no synovial induced destruction of cartilage and bone takes place.
A critical analysis of pathological changes specific for diseases of the SSA-group shows the following common phenomena:
Through ossification of the adjacent fibrous structures, the regular bone borders are overstepped. In diseases of the SSA-group, the pathological ossification takes place exclusively by strict contact with the regular bone, contrary to the heterotopic ossification, like in myositis ossificans for example. We thereby can con-

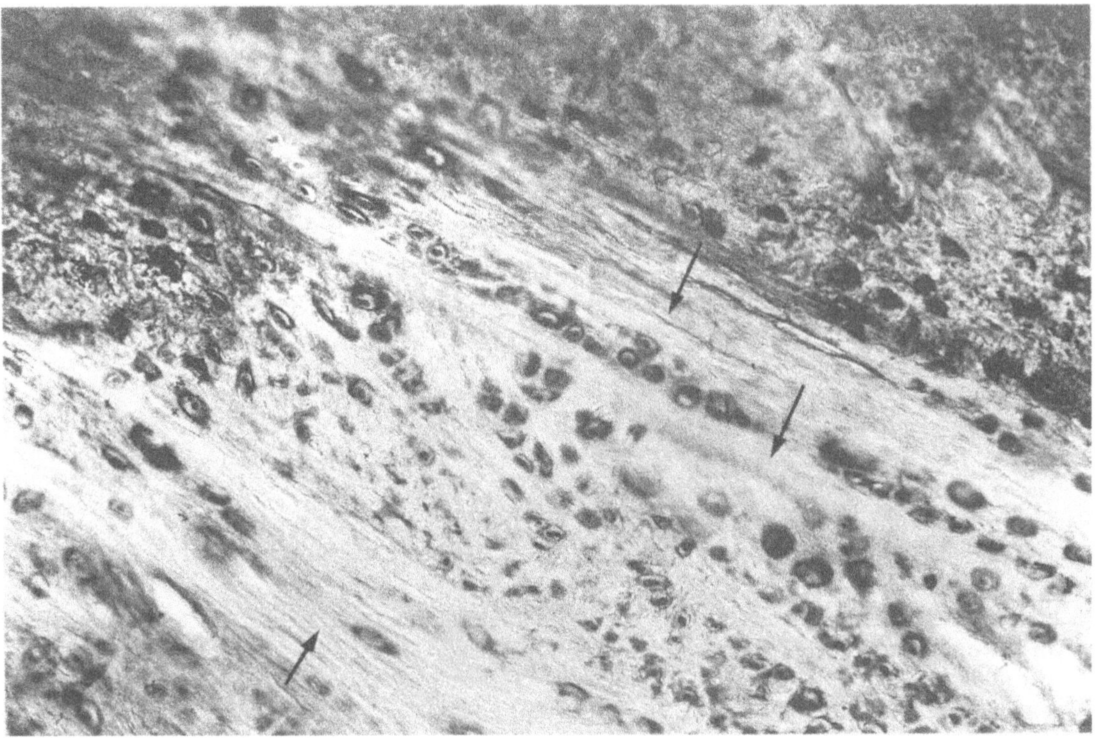

Fig. 6.1 Severe enthesopathy with ossification in the area of hip joint. *Lower and middle half*, chondroid metaplasia of the collagenous tendon tissue; *upper half*, osseous transformation. *Arrows*, remaining collagenous tendon structure

Enthesopathy

sider the ossification in the area of tendinous insertions (enthesopathy) as well as the ossification at the outer bone contours, like in PSA for example, and in the region of the vertebral column in AS as morphologically analogous processes. The different localizations in the area of tendons, capsules, and ligamentous structures, however, share one phenomenon: the ossification courses in the region of radiating collagenous fibres (Fig. 6.1). We never saw evidence of actual or subsided inflammation in the area of these enthesopathic ossification processes of the vertebral column or other localizations! We are convinced that the pathognomonic ossifications and ankylosing processes observable within the SSA-group are in no way consequences of a primary inflammation. Besides that, according to common knowledge and our observations, ossification and ankylosing processes do not belong to the sequelae of non-bacterial inflammatory processes (see p. 199).

Synovitides and periostitides in SSA are, according to our observations, secondary transient accompanying phenomena, which may be indeed clinically impressive, but they are not responsible for the only specific process: the ossification. Anti-phlogistic medication is important to enable patients to benefit from physiotherapy without having to endure too much pain, but it is obvious that they will not exert any influence on the ossification process!

SSA and HLA-B27

AS represents the classical full picture of the SSA with almost obligatory HLA-B27 association in more than 90% of white patients, while in the normal population, the prevalence of the gene is only 8%–10% (Schur 1994; Brown et al. 1996). The level of HLA-B27 association of the different members of the SSA-group in general (but not necessarily) correlates with affliction of the vertebral column and sacroiliac joints. Thus, 60%–90% of patients with REA (including RS) are HLA-B27-positive, however, only in 20%–30% of patients with previous REA, unilateral or bilateral sacroiliitis or syndesmophytes can be detected (Sairanen et al. 1969; Marsal et al. 1981; Leirisalo et al. 1982). In contrast, the frequency of sacroiliitis and syndesmophytes in PSA is in accordance with about 20%–25% occurrence of HLA-B27 which in this disease lies around 20%–35% (Schilling and Stadelmann 1986). Striking in this context, however, is that in PSA, with axial skeleton involvement, the association with HLA-B27 increases to about 60%–90% whereas in PSA with only peripheral joint involvement there is no significant correlation (see p. 215).

There is no doubt that the MHC-I-gene HLA-B27 is the trade mark of the SSA-group. Early observations in monozygotic twins, however, have shown that another component is necessary for the diseases to develop (Arnett 1984; Brown et al. 1997).

Role of microorganisms

Numerous findings bear witness to the role of microorganisms as decisive cofactors for the manifestation. Expressly the bacteria *Klebsiella pneumoniae*, *Chlamydia trachomatis*, *Yersinia enterocolitica*, *Salmonella typhimurium*, and *Shigella flexneri* are accused of potentially triggering the diseases (Sieper and Braun 1995). Brown and coworkers (1997) go even further in their deduction that "the susceptibility to AS is largely genetically determinated but the environmental trigger for the disease is probably ubiquitous".

Role of HLA-B27

The role of the HLA-B27 gene has been largely elucidated: the HLA-type I (HLA-A, HLA-B, HLA-C) molecules serve to present peptides on the cell's surface. They present fragments of proteins that have access to the cytosol. The HLA molecule forms a pocket in that the peptide is deposited. Autologous or "foreign" peptides that are presented by HLA-positive cells may trigger a cascade of immune mechanisms. It is, however, also conceivable that, on the grounds of deficient affinity, HLA-B27 may not be able to bind certain antigens. This might then result in the development of antigen persistence.

Molecular mimicry

For a long time, the role of molecular mimicry in the pathogenesis of AS has been discussed (Ebringer 1983). In this case, the pathogens would deceive the body's defence mechanisms by assimilating their antigenic structures to those of their host. The consequence would be a partial tolerance to the intruder and, finally, the pathogens remaining within the host and causing frequently recurring infections. Molecular mimicry may also cause an alienation of the host towards parts of its own tissue. Several observations are in favour of a cross-reactivity between the antigens of certain pathogens and HLA-B27.

HLA-B27 subtypes

Meanwhile, 20 subtypes of HLA-B27 can be differentiated; some are highly associated with SSA, e.g. B2705 and B2702, others, such as B2709, are not at all related to the disease. Sobao and coworkers report an HLA-B39-gene in a Japanese SSA patient who was negative for HLA-B27 (1999).

At present, other genetic factors are being searched for. Results of these investigations are still being controversially discussed (Gonzalez et al. 1999a).
The specific routes, i.e. those by the HLA-system, all end where a pathological immune process begins, the mechanisms of which are ultimately unspecific. These immune mechanisms are, as is well-known, capable of inducing non-bacterial inflammations.
In other words, the pathogenetic chain, which has so far been assembled by using numerous observations, ends with an item that only offers an explanation for the pathogenesis of inflammatory processes, in particular for synovitides in SSA, that characterize the clinical picture of the REAs and of PSA. These, however, do not differ qualitatively from other, non-bacterial synovitides, as they occur in OA for example.
From what we know today, there is not yet a solid, logically sound link in the chain towards the stigma that distinguishes HLA-B27-associated diseases, namely ossification and ankylosis!
This link might be provided by observations of the effects of bone modelling proteins (BMP), but this poses the question as to how BMP can be activated in the SSAs? The unspecific inflammation does not offer an answer because inflammations of the same quality occur with other diseases but do not induce the formation of new bone.
In the pathogenetic chain of events in HLA-associated diseases of the SSA-group there is thus a link missing between the immunologically induced inflammation and the specific type of ossification. This gap cannot yet be bridged.

6.1 Ankylosing Spondylitis

Synonyms: Bechterew's disease, spondylitis ankylosans, spondylitis ankylopoetica, Morbus Marie-Strümpell, rheumatoid spondylitis.

6.1.1 Definition

"Flagship"

The term "ankylosing spondylitis" (AS) is to be preferred to any of the eponyms, since it is descriptive of the main characteristic of the disease and enjoys international recognition. It has to be emphasized that AS is the "flagship" of the SSA-group. In AS, the pathological ossifications, which not only characterize but also dominate the clinical picture, are the most prominent.
AS is a systemic disorder of connective tissue of the skeleton and some other organs, specifically of the spine and its adjoining skeletal parts with metaplastic and ankylosing changes. Arthritis of the peripheral joints is common, visceral manifestations less so. The disease is distinct from RA, on the one hand, and from degenerative disease of the spine with excessive syndesmophyte formation (hyperostotic spondylosis), on the other.
Clinical as well as morphological variations are such that any single pathogenetic mechanism would fail to explain the different manifestations.

6.1.2 History

Prehistoric findings

Spinal ankylosis has been able to play the role of a fossil in the history of medicine. Prehistoric findings occasionally show skeletal features which have in the past been interpreted as AS but which are, in fact, the result of osteophyte formation in osteoarthritis (OA). However, Ruffer and Rietti (1911, 1912) described the spine of a human skeleton of the third Egyptian dynasty in the third millennium B.C. showing the first definite case of AS. The earliest description of the pathological anatomy of the disease is by the Irish physician Connor who, in 1695, reported an "unusual skeleton", whose vertebrae and ribs, as far as the pelvis, formed one single piece of bone without the interruption of a joint or cartilage. The first clinical descriptions in the 19th century came from England, including the detailed clinical and pathological description by Fagge (1877) of a 34-year-old man with a stiff, kyphotic spine, lack of chest movement, and ankylosis of the hip joints. However, Fagge's claim to priority was forgotten.

Earliest description

In the German literature, the first mention of the disease came from Strümpell, a physician in Leipzig in 1884. He described the cases of three young males who, apart from spinal restriction of movement, had involvement of the joints of the lower limbs and coxitis.

The Petersburg neurologist von Bechterew (Fig. 6.2) added two cases of a similar type (1899a,b). However, the term "Bechterew's disease" is founded on the description of five cases in 1893, probably only one of whom suffered from true AS.

"Bechterew's disease"

In France, Marie and Astie described the disease in 1897. As did the pathologist Leri (1899), they regarded it as a primary infectious and toxic osteopathy with porosis and secondary compen-

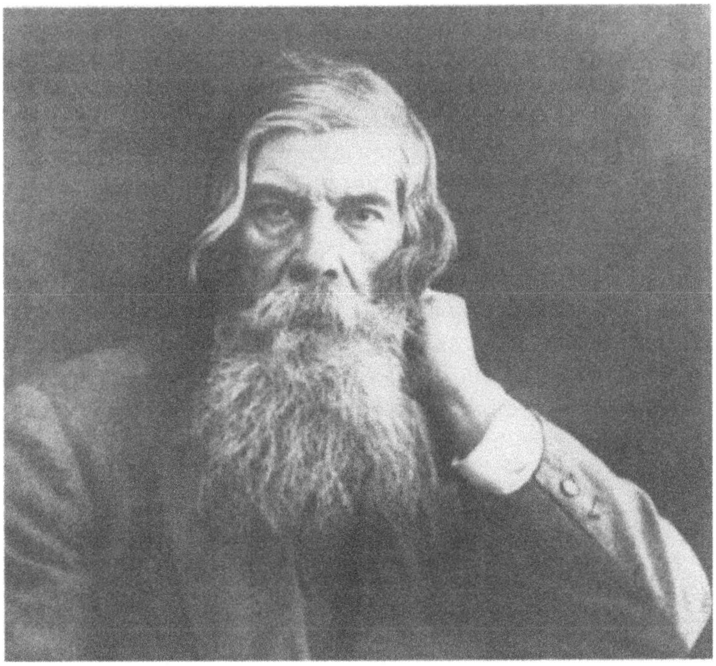

Fig. 6.2

W. von Bechterew, 1857–1927, neurologist in St. Petersburg

"Strümpell-Marie-Bechterew disease"

satory ligamentous ossification considered it to be an entity separate from other forms of "rheumatic" diseases and noted the high incidence among males. Their reports led to the eponym "Strümpell-Marie-Bechterew disease".

Spondylo-arthritic component

The spondylo-arthritic component of AS was particularly noted by Güntz (1933) and also by Klinge (1933). The autopsy performed by Güntz showed an early stage limited to inflammation of intervertebral joints without marked ossification of intervertebral discs. As late as 1943, Oppenheimer regarded AS as "RA" of intervertebral joints and viewed all other pathological features as consequential to this.

Significant contributions in the pathology of AS were made by Cruickshank (1951, 1956, 1960), Hart (1953, 1966), Sharp (1957, 1965), Wilkinson and Bywaters (1957), the Swiss authors Böni and Kaganas (1954) and Aufdermaur (1953). Of leading importance are the investigations of Ball (1971, 1979). Schilling (1974) performed a comprehensive study of 600 patients; the analysis of this material and his interpretation still remain valid within the present-day knowledge of the condition.

6.1.3 Epidemiology

The prevalence of AS varies between 0.1% (van der Linden et al. 1984), 0.9% (Braun et al. 1998), and 1.4% (Gran et al. 1985). The differences arise from the varying frequency of HLA-B27 as fundamental risk factor in the respective population. In 1975, Calin and Fries reported 18% AS diseases among HLA-B27-positive blood donors.

It seems hardly possible to objectify the actual prevalence of AS, as there is a strong possibility of a considerable number of mild and larvate cases hidden behind a lower back symptomatology of unknown origin. Particularly in female patients, the disease generally causes rather few symptoms. The idea that this disease affects in 90% male patients requires, thus, a revision. The disease usually has a symptomatic onset between the ages of 15 and 40 years with a marked accumulation in the 30s.

Genetic factors

Genetic factors play a significant role. Some studies have shown that only 2% of randomly selected B27-positive subjects develop AS, whereas at least 20% of B27-positive relatives of AS patients are at risk (van der Linden et al. 1984). Emery and Lawrence (1967) found bilateral sacroiliitis in 16% of first-degree relatives of patients (Fig. 6.3). As early as 1955, Stecher and Ausenbachs (1955) interpreted this as a predisposition of heterozygotes with an autosomal-dominant gene the penetration of which is weaker in women.

Bilateral sacroiliitis

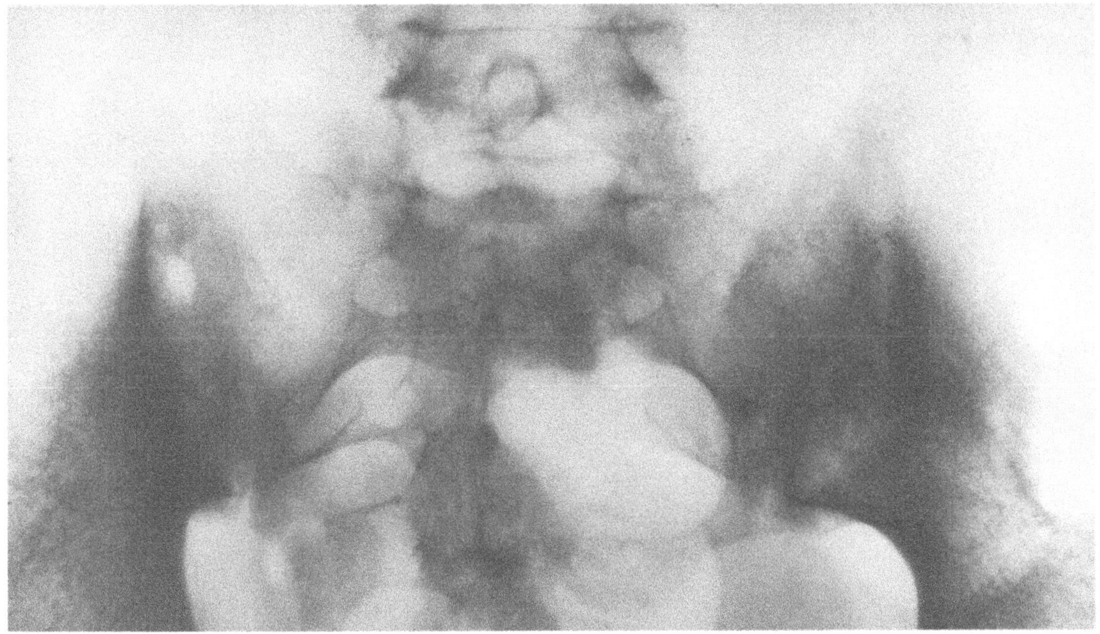

Bilateral sacroiliitis in adolescent ankylosing spondylitis: boy aged 17 years with 3-year history. There is a wide area of involvement

Fig. 6.3
Ankylosing spondylitis

6.1.4 Clinical Manifestations

As the clinical picture of a fully-developed AS is characteristic, the diagnosis can usually be established with certainty and without delay. The New York Criteria, modified by Ball (1993), include the following symptoms which are characteristic for AS:

New York Criteria

1. Lower back pain of at least 3 months' duration, improved by exercise but not relieved by rest
2. Limitation of lumbar spine movement in both the sagittal and the frontal planes
3. Decreased chest expansion relative to normal values for age and sex
4. Bilateral sacroiliitis, grade 2–4
5. Unilateral sacroiliitis, grade 3–4

Diagnosis of AS is definite if the patient suffers from unilateral sacroiliitis grade 3 or 4 or from bilateral sacroiliitis grade 2 or higher, and from at least one of the other clinical symptoms (Ball 1993).

Sacroiliitis is of central importance not only for an early diagnosis by radiological means but also for classifying among the various diseases of the SSA-group. The inflammatory component, corresponding to a narrow articular space and a minimal synovial membrane, is of less importance. Of decisive consequence is, that in sacroiliitis, an analogous process takes place as does in the small joints, in particular as in AS: at first, sacral-hyaline and iliosacral-fibrocartilaginous joint surfaces fuse. This synchondrosis may be followed by enchondral ossification with complete ankylosis (Figs. 6.4, 6.5).

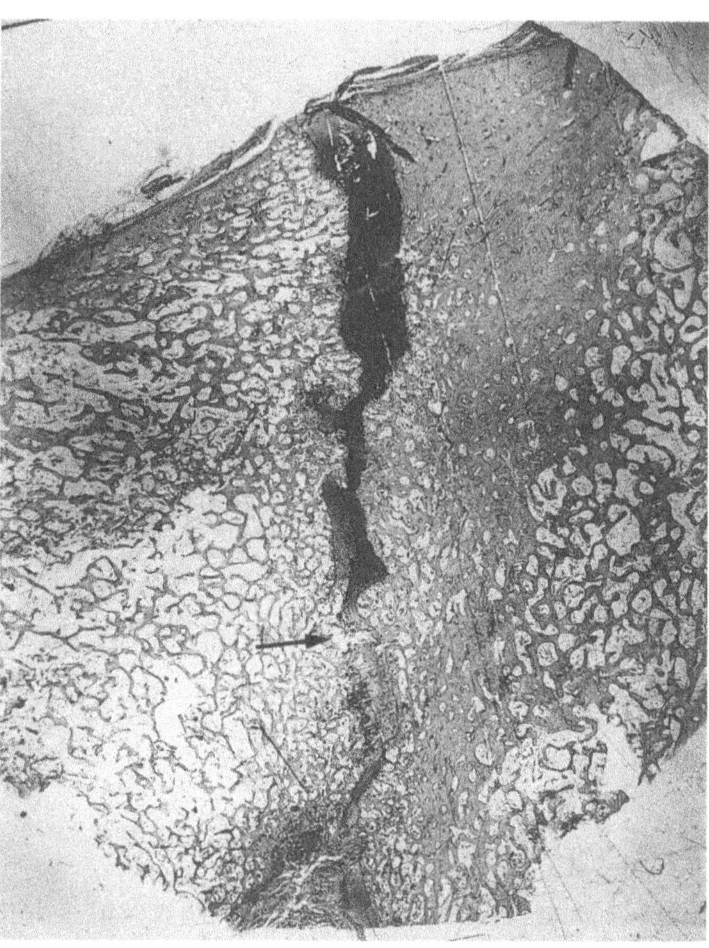

Fig. 6.4
Ankylosing spondylitis

Sacroiliac joint. Complete synchondrosis (*arrow*) without periarticular ossification. (Wurm 1957)

Because of the slowly progressive course and the comparatively benign nature of the lumbar-spine symptoms, AS is often not suspected before a patient is in his 30s. The most common first manifestations are mono- or oligoarthritides occurring in a patient's 20s; their significance as an early symptom of AS, however, is rarely recognized.

6.1.5 Pathogenesis and Pathology

Uncharacteristic arthritides

From our observations of synovial biopsies, we believe that the systemic disease begins before the age of 16 years and that its first clinical manifestations are not ossifications, but uncharacteristic arthritides of the knee and ankle joints. Therefore, too often, most therapeutic measures, which would ideally assist the patient in choosing a suitable occupation, are too late, if they are only taken after the classical lumbar-spine symptoms have lead to the diagnosis.

Pathological ossification process

The pathological process of ossification advances on two "fronts" simultaneously:

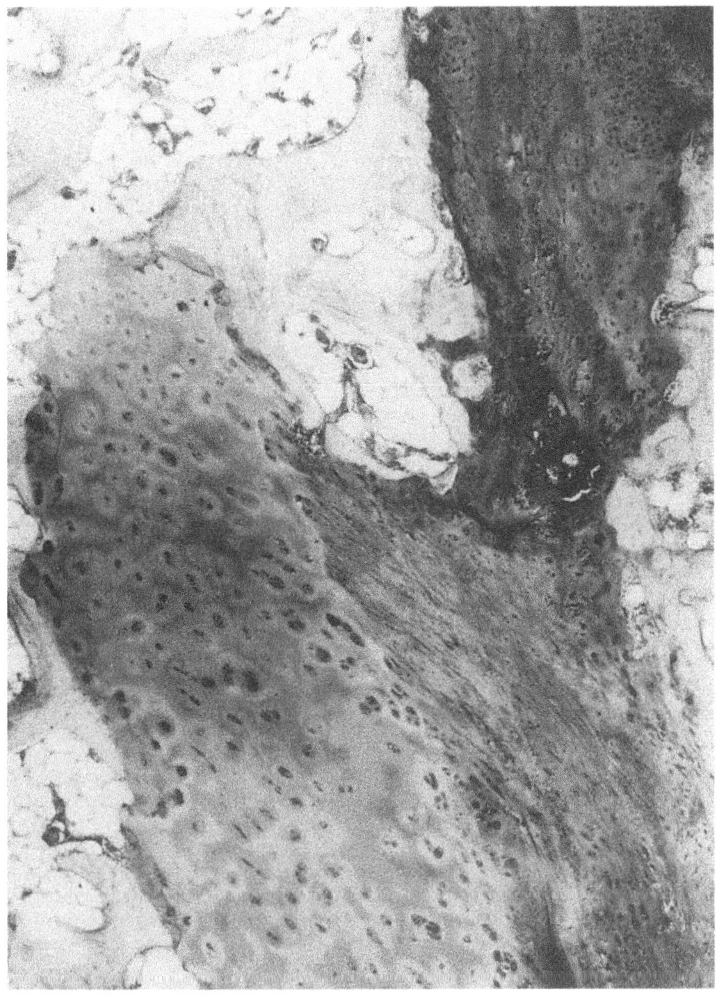

Sacroiliac joint. Enlargement of Fig. 6.4. There is continuity between sacral hyaline and iliac fibrocartilage

Fig. 6.5
Ankylosing spondylitis

1. In areas of tendon insertions (enthesis) by way of direct, desmal ossification due to the transformation of fibroblasts into osteoblasts, and of tendinous collagen tissue into fibrous bone.
2. In areas of contact of bone with hyaline cartilage, such as in the joint or nucleus pulposus by way of enchondral ossification. Apart from this, also in areas of especially strained tendon insertions, chondroid metaplasia of the tight collagenous connective tissue may precede ossification (see p. 193).

Up to the present time, pathogenetic concepts of different authors remain controversial. The term "ankylosing spondylitis" implies that inflammation plays a causal role in the characteristic ankylosing ossification process. But doubts concerning this role were documented as early as 1950 (van Swaay 1950; Ott and Wurm 1957).
The very first beginnings of the formation of syndesmophytes, the transgression of the borders between the cortical bone of the vertebra and the anulus fibrosus are difficult to elucidate: if at all,

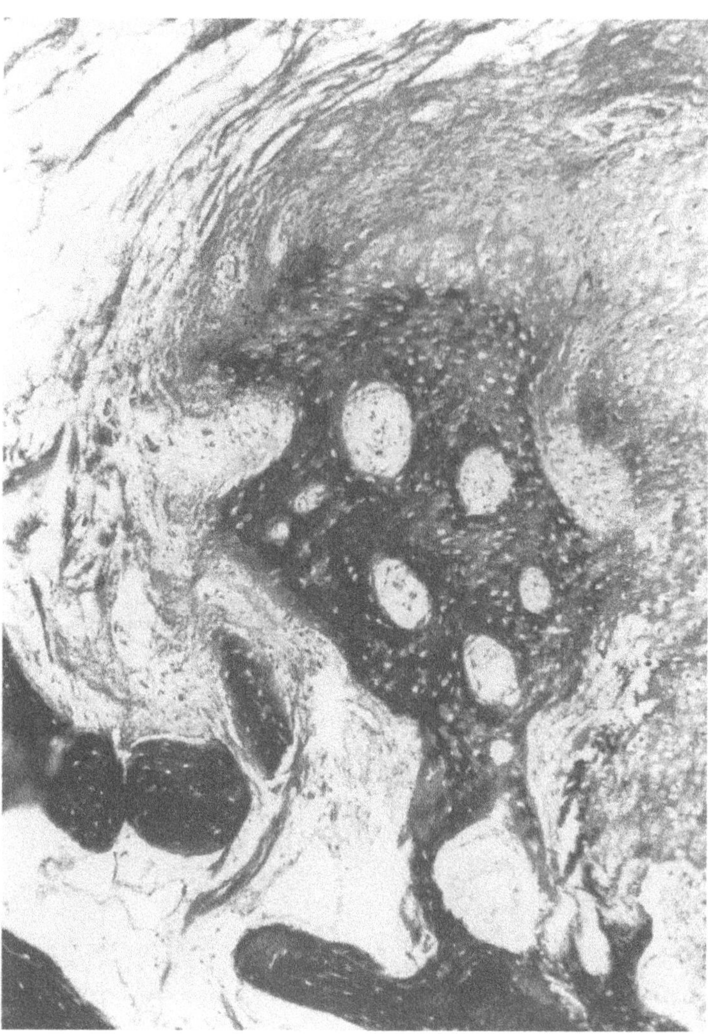

Fig. 6.6
Ankylosing spondylitis

Enthesopathy at the tendon insertion of the greater trochanter. New bone formation near the tendon irradiating into the bone. No inflammatory elements

Non-bacterial inflammation

Enthesopathy

spine biopsies are available only from patients at late- or end-stage disease, and most studies are performed using only autopsy material. Having observed small infiltrations by lymphocytes and plasma cells within foci of ossification, Ball (1979) postulated that some non-bacterial inflammation should trigger the ossifying process and termed the process, which he thought triggered secondary, reparative bone formation, "erosive inflammation".

The fact that our findings do not substantiate Ball's findings is not in itself an absolute proof against his theory. If, however, we observe ossification in AS under the general aspect of enthesopathy, characteristic for diseases of the SSA family, as is in accordance with Ball's concept, we can acquire some understanding of the pathogenesis of syndesmophyte formation by studying analogous processes in the transitional zone between bone and tendon (Fig. 6.6). The anatomical situation at tendon insertions and at the area of contact between cortical bone and periosteum is

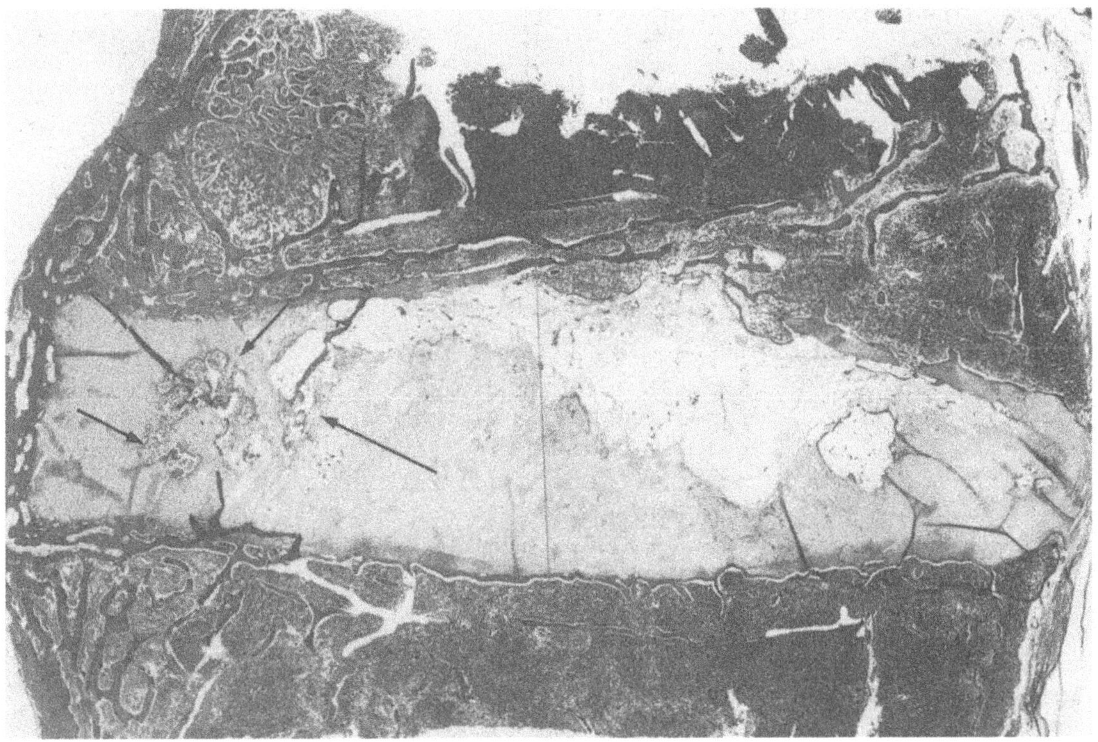

Lumbar spine. Narrow syndesmophyte and early enchondral ossification (*arrows*) of nucleus pulposus. Dissolution of bony endplates and osteoporosis

Fig. 6.7
Ankylosing spondylitis

analogous to the border between vertebra and anulus fibrosus. In all these cases, the framework of bone and adjacent tissues consists of the same collagen type I. In numerous biopsies of patients with psoriatic arthritis (PSA) and with Reiter's syndrome (RS; see pp. 212), we have had the opportunity to study the enthesopathic process at various developmental stages. As outlined above, the basic mechanism is desmal ossification. When coming into contact with the adjacent cartilage, such as the nucleus pulposus, cartilage tissue undergoes secondary, enchondral ossification.

Desmal ossification

Judging from our observations, we believe that the impetus of ossification is the activation and hyperplasia of fibroblasts at the border of fibrous bone. As the fibroblasts migrate closer to the surface of the bone, they transform into osteoblasts. The osteoblasts then deposit into the collagen network which attaches fibrous tissue and bone to each other, and form new fibrous bone (see p. 180). The enthesopathic process is thus characterized by the transgression of the contour of the bone, brought about by metaplasia of collagen tissue into fibrous bone. An osteophyte formed by lamellar bone gives evidence of its advanced age, as after a period of time, the primary fibrous bone matures into compact bone.

Metaplasia of collagen tissue into fibrous bone

The term "syndesmophyte" was coined by Forestier and Robert (1934) who interpreted this radiological appearance as an ossification of ligaments. Van Swaay (1950) and Ott and Wurm (1957) showed, however, that ossification usually involves the anulus fibrosus (Fig. 6.7).

Formation of syndesmophytes

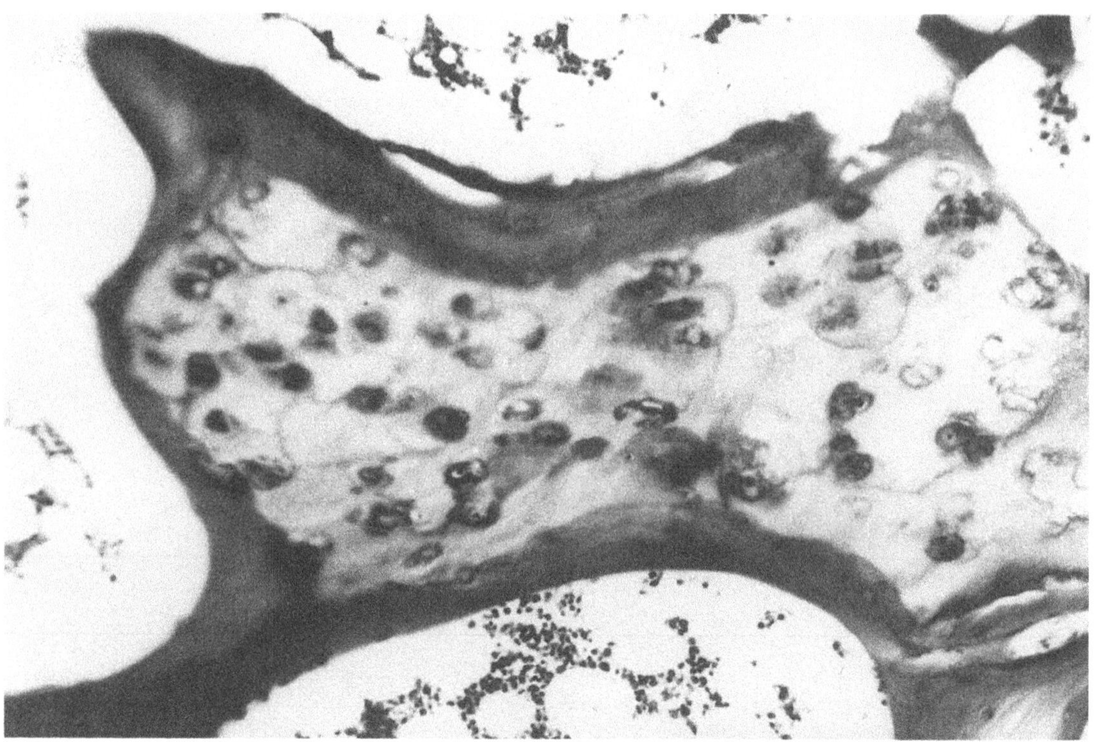

Fig. 6.8
Ankylosing spondylitis

Thoracic spine. Remnants of nucleus pulposus surrounded by seams of bone

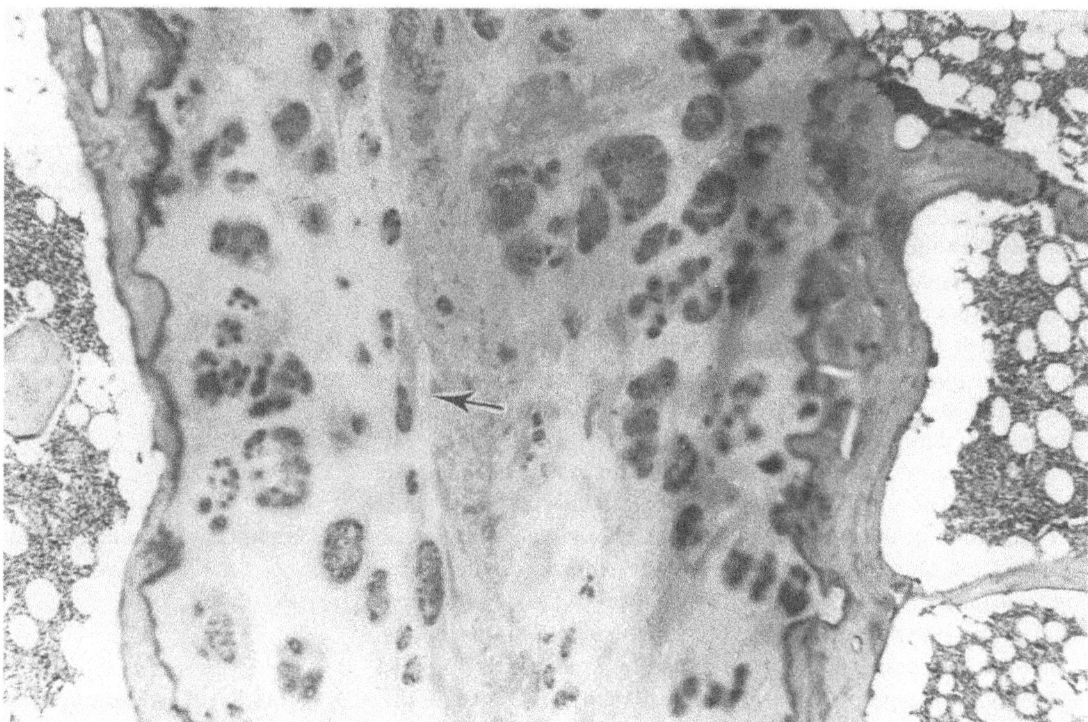

Fig. 6.9
Ankylosing spondylitis

Thoracic intervertebral joint. Central coalescence of cartilaginous surfaces (*arrow*) surrounded by clusters of chondrocytes

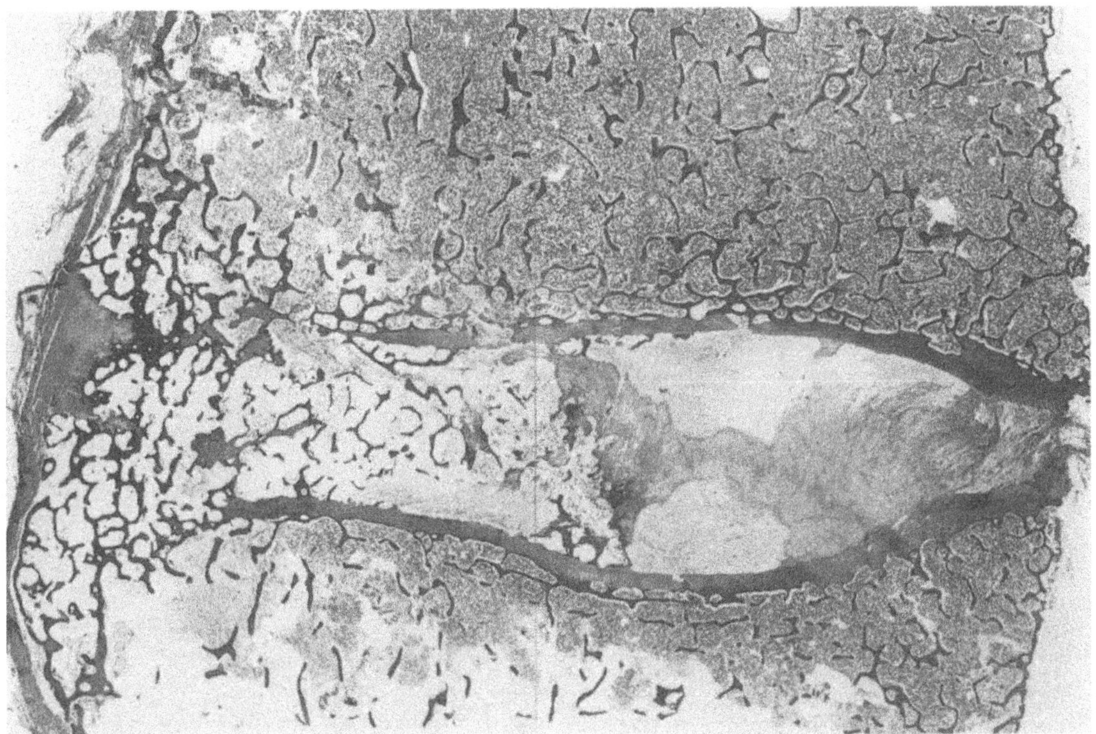

Lumbar spine. Osseous transformation of anterior half of intervertebral disc. Marked osteoporosis

Fig. 6.10
Ankylosing spondylitis

Ossification of the peri-vertebral connective tissue lying beneath the adjoining ligaments occurs less frequently, with the anterior longitudinal ligament only exceptionally undergoing ossification. This latter type of involvement resembles spondylosis hyperostotica.

Destruction of end plate

After destruction of the vertebral end plate and desmal ossification of the anulus fibrosus, the syndesmophytes move towards each other to form a bridge-like structure, initially sparing the nucleus pulposus but encasing it like a "shell" (Ball 1979; Figs. 6.8, 6.9).

Enchondral ossification of nucleus pulposus

As the disease progresses, enchondral ossification of the nucleus pulposus begins, starting from the lateral front of the syndesmophyte (Fig. 6.10). This paves the way for the ossification of the entire intervertebral disk. The prerequisite for the ossification of the nucleus pulposus is the completed formation of the "bridges" which connect the vertebral bodies to one another (Fig. 6.11).

Ball explains the growth of the syndesmophytes to be caused by recurrent inflammations, a notion which we cannot confirm by our findings. We believe that, here as well as in other areas (see p. 189), desmal ossification proceeds according to the type of enthesopathy without any inflammatory challenge. According to the laws of enthesopathy, individual or several segments may ankylose, even leading, in extreme cases, to an immobile column of bone.

Bamboo spine

The so-called bamboo appearance is brought about by the straightening out of the anterior vertebral lips, squaring of the bodies, and alteration of the spinal contours by rings of syndesmophytes (Figs. 6.12–6.14). The ensuing loss of movement is as-

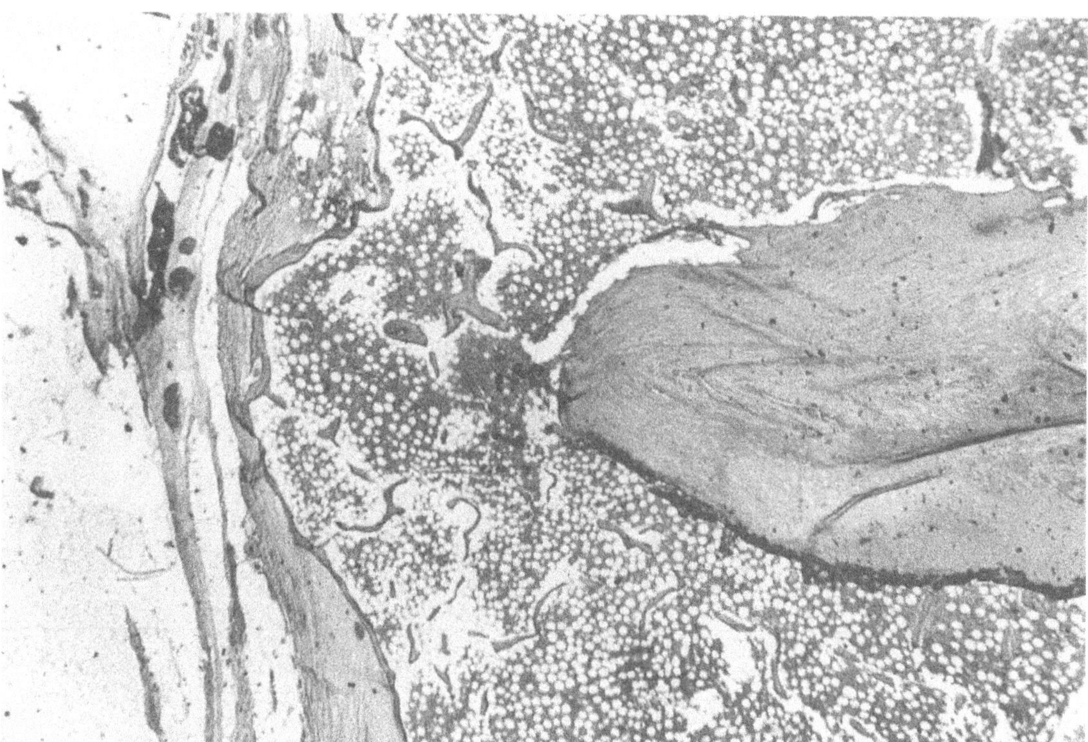

Fig. 6.11
Ankylosing spondylitis

Ossification of the margin of the anulus has led to bony continuity of the thoracic spine

Osteoporosis

sociated with osteoporosis of varying severity (Fig. 6.15). Fortunately, such extreme courses of the disease have become rare, which is probably due to more patients receiving methodical physiotherapy at the earlier stages of the disease. Antiphlogistic medication is ineffective in the treatment of ankylosing processes, but it is plausible that osteoblastic processes may be influenced by cytostatic substances.

Intervertebral joints

The ossification of apophyseal, intervertebral joints proceeds according to principles different from those outlined above, due to their being synovial, diarthrotic joints. In these, the desmal contact zone is limited to the joint capsule. Here, desmal ossification occurs according to the laws of enthesopathy in the same way as it does between the margin of the vertebral body and the anulus fibrosus, the difference being that the ossified tissue surrounds the joint with the synovial membrane and the two cartilaginous surfaces (Fig. 6.16). This results in a situation which is comparable to that of the ankylosing of finger joints in PSA. It is plausible that, in AS, as in PSA (see p. 228), the synovial membrane of intervertebral joints responds to the ossification of the capsule by slight inflammatory reactions. Ball described slight infiltrations by lymphocytes and plasma cells. Even after complete ossification of the capsule, articular cartilage may survive. A fusion of both cartilaginous surfaces takes place after the ossification of the intervertebral joint capsule. How frequently also the cartilage is a victim of ossification cannot be estimated from isolated observations. Whether the ossification of intervertebral joints depends on the ankylosing of the corresponding vertebral segment,

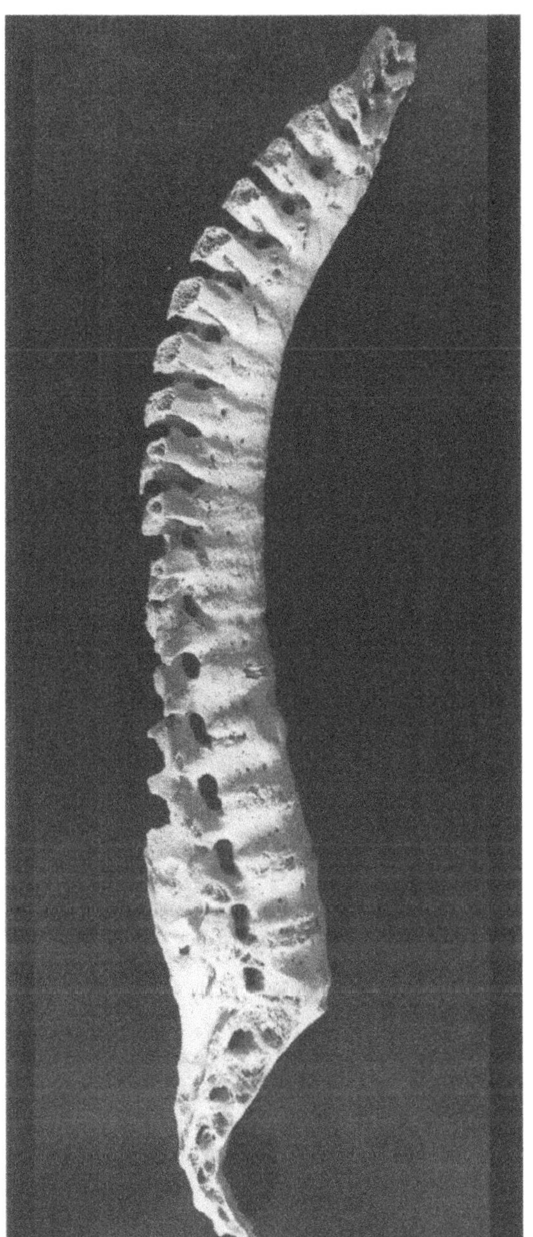

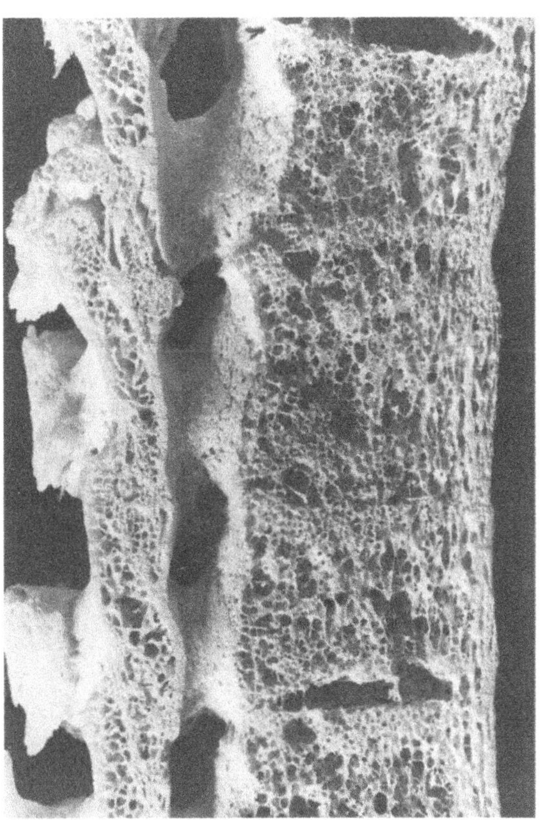

Left: Total ankylosis of vertebral column and of the small joints ("bamboo-spine"; macerated specimen)
Right: Total spinal ankylosis. All segments show bony union (macerated specimen)

Figs. 6.12 and 6.13
Ankylosing spondylitis

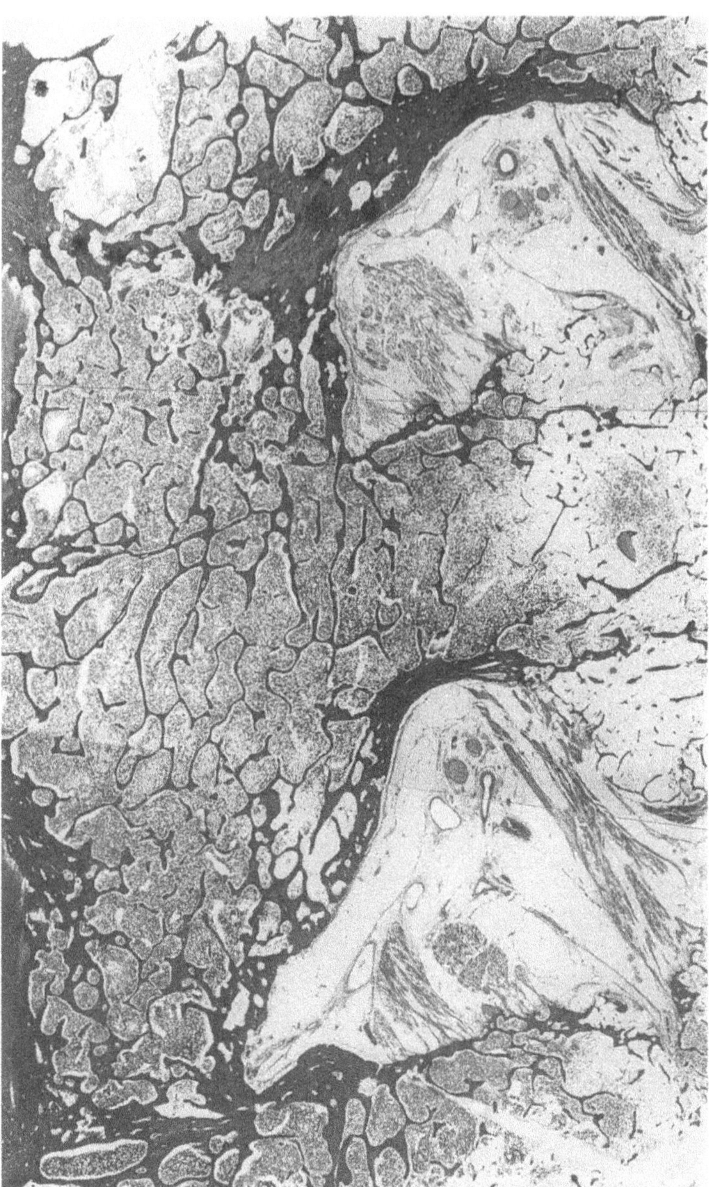

Fig. 6.14
Ankylosing spondylitis

Ankylosis of three thoracic vertebrae with bony continuity to the pediculi arcus vertebrae

or whether it occurs independently, used to be a controversial issue. Ball's report, however, of the ossification of the capsule of an intervertebral joint without the corresponding vertebral segment being ankylosed, should suffice to confirm the concept of an autonomous process.

Costovertebral joints

The anatomical situation of costovertebral joints corresponds to that found in the intervertebral joints. The ossification process can thus proceed in the same fashion as it does in the apophyseal intervertebral joints. The articular cartilage may also be preserved in a "bony shell" (Fig. 6.17). Ossification of the costovertebral joints, however, causes further complications for the patient by restricting breathing. In extreme cases, total ossification of the costovertebral joints may transform the thorax into

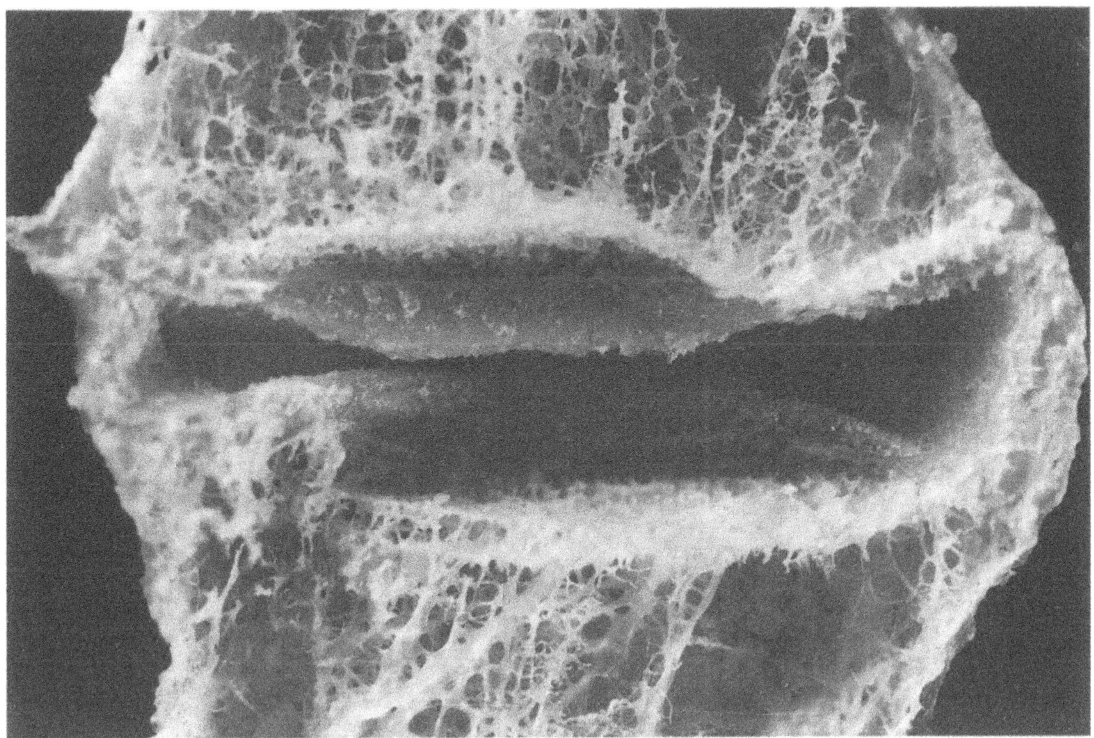

Syndesmophyte formation between two vertebral bodies, sparing the central portions of the anulus fibrosus and nucleus pulposus. Advanced osteoporosis (macerated specimen)

Fig. 6.15
Ankylosing spondylitis

a "cage" (Fig. 6.18). This not only renders thoracic respiration impossible, but also leads to chronic pulmonary hypertension and ultimately to cor pulmonale with the respective consequences.

Osteolytic processes

The insidiously slow course of AS may in some cases be painfully complicated by intercurrent lesions in the vertebral discs, the so-called Andersson lesions or spondylo-discitis (Dihlmann and Delling 1983). Even at an early stage of the disease, destructive lesions of the anterior aspects of vertebrae of the lumbar region may be apparent and have sometimes been termed "spondylitis anterior". Further osteolytic lesions of the intervertebral spaces may take the form of spondylitis marginalis or spondylo-discitis (Fig. 6.19). While anterior spondylitis affects longer segments of the vertebral column, spondylo-discitis is usually limited to one segment (Fig. 6.20).

"Spondylitis anterior"

"Spondylo-discitis"

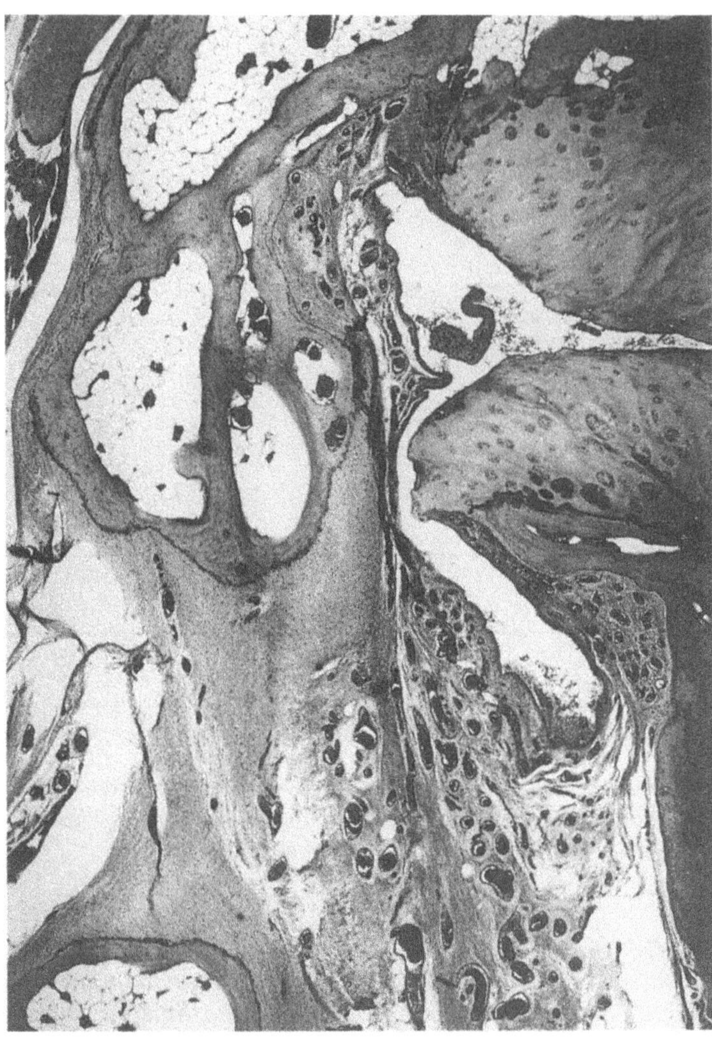

Fig. 6.16
Ankylosing spondylitis

Ossification in the capsule of an intervertebral joint. (Wurm 1957)

Spondylo-discitis may also be the cause of neck pain in patients with AS. Radiographic findings are seen in 1%–28% of patients, usually within the first 10 years after the onset of AS (Hardin and Halla 1993). The more destructive the lesion is, the more likely will there be extensive spinal ankylosis, too (Dihlmann 1979). It is not clear whether a truly inflammatory process is the basis of these osteolytic lesions, judging from findings documented to date. By radiology and at autopsy, loss of vertebral marginal structures and sclerosis of adjoining bone have been found (Fig. 6.21). We have observed there breaks in cortical bone and new formation of bone in connective tissue and in scar tissue.
In two cases, we observed lines of acute fibrinous exudate and an infiltrate of neutrophils beneath the anterior longitudinal ligament in the lumbar region. The cortical bone of the anterior margin had been eroded and breached in places. We are under the impression that such acute exudative inflammatory changes are discrete and evanescent in nature but they would appear to pro-

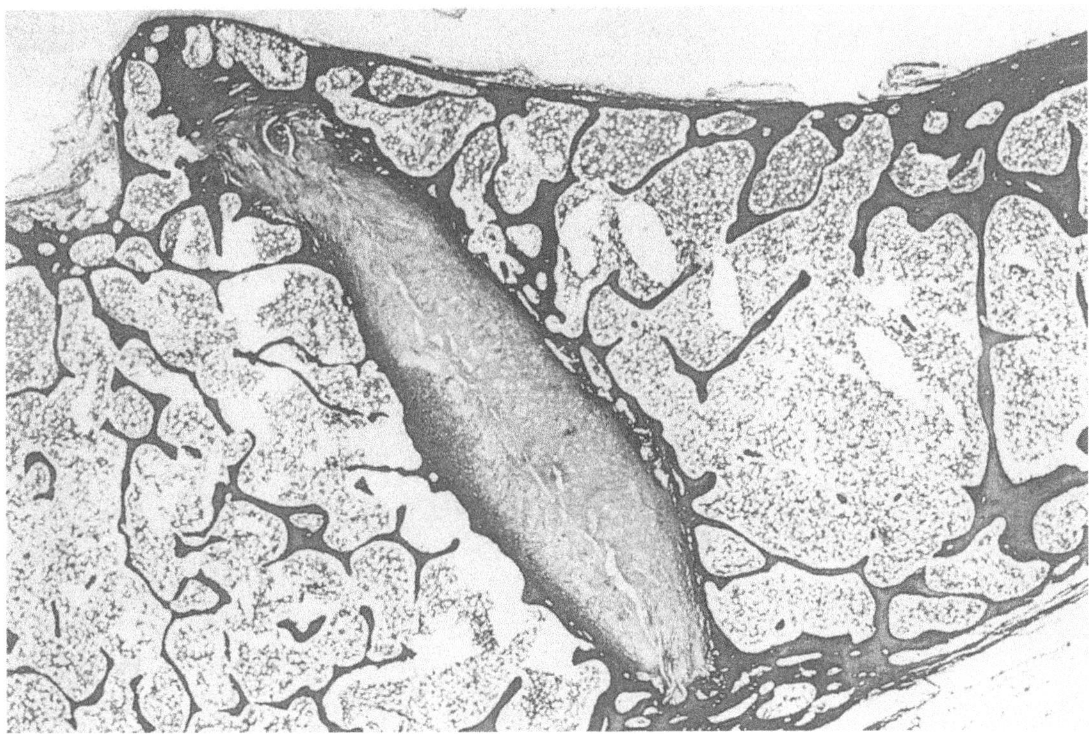

Costovertebral joint. Lateral ossification with central continuity of cartilaginous surfaces ("bony shell"). (Aufdermaur 1953)

Fig. 6.17
Ankylosing spondylitis

vide some evidence for the inflammatory nature of the osteolytic processes and to justify the term "spondylitis anterior". The fact that we are able to observe clinically inconspicuous bacterial superinfections (CLBS; see p. 395) in 13.5% in RA as well as in 8.8% in OA, gives rise to consider also transient haematogenic infections as being the cause. Therefore, we believe that these inflammatory processes in the region of the vertebral bodies are secondary bacterial affections and even though belong to the AS. The question, whether inflammatory mechanisms are an etiological factor in the development of AS, as is implied in the term spondylitis, needs to be thoroughly discussed. A remarkable lack of knowledge is apparent in many conflicting hypotheses regarding the role of inflammation in the pathogenesis of ankylosing processes. This lack of understanding and the wide variety of theories do not at least result from the fact that most morphological studies are performed on bioptic material of patients with late- or end-stage disease when possible inflammatory activity can no longer be detected.

Bacterial superinfections

Ankylosing spondylitis and inflammation

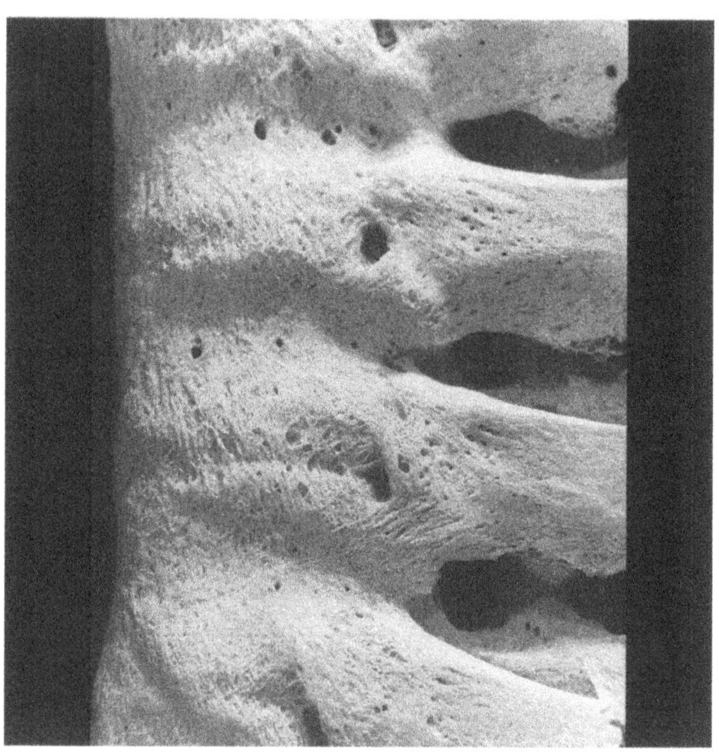

Fig. 6.18
Ankylosing spondylitis

Total ankylosis of vertebral bodies and costovertebral joints in the thoracic region. Note state of complete ossification

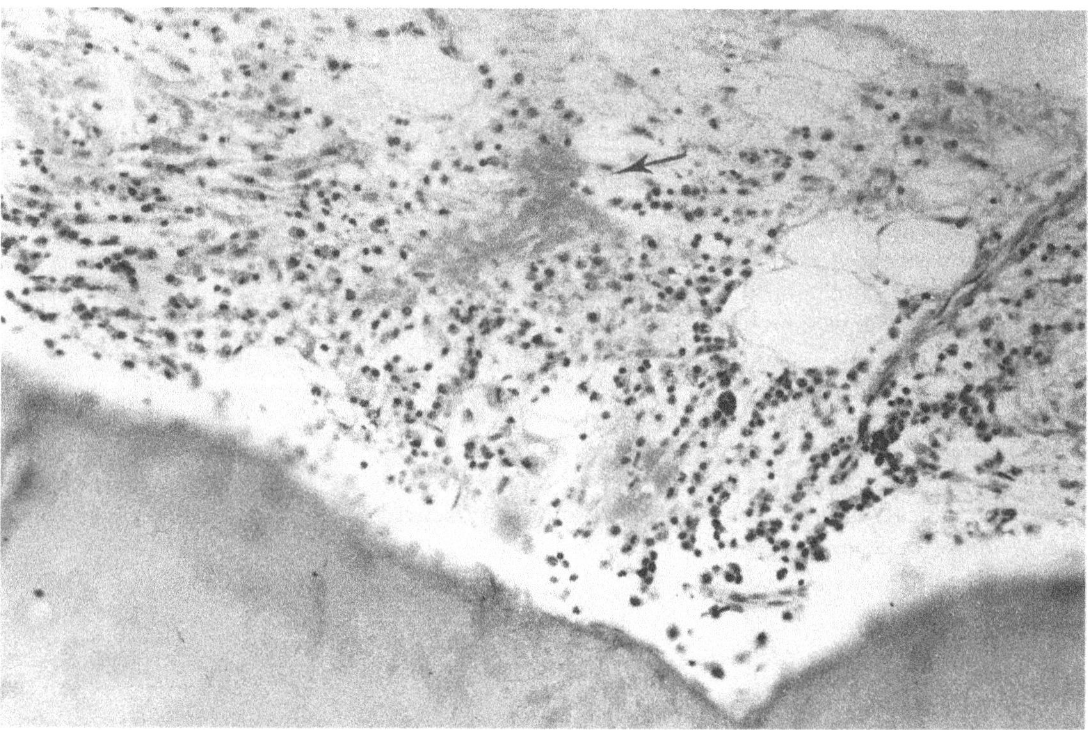

Fig. 6.19
Anterior spondylitis

Fibrin (*arrow*) and neutrophil infiltration in contact with the anterior vertebral margin

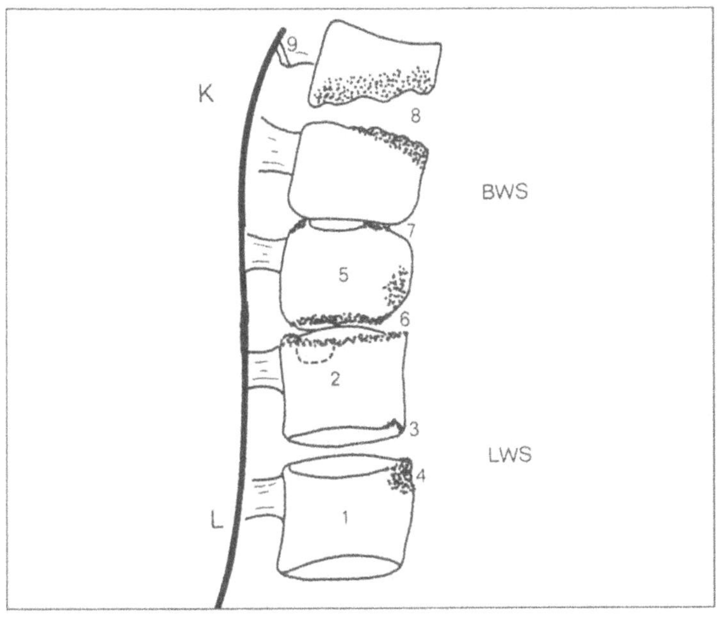

Scheme of disco-vertebral destruction (according to Schilling 1974): *1*, anterior spondylitis (anterior margin becoming convex); *2*, anterior spondylitis (straightening of anterior margin); *3*, marginal spondylitis (marginal erosion); *4*, marginal spondylitis ("shining corner"); *5*, barrel vertebra; *6*, discitis; *7*, discitis; *8*, spondylo-discitis; *9*, spontaneous fracture through apophysis with segmental collapse in spondylo-discitis

Fig. 6.20

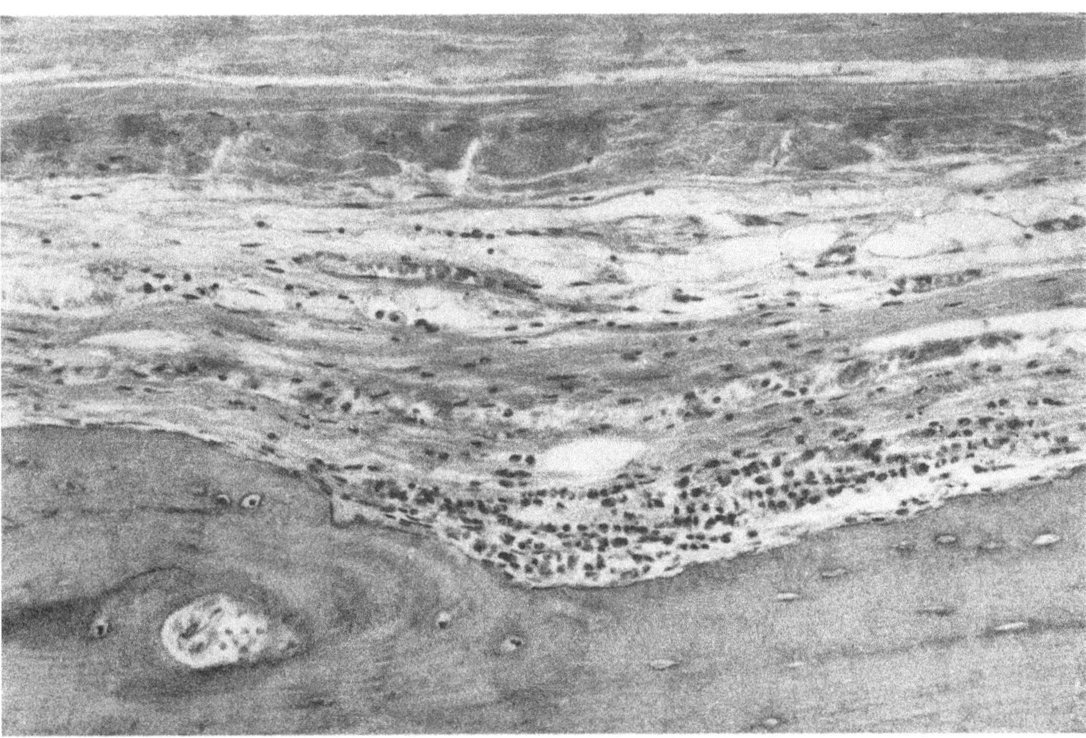

Prevertebral neutrophil infiltration in close contact with the eroded anterior vertebral margin

Fig. 6.21
Anterior spondylitis

In studies designed to substantiate the theories of an inflammatory pathogenesis of AS (Ball 1971, 1983; Bluestone 1985; Aufdermaur 1989), small aggregates of lymphocytes and plasma cells were found, some authors also report finding few neutrophils (Ball 1971). The interpretation of these findings needs to be commented on: from what we know today, lymphocytes and plasma cells are not primarily elements of inflammation, but are elements of local antigen processing and antibody production, and they themselves have no tissue-destroying potency. Even in general pathology, there is no single example of lympho-plasmocytic infiltrations which trigger or cause bone destruction or act as impetus for ossification. It is, however, feasible that tissue antigens arising from ossification processes in the course of local immune reactions attract lymphocytes and plasma cells. This is a non-specific immunological phenomenon not uncommon in different types of tissue disintegration. On the other hand, focal bacterial inflammations cannot only destroy bone within very short periods of time, but can also, after restoration, induce ossification. Bone is destroyed enzymatically by proteases released from neutrophils. Focal bacterial infections, however, have not been observed in areas of ossification in patients with AS, and, in any case, would not serve to explain the systemic enthesopathic bony metaplasia in patients with AS or other forms of SSA. The very few neutrophils, which Ball found among plasma cells and lymphocytes in some of his cases, cannot explain bone destruction. Studying enthesopathic ossification processes in other members of the SSA-group, particularly in PSA, we have never seen any infiltration by lymphocytes, plasma cells, histiocytes, or neutrophils, nor any other signs of present or past inflammation (see p. 182). On the other hand, we have not observed basically bony ankyloses in non-bacterial joint lesions in any other disease. Therefore, ossification cannot be explained as a consequence of immunologically induced inflammations. Consequently, we must speculate whether pathological gene expression controls the processes of ossification in patients possessing the HLA-B27 gene.

Immune phenomena

Role of infection in ankylosing spondylitis

Although to date we have not found any plausible reason for thinking that the ossification in AS is inflammatory in origin, there can be no doubt that there must be a component apart from the genetic disposition to trigger the onset of the disease.

Despite the almost obligatory association of AS with HLA-B27, only about 20% of the carriers of this genetic trait develop the disease.

"Triggers"

This fact, together with the observation of discordance between monozygotic twins (Arnett 1984), supports the concept that environmental factors act as triggers. Indeed, the implication of Yersinia, Shigella, Salmonella, Campylobacter, and Chlamydia in the initiation of reactive arthritides (REA) in HLA-B27 carriers supports the idea that, in a similar way, bacteria play a significant role in the pathogenesis of AS. In this context, it is of interest to consider some different hypotheses. The "cross-tolerance" or "molecular mimicry" hypothesis infers that development of disease is a consequence of structural homology between Klebsiella antigens in the case of AS (and other organisms in the case of

Different hypotheses

REA) and a part of the sequence of the heavy chain which determines HLA-B27 specificity (Ebringer 1983; Woodrow 1988). On the other hand, there is the "modifying factor" hypothesis that a plasmid-like structure originating in Klebsiella and other gut organisms gains entry to the genome of the cells of affected individuals, thereby coding for a product which becomes associated in the cell membrane with B27 molecules and thus providing a target for T cell cytotoxicity (Geczy et al. 1985). Another hypothesis is the "arthritogenic peptide theory". This theory postulates that the repertoire of peptides presented by HLA-B27 has to change during bacterial infection (Gonzalez et al. 1999b). It is suggested that this results in the breaking of tolerance to the shared epitope, leading to disease via an autoimmune mechanism.

Peripheral joints

AS predominantly affects joints of the lower extremities, primarily the knee joints. The synovial membrane is considerably enlarged compared to its normal size due to an excessive hyperplasia of villi – mainly of long and narrow ones (Fig. 6.22). Depending on the degree of inflammatory irritation, the lining cells are flat to cuboid. The synovial stroma cells are not proliferated as they are in RA (see p. 89). The lympho-plasmacellular infiltration in itself is not characteristic, it only reflects the systemic immunological process (see above). In AS, the synovitis itself is not destructive.

Especially with AS, a biopsy of the synovial membrane is of utmost importance for an early diagnosis of the disease. When examining biopsies taken from adolescents with unspecific and unexplained knee complaints, we found features characteristic of SSA (synovial villi and their blood vessels; Fig. 6.23; see p. 181). An incipient AS may thus be diagnosed years before any of the classical symptoms appear and therapeutic strategies can promptly be initiated.

Viscera

Visceral disease is an occasional accompaniment of involvement of the axial skeleton and proximal joints in the course of AS.

Cardiac manifestations

Signs of aortic insufficiency have been observed in about one-half of the cases. Characteristic pathological anatomical features are observed which may be summarized as a fibrosis of the valve ring. There is a preference for the aortic valve but similar changes are, although rarely, seen in the mitral valve. Morphological markers such as the Aschoff type of granuloma are absent, as are fibrinous vegetations or the rheumatoid type of necrosis. However, the presence of fibrous scarring and secondary adhesions with occasional ossification of the fibrous ring are characteristic and the process may extend to the valvular tissue. The valves are of increased thickness with rolled edges. Although there may be small points of adhesion between opposing valves, the extensive adhesions of margins which is one of the sequelae of rheumatic fever (RF) is not seen. In the neighbourhood of fibrotic foci, blood vessels show a hypertrophied media and endothelial hyperplasia. The mitral valve undergoes vascularisation.

Fibrosis may become extensive in the myocardium and may interfere with the conduction system and lead to heart block. Only the final fibrotic stages have been observed to date, while the more florid phase, which might have given clues to pathogenicity, has not yet been viewed.

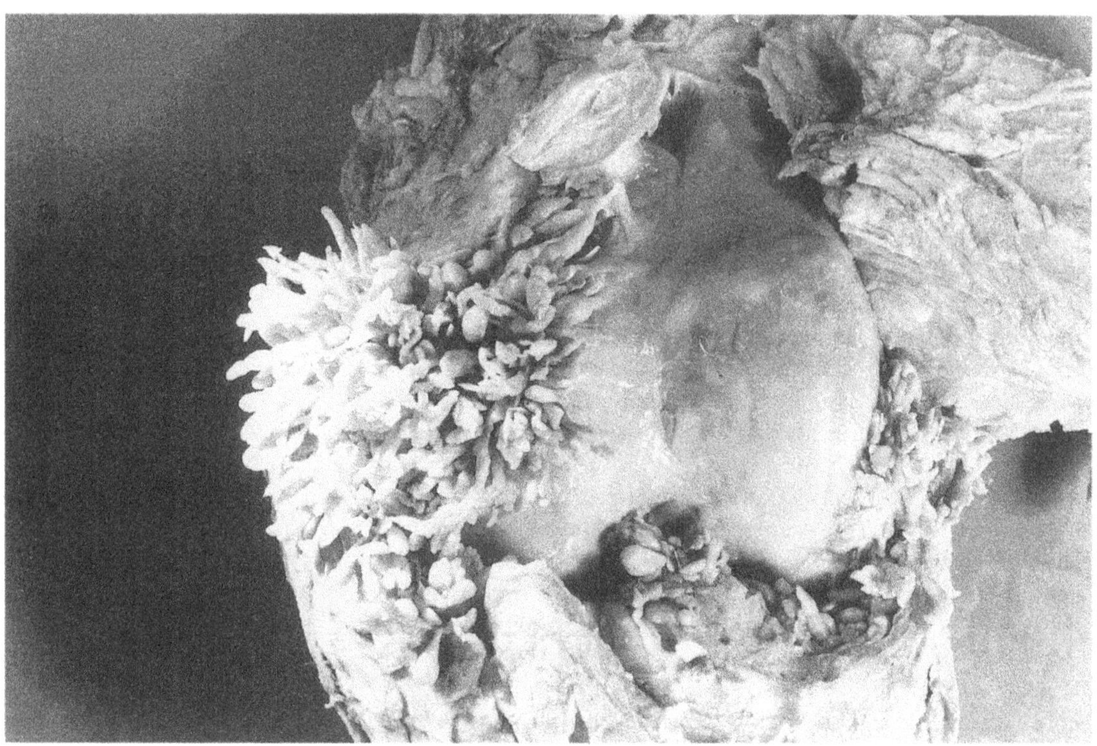

Fig. 6.22
Ankylosing spondylitis

Cauliflower-like hyperplasia of synovial villi with almost intact articular cartilage of knee joint

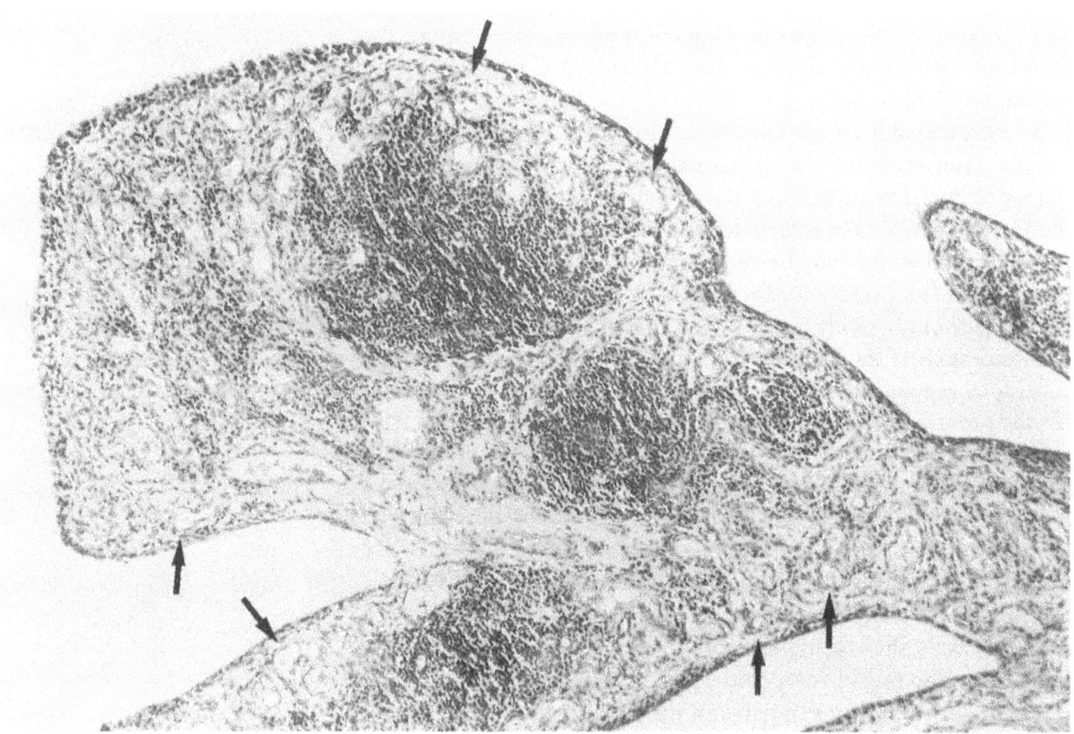

Fig. 6.23
Ankylosing spondylitis

Typical picture of the synovial membrane (knee joint): single- or double-staged lining cell layer, abundant development of thin-walled blood vessels (*arrows*), in between focal lymphocytic infiltration, sparse plasma cells

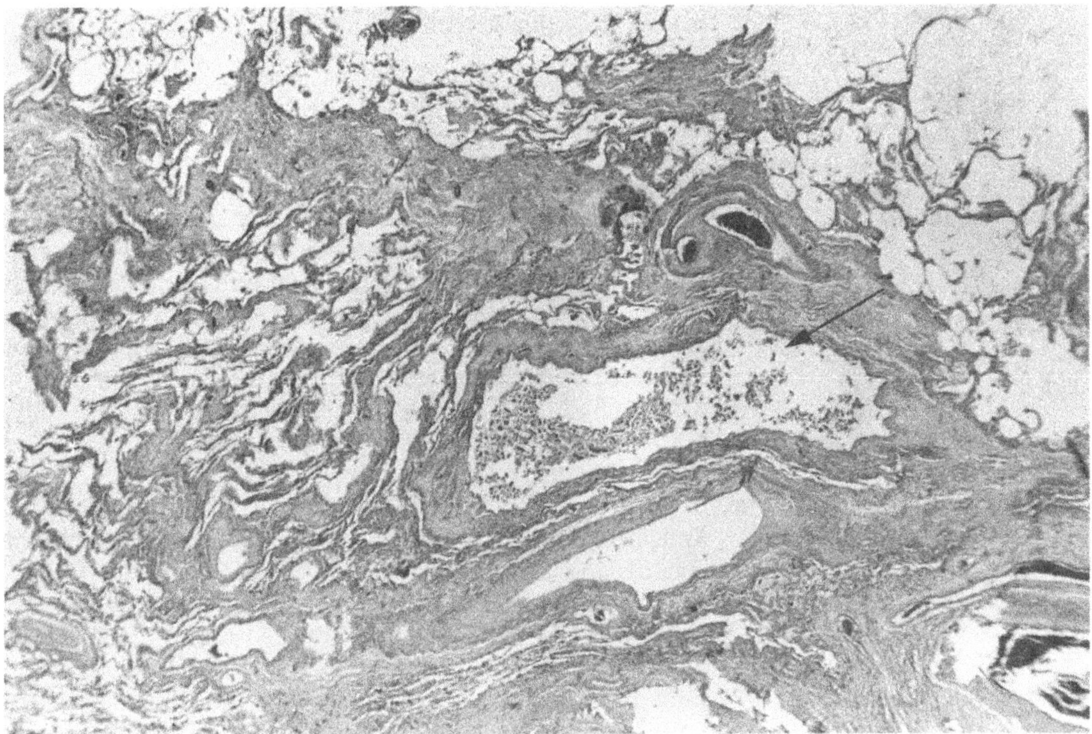

Fibrosis of right upper lobe of lung (*arrow*, bronchus)

Fig. 6.24
Ankylosing spondylitis

Pulmonary manifestations

Of clinical significance in the process of ankylosis is the interference with respiration, occasioned by the involvement of costovertebral joints which play a part in respiration. The virtual fixation of the thorax leads to over-inflation of the lung and chronic emphysema. This may result in pulmonary hypertension and cor pulmonale (see p. 197).
Another complication, cystic fibrosis of the upper lobes of the lung, has been described for the first time by Riemann and coworkers (1974; Fig. 6.24).
With a view to pathogenesis and pathology of AS, many questions are still unsolved. One of the most interesting areas of research in the fundamental mechanisms of AS and other members of the SSA-group remains: the interplay between microorganisms und major histocompatibility complex (MHC). The increased knowledge of the molecular biology of the MHC and the immune response to bacteria has sharpened the focus of inquiry. There are a lot of phenomena, which are specific for the SSA family and which are asking for explanation, e.g. the predilection for the sacroiliac joints and enthesis and the tendency to transgression of the border between bone and soft tissue. These are processes that cannot be fully explained by immunological inflammatory mechanisms.

6.2 Reactive Arthritides

6.2.1 Definition

Asymmetric affliction

Reactive arthritides (REA) are acutely occurring, painful arthritides which progress predominantly mono- or oligoarticularly. In contrast to RA, the joints are afflicted asymmetrically. The joints of the lower extremities, particularly the knees and ankle joints, are most often affected. The term REA implies a temporal and causal association with a previous infection by certain microorganisms (see below). In general, the latent period between infection and the subsequent arthritis is 1–2 weeks.

6.2.2 History

First clinical description

Sydenham (1701) has already alluded to the connection between enteritis and arthritis. But the first clinical description of REA goes back to the German hygienist Reiter, who in 1916 reported about an officer who, following septic urethritis with haemorrhagic diarrhoea, became ill with conjunctivitis and arthritis. In the same year, the French military doctors Fiessinger and Leroy (1916) observed the same symptomatology in four soldiers. Since then the Reiter-Fiessinger-Leroy triad consisting of arthritis, urethritis, and conjunctivitis has established itself as a prototype of REA, under the short designation Reiter's syndrome (RS). While all its relevant clinical features fit in with the framework of REA, RS does deserve a special position due to several particularities regarding etiology, clinical course, and prognosis (see p. 211).

Reiter-Fiessinger-Leroy triad arthritis

6.2.3 Clinical Manifestations

REA generally is taking a self-limiting course. The acute arthritis disappears after 3–5 months, sometimes only after 1 year, rarely does it become chronic. A chronicity probably develops by passing through an immune reaction. Approximately two-thirds of patients with acute Yersinia arthritis have exhibited mild joint symptoms as late as 4–5 years after infection (Aho et al. 1976; Kalliomäki and Leino 1979; Marsal et al. 1981).

Diagnostic criteria of reactive arthritis

In the last few years, the disease picture of REA has acquired an increasingly sharp profile characterized by the following summarized diagnostic criteria:

1. REA is triggered by a preceding enteral or urogenital (possibly sexually transmitted) infection. Thereby, *Yersinia enterocolitica*, *Shigella flexneri*, Salmonella, Campylobacter as well as Chlamydia are in the forefront.
2. Within an average time-scale of 1–2 weeks (in RS up 4 weeks), an acute mono- or oligoarticular arthritis with asymmetrical joint affliction, mainly of the lower extremities, occasionally also accompanied by an enthesopathy with involvement of tendons and their insertions follows.
3. Sacroiliac joint changes are found in 3–20% of patients with acute REA (Ahvonen 1972; Thomas et al. 1975; Leirisalo et al.

1982). Radionuclear examinations may reveal abnormal sacroiliac joint uptake in as many as 75% of patients (Russel et al. 1977). One may note paravertebral ossification around the lower three thoracic and upper lumbar vertebrae.
4. Patients with REA are negative for rheumatoid factors and antinuclear antibodies (ANAs); they lie in the normal range of the healthy population.
5. Extra-articular manifestations occur (e.g. ocular and mucocutaneous symptoms).
6. The course of the disease is generally self-limiting (3–5 months, occasionally up to 1 year, more rarely chronic). An exception in this connection is chronic RS (see p. 211).
   But approximately two-thirds of patients with acute Yersinia arthritis have exhibited mild joint symptoms as late as 4–5 years after infection.
7. There is a strong association with the histocompatibility antigen HLA-B27 (in about 60%–80% of patients; Sairanen and Tiilikainen 1975; Leirisalo et al. 1982; Calin 1984). The prevalence of HLA-B27 depends on ethnicity, in non-white populations it occurs more rarely.

6.2.4 Pathogenesis

Antigens of causative organisms

Whilst with acute septic or bacterial arthritis (BA) haematogenic colonization of the causative organisms occurs in the joints, it is a fundamental characteristic of REA that the causative organisms cannot be detected within the inflamed joint. Antigens of Chlamydia, Shigella, and Salmonella, however, have been identified in the synovial membrane as well as in the synovial fluid (Leirisalo et al. 1982; Keat et al. 1983; Taylor-Robinson et al. 1988; Granfors et al. 1989).

Nanagara and coworkers (1995) investigated the synovial membrane of six patients with Chlamydia-induced arthritis. In all six patients, they found atypical reticular bodies in the fibroblasts and macrophages as evidence of persistent infection. The observation of Zhang and colleagues (1996) is also interesting. They succeeded in preventing the onset of arthritis in Lewis rats infected with *Yersinia enterocolitica* by prophylactic administration of antibiotics.

Circulating immune complexes

There can be no doubt that the basis of REA is an immune mechanism triggered by a reaction of circulating antibodies with antigenic deposits in the synovial membrane. Briem and coworkers (1980) discovered circulating immune complexes in 13 out of 14 patients with enteritis complicated by REA but only in 26 out of 44 patients without joint symptoms. On the other hand, the cross-reactions of antibodies against bacterial antigens with tissue antigens must be taken into consideration. Thus, the presence of apparent cross-reactivity between antigenic components related to HLA-B27 and material derived from several gram-negative bacterial strains including Klebsiella, Shigella, and Yersinia species have been demonstrated (Bohemen van et al. 1984).

Distinction from rheumatic fever

It would seem obvious to classify RF (see p. 10) among the REA due to their temporal correlation with a preceding infection by streptococci A having been confirmed. Also no infecting organism can be detected in the joints. In RF, however, there is no association with HLA-B27 and the focus of the disease is not in the joints but in the myocardium and endocardium. In contrast to the HLA-B27-associated arthritides, the pathomechanism of RF has largely been elucidated. The fleetingly occurring arthritides and polyserositides are induced by immune complexes, whereas the processes in the myocardium and endocardium, which under certain circumstances can be life-threatening, are caused by cross-reacting antibodies and autoantibodies (see p. 12; Fassbender 1963; Kaplan 1963; Kaplan and Suchy 1964; Williams 1986).

Distinction from Lyme disease

Lyme disease (see p. 243) can also not be included in the REA, although a connection with a preceding Borrelia infection is not disputed. However, on the one hand, the temporal correlation between infection and subsequent arthritis is extremely variable and, on the other hand, the infective organism, the *Borrelia burgdorferi*, is detectable in synovial fluid and in synovial tissue (Valesova et al. 1989). As in the case of RF, there is no association with HLA-B27 in Lyme disease. Moreover, the infection pathways are different from those of REA (throat in RF, skin in Lyme disease).

6.2.5 Pathology

No destruction of joint structures

It is morphologically extremely interesting, particularly with respect to the joint destruction in RA, that in arthritides, which are characterized by high-grade immunologically induced inflammation, however, destruction of articular cartilage and articular bones does not occur. This is also conform with our experience in other non-bacterial induced arthritides. The hereby released cytokines and enzymes are paralyzed by inhibitors of the synovial fluid without any destructive effect to the articular surface (see p. 85).

We are convinced that even in the rare cases with description of joint damage episodes of self-limiting haematogenous bacterial superinfections can be expected. We were able to observe this in RA in 13.5% and in OA in 8.8% of cases (see p. 395).

Synovial processes in reactive arthritis

If the suspicion of a REA is to be confirmed by a synovial biopsy, we consider this to be an equation with two unknown factors. Otherwise than in RA, OA, or BA (see above), we could not find any morphological features in the synovial tissue that would sustain the diagnosis "REA" by themselves. Therefore, we studied biopsies taken from patients who had been clinically and indisputably diagnosed with REA. We tried to find pathological characteristics that could be assigned to this disease, as we have done for other SSA diseases. Approximately 0.56% of tissue taken from patients with rheumatic diseases and sent to us is from patients with unequivocally clinically diagnosed REA. In the period from 1989 to 1998, 130 of our cases have fulfilled the clinical criteria. An analysis of the biopsies lead mainly to the following aspects: First, we did not once observe in the synovial tissue from patients with unequivocally clinically diagnosed REA a proliferation of

synovial stroma cells (as in RA), not once the development of "glass villi" (as in OA; see p. 340), and never stronger fibrin exudation or neutrophil infiltration (as in BA). On the other hand, REA is a principally self-limiting disease. In this case, this means: it must be taken into account that the morphological features obviously reflect the different stages, i.e. "blooming", possible fully developed disease, and healing.
The following variables are to be reckoned with:
1. The degree of the inflammatory irritation present is reflected in the height (e.g. multi-layered) of the lining cell layer and in the form of its cells.
2. With duration and intensity of the disease, the formation of new synovial villi increases.
3. With the duration of the disease, also the new formation of collagen fibres and blood vessels in the villous stroma increases.
4. The immune process is manifested by infiltrates consisting of lymphocytes and plasma cells.

Histological characteristics

Taking these variables into account, the following characteristics of REA synovitis emerge: in most cases, a significant synovial hyperplasia is observed in the stage of blooming and in the stages of full development and healing. The number of newly formed villi corresponds to that formed in RA. The villi, however, are shorter and coarser. In some early cases, the lining cell layer is multi-staged, its cells are cubic to cylindrical. Fibrin is seen, if at all, in early cases in the form of discrete stripes that – depending on the age of the exudation – lie between the lining cells or are incorporated into the adjacent stroma. In contrast to BA, fibrin is not lamellated and does not contain neutrophils. At all stages, the villous stroma is infiltrated by lymphocytes and plasma cells. At the early stages, the infiltration is diffuse, 80% of the infiltrate consists of plasma cells (Fig. 6.25). At later stages, focal accumulations of lymphocytes aggregate around small blood vessels, a picture that bears resemblance to the accompanying synovitis in OA (Fig. 6.26). The fibre density in the collagen framework in the synovial stroma increases with duration of the disease, at the same time newly formed vessels occur, the wall of which increases in thickness. A proliferation of synovial stroma cells, as it is typical of RA, is not seen in REA. The number of blood vessels and the thickness of their walls give thus an insight into the duration of the disease. Peripheral blood vessels with thin walls, as we described them as characteristic for PSA and various diseases of the SSA-group, were not observed. We think that the most impressive feature is the reactiveness of the lining cell layer as a mirror of the inflammatory process.
In summary, by differentiating from other synovitides and by emphasising some features, some contours emerge that characterize the synovitis in REA and that justify taking a biopsy.

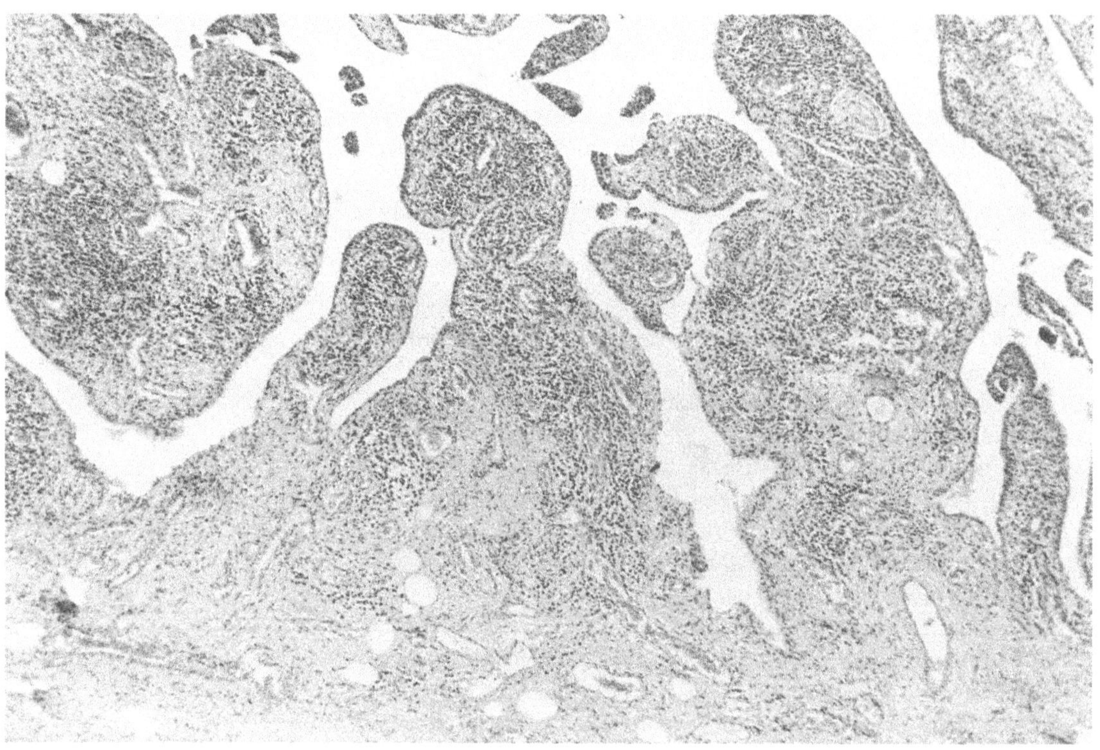

Fig. 6.25
Reactive arthritis

Knee joint. Early stage. Hyperplastic synovitis with dense, mostly plasmocytic infiltration of synovial stroma

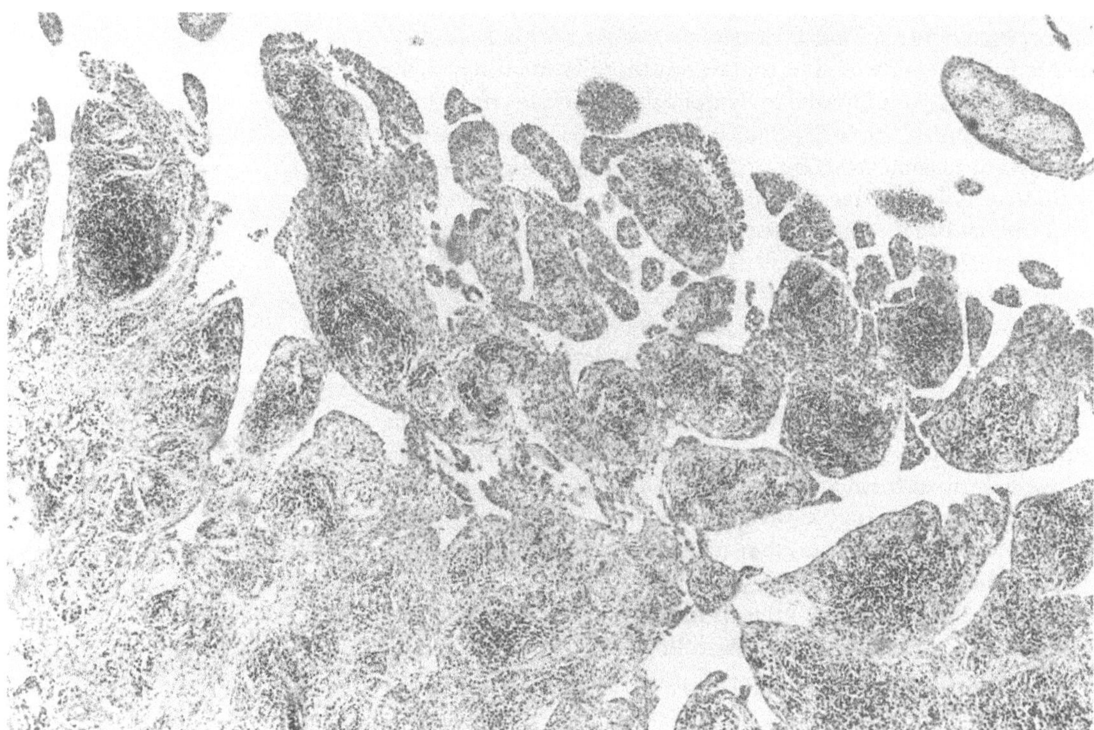

Fig. 6.26
Reactive arthritis

Knee joint. Later stage. Hyperplastic synovitis with mostly lymphocytic infiltration of synovial stroma

6.2.6 Reiter's Syndrome

Reiter's syndrome (RS) takes a special place amongst the REA in as far as the arthritis is mostly not short-lived but in over 2/3 of the patients becomes resident or chronic (chronic RS).

6.2.6.1 Epidemiology

In 1%–3% of individuals, RS develops with an enteric or urogenital infection (Briem et al. 1978; Keat et al. 1978; Eastmond et al. 1982). Approximately 60–80% of them are HLA-B27 positive (Keat 1983; Arnett 1987), patients with chronic RS with axial involvement are about 90% positive for HLA-B27. RS is a rheumatic disease which tends to affect young adults (especially young males), but no age-group is exempt. It must be borne in mind that the full syndrome may be diagnosed with difficulty in females. Helpful in this context is the discrimination between the two forms of the disease (Keat 1983; Philipps 1988):

HLA-B27

Two forms of disease

1. The epidemic or post-dysenteric RS which usually occurs after an attack of dysentery; in this form, the male-to-female ratio is nearly 1:1.
2. The sporadic, endemic or post-venereal RS, which is more dominant in males. This may relate to the fact that the disease in females is "camouflaged" as it progresses and thus cannot be detected.

For several reasons, the incidence and prevalence of RS are difficult to assess: The enteric and venereal features may be minimal, and the non-specific but clinically significant features, such as eye disease, keratodermia or cervicitis (in females) may be overlooked. This may lead to patients being diagnosed with AS, who, in fact, have sacroiliitis and spinal disease as a secondary manifestation of RS.

Keratodermia and cervicitis

Sacroiliitis

Although described as a classical triad, the clinical picture in RS can often be incomplete, conjunctivitis and less often urethritis may be absent.

Diagnostic criteria

The Subcommittee on Criteria for RS of the American College of Rheumatology's Diagnostic and Therapeutic Criteria Committee defines RS as "an episode of peripheral arthritis of greater than 1 month's duration in association with urethritis or cervicitis" (Willkens et al. 1981).

Calin (1984) regards REA associated with Yersinia, Salmonella, Shigella, and other microorganisms as "Formes Frustes" of RS. He defines RS as "seronegative asymmetric arthropathy (predominantly lower extremities) plus one or more of urethritis-cervicitis, dysentery, inflammatory eye disease, mucocutaneous disease (balanitis, oral ulceration, keratodermia)".

"Formes Frustes" of RS

6.2.6.2 Clinical Manifestations

From several days up to 4 weeks after a non-specific urethritis (in females cystitis or cervicitis) and enteritis, an acute arthritis with

Mono- or oligoarticular affliction

Big toe

Uveitis

joint swelling, over-heating, and redness starts. The manifestation is according to that in REA mono- or oligoarticular asymmetrical with a predilection for the lower extremities. Particularly affected are the knees, ankle joints, and fore-feet. A noticeably frequent first localization is the big toe joint (a "sausage digit" or dactylitis is a typical lesion). Only soft tissue swellings are found radiologically in the early stages. Further clinical symptoms which often develop mildly, or may even be completely absent, are besides a mostly bilateral conjunctivitis particularly keratodermia (mostly on the soles of the feet) and balanitis. Uveitis occurs in 15% of patients with recurring disease (Amor and Toubert 1993). The complete clinical picture of RS develops in only about 1/3 of the patients (Cush and Lipsky 1993).

Chronic Reiter's syndrome

Enthesopathy

Iliosacral joint

Spondylitis

Paravertebral ossifications

The healing of acute arthritis is often rather delayed (approximately after 4–12 months). In more than two-thirds of the cases, it resides or turns into chronic RS; during the latter, the axial skeleton as well as hand and finger joints (often in the form of diffuse swelling as "sausage finger", dactylitis) are also affected. Radiologically, indications of joint destruction combined with new bone formation (analogous to bone processes in PSA; see p. 221) are seen as well as calcifications in tendons and ligaments (see p. 216). Also ankle pains in the region of insertion of the plantar aponeurosis at the calcaneus and the insertion of Achilles' tendon, as signs of enthesopathy, and deep-seated back pain, associated with the often co-occurring iliosacral joint disease, indicate that RS belongs to the SSA, which are characterized by common, serological, morphological, and clinical phenomena (see p. 178). Approximately half of the patients with chronic RS develop sacroiliitis and at least 40% of them develop spondylitis (Schilling 1987). Thereby, it is valid that the longer the duration of the disease the higher the frequency of sacroiliac involvement. Analogous to PSA, isolated paravertebral ossifications ("non-marginal" syndesmophytes; see p. 214) can develop in the region of the hip vertebrae, spanning the disc cavity. In Reiter's spondylitis, however, they often have a rougher morphology than in psoriatic spondylitis. Involvement of the cervical spine is uncommon. In persistent disease, bony ankylosis is common in the axial skeleton but only rarely observed in peripheral joints.

6.2.6.3 Pathology

Periosteal bone formation

The morphological characteristics of the synovial and bone processes in the SSA (see p. 180) can also be detected in RS. We therefore believe that the joint destruction with periosteal bone formation in chronic RS is based on the same mechanism as in PSA (see p. 224) and other SSA.

In bioptic material taken from synovial tissue of patients with RS, we saw the same changes we described for REA (see p. 209). The main characteristic is an unusual new formation of numerous thin-walled blood vessels, predominantly in the vicinity of the lining cell layers of narrow villi. While the lining cells may exhibit a significant proliferation, there is no reaction of the synovial stroma cells. The intensity and the composition of the lym-

pho-plasmacellular infiltration depends on the degree of the activity of the disease at any given time. Neutrophils are not observable. In cases of chronic or resident RS, the density of collagen fibres in the synovial stroma increases.
RS is in fact the prototype of the REA. Nevertheless, its specific symptomatology, i.e. the triad arthritis, urethritis, and conjunctivitis, as well as its severe clinical course grant to RS a special position within the group of diseases. It becomes evident that the individual members of the SSA family do each have their own profile, but they still share specific characteristics, such as the potential involvement of the axial skeleton and the association with HLA-B27. An important contrast of the enterogenous REA towards RA is that REA takes its course without joint destruction.

6.3 Psoriatic Arthritis

Synonyms: psoriatic arthropathy, (osteo)arthropathia psoriatica.

6.3.1 Definition

Five forms of psoriatic arthritis

Due to the manifestation of the joint process, Moll and Wright (1973) distinguished five forms of psoriatic arthritis (PSA) which in the meantime have been further differentiated:

Pattern of joint involvement

1. Asymmetrical oligoarticular arthritis is the most characteristic pattern of joint involvement in psoriasis. Distal interphalangeal (DIP), proximal interphalangeal (PIP), metacarpophalangeal (MCP), and metatarsophalangeal (MTP) joints are usually involved.
   Included in this subgroup are patients with "sausage-shape" fingers or toes (dactylitis) as a result of flexor tendon sheath involvement and those with monarthritis involving other than DIP joints.
2. Symmetric polyarthritis in association with psoriasis. In contrast to RA, there is a persistent seronegativity, a higher frequency of DIP joint involvement, a tendency of bony ankylosis of the DIP and PIP joints (Fig. 6.27), and often an association with sacroiliitis. **Ankylosis**
3. Predominant involvement of DIP joints in the absence of other joint involvement is regarded as "classical" PSA (Green et al. 1981; Scarpa et al. 1984; Biondi Oriente et al. 1989). There is a strong association with psoriatic nail changes.
4. Arthritis mutilans, due to osteolysis of the phalanges, metacarpals or metatarsals, leads to severe deformities. It occurs in about 5% of patients with PSA and is often associated with sacroiliitis. **Arthritis mutilans**
5. Axial involvement in PSA usually becomes manifest after several years of peripheral joint disease and provides the reason for including this disease in the SSA (see p. 178). The most important features are sacroiliitis and spondylitis. Classical "marginal" syndesmophytes, like in AS (see p. 193), but in most cases, atypical "non-marginal" syndesmophytes, which occur by calcification in the adjacent spinal ligaments **Axial involvement** **Sacroiliitis and spondylitis** **Syndesmophytes**

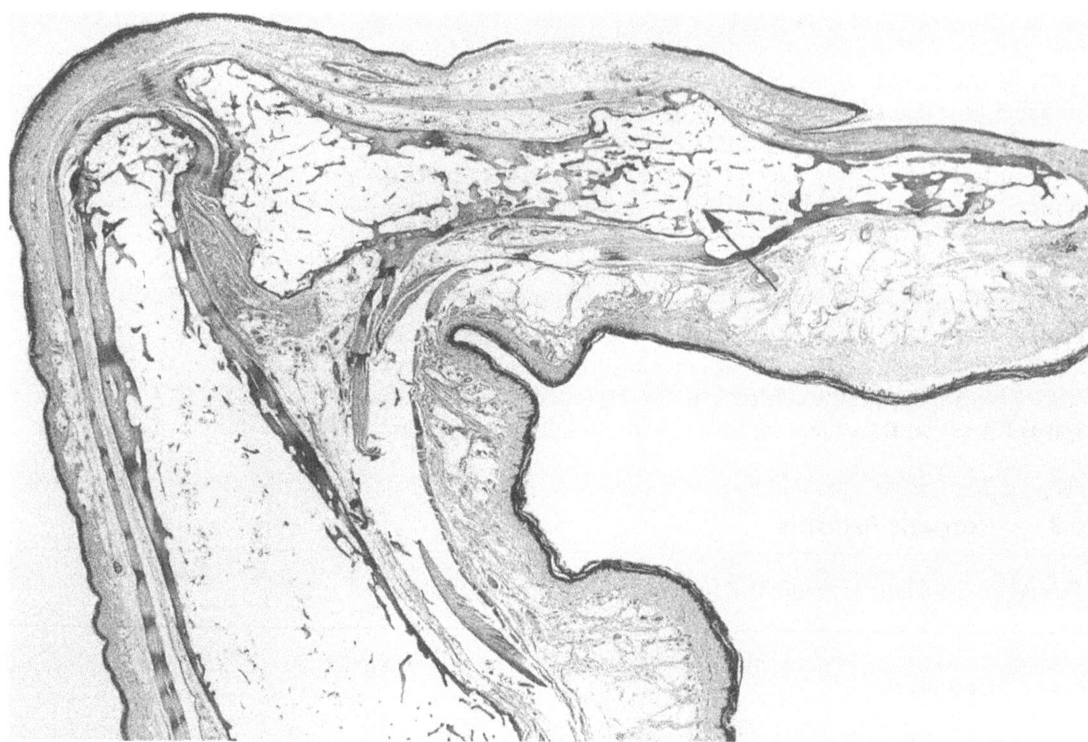

Fig. 6.27
Psoriatic arthritis

Finger joint. Bony ankylosis of the distal interphalangeal joint (*arrow*). The subchondral bone lamella break through into the proximal interphalangeal joint with fibrous ankylosis. New bone formation in the region of the cortical bone. Severe osteoporosis

and thus proceed without spinal contact (paravertebral ossification), can be seen also without an associated sacro-iliitis. The syndesmophytes in PSA can also appear in both forms.

6.3.2 History

First descriptions

For a long time, psoriasis was considered as a form of leprosy whereby the deformity of the distal phalanges, which accompanies this disease, contributed to this assumption. It is not certain therefore whether the descriptions by Willan (1808) and Alibert (1810, 1818), who were the first to report a relationship between psoriasis and arthritis, meant the same as that designated as "psoriasis arthritique" by Bazin (1860). In 1888, Bourdillon described in detail 36 cases of psoriasis associated with peripheral arthritis. The association between psoriasis and AS was mentioned for the first time in 1928 by Zellner and in 1935 described by Coste and Forestier.
Detailed clinical-radiological and serological studies led in the course of time to a differentiation between different types of PSA (see p. 213).
The discovery of a rheumatoid factor by Waaler (1940) facilitated the differentiation of PSA, which in general is seronegative, from RA and opened up the possibility for Bauer et al. (1941) to

illustrate a typical profile for the joint process in PSA thus distinguishing it from that of RA. Thereby they emphasized the tendency to osteolysis and mutilant deformity of the distal phalanges in PSA.

6.3.3 Epidemiology

Psoriasis vulgaris is a widespread skin disease, affecting 1%–3% of adults of Western European, East Indian or Asian descent, but rarely affecting African-Americans, suggesting that genetic susceptibility factors play an important role in the expression of both the skin disease and the arthropathy (Smiley 1995). Approximately 6%–20% of these patients develop PSA. The male-to-female ratio is 1:1.04 and is thus not very different from that of psoriasis vulgaris with 1:1.4 (Wright 1985).

6.3.4 Clinical Manifestations

The skin disease precedes the arthritis in 60%–75% of patients (Greif et al. 1985; Arnett 1989), on average by 8 years. In about 20%, the order of the manifestation is reversed, whereby it can no longer be clarified whether minimal symptoms of psoriasis had already existed at an earlier time but had not been diagnosed.

First manifestations of psoriatic arthritis

There is a greater percentage of patients with juvenile onset presenting with arthritis before psoriasis. The simultaneous onset of skin and joint disease, however, is rare. The first manifestation of PSA is possible at any age. An accumulation is found in the group aged between 30 and 50 years (Greif et al. 1985), women often being affected at an earlier age. Patients with severe deforming arthritis (mutilant arthritis; see p. 213) usually had a juvenile onset of PSA (Shore and Ansell 1982; Rose and Belsky 1989; Southwood et al. 1989).

Inheritability

HLA-B27

HLA-BW38

In family studies, it has been noted that psoriasis and PSA are increased in families of patients with PSA. Moll and Wright (1973) found an 80%–90% chance of inheritability in a first degree relative of a PSA patient. This suggests a common genetic predisposition. However, compared with the strong association of AS and RS with HLA-B27, in PSA the HLA-B27 associations are less distinct. The increased prevalence of HLA-B27 in PSA is linked to the presence of sacroiliitis and/or spondylitis, while peripheral PSA may be associated with HLA-BW38 (Espinoza et al. 1982). According to the studies of Wright (1985), 60%–90% of PSA patients with sacroiliitis and syndesmophytes (see Figs. 6.3, 6.7) are HLA-B27-positive whereas 60%–80% of PSA patients with sacroiliitis without syndesmophytes are also positive. Sacroiliitis occurs in 20%–40% of patients with PSA (Lambert and Wright 1977). If sacroiliitis is absent while syndesmophytes are present, HLA-B27 is detectable in 43% of the cases, whereas in PSA patients with only peripheral joint involvement no association with HLA-B27 exists.

Common features with RA

PSA also deserves the designation "chronic polyarthritis" since it has the following features in common with RA:

1. Both diseases are systemic, the processes not being restricted to the joints.
2. Both diseases can proceed intermittently into a chronic state.
3. The joint processes are non-bacterial.

Profile of psoriatic arthritis

Since the name-giving psoriatic skin changes are often minimal and frequently overlooked, the following points can sharply distinguish the profile of PSA with respect to that of RA:

1. PSA, in contrast to RA, proceeds strictly seronegatively.
2. PSA has, in general, an asymmetrical joint involvement pattern different from that of RA with inclusion of the distal finger and toe joints. Typical for PSA is the affection of all joints of a finger and of a toe. A both interesting and plausible explanation for the fact that PSA predominantly affects the distal interphalangeal joints was put forward by Fourniè (1998). Under the aspect of enthesopathy as the basic pathogenetic mechanism in PSA, he reminds us that numerous tendinous insertions surround the tips of fingers and toes like a net. This net encompasses the DIP joint, a joint which is fibrous rather than synovial in nature (Fournié et al. 1989, 1992; Fournié 1993). Moreover, the soft tissue of single fingers and toes can swell to the form of "sausage-shape" dactylitis (see p. 229).
3. PSA, in contrast to RA, has a tendency towards osteolysis and osseous ankylosis of the finger and toe joints.
4. In contrast to RA, ossification also occurs in PSA in the capsule area outside the joint space and also in the region of ligament and tendon insertions at the vertebral column and body periphery (see p. 220), common areas are the calcaneus, the trochanters, and ischial tuberosities (see Fig. 6.6).
5. PSA associated with HLA-B27 can attack the vertebral column. Characteristic thereby are the paravertebral ossifications and sacroiliitis. In RA, the participation of the vertebral column remains restricted to the cervical spine, whereby the destabilizing and destructive components are prominent (see p. 107).
6. In contrast to RA, rheumatoid necroses ("rheumatoid nodules") never occur in PSA.

Distal finger and toe joints

Osteolysis and osseous ankylosis

Enthesopathy

Sacroileitis

Nail changes

Moreover, in PSA, typical nail changes may appear, such as indentations, onycholysis, subungual keratotic fragments (debris), and macular, yellow discoloration of the nail. Up to 80% of PSA patients suffer from nail changes, but only 15–30% of patients with no joint involvement. Typical X-ray findings of finger and toe joints of patients with PSA are the simultaneously occurring bone destruction and new bone formation, mutilation, ossifying periostitis as well as osteolytic defects.

Osteolytic defects

A further characteristic hallmark is the osseous ankylosis in fingers and toes.

6.3.5 Pathogenesis

The cause of PSA is a combination of genetic susceptibility and exogenous factors (Reveille 1993). In the latter category, increasing evidence has pointed to microbial antigens as triggers for PSA. Li and colleagues (1994) have recently shown gram-positive bacterial cell wall peptidoglycan to be present in joint tissues of patients with PSA. Rahmann and coworkers (1990) found increased levels of antibodies in the blood to gram-positive bacterial peptidoglycans in patients with PSA.
Despite our observations that starting as well as crucial point in understanding PSA is to search in the bone tissue, this process, however, can secondarily trigger a synovitis, which is responsible for the actual manifestation. In view of the extremely painful dactylitis triggered by the periosteal proliferation, the synovial joint inflammation itself becomes less important.

6.3.6 Pathology

Corresponding to the clinical-radiological peculiarities, PSA demonstrates also a morphological profile which diverges from other joint diseases. Following our observations, morphological characteristics are found in synovial tissue as well as in joint cartilage and juxta-articular bone.

Synovial membrane

As PSA is a member of the SSA family, the alterations of the synovial membrane in PSA are much the same as those observed in other types of SSA. In contrast to the alterations in RA and OA, the following morphological features are characteristic for PSA: the synovial villi are longer and thinner. Depending on the process' activity, the lining cells may be either high-cylindrical and multi-layered or inconspicuously flat and single-layered. A multi-layered proliferation of the lining cells is transitory and merely an expression of an actual but uncharacteristic inflammatory reaction which is observable in every joint disease. The fibrosis of villous stroma is denser than in OA but not as compact as in RA.

Increased vascularisation

From our observations, the pattern of vascularisation is the most reliable feature (Fassbender and Fassbender 1992; Fassbender 1994). Within the synovial stroma, mainly in the periphery, close to the lining cell layer, there is an unusually high number of narrow, thin-walled blood vessels (Figs. 6.28, 6.29). These can best be seen in the early stages of synovitis. We presume that after each episode of inflammation these vessels either disappear or are reduced in number and become coarser due to the ensuing increased density of collagen fibres (Fig. 6.30). Thus, diagnosis becomes more difficult. Danning and coworkers (1998b) believe that increased expression of $\alpha_v\beta_3$ integrin is one explanation for the neovascularisation during the early phases of PSA. Fearon and coworkers (1998) believe that the increase in blood vessels within the villi, compared to patients with RA, is due to higher levels of TGF-β1 and increased VEGF expression in the synovial membrane. These thin-walled, newly formed blood vessels adjacent to the lining cell layer should not be confused with the coarser blood vessels that form after the infection has ceased.

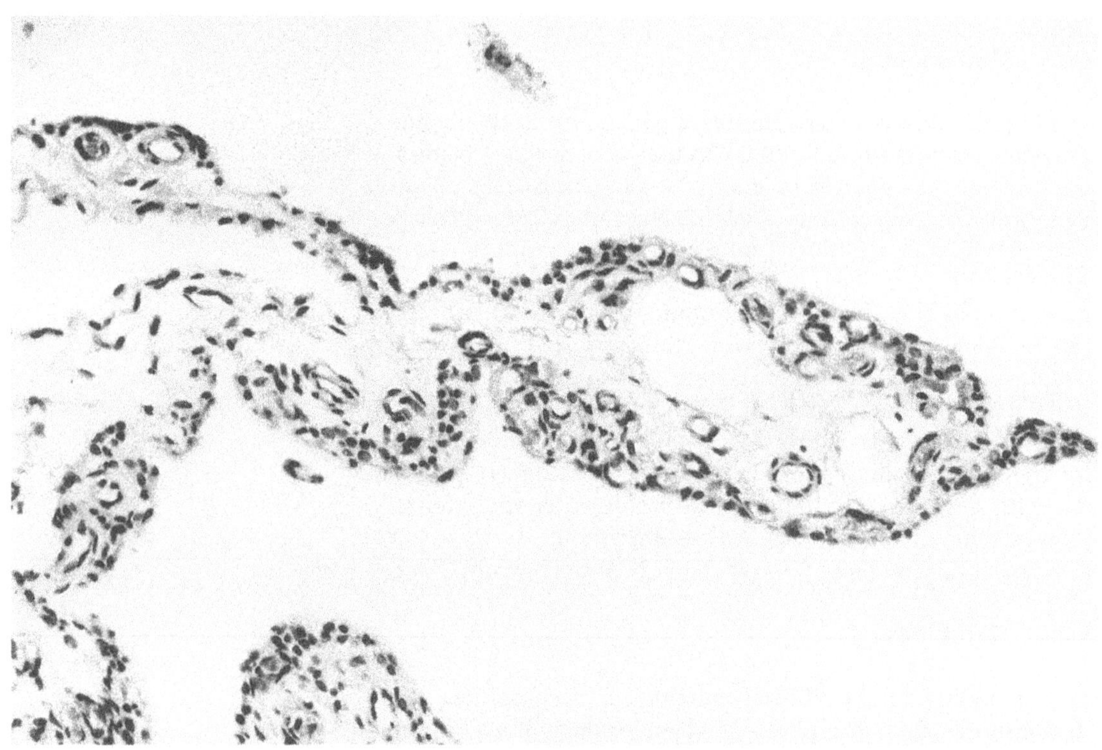

Fig. 6.28
Psoriatic arthritis

Knee joint. Narrow synovial villus with delicate stroma and numerous small blood vessels beneath the lining cell layer. Duration of disease 11 months

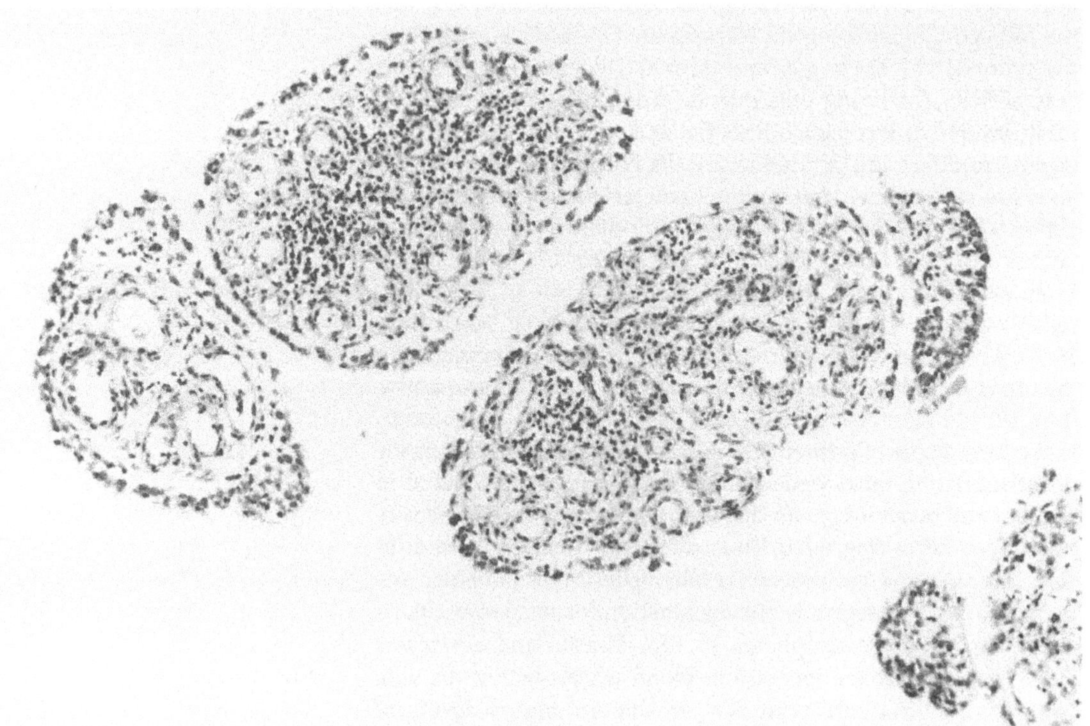

Fig. 6.29

MCP joint. Hyperplastic synovitis. Single- to double-staged lining cell layer with numerous thin-walled blood vessels in its neighbourhood. Duration of disease 8 months

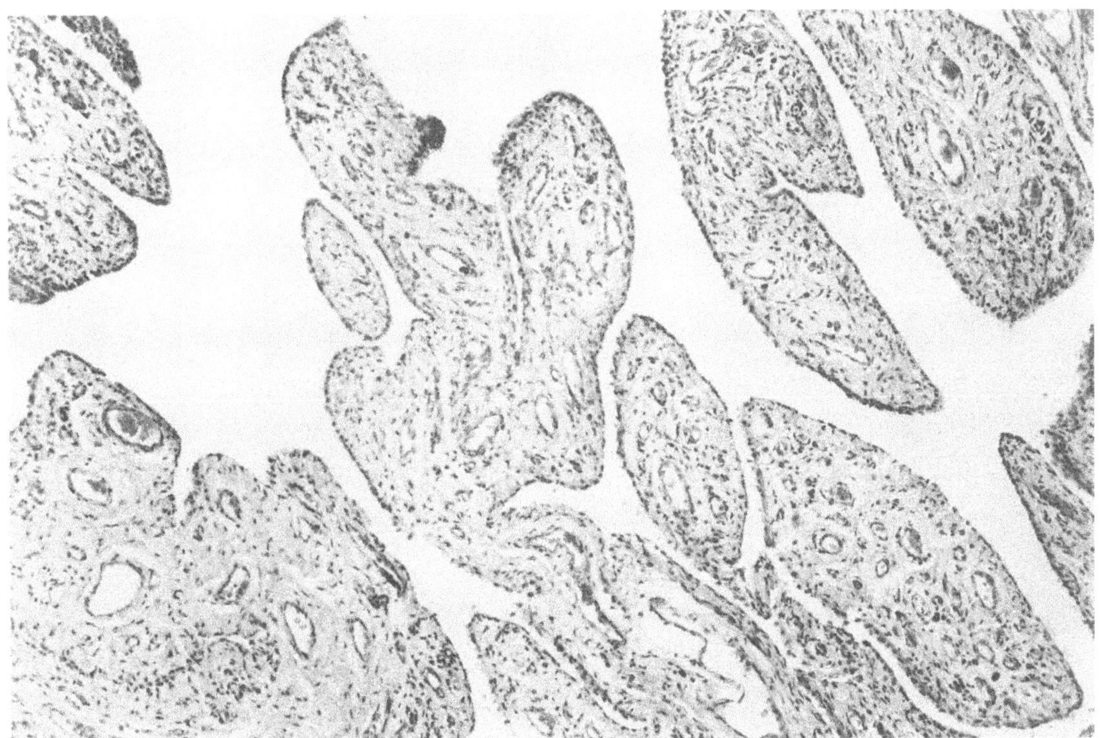

Knee joint. Hyperplastic synovitis. Flat, single-staged lining cell layer beneath multiplied but enlarged blood vessels. Duration of disease 6 years

Fig. 6.30
Psoriatic arthritis

Lymphocytes

The infiltration of the villous stroma by lymphocytes is generally of medium density. In between, plasma cells are often found. Occasionally, lymphocytes can aggregate focally. True lymph follicles with germinal centres, however, are never observed (Fig. 6.31). In rare cases, we found proper lawn-like aggregates of plasma cells. Neutrophils are not a part of the inflammatory cell components of PSA.

Cytokines

Danning and coworkers (1998a,b) compared cellular infiltrations of synovial membrane biopsies of patients with RA and patients with PSA. They found no differences either in the amount or in the composition of lymphocytic infiltrations; also, the distribution and the amount of critical pro-inflammatory cytokines, such as TNF-α, IL-1α, and IL-1β, were similar in the synovial membranes of both groups. T cell activating monokines such as IL-12 and IL-15 were found in the lining cell layer and in the stroma of the synovial membrane; these again were comparable in both groups. High levels of lymphocytes of the subgroups CD28 and CD69 and lower levels of CD25 lymphocytes were found in both groups. These findings are also in accordance with our observations.

The oncogene c-myc is more often expressed in both the skin and the synovial cells of patients with PSA than in normal skin and synovial cells. Gladman (1992) found in the synovial membrane of patients with PSA c-myc in 98% and in 88% in the psoriatic skin, in contrast to normal skin in 62%.

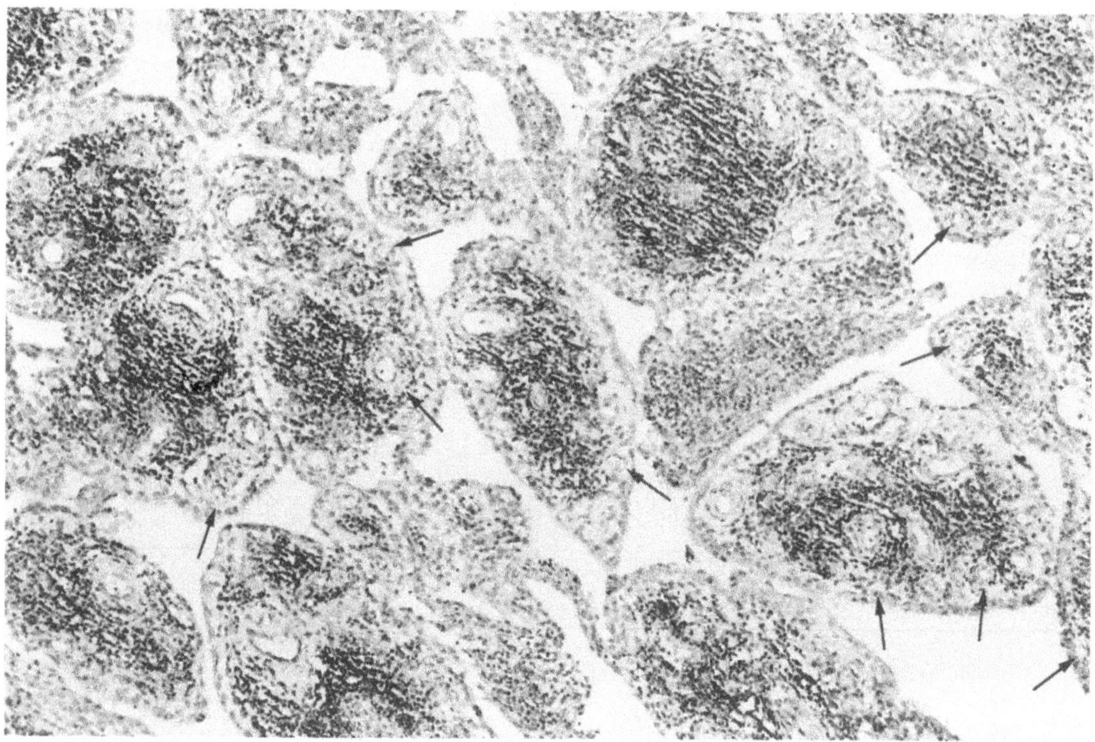

Fig. 6.31
Psoriatic arthritis

Ankle joint. Florid, high-grade hyperplastic synovitis. Lining cell layer single- to double-staged, beneath densely lying, thin-walled blood vessels (*arrows*). Duration of disease 6 years

It has to be emphasized, however, that in the course of the disease, processes within the synovial membrane lose their morphological characteristics. The lining cell layer, for example, appears mostly flattened and single-staged. Collagen fibres increase, the villous stroma becomes slightly fibrotic, and the typical thin-walled blood vessels decrease in number and may eventually disappear. Infiltration by lymphocytes and plasma cells may persist in the early as well as in the later stages. Considering that cells proliferating from the stroma in patients with RA can, by releasing proteases, destroy cartilage and bone, we wish to emphasize that we never observed the slightest proliferation of synovial stroma cells in patients with PSA.

Bone process in psoriatic arthritis

The clinical and radiological changes, particularly in areas near the phalangeal joints, i.e. osseous ankylosis, osteolysis, and ossification in the capsule region outside the joint cavity, would predict a bone process of a special kind which differs qualitatively from other joint diseases.

We examined juxta-articular bone tissue from 168 patients with PSA and could detect an unusual process in the spongy and cortical bone, the stepwise progress which we divided into four phases (Fassbender 1979, 1986b):

First phase

Loss of aggrecan and calcium apatite

The first phase is characterized by a focal loss of the aggrecan and calcium apatite substance in the lamellar bone of the spongiosa. The exposed collagen fibre network is preserved and still mirrors the original pattern of the bone structure. The delineation between the intact bone and the demasked collagen fibre

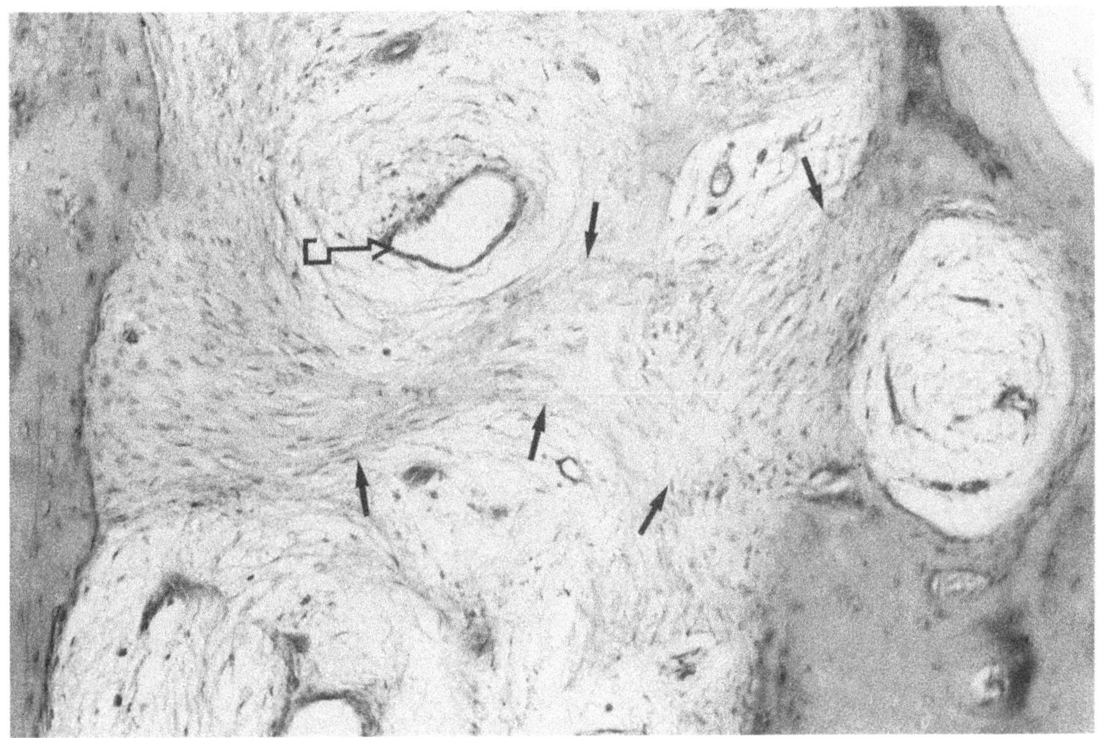

Finger, distal phalanx. Proteoglycan- and calcium apatite-loss zone in the area of spongy bone. The preserved collagen fibre clusters mark the original spongiosa structure (*arrows*). On both sides, proteoglycan-containing trabeculae are still preserved. *Open arrow* indicates an expanded vessel as the remains of a Haversian canal

Fig. 6.32
Psoriatic arthritis

network is sharp. The exposed collagen fibres are initially still fine. However, in the course of time, they become coarser under the deposition of fibrocytes. Instead of Haversian canals one sees expanded blood vessels which also have survived the process (Fig. 6.32).

Second phase

The loss of the proteoglycan-containing interstitial substance of these circumscribed bone sections is not disregarded by the surrounding connective tissue. The sharply defined areas resulting from loss of aggrecan are reactively settled by osteoblast chains (Figs. 6.33, 6.34). The osteoblasts position themselves between the remaining collagen bundles and use these as a so-to-speak building frame for the remodelling which subsequently starts.

Remodelling

Depending on the age of the osteoblast chains, newly formed osteoid is found here which smoothly covers the rough disrupted surface between the fibres. Also in this second phase, not the slightest evidence of an inflammatory reaction is found.

Third phase

The third phase is characterized by the new formation of fibrous bone in the region of the aggrecan loss zones. In contrast to the specific structural pattern of the original lamellar spongiosa, this newly formed bone shows an unarranged matrix. The bone cells of this fibrous bone, in contrast to the lamellar bone, are larger and tend to be round. The preserved collagen fibre frame indeed functions largely shaping in bone remodelling. In fact, however,

New formation of fibrous bone

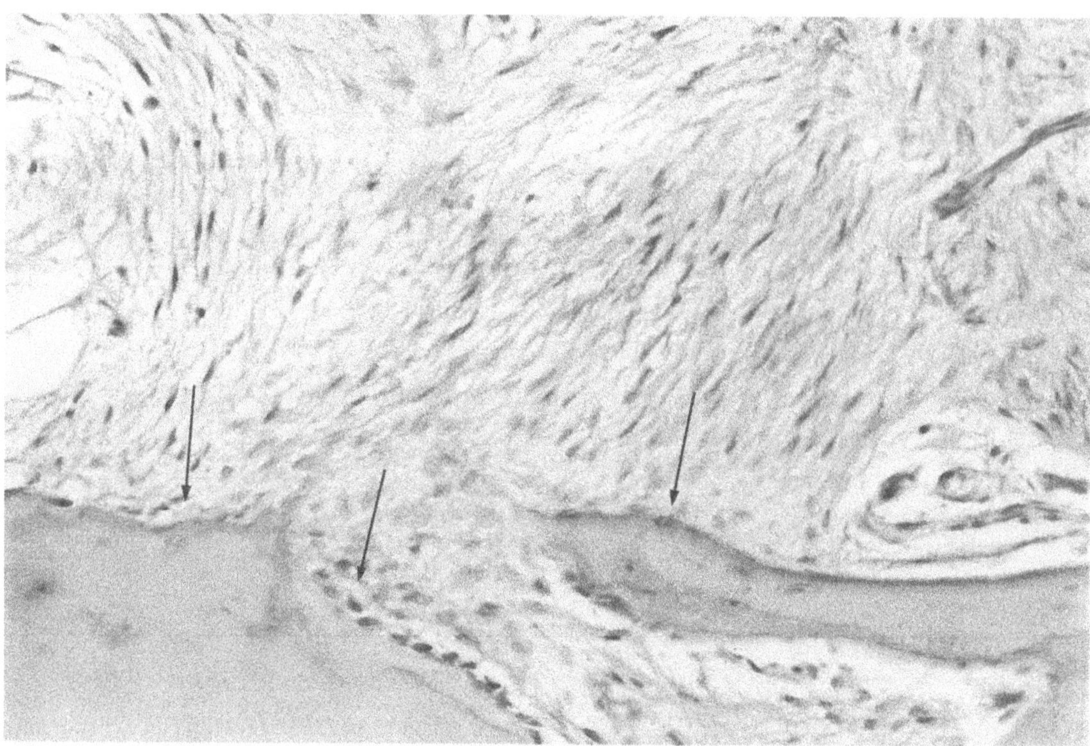

Fig. 6.33
Psoriatic arthritis

Finger, middle phalanx. Deposition of osteoblast chains (*arrows*) in the area of proteoglycan loss zone. Among this, a collagen fibre clump, which remarks the original spongiosa development

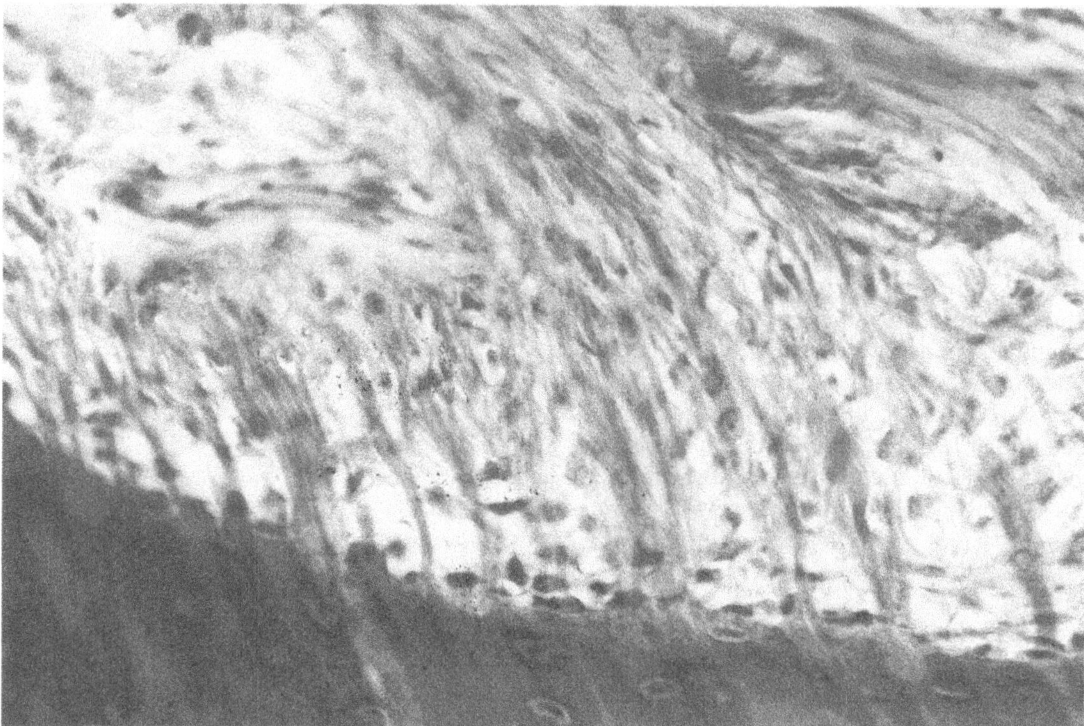

Fig. 6.34
Psoriatic arthritis

Finger, end phalanx. New bone formation at the outer surface of the cortical bone in the region where the loss of proteoglycanes and calcium apatite has occurred. Osteoblast chain between the preserved collagen fibres

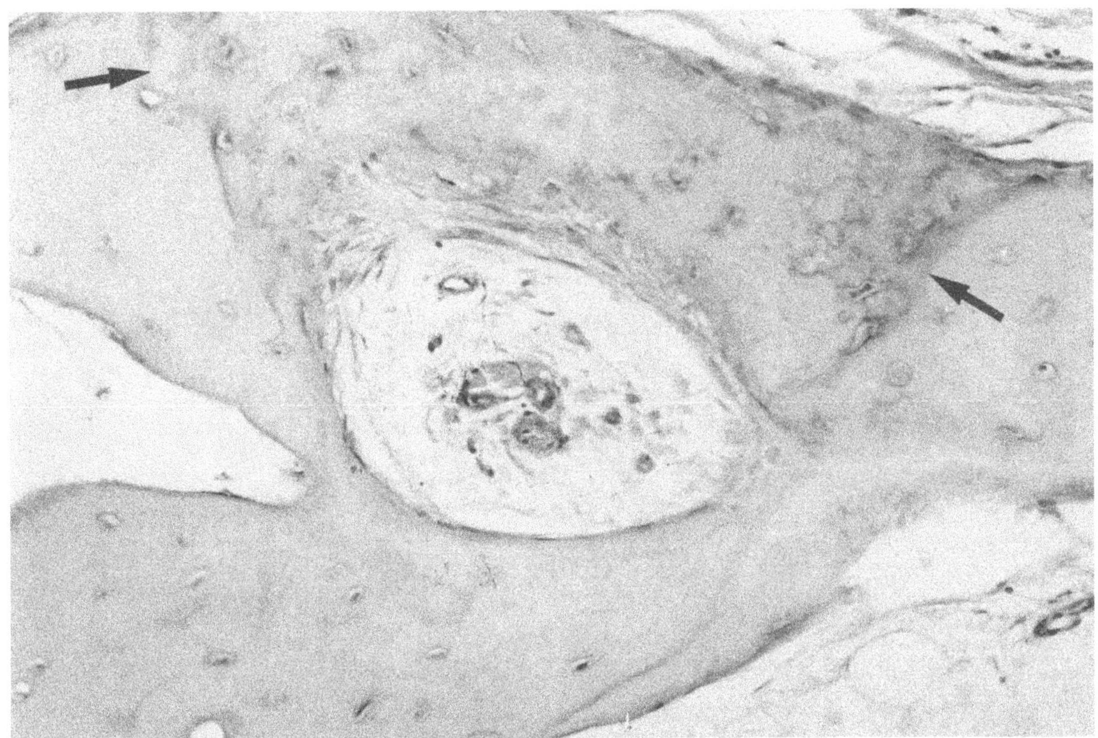

Finger, distal phalanx. Rough remodelling of the spongiosa structure through newly formed fibrous bone between the spongiosa residue. The *arrows* mark the delineation between old lamellar und newly formed fibrous bone

Fig. 6.35
Psoriatic arthritis

these newly formed fibrous bone areas are significantly coarser and bulkier and only a caricature of the genuine structure (Fig. 6.35).

Fourth phase

Probably the aggrecan loss described above and the new fibrous bone formation processes occur in rare and probably short episodes, since we saw situations in which neither an indication of acute collagen fibre unmasking, osteoblast activity, nor the formation of new fibrous bone were observable, but only a gravel-like, pagetoidal course of disordered fusion lines and an irregularly arranged surface indicating a partial or completely healed condition. These pagetoidal final stages, however, achieve neither qualitatively nor quantitatively the structure of the original spongy or cortical bone. The provisional fibrous bone will, in the course of time, be remodeled into definite lamellar bone. The irregular path of the fusion lines remains as a witness of the newly formed bone and the remodelling process. On the other hand, these gradually progressing processes can lead to a negative balance in the bone structure and can result eventually in osteolyses (Fig. 6.36).

Pagetoidal final stages

Since phases I and II (fibre unmasking and remodelling) are probably of short duration, histological examinations are most likely to encounter the longer lasting phases III and IV. In cases of doubt, the following characteristics verify the diagnosis: smooth, round spongiosa break-offs and polarization optical proof of bone remodelling whereby the trabeculae, in addition to

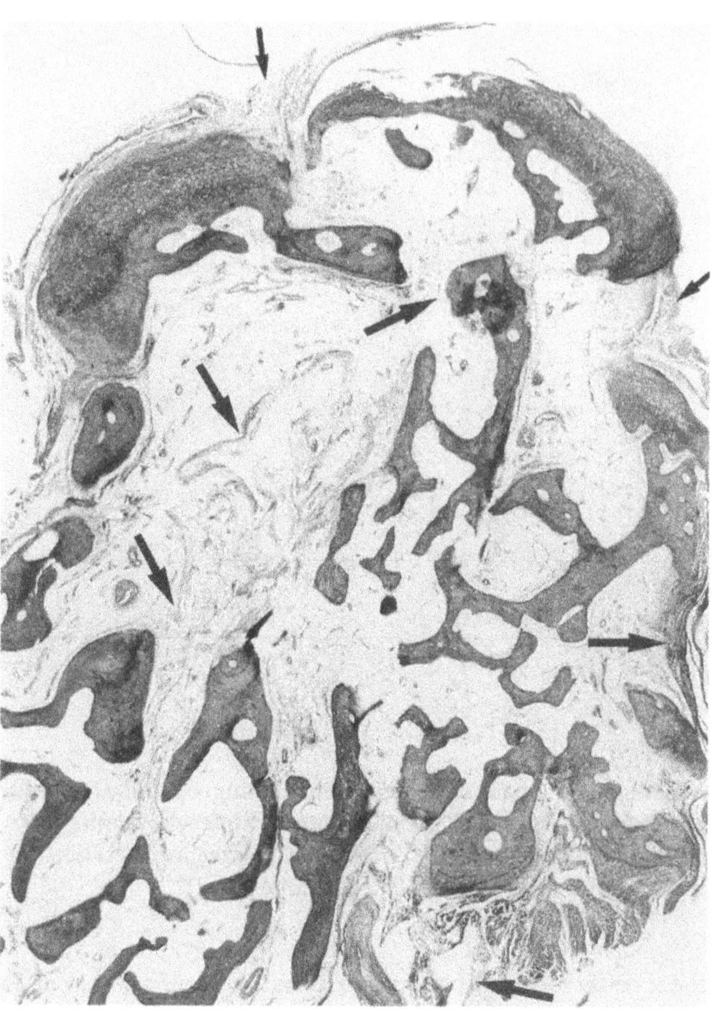

Fig. 6.36
Psoriatic arthritis

Finger, end phalanx. Psoriatic osteolysis. Focal break-offs of the spongiosa trabeculae and destruction of the cortical bone (*arrows*)

the old lamellar bone, contain newly formed fibrous bone areas. It is of importance, however, that in these areas, all indications of an acute or expired inflammation are excluded.

Cortical bone

In cortical compact bone, the process is quite different. In a few cases, we have had the opportunity to investigate abarticular corticalis from patients with PSA and RS in the initial stages. So, we could observe proliferation of the periosteum during a highly active stage: between the outer surface of the corticalis and the periosteum, we found an approximately 1–3 mm zone of densely packed cells (Fig. 6.37). These cells increase in number proceeding from the periosteum on the guideline of collagen fibres and at first exhibit the characteristics of fibroblasts. But, towards the cortical bone, they increasingly undergo transformation into osteoblasts, forming a compact cell layer between periosteum and cortical bone, a cambium layer (Fig. 6.38). In this way, duplicates of the external cortical contour may be formed, occasionally also bud-shaped forms or fierce formations of new, bizarrely shaped fibrous bone may develop (Fig. 6.39), the latter are almost pathognomonic.

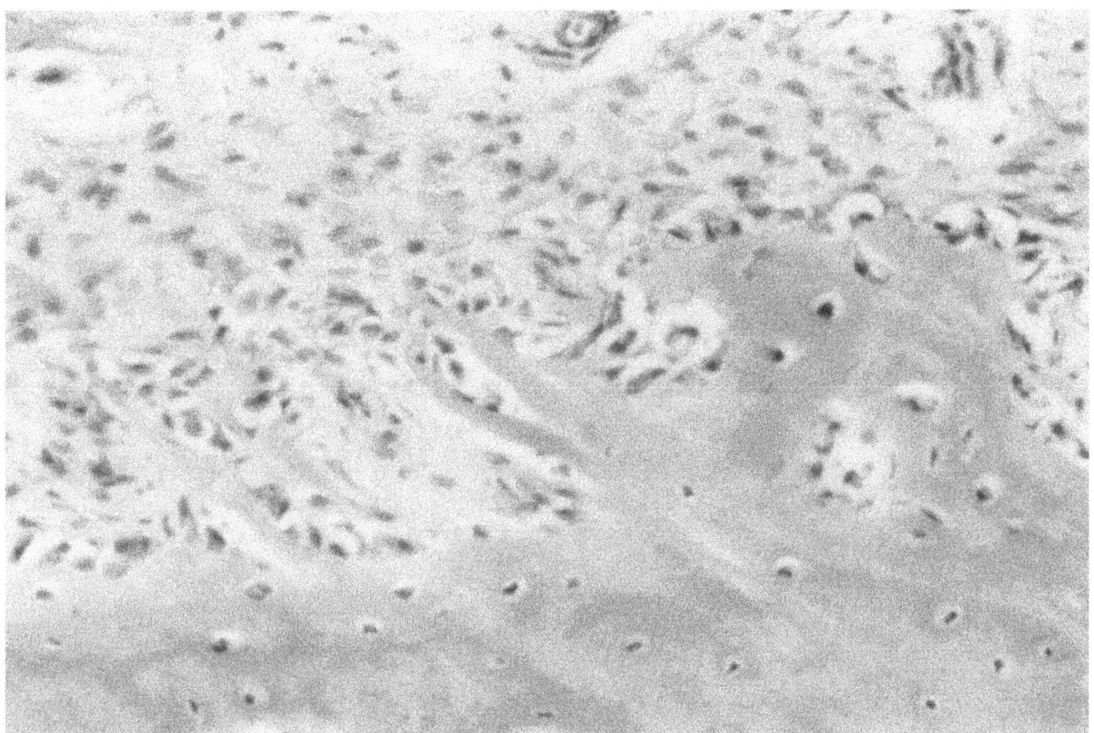

Finger, proximal phalanx. New fibrous bone is being formed by multi-layered, proliferated osteoblasts situated between periosteum and cortical bone

Fig. 6.37
Psoriatic arthritis

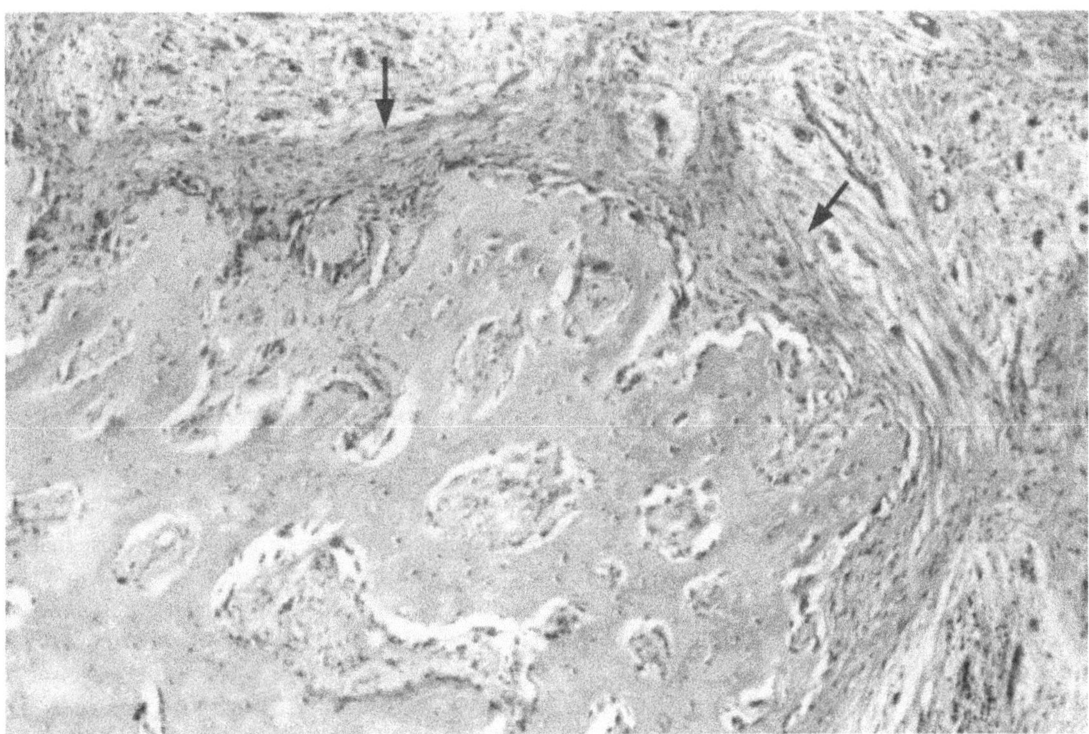

Femoral bone. Osteoblast proliferation between cortical bone and periosteum with bizarrely-shaped new formation of fibrous bone (*arrows*) (cambium layer; 35-year-old male)

Fig. 6.38
Psoriatic arthritis

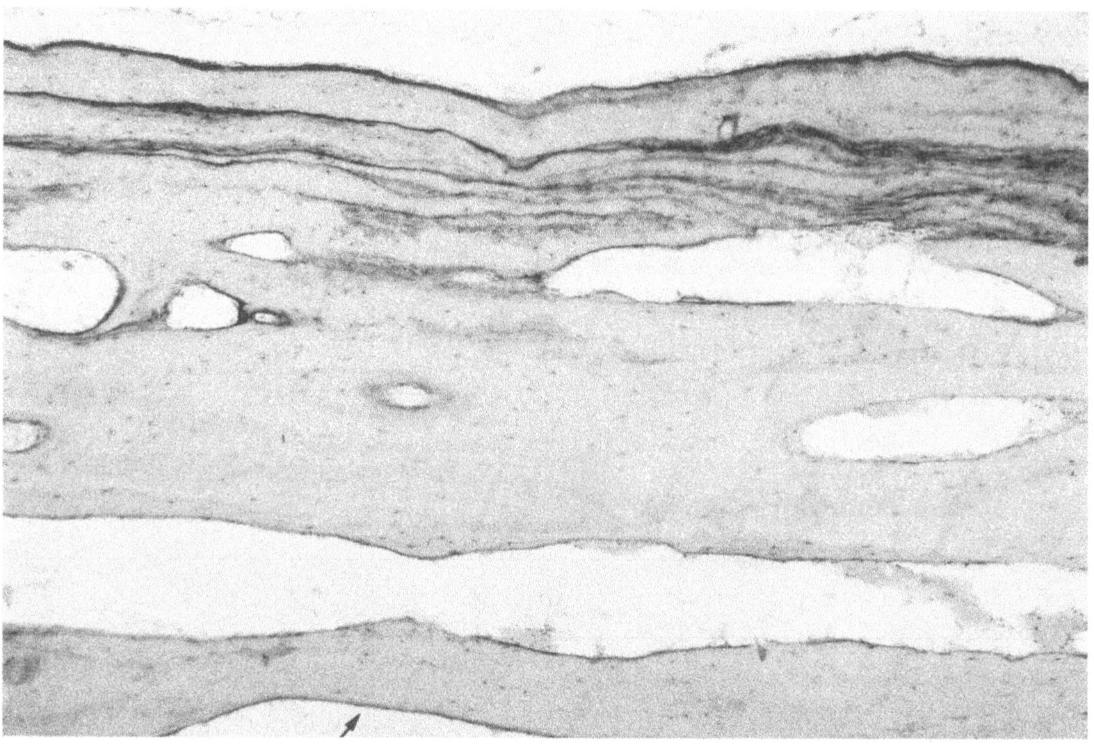

Fig. 6.39
Psoriatic arthritis

Finger, middle phalanx. Traces of formation of new fibrous bone that has developed at different times above the cortical bone (*arrow*)

Bone modelling proteins

As our observations serve to exclude an inflammatory cause of the pathological formation of new bone in PSA and other SSA, we believe that bone modelling proteins (BMP) play a role in the osteoblastic transformation process. We could identify e.g. analogous benign new formation of fibrous bone in the shoulder girdle and pelvic girdle of BMP-6 transgenic mice (Märker-Hermann et al. 1997). The cambium layer contains neither lymphocytes, plasma cells, macrophages, nor neutrophils. It is the prototype of ossification without any interfering inflammation mechanism and characteristic not only of PSA but also of the ossifying processes in SSA (see p. 180).

Also the surrounding bone marrow tissue is loosely structured, transparent, and without any fibrosis indicative of an expired inflammation. Moreover, an enzymatic degradation by osteoclasts or damage via an inflammatory mechanism would never selectively deplete the proteoglycans and leave the collagen fibre framework of the bone intact. We have no doubt therefore that, in this case, a bone process of a special kind progresses, in which no inflammatory or immunological elements can be identified. Analogous changes we find also in the bone tissue from patients with RS.

Morphological background

The irregular and excessive new bone formation offers an explanation for the radiological phenomena (including the capsular ossification) which appear in the region of the phalanges, particularly in PSA and RS. The remodelling processes at the diaphyseal corticalis cause inflammation of the surrounding soft tissues

and are the reason for the dactylitis ("sausage finger" and "sausage toe") in both these diseases.
Two questions remain to be answered:
1. How do bony bridges (ankyloses) between articular cavities develop in patients with PSA and other SSA?
2. How does arthritis develop in PSA and other members of the SSA family?

Pathogenesis of ankylosis

Our studies confirm Ball's clinical concept, dating from 1971, which states that one pathogenetic mechanism is common to all the skeletal processes in the SSA-group, namely the enthesopathy. Enthesis designates a transitional zone, where sinews and bony tissue are interwoven. Such transitional zones also exist between cortical bone and periosteum, between bone and articular cartilage, as well as between vertebrae and anulus fibrosus.
Bone and adjacent tissues, with the exception of articular cartilage, are basically made of collagen type I fibres. With the help of microscopic studies done with polarization technique, these fibres can be visualized radiating into the respective adjacent tissue. Of decisive importance for the progress of the process is the proliferation of regional fibroblasts and their transformation into osteoblasts. With varying degrees of intensity, the osteoblasts begin to form fibrous bone. Hereby the collagen fibres radiating into the neighbouring tissue serve as a guiding structure. Primary structure borders between tissues, such as between bone and collagenous connective tissue, are thus transgressed without any inflammatory interference. Therefore, zones of ossification form in areas of tendon insertions, and bone remodelling develops along the remaining collagen fibre framework within the spongiosa. These processes duplicate when bony structures stand face-to-face, as they do in the following cases:

Osteoblastic transformation

- Finger joints
  The formation of new bone leads to a bridging of the interarticular space and to osseous ankylosis.
- Vertebral column
  Here, the process begins with an attack of ossification at the margins of the vertebral body and proceeds to move vertically to the collagen fibres of the anulus fibrosus. The same type of transformation takes place between the margin of the neighbouring vertebra and the anulus fibrosus. The so-called fronts of ossification of one upper and one lower vertebra converge until an initially thin "clasp" of spongy bone is formed. At the inner surface of these marginal syndesmophytes, areas of new horizontal ossification "fronts" arise, which as they approach each other bring the nucleus pulposus into the ossifying process, resulting in the more or less total ossification of the vertebral body (see Fig. 6.18).

Osseous ankylosis

One explanation for the fact that the anulus fibrosus is the first site of ossification is obvious from the direction of the collagen fibres, the other explanation is that it consists of the same type of collagen as bone (collagen type I).
According to our findings, a morphological analysis of all the pathological ossification processes specific for the SSA-group re-

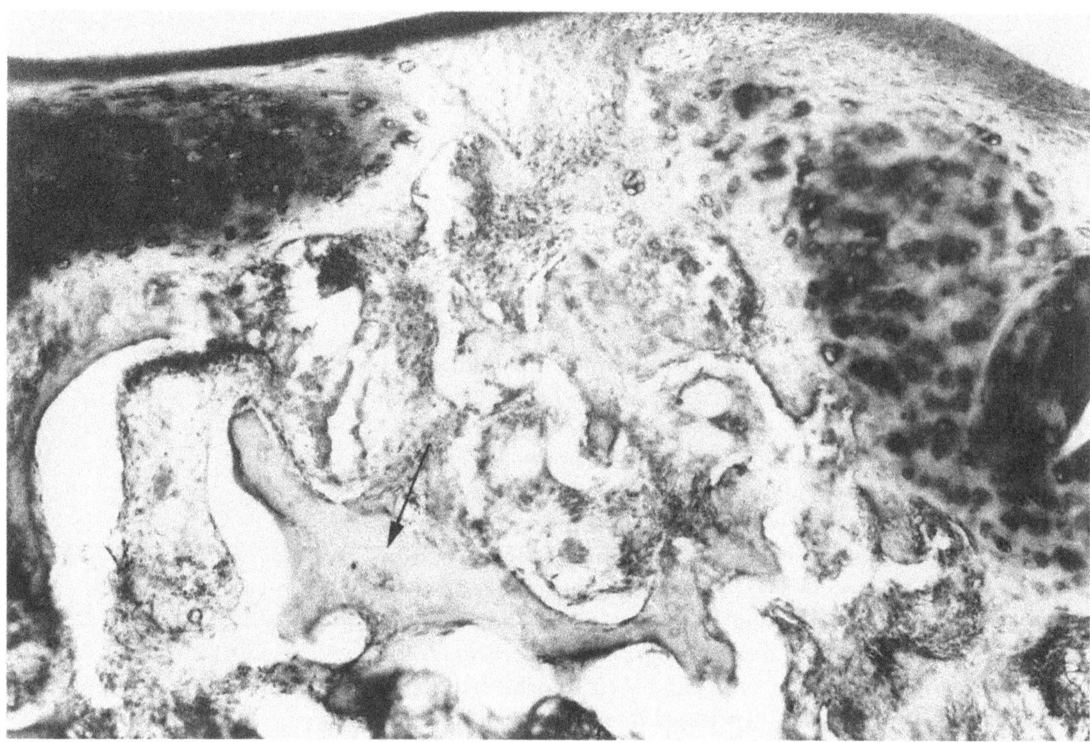

Fig. 6.40
Psoriatic arthritis

In the centre of the picture, subchondral bone that is broken through can be seen. In this region, there is collagenous fibre tissue (articular surface of the metatarsophalangeal joints). At the *right* side, remnants of articular cartilage. At the bottom left, remains of the spongiosa (*arrow*). In this region, articular cartilage has been substituted by fibrous cartilage

veals that they can be attributed to excessive, pathological ossification in bordering zones between bone and respective adjacent tissue. The ossification comes about in two forms (see p. 180):

Ossification in two forms

1. In loose tissue, such as the periosteum, by the proliferation of osteoblasts and the development of new fibrous bone.
2. In tight tendinous tissue, such as the Achilles' tendon, initially by chondroid metaplasia of collagen tissue and later by ossification. This enthesopathic process takes its course analogously in PSA and AS (see Fig. 6.1).

Pathogenesis of synovitis

What remains to be clarified is the question of the origin of the synovitis, that, long before the specific bone processes become apparent, characterizes the clinical symptomatology of arthritis. The morphological similarity between the synovitis in PSA and that in other members of the SSA family suggests that the synovitis in PSA is most likely a concomitant phenomenon caused by a systemic immunological disorder. On the other hand, according to our observations, it could be argued that the spreading of the primary, non-inflammatory bone lesion into the articular space causes inflammatory reactions in the synovial membrane (Fig. 6.40). The irritability of the synovial membrane is obvious, we observed that even the slightest trauma may induce reactive hyperplasia of the villi. If the synovitis is triggered by a mechanical cause, the inflammation in PSA could be considered to be analogous to the synovitis accompanying OA or following intra-articular injuries, that is, the inflammatory mechanism in PSA would be a reaction to structural damage in cartilage or bone and to the ensuing biochemical consequences. Depending on the degree and activity of the disease, the synovial membrane in PSA may contain lymphocytes and plasma cells. This, however, is not conducive to an answer because lymphocytes, plasma cells, and even sometimes true lymph follicles are also seen in the synovial membrane in patients with OA or synovitis following intra-articular injuries, both of which certainly do not result from immunological reactions. At the present time, the problem of the origin of synovitis in PSA, whether it arises from immunological reactions as it does in REA, or whether it is induced by mechanical processes spreading from adjacent bone, remains to be investigated. Whatever the origin of joint destruction may be, the morphological features do not offer anything indicative of either mechanism.

From what we know today, two possible mechanisms responsible for the joint destruction ought to be taken into consideration: the enzymatic degradation of cartilage and bone by proteases released by neutrophils, as is the case in BA (see p. 386), and destruction caused by the invasion of "aggressive" proliferated synovial cells and their proteases, as is the case in RA. No evidence of either mechanism is found in the synovial membrane of patients with PSA: we never observed synovial aggression upon cartilage. Nor did we see caving in of granulation tissue into cartilage, bone or marrow space – which would be present were the destructive lesions inflammatory in origin – nor infiltration of synovial tissue by neutrophils, the enzymes of which can destroy cartilage and bone, as they do in BA. Even though the mechanism that triggers the synovitis in PSA cannot yet be identified, any claim that the synovitis may be responsible for the destructive lesions characteristic of PSA is certainly to be dismissed. Consequently, antiphlogistic medication, while it may well influence the inflammatory processes, will be ineffective in controlling the bone process. On the other hand, it is plausible that cytostatic substances seem to be a promising therapeutic option as they influence the proliferation of osteoblasts. While the bone lesions can be visualized with the help of radioactive isotopes, they cause pain only when they encroach on the periosteum and induce secondary inflammation of neighbouring soft tissues ("sausage finger"; see p. 213).

Cytostatic therapy

Scintigraphic studies

The skeletal scintigraphic studies of Holzmann and coworkers (1978, 1982), Haydl and coworkers (1984) as well as Hahn and coworkers (1985) who used ^{99m}Technetium can offer elucidation on the connection of bone processes and arthritis in PSA. Holzmann and coworkers found in 3% of patients with PSA not only an accumulation of the tracer in the area of manifest joint processes, but also in the neighbourhood of clinically intact joints and, moreover, also in the skeletal system distant from the joints as well as in the area of the cranium and the ribs. Haydl and coworkers (1984) describe corresponding findings in the vertebral column in 60% of their patients with PSA. Their results

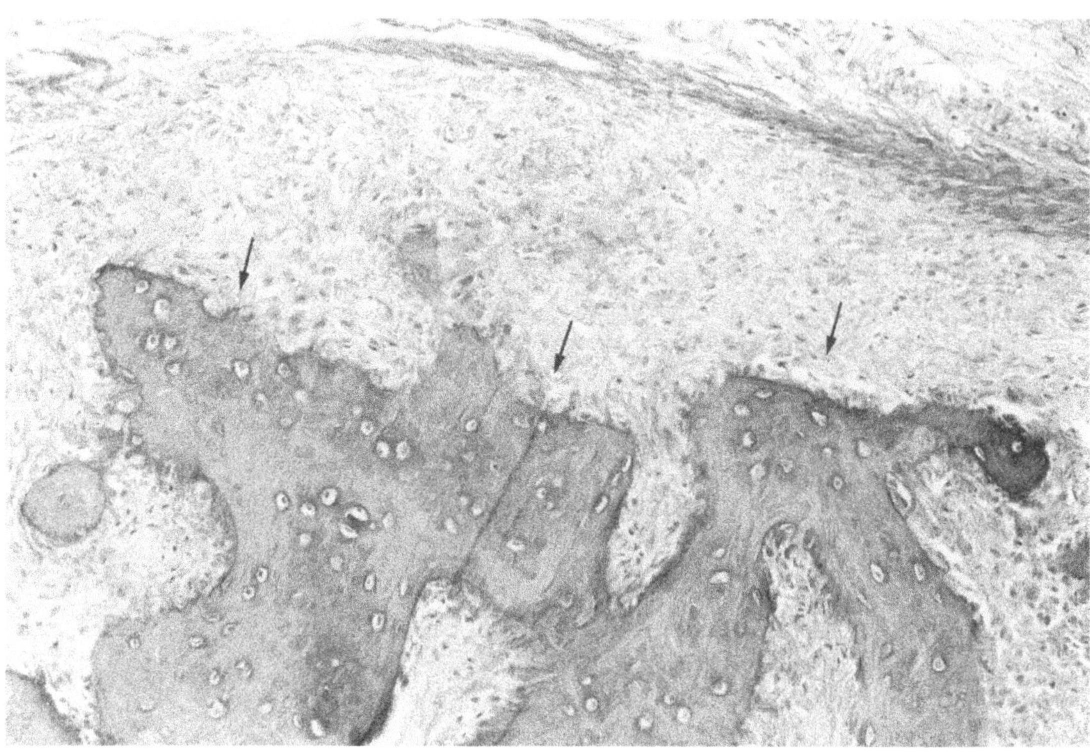

Fig. 6.41

Spondarthritis hyperostotica pustulo-psoriatica. Sternoclavicular joint. Highly florid osteoblast proliferation in the cambium layer (*arrows*) between cortical bone and periosteum with bizarrely-shaped new formation of fibrous bone (14-year-old female)

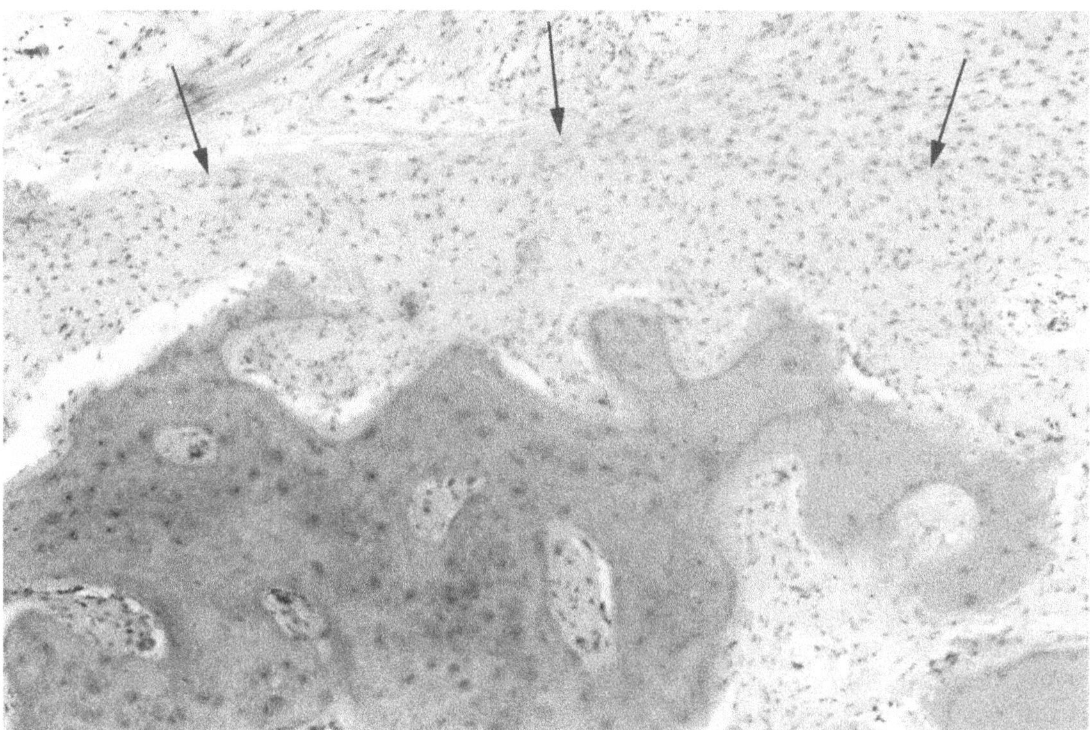

Fig. 6.42
Psoriatic arthritis

Sternoclavicular joint. Cambium layer of proliferated fibroblasts transformed into osteoblasts (*arrows*) with bizarrely-shaped new formation of fibrous bone (14-year-old female)

correlate with our findings in that extraarticular pathological processes were detected. The concentration of radionuclides can be explained by the osteoblast proliferation and new bone formation.

Taking into account our observations and these findings, we recommend the term "osteoarthropathia psoriatica" which includes the generalized bone process, which, only by spreading to the neighbouring joint, causes a secondary synovitis.

Erosions of subchondral bone lamella

Erosions of the subchondral bone lamella and partial transformation of hyaline articular cartilage into fibrous cartilage of low cell density are evidence of the bone process extending from the medullary space into the articular cavity. That collagen type I fibres permeate bone and penetrate into the layer of fibrous cartilage can be documented microscopically at numerous sites using the polarization technique.

"Spondarthritis hyperostotica pustulo-psoriatica"

In 1975, Köhler and coworkers described a painful sternoclavicular hyperostosis in patients with PSA. In 1981, Sonozaki and coworkers mentioned an "ostitis" in the frontal region of the upper thoracic aperture that was similar to AS and accompanied by a palmoplantar pustulation (PPP). Altmeyer and Holzmann (1984) found scintigraphic evidence of remodelling processes in the sternoclavicular region in a large number of PPP patients.

Schilling and coworkers (1986) described these dermal and osseous processes in nine patients and summarized this syndrome with the somewhat complicated term "spondarthritis hyperostotica pustulo-psoriatica" (SHPP). All patients were negative for HLA-B27. There was no ankylosing tendency. From six of these patients, we could study histologically the surgically removed tissue from the sternoclavicular region (Figs. 6.41, 6.42). The changes corresponded to the phases III and IV, as described above in the psoriatic bone process. Together with Schilling, we are convinced that SHPP has to be classified in the overall picture of psoriasis.

6.4 Arthropathy with Inflammatory Bowel Disease

6.4.1 Definition

The definition of inflammatory bowel disease (IBD) comprises ulcerative colitis (UC) and Crohn's disease (CD, also called granulomatous ileocolitis). Both diseases have comparable rheumatologic and other associated features that cannot be easily differentiated.

6.4.2 History

Samuel Wilks (1824–1911) and Walter Moxon (1836–1886) were the first to mention a case of UC. It is William Henry Allchin (1846–1912), however, to whom we are indebted for the first portray of the clinical signs and symptoms. He also described in detail an autopsy on a patient with extensive ulcerations in the colon (Otto et al. 1976). Allchin's statement: "The etiology of the case is doubtless most obscure" remains valid until the year 2000.

The history of CD begins in 1923 with Moschowitz and Wilensky describing "non-specific granuloma of the intestine" (Crohn 1949). In 1931, Mock spoke of an "infective granuloma with non-specific chronic tumour-like productive inflammations of the gastrointestinal tract" (Crohn 1949).

In 1932, Crohn, Ginsburg, and Oppenheimer described a disease affecting the terminal ileum, a regional ileitis. They believed it to be limited to the terminal ileum. Soon afterwards, though, comparable clinical signs and morphological findings were also observed in other portions of the intestine (Crohn 1949).

Peripheral arthritis

The association between colitis and arthritis was first described by White in 1895. This group of diseases enters the rheumatological context because in 10%–20% of all patients the joints are co-diseased (Moll 1985; Arnett 1989).

6.4.3 Epidemiology

Males and females are equally affected at all ages. Between 10% and 20% of UC and CD patients suffer from arthritis, the inflammatory activity of which corresponds to that of the intestinal disease, and which generally occurs simultaneously with or subsequent to a flare-up of the intestinal disease. Fifteen percent of UC and CD patients suffer from sacroiliitis, only 3–6% from spondylitis. In contrast to the peripheral arthritides, these axial lesions often precede the intestinal disease. The intensity of the enteral inflammatory processes and that of the axial lesions do not correspond. HLA-B27 association is rated at between 40% and 85% and is highest in patients with involvement of the central skeleton, lowest in patients with sole involvement of peripheral joints.

6.4.4 Clinical Manifestations

Intestinal manifestations

Clinically, CD and UC are characterized by abdominal pain, diarrhoea, and intestinal haemorrhage.

Extra-intestinal manifestations

In about 25% of patients, IBD is accompanied by extra-intestinal manifestations (e.g. secondary amyloidosis and anterior uveitis which is associated with HLA-B27, and axial involvement). Erythema nodosum occurs more often in CD, pyoderma gangrenosum more often in UC. Arthritis, occurring with IBD, has the following characteristic features:

1. In most cases, arthritis starts after the beginning of an intestinal illness.
2. The arthritic attacks are related temporally to flare-ups of the bowel disease.
3. The attacks of arthritis are followed by complete remission of synovitis.
4. Rheumatoid factors are absent.

It involves highly acute and painful mono- and oligoarthritides, affecting peripheral joints in an asymmetric pattern, and favouring the lower extremities. In about half of the patients, the arthritis often disappears a few days up to weeks after waning of the gut disease. In about 20% of IBD patients, joint attacks persist, however, for longer than 1 year.

Joint involvement

The following joints are afflicted in IBD in decreasing order of frequency: knee, ankle, elbow, proximal interphalangeal joint of a finger, wrist, shoulder, and metacarpolphalangeal joints. The process progresses non-destructively and there is, in general, no permanent joint damage.

Bacterial superinfections

In about 25% of patients, clinical or radiological residues are alleged to be detected. However, because of the known tendency of CD to cause septic arthritides of the hip it must be considered in these cases whether the damage is due to previous clinically latent bacterial superinfections (see p. 386).

Axial involvement

HLA-B27

The IBD gets into the context of the SSA (see p. 178) due to the observation that in about 10–15% of all patients a sacroiliitis with or without spondylitis occurs (Moll 1985). The true prevalence could be higher because of silent axial involvement. About half of the patients with spine involvement are HLA-B27-positive (Arnett 1989). The association is, however, less dominant than in other SSA (see p. 183). Involvement of the axial skeleton in IBD does not develop parallel to the gut disease characteristics and is completely independent of the peripheral arthritis. A spondylitis can precede the intestinal manifestations even by years. The clinical picture as well as the male-to-female ratio with a general male predominance corresponds mainly to AS (see p. 183).

The IBD does not only affect the intestine and the skeleton, iridocyclitis, conjunctivitis, and, rarely, episcleritis, aphthous stomatitis, and other cutaneous lesions, such as erythema nodosum (see above), broaden the spectrum of pathological phenomena.

6.4.5 Pathology

Intestinal lesions in Morbus Crohn

CD is characterized by non-caseating epithelioid granulomata which can attack all layers of the intestinal wall in the region of the ileum and colon (Fig. 6.43).

These granulomata are also found outside the intestinal wall, in the synovial membrane as well as in lymph nodes, liver, uveal tract, and skeletal musculature (Lindstrom et al. 1972; Fraya et al. 1975; Hermans et al. 1984; Mohr 1984) and give rise to confusion with sarcoidosis.

Synovial membrane

In contrast to CD, the morphologically specified ulcerative reactions in UC restrict themselves to the mucosa and submucosa of the colon. In both forms of IBD, the histological picture of the synovial membrane is not characteristic. In joint biopsies taken from patients with CD, we observed the same synovial changes we saw in biopsies taken from PSA and AS patients: thin villi of medium length with loosely fibrosed stroma. Typical are numerous small, thin-walled vessels, predominantly at the margins of the villi (Fig. 6.44). Extent and composition of a cellular infiltration depend not only on the activity of the local and the systemic process but also on therapeutic measures. That there is never any proliferation of stroma cells frequently

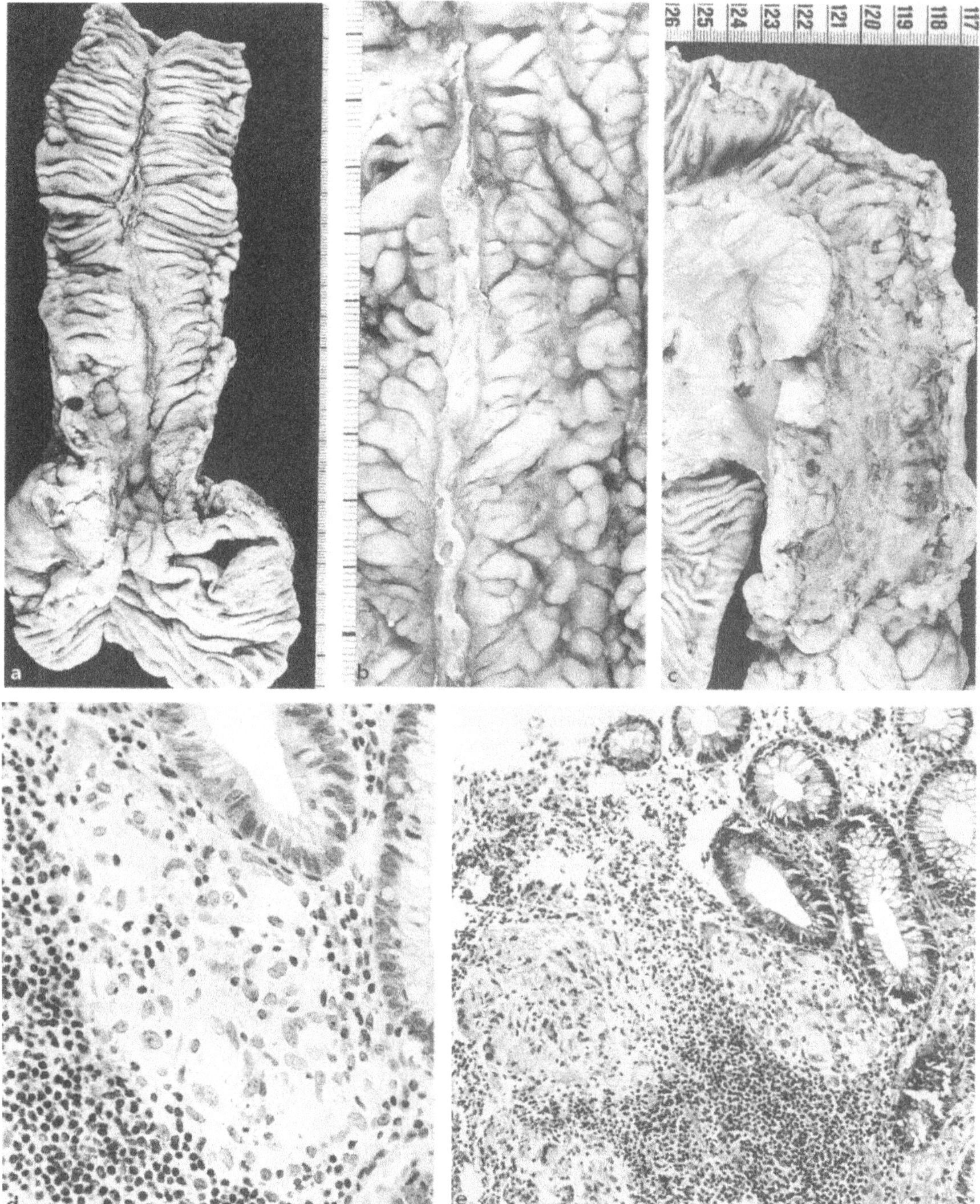

Fig. 6.43 a–e
M. Crohn

Ileocecal region. **a–c** Ileum with large, longitudinal ulcus, numerous polypi and pseudopolypi ("pavement-like picture"). **d,e** Epithelioid cell granulomata in the mucosa of the ileum. (Otto and Remmele 1996)

contrasts sharply with the substantial hypertrophy of the lining cells.

Unfortunately, no separated data are available concerning synovial biopsies from UC patients with or without HLA-B27. Thus, no comment can be made to the question of whether or not the synovial changes correspond to those in other forms of SSA (see p. 181).

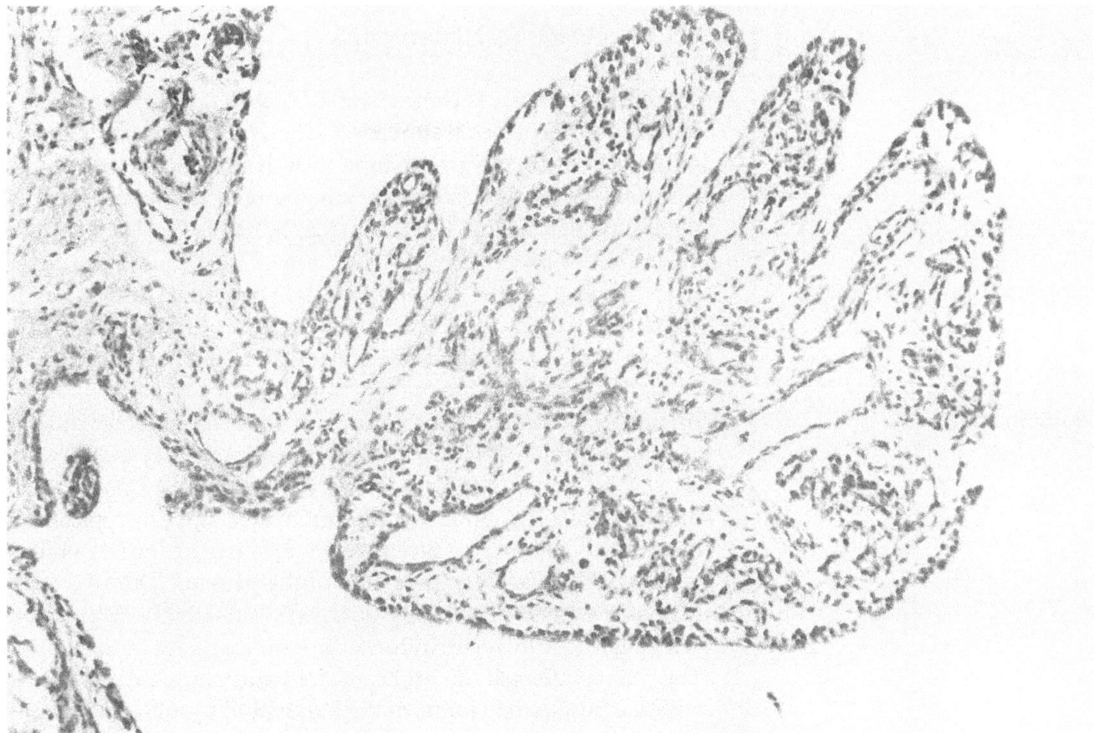

Formation typical for SSA: single-staged lining cell layer, sizeable development of thin-walled blood vessels. Sparse lymphocytic infiltration

Fig. 6.44
M. Crohn

6.5 Whipple's Disease

Synonym: Morbus Whipple.

6.5.1 Definition and History

Multisystemic disease

Whipple's disease (WD) is a rare disease. It is triggered by bacteria and is multisystemic, but the small intestine is always affected. WD was first described by the American pathologist George Whipple (1907): a 36-year-old patient with severe weight loss, low fever, and persisting cough was ill with steatorrhoea, anaemia, and polyarthritis.

6.5.2 Epidemiology

This disorder is most common in white males between 40 and 60 years of age. The male-to-female ratio is 9:1. The disease is usually sporadic, but has been noted in siblings. Many patients are farmers and live in rural areas. Prolonged exposure to animals or birds may have etiological significance (Rubinow 1986). The data are yet too few to reliably deduce epidemiological hypotheses. Until 1986, that is approximately 80 years after the first description, only 250 cases were known (Rubinow 1986).

6.5.3 Clinical Manifestations

The clinical picture is characterized by chronic diarrhoea, that in 80% is the form of steatorrhoea. The clinical course is distinguished by increasing adynamia as well as marked weight loss. Clinical signs include scaling erythemas and a greyish hyperpigmentation of the skin. If left untreated, the disease leads to marasmus and is eventually fatal.

Polyarthralgia and myalgia

It is because of the intermittent polyarthralgia and myalgia, which precede the characteristic symptoms, that WD has been classed with the indistinctly defined group of rheumatic diseases.

Joint involvement

Rheumatic manifestations occur in 60–90% of patients with WD (Amor and Toubert 1993). Thereby, the joint disease may precede for several years up to decades the clinical onset of the enteritic disease. Thus, the joint symptoms, which appear typically at intervals of a few hours and several days, are the initial manifestations of the disease in over 50% of the patients with WD. Rarely do these attacks last a long time. The joint attacks extend from arthralgias to polyarthritides with swelling, pain, and redness. The joints affected in order of frequency are knees, ankles, wrists, elbows, small joints of the hands, and shoulders (Rubinow et al. 1981).

The joint process regresses with antibiotic treatment. Untreated arthritides, the character of which could not be recognized before the onset of WD, can be misinterpreted as atypical RA.

Axial involvement

The significance of a systemic component is also indicated from the observation of an only slightly increased prevalence of HLA-B27 in patients with WD (30% according to the studies of Dobbins 1987), suggesting an association with AS or sacroiliitis, even in the absence of concomitant spondylitis (Rubinow 1986).

Sacroiliitis

Thus, a relationship between WD, HLA-B27, and axial involvement is to be judged controversially. Some studies suggest a relationship (Canoso et al. 1978; Khan 1982), others found that HLA-B27 was equally common in patients with and without sacroiliitis (Feurle 1985). It is certain that axial involvement in WD is far less frequent than in peripheral arthritis. Amor and Toubert (1993) report that only four from a group of 95 patients with WD suffered from spondylitis or sacroiliitis.

6.5.4 Pathogenesis

Rod-shaped, gram-positive bacteria

The hypothesis that WD is triggered by an infection was confirmed by the identification of rod-shaped, gram-positive bacteria and their metabolites. These bacteria had earlier been observed electron-microscopically. Based on studies by Wilson and coworkers (1991) and by using the PCR-technique on a small rRNA-subunit of the bacterium, Relman and coworkers (1992) demonstrated a previously unknown, and to date unique, sequence, 1,321-bases-16S-rRNA, in patients suffering from WD.

Tropheryma whippelii

The bacterium was then identified and named *Tropheryma whippelii* gen.nov.sp.nov. These results were confirmed by studies performed by Meier-Willersen and coworkers (1993).

From these findings, doubt can no longer exist about the essential role of a bacterial infection, which is also confirmed by the success of anti-bacterial therapy. WD is therefore probably a form of REA caused by an intestinal infection.

Reactive arthritis

The disease is based on an insufficiency of the macrophage system and also possibly of the immune defence system. This defect expresses itself in the incomplete degradation of the phagocytosed microorganism. Only due to the insufficiency of the body's defence mechanism do the haematogenically colonized bacterial instigators achieve their pathogenic quality.

Insufficiency of defence

Frequent opportunistic infections might be caused by immune deficiencies in patients with WD.

6.5.5 Pathology

SPC cells

Diagnostic key fossil of WD are PAS-positive sickle-form particles containing cells (SPC cells), detected in biopsies of the small intestine.

The mucosa of the small intestine may exhibit berry-like swellings, the serosa is fibrosed and reddened. Beneath the serosa a network of congested lymph vessels can be seen. The villi of the small intestine appear bulb-shaped and enlarged. In the mucosa as well as in deeper wall layers, pathognomonic SPC cells with intense cytoplasmatic PAS-reaction, caused by lysosomes containing bacteria and bacterial metabolites, are seen electron-microscopically.

Electron-microscopical findings

SPC cells have been found in all organs studied: liver, lymph nodes, spleen, pancreas, heart, lungs, synovial membrane, serosal membrane, and in the central nervous system. Occasionally, epithelioid-cell granulomata are found in the mucosa of the small intestine, in lymph nodes, liver, spleen, lung, and/or in skeletal muscle of patients with WD, the etiology of which is unknown. SPC cells may persist for a long time, even after antibiotic therapy (Meier-Willersen et al. 1993).

Synovial process

The changes revealed by light-microscopy in the synovial membrane correspond to the degree of joint affliction. At the peak of the attack, proliferation of the lining cells, new formation of blood vessels, and, in particular, neutrophil infiltration within the membrane are observed. Only a few lymphocytes are found after the fading of the acute process. The diagnosis is confirmed by the detection of foamy vacuolated macrophages (SPC cells) containing discretely PAS-positive granules (Fig. 6.45). The joint process is not destructive!

PAS-positive granules

In view of the rarity of WD, no extensive survey has yet been reported, so that the question of whether the WD belongs to the SSAs (see p. 178) cannot be unequivocally answered.

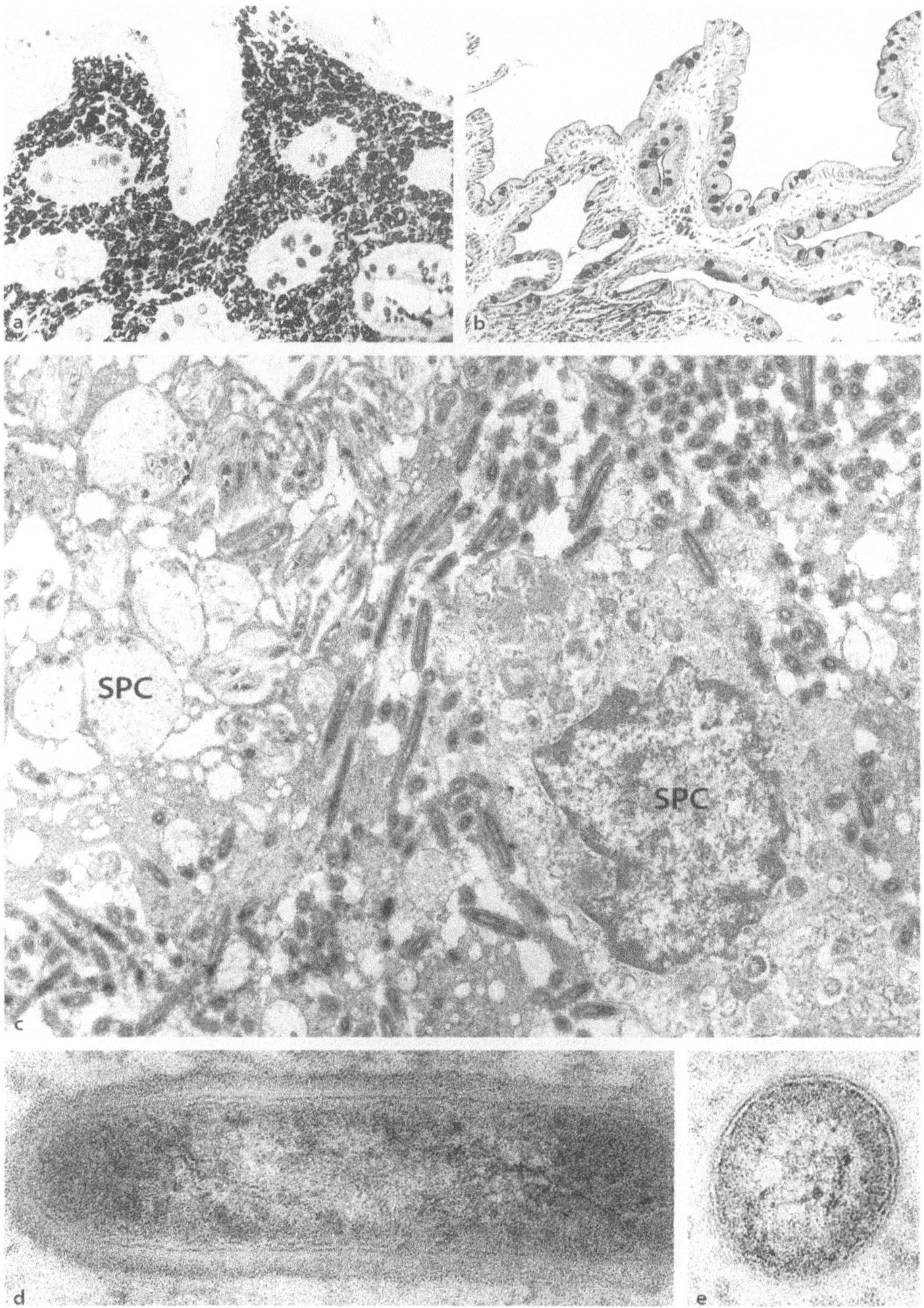

Fig. 6.45 a–e
M. Whipple

a Masses of PAS-positive *SPC* cells in the mucosa of the ileum. **b** Mucosa after a course of antibiotic therapy for several weeks. The *SPC* cells have almost completely disappeared. **c** *SPC* cells with phagolysosomes in the mucosa of the ileum. Numerous, extracellularly situated "Whipple bacteria". **d,e** Longitudinal and cross-section through the "Whipple bacterium". (Otto and Remmele 1996)

7 Behçet's Syndrome

7.1 Definition

Multisystemic disease

Behçet's syndrome (BS) is a chronically-residing multisystemic disease which is characterized by a triad of chronic stomatitis aphthosa, recurrent genital ulcerations, and uveitis. New, internationally agreed diagnostic criteria were elaborated by the International study group for Behçet's disease (1990): "Recurrent oral ulcerations plus any two of the following symptoms: genital ulceration, typical defined eye lesions, typical defined skin lesions."

7.2 History

The syndrome was described for the first time in 1937 by the Turkish dermatologist Behçet. The indication from Feigenbaum (1956) is, however, interesting that already in Hippocrates' third book about the endemic diseases, a description of this disease picture can be found (Behçet 1937).

7.3 Epidemiology

Prevalence

BS mainly spreads in the eastern Mediterranean countries as, for example, in Turkey with a prevalence rate of 38:10,000 (Yurdakul et al. 1988) and in Japan where its prevalence is 1:10,000 (Hirohata et al. 1975). According to Hamuryudan et al. (1997), the prevalence is 1:300,000 in Northern Europe. Men and women are equally affected. The uveitis in the context of BS is said to be the most frequent cause of blindness in Japan (Shikano 1966).

Genetic predisposition

Japanese and Turkish authors (Ohno et al. 1973; Yazici et al. 1980) report about a three- to sixfold higher association of HLA-B51 in BS, compared to the normal population, whereas HLA-B27 was only observed with simultaneously occurring sacroiliitis and/or spondylitis. It has been suggested that HLA-B27-positive patients with BS are at risk to develop mild sacroiliitis and/or spondylitis (Empey and Hale 1972). Nevertheless, no consistent increase in

Sacroileitis

HLA-B51

HLA-B27 has been noted. A more severe clinical course of BS seems to be associated with the presence of HLA-B51 (O'Duffy 1990).

7.4 Clinical Features

The onset of the disease is usually between puberty and the third decade of life. The disease advances progressively in attacks, the particular symptoms develop episodically within longer periods of time. When taking the history, all symptoms should therefore be gathered and then assessed cumulatively.

Aphthous oral ulcerations

Aphthous or herpetiform oral ulcerations occur in over 95% of patients. Ulcers may be located anywhere within the mouth or pharynx. Their size ranges from a few millimeters (herpetiform) to several centimeters in diameter. Oral ulcerations are often deep; they soften and disappear after 1 to 2 weeks but tend to be recurrent and may leave scarring.

Genital lesions

In males, the genital lesions take the form of painful, punched-out ulcers on the scrotal skin or rarely on the glans penis. In contrast, the vaginal ulcerations in women may go entirely unnoticed by the patient. The overall frequency of these lesions in reported case series is 80%–90% (Hamuryudan et al. 1997).

Eye affection

The eyes are affected at some time in the course of Behçet's disease in 50% of patients, but generally become symptomatic some years after the onset of aphthous stomatitis. The typical lesion is recurrent unilateral or bilateral iritis with a purulent collection in the anterior chamber (hypopyon). But conjunctivitis, episcleritis, keratitis, iridocyclitis, and optic neuritis also have been observed. Uveitis is believed to be a sequel of vasculitis.

Cutaneous involvement

Cutaneous involvement occurs in 70%–80% of patients as nodular lesion of the lower extremities resembling erythema nodosum or as pathergic erythema, a form of hypersensitivity with pustule formation within 24 h at sites of trivial trauma (e.g. needle puncture; Medsger 1986).

Central nervous system involvement

Central nervous system involvement occurs in 1%–15% of patients, manifesting as brain stem or pyramidal signs.
Meningoencephalitides were observed in approximately 30% (O'Duffy and Goldstein 1976); mortality of "neuro-Behçet" is estimated to be around 40%.

Gastrointestinal bleedings

Gastrointestinal bleedings, from ulcerations in the oesophagus or duodenum or from ulcerations brought about from enteritides, may cause the course of the disease to take a dramatic direction and thus obscure its true nature. Twenty-five percent of patients develop thrombophlebitides.

Joint involvement

The joint involvement accounts for, besides the pathognomonic triad in 40%–50% of patients, the most frequent comanifestations of BS (Yurdakul et al. 1983). It is mainly a question of arthralgia, rarely, however, real arthritides. The joint process frequently recurs. The episodes can last several weeks and more seldom up to several years. The joint attack is monoarticular or often asymmetrically oligoarticular, preferring the knee, ankle, hand joints, and elbows. The small joints, in contrast, are seldom affected.

7.5 Pathology

Although to date not all phenomena of BS, such as meningoencephalitis or synovitis, can be attributed to one and the same pathogenetic mechanism, vascular processes do seem to be the cause common to all significant manifestations: leucocytoclastic and lymphocytic vasculitides are found in acute skin lesions. Depending on age and extent, oral ulcerations are surrounded by a wall of lymphocytic and monocytic aggregations that infiltrate the basal cell layer of the mucosa. Similar perivascular inflammation at times, with frank necrosis of vessel walls, occurs in the skin and vulva, retinal vessels, and brain (McMenemey and Lawrence 1957; Shikano 1966). In these processes, a tendency to develop thrombi due to a state of hypercoagulability seems to be of decisive importance. Occlusions and aneurysms of large systemic arteries can cause life-threatening or fatal illness from limb ischaemia, stroke, renovascular hypertension or aortic aneurysm (Shimizu et al. 1979). BS is virtually alone among the vasculitides as a frequent cause of fatal aneurysms of the pulmonary arterial tree (Davies 1973; Grenier et al. 1981). The affinity to the vascular system also extends to the venous system. Phlebitis of major veins can result in such divergent syndromes as Budd-Chiari syndrome, vena caval occlusion, and, in the case of the dural veins, the syndrome of benign intracranial hypertension (Shimizu et al. 1979; Pamir et al. 1981).

Vascular processes as common causes

Occlusion and aneurysm

Venous system

Synovial membrane

The morphological changes in the synovial membrane are uncharacteristic. Depending on the activity of the process, discrete fibrin exudate and a few covering cell proliferates are found. The content of lymphocytes and plasma cells varies. Solitary neutrophils appear only occasionally in the synovial membrane. From our observations a fleeting arthralgia with minimal synovitides must also be taken into consideration. Proliferation of the synovial stroma cells does not occur. Correspondingly, reports of occasional joint destruction are to be considered sceptically since neither sufficient enzyme activity of the neutrophils nor aggressive synovial cell formation are available to promote cartilage or bone degradation. On the other hand, bacterial superinfections are, in our experience, not rare in already existing joint diseases (see p. 395).

The pathogenesis of BS remains until today unclear. It might not have a primary autoimmune basis. Perhaps, because no specific autoantibodies or clear-cut abnormalities in B cells have been demonstrated, more attention has been given to aberrations in T cell function (Yazici et al. 1999).

8 Lyme Disease*

8.1 History

Lyme arthritis was recognized in November, 1975, because of an unusual geographic cluster of children with inflammatory arthropathy in the region of Lyme, Connecticut, USA (Steere et al. 1977a). This discovery and identification provided an interesting new disease entity which augmented rheumatology. Its clear etiology can contribute to the pathogenetic understanding of acute and chronic joint disease in general. Lyme disease is part of a complex multi-system, tick bite-borne disease. Its dermatological and neurological components were already known from the beginning of the 20th century as consequences of tick bites under the terms erythema chronicum migrans (ECM) and meningopolyneuritis (Afzelius 1910; Garin and Bujadoux 1922; Bannwarth 1941). The type of joint involvement in young people was reminiscent of a juvenile chronic arthritis (JCA). Steere and colleagues (1976) in their first report of the disease, had, however, recognized that it was an epidemic form of arthritis and that it was probably transmitted by an arthropod vector.

Type of joint involvement

8.2 Epidemiology

In 1982, Burgdorfer and associates isolated the spirochaete that now bears his name from *Ixodes dammini* collected on Shelter Island, New York, USA, and linked it serologically to patients with Lyme disease. Within months of its discovery, this organism was cultured from blood, skin, and cerebrospinal fluid of patients with Lyme disease (Benach et al. 1983; Steere et al. 1983). With good reasons, Malawista et al. (1984) emphasize that Lyme disease presents an unique human model of an infectious etiology of rheumatic diseases. The effect of an antibiotic therapy stresses the causal role of the germ. The first epidemiological investigations (Steere et al. 1977a) showed a topographical incidence in three rural communities of the US state of Connecticut (Lyme, Old Lyme, Haddam) and a characteristic onset between May and

**Synonym:* Borrelian infection

November. Retrospective researches and later supplementary observations then revealed an association between the arthritis and a previous ECM in addition to neurological and cardiac disturbances. Lyme borreliosis occurs with similar frequencies in males and females in the USA, and affects people of all ages. A bimodal age of distribution of cases in the USA has been described with highest rates in children aged 5–9 years and in adults over 30 (Nadelman and Wormser 1998).

8.3 Pathogenesis

The identification of the causative agent made the integration of the arthritic, dermatological, neurological, and cardiac manifestation into a combined complex disease picture possible. The spirochaete of the Borrelian group was transmitted by the bite of a tick of the genus *Ixodes ricinus*, already known in Europe as the cause of ECM (Steere et al. 1983). We are indebted to the work of Steere and his group for the detailed elucidation of all aspects of Lyme disease based on the thorough analysis of a great number of patients. The observations of Herzer and colleagues (1986) suggested some variations in the transmission and course of Lyme disease in Europe, on the evidence that in spite of decades of knowledge of ECM, there had never been an associated arthritic component. While in North America the most important reservoir for *B. burgdorferi* is the white-footed mouse, in Europe a variety of small mammals and some birds can harbour the germ. Recombinant DNA technology has subsequently shown that the outer surface proteins of the *B. burgdorferi* found in Europe and North America are heterogeneous. This can account for the different clinical manifestations in Europe and North America and for the higher incidence of arthritis in the USA (Schoen 1988).

Spirochaete of Borrelian group

Pathogenetic considerations

1. There is no doubt about the causal role of *B. burgdorferi*. Its identity is confirmed parasitologically and immunologically. In addition, there is electron-microscopic evidence of the causative agent in skin biopsies, the synovial fluid, and in the synovial tissue of patients with Lyme disease (Valesova et al. 1989).
2. The slight rise of ESR is evidence against the direct release of an intensive inflammatory process by the infecting agent.
3. At the onset of the illness, in the stage of the ECM, circulating immune complexes occur in many patients (Hardin et al. 1979a,b). The presence of a raised IgM-titre and cryoglobulin containing IgM at this point predict subsequent nervous system, heart or joint involvement (Steere et al. 1977b, 1979a).
4. In the later phase of the joint, disease process, the IgM-level returns to normal. At this point the immune complexes and cryoglobulins disappear from the serum. In contrast, the IgG-antibodies reach their highest titre and can persist for years after clinical recovery.

Genetic disposition

5. Investigations of Steere and colleagues (1979b,c) show the significance of genetic disposition for the full development of the disease complex. Thus, 67% of patients with severe forms like meningoencephalitis or chronic arthritis evinced the B cell al-

loantigen DR2; in the shorter milder forms it occurs in only 36%.

6. According to Steere and colleagues (1977b) the cell content of the synovial fluid lies between 2,100 and 72,250 per mm^3, with a median of 24,250. Neutrophils are said to predominate. There is, thus, no basic difference from the cell content of synovial fluid in rheumatoid arthritis (RA). From our observations, however, we are convinced that the very high cell content is evidence of a clinically latent bacterial superinfection comparable to that which we found for example in RA in 13.5% of cases (see p. 395).

8.4 Clinical Manifestations

ECM

Lyme disease may take two different courses: the stages of the disease may either merge into each other, or be divided by symptom-free intervals. The early manifestation is the ECM that occurs 3–32 days after a tick bite in 90% of the patients. The ECM may be followed by neurological, cardiac or joint abnormalities, all of which occur weeks or months after and which may worsen at later stages of the disease. The ECM typically begins as a red macule or papule at the site of a tick bite after 7–10 days. The rash expands over days to weeks on the trunk in an annular form and can vary in diameter between 1 and 50 cm, presumably as the spirochaetes spread centrifugally through the skin. It can persist for some weeks without treatment and can reappear in subsequent attacks of arthritis. The patient feels tired and ill.

Variant of pathogen

Borrelial lymphocytoma

An Eurasian variant of the pathogen, *B. afzelii*, may, by typical skin manifestations, complicate the clinical picture of Lyme disease: the Borrelial lymphocytoma at the early stages, and chronic, atrophying acrodermatitis [acrodermatitis chronica atrophicans (ACA)] at the end stage. Borrelial lymphocytoma, principally caused by *B. afzelii* and *B. garinii* (Picken et al. 1997), is a tumour-like nodule which typically appears (in European patients) on the pinna of the earlobe, in the scrotum or on the nipple or areola of the breast (Stanek et al. 1996). Lesions resolve spontaneously or disappear within a few weeks after antibiotics. *B. garinii* exhibits a particular neurotropy (Nadelman and Wormser 1998).

Acrodermatitis chronica atrophicans

ACA, a late complication of Lyme disease, is caused by *B. afzelii*, a genospecies of *B. burgdorferi* which only occurs in Eurasia. This characteristic skin manifestation develops insidiously on a distal extremity, characterized by a swollen, bluish-red appearing skin lesion with ultimately atrophy. One-third of patients have an associated (usually sensory) polyneuropathy. *B. burgdorferi* has been recovered from skin biopsy specimens of ACA lesions of more than 10 years' duration (Steere 1989).

The demand for an isolation of the germ in culture for the diagnosis of an infectious disease could not be fulfilled in most case-series of Lyme borreliosis despite the fact that *B. burgdorferi* can be readily cultured in vitro (Nadelman and Wormser 1998).

Neurological complications

During the course of weeks or months 15% of patients in the USA infected develop neurological complications like meningitis and meningoencephalitis as well as motor and sensory neuro-tides ("neuroborreliosis"). These disappear without trace some further months later.

Carditis

The carditis due to *B. burgdorferi* typically develops weeks to months after infection and is usually manifested by fluctuating degree of atrioventricular block which may cause the patient to complain of dizziness, palpitations, dyspnoea, chest pain or syncope (van der Linde and Ballmer 1993). Before the widespread use of antibiotics for ECM, carditis was reported in 8% of patients in the USA (Steere 1989). In more recent series, the incidence has been lower, in both the USA (<1%; State of Connecticut, Department of Public Health 1993; Gerber et al. 1996) and in Europe (<4%; van der Linde and Ballmer 1993).

Lyme arthritis

The clinical features of Lyme arthritis are fundamentally similar in Europe and North America (Steere 1989). Within a period of a few weeks up to 2 years, about 60% of patients develop joint symptoms of various kinds. In the early stage of the disease there is migratory musculoskeletal pain in joints, tendons, bursae, muscles or bones often without joint swelling. The pain tends to affect only one or two sites at a time and usually lasts a few hours to several days in a given location. Equally characteristic is the frequent and early occurrence of Baker's cysts. In the late phase of the disease, clear arthritis develops (Steere et al. 1977c, 1980), usually characterized by intermittent attacks of asymmetric joint swelling and pain primarily in large joints, predominantly in the knees though in general both large and small joints can be affected. This late form of joint involvement can occur not only as a single event, but also as intermittent attacks persisting for days or months, and followed by complete remission. However, the illness can also recur after some years (Steere and Malawista 1985). In about 10% of patients with Lyme arthritis, especially those with HLA class II antigen DR4 or DR2, involvement in large joints can become chronic. Thereby joint space narrowing and marginal erosions are observed (Rahn and Malawista 1993). Herzer (1990) saw in the localization of these erosions at the junction between vascular and avascular tissue, as well as in the region of tendons and ligaments, a preferred site for antigen deposition and antigen persistence, respectively. In occasional cases, a symmetrical polyarthritic joint involvement has been reported.

Laboratory findings

In general, the ESR is only slightly raised. There is no evidence of rheumatic factors and HLA-B27. Between the 3rd and 8th week after the onset of the illness specific IgM-antibodies against Borrelia are present. Specific IgG-antibodies, however, develop slowly and reach their highest titre some months later when arthritis is present. At this point no further significant increase of IgM-antibodies is to be expected. IgM und IgG titres $\geq$1:64 were regarded as positive (Herzer et al. 1986).

Joint destruction

It is the destructive component of chronic Lyme arthritis that gives it its serious profile. But as cartilage and bone erosions occur in only about 10% of patients with Lyme arthritis, the question arises as to the nature of the destructive mechanism. If the joint destruction in Lyme arthritis would be an integral constituent as in RA, then it is difficult to understand why erosions are reported in only a small percentage of cases. Furthermore, if it were comparable to the processes in RA, Lyme arthritis would

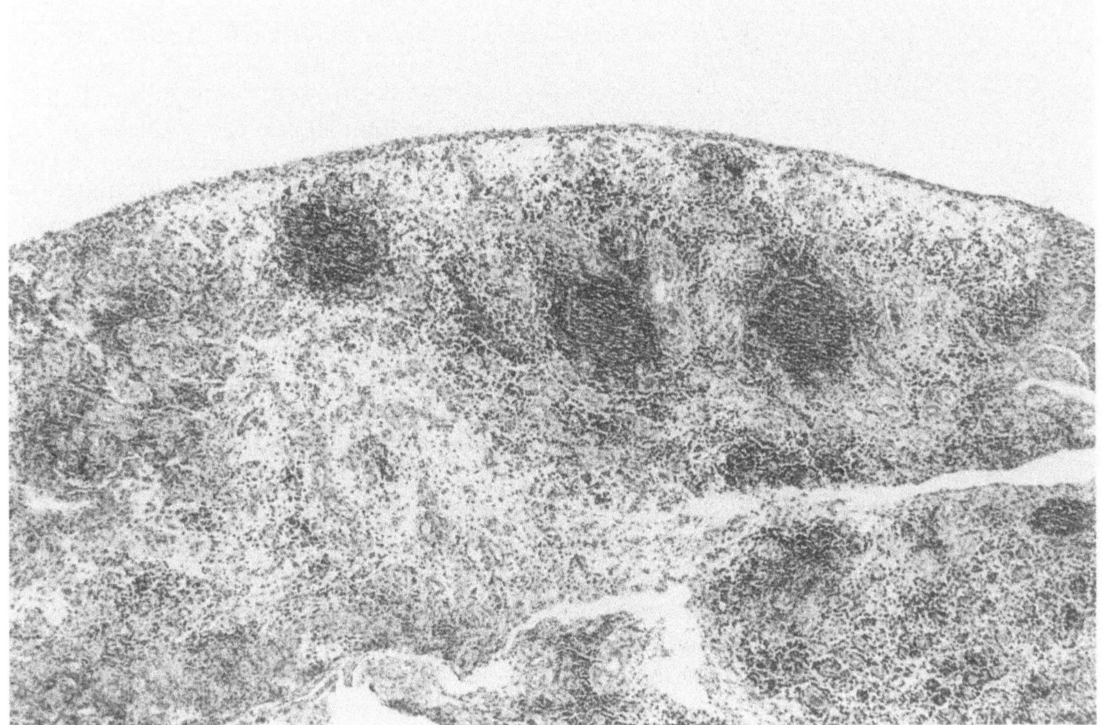

Five months' duration of the disease. Plump synovial villus, lining cell layer single-staged with flat to cuboidal cells. In the synovial stroma, focal accumulation of lymphocytes surrounding small blood vessels and diffuse plasma cell infiltration. Blood vessels without pathological findings

Fig. 8.1
Lyme disease

not be limited to relatively discrete changes like joint space narrowing and marginal erosions.

8.5 Pathology

In order to gain an understanding of the dynamics of the synovial processes, histological examinations of a large amount of synovectomy material would be necessary. However, the rare incidence and low destructive power of Lyme arthritis give rise at most to biopsies, and only rarely to surgical procedures. The biopsy findings are reported as "villous" hypertrophy, vascular proliferation, and a heavy infiltration of mononuclear cells, including plasma cells (Fig. 8.1; Steere et al. 1977c, 1980; Johnston et al. 1985). They agree with our own findings in six patients with Lyme arthritis. These changes are, however, quite unspecific. The same histological picture can be found in various non-bacterial synovitides, even in osteoarthritis (OA).

Demonstration of pathogenic organisms

The reliability of methods other than culture to detect spirochaetes in tissue specimens is open to question. For example, although forms resembling *B. burgdorferi* can be identified by silver impregnation histochemical staining, spirochaetes can be difficult to distinguish from elastic tissue fibres or procollagen fibres and other artifacts. Monoclonal antibody staining and polymerase chain reaction (PCR) techniques to detect DNA sequences specific for *B. burgdorferi* in clinical specimens, even if positive, cannot distinguish between live and dead organisms, and results may persist as positive after clinical cure (Nadelman et al. 1997). As culture and PCR require a great deal of time and are rather expensive, they are not suited for routine diagnosis. The infection is diagnosed serologically, by detecting specific antibodies (IgM, IgG). In routine patient management, the diagnosis of ECM in locations endemic for Lyme borreliosis is purely clinical. Culture is virtually 100% specific and appears to be more sensitive (57–86%; Kirkland et al. 1997; Tugwell et al. 1997) than serology (about 50% in the USA and <50% in Europe; Asbrink et al. 1986; Strle et al. 1999). *B. burgdorferi* can be detected by PCR in the synovial fluid of up to 85% (Nadelman and Wormser 1998).

Role of bacterial superinfection

The fact that in only about 10% of cases of Lyme arthritis localized cartilage and bone destruction occurs suggests there may be a complication of the actual Lyme process by a clinically latent bacterial superinfection with enzymatic degradation of the cartilage by dense masses of neutrophils (see above).

Role of synoviogenic enzymes

On the other hand, already since the in vitro investigations of Harris et al. (1975), it has been recognized that synovial cells have the ability to produce collagenase in various diseases. Its effectiveness, however, due to inhibitors in the synovial fluid, prerequisites a cell attachment with the cartilage or bone substrate, as occurs in RA (see p. 105).

Joint process

If the clinical facts are compared with the joint phenomena of Lyme arthritis, two completely different joint processes can be distinguished:

1. Arthralgia and myalgia
   The circulating immune complexes would be expected to give rise to low-grade, exudative synovitides. Unfortunately, there is no histological evidence of this stage. There is a certain parallel here to rheumatic fever (RF), where there are also short-termed exudative synovitides which are correlated with the circulation of immune complexes. In RF, however, this type of joint process becomes never chronic and above all there is no destruction.
2. Chronic arthritis
   Difficulties arise in the evaluation of the chronic arthritic course in the late stage of the illness. In this phase, circulating immune complexes are no longer found. The IgM-antibodies are replaced by IgG-antibodies. This altered immunological constellation in the late phases corresponds to a joint process totally different from that in the early phases. Its similarity with RA, apart from the rheumatoid factors of RA for which there is no evidence in Lyme arthritis, has often been stressed. The chronicity of an inflammatory, non-bacterial disease, like RA, and also of the seronegative spondylarthritides (SSA) presupposes a superimposed systemic "motor" which keeps the local process going, respectively giving rise to subsequent recurrences. This supposition basically applies to the late form of Lyme arthritis. The fact that in cases of chronic Lyme arthritis *B. burgdorferi* were found both in the synovial fluid and

in the synovial membrane suggested a persistence of the infective agent. In addition, persistence of partial Borrelia antigens is to be expected. This theory is supported by the effectiveness of antibiotic therapy in this stage. Alternatively, the high association of the severe chronic forms with the B cell alloantigen DR2 is evidence for the role of a genetic disposition in the chronic arthritic course of the disease.

Myocardial biopsy

Myocardial biopsy is not often done in patients with acute myocarditis but in anecdotal cases spirochaete-like forms have been associated with a local inflammatory response (van der Linde and Ballmer 1993). *B. burgdorferi* has been recovered in culture from the myocardium of several European patients with congestive heart failure, including two with acute myocarditis and one with chronic cardiomyopathy (Stanek et al. 1990)

Pathogenetic position of Lyme arthritis

To place Lyme arthritis in the spectrum of the infection-dependent arthritides is difficult. On the one hand, in Lyme arthritis, spirochaetes are reported both in the synovial fluid and in the synovial membrane (Schmidli et al. 1988). Accordingly, Lyme arthritis would be classified as an "infectious" arthritis, which also agrees with the frequent joint attacks. On the other hand, the pattern of incidence of Lyme arthritis most closely resembles that of the post-infectious reactive arthritides (REA) respectively of the seronegative spondarthritides (SSA) although the characteristic involvement of the iliosacral joints in this disease group is not a characteristic of Lyme arthritis. A further important difference is the lack of an association with the genetic marker HLA-B27. Therefore, at the present time, Lyme arthritis would be classified between an infectious and a reactive arthritis.

9 Systemic Lupus Erythematosus

9.1 Definition

Systemic immunodisease

Systemic lupus erythematosus (SLE) is a systemic immunodisease of the connective tissue in which mainly the skin, joints, kidneys, nervous system, and serosal membranes are affected. SLE owes its inclusion in the heterogeneous group of "rheumatic" diseases to the joint involvement which does not, however, constitute the main focus of the disease. On the other hand, the rheumatic cycle is enriched by SLE, a disease in which there is no doubt about the pathogenetic importance of the autoantibodies which, in other diseases, are often only a doubtful or meaningless epiphenomenon. Typical features of SLE are antinuclear antibodies (ANAs) which occur in 90% of the patients.

9.2 Epidemiology

The prevalence of SLE varies throughout the world. In North America and northern Europe, for example, it is about 40 per 100,000 population (Mills 1994). The annual average incidence of SLE in the USA has been estimated to be 27.5 per million population for white females and 75.4 for black females (Rothfield 1993). The black population, Chinese, and some Indian tribes are affected more often than the white race. Women are nine times more likely to be affected than men. Amongst Rothfield's 433 patients with SLE, 90% were female. The onset of the disease has been observed in patients between the ages of 2 and 97 years. SLE manifests itself mostly between the ages of 20 and 30 years.
Intrauterine infection is possible, the disease may then manifest in the neonate as neonatal SLE.

9.3 Etiology

The cause of the disease is still unknown. At present, it is assumed that genetic defects lead to an imbalance of B and T lymphocytes. An increased proliferation and secretion of B lymphocytes would then lead to an increased production of immunoglobulins. For this, an intensified function of T-helper cells and probably also of the T-suppressor cells seems to be responsible. It seems likely that this intrinsic defect is subject to external factors (Mills 1994; Dayal and Kammer 1996). Only single causative and facilitating factors are known. Thus, UV light triggers a rash in the area of exposed skin regions. Infections and certain drugs can lead to exacerbation of SLE. The obvious predilection for the female sex suggests the importance of endocrine factors. The participation of genetic factors is indicated by the increased occurrence of connective tissue disorders (including SLE, dysgamma-globulinaemia, autoimmune phenomena, and abnormal cellular immune responses) in approximately 10% of the relatives of SLE patients, as well as a 67% concordance rate of SLE in identical twins (Schur 1986). An increased prevalence of certain HLA-markers has also been reported in some lupus patients (B8, DR2, DR3, Drw52, DQw1, and DQw2). Also the possible role of viruses causing SLE is discussed.

Genetic factors

9.4 Pathogenesis

SLE thus appears to us today as a multisystemic disease in which, through the interaction of genetic, endocrine, and exogenous factors, a mosaic of autoantibodies arises. In the foreground stand the antibodies against components of the cell nucleus, such as antibodies against double-stranded DNA, against small nuclear ribonucleoproteins, and against proliferating cell nuclear antigens (Tan et al. 1981; Zvaifler and Woods 1985). Nuclear antigens, Ro/SSA-and La/SSB-antigens, have been detected in SLE patients, the sensitivity of which, however, is only between 30–35% (Schneider and Specker 1996). Antibodies against cytoplasmic antigens also seem to play a role in SLE (Hiepe et al. 1996). Antiphospholipid antibodies can be detected in approximately 30% of patients with SLE (Mills 1994).

Formation of immune complexes

The pathogenetic significance of the autoantibodies begins with the formation of immune complexes which can arise in the circulation as well as on the surface of tissue structures. A clearing defect in SLE patients hinders the elimination of immune complexes thus enabling them to exert their pathogenetic activity.

Role of immune complexes

In contrast to rheumatoid arthritis (RA), for example, in which three different pathomechanisms (exudation, primary necrosis, and tumour-like proliferation) characterize the overall disease picture, the SLE mechanism with its variations and gradations is mainly determined by immune complex formation and its consequences. Immune complexes acquire pathological significance by fixation and activation of complement, particularly in the mesangium and basement membrane of kidney glomeruli, in the small arteries of the brain, in the capillaries of the choroid plexus, in the vessel network of serosal skins, and in the vessels of the dermal-epidermal junction.

The overall pathological concept of SLE shows a certain analogy to the experimental immune complex-mediated serum sickness of rabbits. The human disease, however, becomes more complicated, since in SLE, different antibody constellations must be taken into account, and these also correspond to a various manifestation pattern of the disease. Thus, patients with antibodies against double-stranded DNA, hypocomplementaemia, and glomerular nephritis have a bad prognosis, whereas high titres against anti-nuclear ribonucleoprotein are usually correlated with Raynaud's phenomenon, finger swelling, polyserositis, and with a milder progression. Since besides different nuclear antibodies, cytoplasmic antibodies can also occur in SLE, a mosaic of pathogenetic factors result which, for each constellation, determine the disease profile in each single case.

It is not clear how the individual immune complexes exert their action, the more as deposits of immune complexes are also found in regions of intact skin in SLE patients. It thus seems that the immune complexes fixed at the dermal-epidermal junction require an additional irritation (e.g. sun radiation) in order to act pathologically.

Impediments in pathogenetic explanation

There are indeed several animal models available for the study of the pathomechanism of SLE in which phenomena similar to SLE develop, but still many questions about the genesis of the human disease remain open. This is, amongst other reasons, due to the fact that the complex disease picture of SLE, in contrast to for example RA, gives no reason for surgical intervention and thus, apart from skin excisions, kidney biopsies, and sparse synovial biopsies, not enough tissue is available for pathological analysis. Even the very informative kidney biopsies cannot routinely be performed due to technical and ethical reasons, and therefore no definite statements about the incidence of kidney attack and about its particular type can be made. It also has to be taken into consideration that all kidney lesions underlie a dynamic process in which a single tissue biopsy secures only an instantaneous record. Therefore it is, for example, obvious that the sclerosis of an artery corresponds to the final stage of an expired arteritis which, in contrast to sclerosis, can definitely be the manifestation of immune complex damage.

Very valuable of course are large numbers of autopsies (Ropes 1976; Haupt et al. 1981). They offer, on the one hand, a complete insight into the entire scope of the SLE process, but, on the other hand, it must be taken into consideration that there are pictures of the condition which, in general, reflect late stages of the disease in which specific acute processes have waned. Thus, only a very widely meshed network of pathological facts is available for the study of SLE besides the animal models and numerous immunological data.

9.5 Clinical and Pathological Manifestations

The disease may manifest in three different forms: the most common is discoid lupus (DLE; cutaneous manifestations only), then follows the subacute-cutaneous form (SCLE), and, finally, the systemic form (SLE).

Discoid lupus

Lesions of discoid lupus were found by Rothfield (1985) in 19% of her 365 SLE patients, often already prior to the onset of the systemic disease. These lesions develop most often in the form of

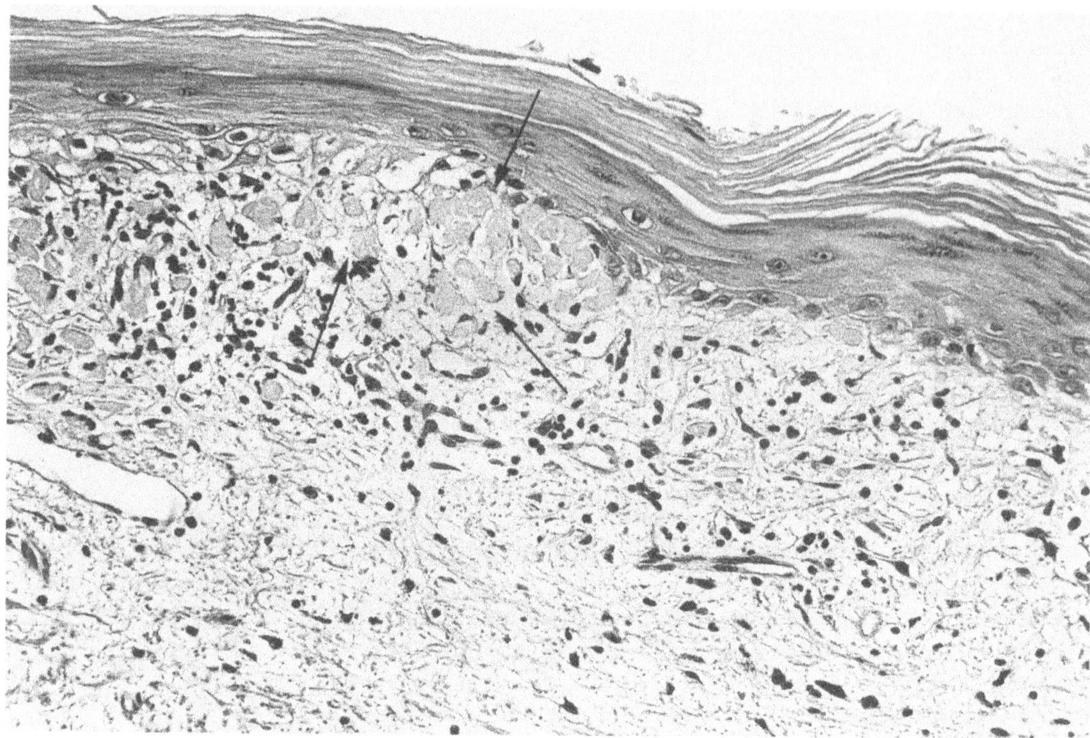

Fig. 9.1
Systemic lupus erythematosus

Skin. Liquefaction of the basal layer. Oedema of the upper dermis. Precipitation of fibrinoid material in the subepidermal zone (*arrows*)

sharply defined papillae and plaques with erythema, oedema, and central elevation of the butterfly area on the face, and also on the scalp, ears, and forehead. Rothfield describes three stages of development of the discoid lesion: erythema, hyperkeratosis, and atrophy. The process burns out leaving atrophic, often pigment-free scars.

Skin

The skin changes, which have given the name to the disease, are present in about 85% of the SLE patients according to the investigations of Rothfield (1985; Fig. 9.1). (Thus, however, the question arises as to the certainty with which SLE patients without skin phenomena can be diagnosed at all.)

Butterfly rash

The typical erythematous butterfly rash is found, according to Rothfield (1985), in about 50% of patients at the time of diagnosis. The slightly oedematous lesion above both cheeks and nose is mostly the first manifestation of the systemic disease, which often is triggered by exposure to the sun. With immunofluorescent techniques, ribbon-like deposits of IgG, IgM, and complement factors can be detected in the dermal-epidermal junction in all skin phenomena of SLE, the so-called lupus-band-test. It remains, however, still open whether circulating immune complexes are trapped here in the region of the dermal-epidermal junction or whether immune complexes are formed there in situ. A less frequent form of SLE rash is the erythematous maculopapular eruption which can occur in the whole body and is provoked by sun radiation.

Lupus profundus or relapsing nodular, non-suppurative panniculitis is a rare manifestation form of SLE, in which subcutaneous indurated nodules develop. Rothfield (1985) saw this form, however, only twice amongst her 365 SLE cases.

Lupus profundus

In about 20% of patients, vasculitic skin lesions occur in the form of a palpable purpura, particularly on the extensor side of the forearms and at the finger-tips (Rothfield 1985). Small-vessel inflammatory angiopathy predominantly affects the kidneys and more infrequently the heart, the lungs, the gastrointestinal tract, and the central nervous system (CNS). Histologically, it corresponds to the picture of a leucocytoclastic vasculitis, thrombosis, and fibrinoid necrosis (Belmont et al. 1996). Ropes (1976) saw mucosal lesions, particularly at the roof of the mouth, in 41% of her SLE patients. Rothfield (1985) found nasal mucosal ulcers in 20% of her SLE cases.

Vascular lesions

Whilst the main processes of SLE are only pathognomonic, the participation of the kidneys which has to be considered for 70%–80% of the patients (Rothfield 1985) can mean grave danger for the patients. The pathogenetic mechanism is here, too, the deposition of immune complexes in the capillaries and mesangium of the glomeruli. Glomerulonephritis in SLE is the prototype of autoimmune diseases. Autoantibodies are directed against various components of the cells' nuclei and cytoplasm. The formation of immune complexes triggers the complement cascade and leads to the activation and release of inflammation mediators, such as adhesion molecules, cytokines, and growth factors.

Kidneys

The kidney biopsy gives the best insight into the pathological process since here the structures of the glomeruli are uniform and distinct and the histological changes can be unequivocally classified.

From the pathological viewpoint, six types of glomerulus lesion can be differentiated, some of which are only marginally different and also have a different importance.

The WHO classification, modified after that of Churg und Sobin (1982), differentiates the following morphological types of glomerulonephritides (Table 9.1):

Normal glomerula

Class I: "Normal glomerula": this includes findings in glomeruli that are either completely normal on light- or electron-microscopical or immunohistological examination (Ia) or that appear normal on light-microscopy and show mesangial deposits on immunohistological or electron-microscopic observation (Ib).

Slight or moderate mesangioproliferative glomerulonephritis

Class II: "Slight or moderate mesangioproliferative glomerulonephritis": typical features of this class are slight (IIa) or moderate (IIb) mesangial broadening with or without an increase in cells. The depositions in the mesangium are exclusively visible by immunohistological or electron-microscopic means (Figs. 9.2, 9.3). Slight to moderate proteinuria and haematuria without restriction of excretory renal function is common with this lesion.

Focal segmental glomerulonephritis

Class III: "Focal segmental glomerulonephritis": in this form, less than 50% of the glomerular tufts are seen, by light-microscopy, to be affected by segmental proliferation of mesangial cells and

Table 9.1. Modified WHO classification of lupus nephritis (Churg and Sobin 1982)

Class I	Normal glomeruli (by LM, IF, EM)
Class II	Pure mesangial alterations a) Normal by LM, mesangial deposits by IF and/or EM b) Mesangial hypercellularity and deposits by IF and/or EM
Class III	Focal segmental glomerulonephritis a) Active necrotizing lesions b) Active and sclerosing lesions c) Sclerosing lesions
Class IV	Diffuse glomerulonephritis (severe mesangial, endocapillary or mesangiocapillary proliferation, and/or extensive subendothelial deposits) a) Without segmental lesions b) With active necrotizing lesions c) With active and sclerosing lesions d) With sclerosing lesions
Class V	Membranous glomerulonephritis a) Pure membranous glomerulonephritis b) Associated with lesions of category II (a or b) c) Associated with lesions of category III (a, b, or c) d) Associated with lesions of category IV (a, b, c, or d)
Class VI	Advanced sclerosing glomerulonephritis

LM, light-microscopy; *IF*, immunofluorescence; *EM*, electron-microscopy.

capillaries with loop-shaped necroses, whereas the majority of the glomerular tufts are normal. Immunofluorescence reveals immunoglobulins and C3 in the mesangium of all glomeruli of the tuft. Fine scattered granules may be found along the glomerulary loops in the areas of proliferation. The deposits are scattered and are not found in all capillary loops. One sees electron-dense deposits in the subendothelial, subepithelial, and intrabasement areas. The disease progresses with remissions. The patients are not threatened with kidney insufficiency.

Severe diffuse glomerulonephritis

Class IV: "Severe diffuse glomerulonephritis" with severe clinical progression, in which more than 50% of the glomerular tufts are affected. In this class, high-grade, diffuse, endocapillary, mesangioproliferative, and/or membranoproliferative glomerulonephritides with segmental necroses are observed. Nephrotic syndrome with proteinuria and haematuria occurs. Under immunohistological aspects, this is a "full house pattern" with mesangial and/or in the capillary walls located depositions of C1q and C3 complement as well as of IgG, IgM, and IgA, fibrin and fibrinogen. The damage to the glomeruli seen in class III and IV comprises approximately 50–60% of all SLE-associated glomerulonephritides.

Membranous glomerulonephritis

Class V: "Membranous glomerulonephritis": the number of mesangial cells increases slightly but they do not proliferate. The

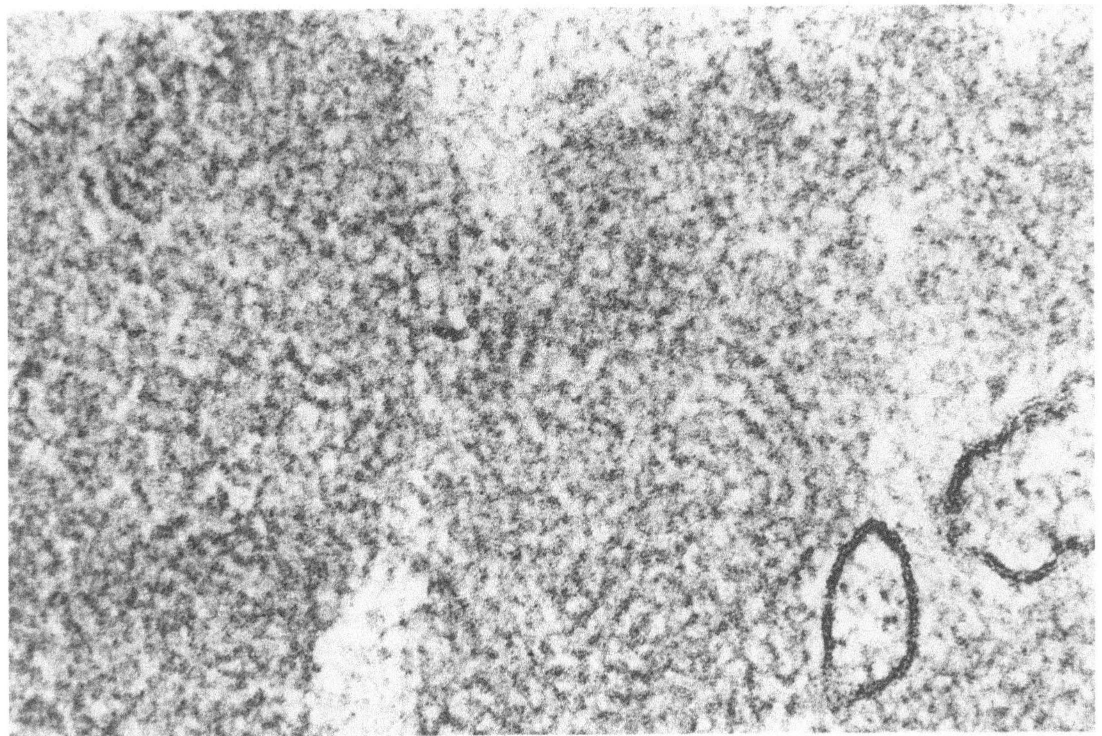

Mesangially localized, electron-dense deposits with fingerprint-like structure as frequently seen in lupus nephritis. (Electron micrograph, 1:36,500; courtesy of J. Kriegsmann, Department of Pathology, University of Mainz)

Fig. 9.2
Systemic lupus erythematosus

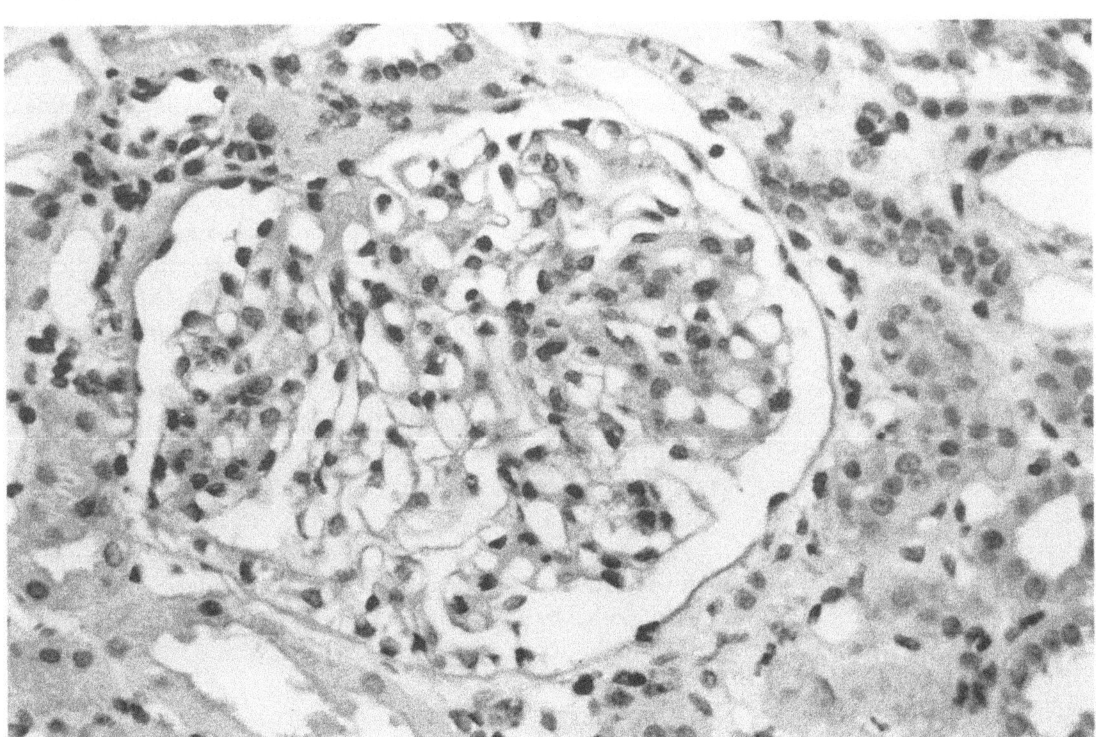

Lupus nephritis. Glomerulus with mesangio-proliferative glomerulonephritis with moderate proliferation of mesangial cells and low accumulation of the mesangial matrix. (Courtesy of J. Kriegsmann, Department of Pathology, University of Mainz)

Fig. 9.3
Systemic lupus erythematosus

broadening of basal membranes is even and band-shaped. Coarsely granulated depositions of IgG, IgM, IgA, and C1q, C3, and C4 along the basement membrane are clearly shown by immunofluorescence. Patients with this form have pronounced proteinuria, more rarely also a slight haematuria. The prognosis of the membranous lupus nephritis is good.

Advanced sclerosing glomerulonephritis

Class VI: "Advanced sclerosing glomerulonephritis": with no knowledge of the results of previous biopsies, these findings alone often do not allow conclusions as to the primary type of glomerulonephritis. In order to definitely evaluate the chronicity and irreversibility of the process, the extent of the atrophy of the tubuli as well as that of interstitial fibrosis should be taken into account also in these cases.

Tubular lesions

In 20–50% of SLE patients, immune complexes can be detected on the basement membrane of the kidney tubuli and in the interstitium by immunofluorescence and electron-microscopy (Mèry et al. 1973; Breutjens et al. 1976). They can be accompanied by interstitial fibrosis and single mononuclear cell infiltrates. The detection of complement factors (C5–C9), which are responsible for membrane damage, indicates their pathological importance (Biesecker et al. 1981). Tubular atrophy and interstitial fibrosis are signs of the chronicity (Helmchen 1996).

Zvaifler and Woods (1985) see the preference of specific kidney areas for immune complex deposition in an impaired mesangial function, which can lead to a reduction of the clearance of complexes or to an incomplete removal of deposited material from the subendothelial space. The consequence in every case is an increase in glomerular deposits.

Role of immune complexes

What eventual role the immune complexes play is not yet finally clear. Rothfield (1985) refers to the parallel between the symptomless deposition of IgG in the mesangium and the IgG deposits in non-affected skin areas in patients with active SLE. In both cases, the deposits are without pathological significance. On the other hand, however, in SLE, the fixation of immune complexes is obligatory for mesangial proliferation. In these cases, a correlation exists between the amount of IgG and the degree of proliferation (Hill et al. 1978).

Central nervous system

In about 20–25% of SLE patients, the participation of the central nervous system can evoke different neuropsychiatric complications, the nature of which obviously depends on the localisation of the vascular process, and can thereby, under certain circumstances, give a dramatic "turn" to the disease picture. Whereas skin and kidney changes are accessible to biopsy examination, the detection and assessment of possible changes is, in this case, only feasible by post-mortem examination, which makes any correlation between actual clinical symptoms and pathological changes impossible.

Neuropsychiatric manifestations

The prevalence of neuropsychiatric involvement is up to 50%, the lethality is reported to be up to 20% (Harten 1996), thus, neuropsychiatric manifestations are among the most frequent and severe complications in SLE patients. Feinglass and coworkers (1976) documented 10 different neuropsychiatric manifestations in 140 SLE patients. The phenomena are indeed very different, but they give a clear indication that the CNS manifestations are mainly caused by SLE-characteristic deposits of immune complexes in the vessels of the anastomosis.

The neuropathological findings of Ropes (1976) and Ellis and Verity (1979) correspond also to that. In 23 SLE patients who died from seizures, they found microembolizations of small arteries in 61%, vasculitides in 35%, and intracerebral haemorrhages in 22%.

Unspecific infiltrates in the intima and adventitia of predominantly small leptomeningal and cortical arteries may be seen. A proliferation of the intima with subsequent formation of thrombi may follow. LE cells are pathognomonic. There are unstructured, basophil inclusions in the cytoplasm that originate from antigen-antibody reactions and subsequent damage to the nuclei. The homogenized nuclei can then be taken up by macrophages (Roggendorf 1995). Ropes (1976) describes numerous microinfarcts in the brain of a patient with chorea. Several small arteries were blocked with necrotic material. Apart from that, in some cases with neuropsychiatric manifestations, the search for a pathological substrate was negative.

Overall, it can be said that a lot of clinical phenomena and also the described morphological changes can be reduced to the SLE-characteristic vessel processes which consist of the deposition of immune complexes in small blood vessels.

Vascular lesions

The vessels show degenerative and proliferative changes similar to those in hypertensive encephalopathy and thrombotic thrombocytopenic purpura (Johnson and Richardson 1968; Ellis and Verity 1979). The intima and media of the small arteries are thickened. Fibrinoid necrosis and cellular infiltrates in the wall of small and middle-sized vessels, which occur also in other systemic lesions in SLE, are, however, very rare in the CNS. To explain the neuropsychic processes in SLE as brought about by the vasculitides characterizing the disease, suggested itself. These expectations, however, were only fulfilled to a very limited extent.

The brain processes triggered by the immune complexes are by themselves, however, neither clinically nor neuropathologically pathognomonic for SLE.

A significant discrepancy often exists between the neuropathological findings and the clinical symptoms. Whilst, in some cases, the microvascular processes correspond to the clinical manifestations, only minimal changes are found at post-mortem examination in patients with pronounced SLE encephalopathy. A series of studies on autoptic material found instead of the vasculitic changes, that were expected, completely different changes such as multi-focal embolizations of small (<100 μ) arteries, in some cases accompanied by microhaemorrhagia. These non-inflammatory, so-called lupus vasculopathies are characterized by proliferation of the endothelium, obliterating fibrosis of the intima with hyalinization, and also thrombosis (Hanly et al. 1992). Also surprising was the discovery of clinically undetected intracerebral infections (up to 10%) causing the neuropsychiatric symptoms of SLE. It can be deduced that autoptic findings often do not show typical vasculitic tissue damage that can be explained by deposits of immune complexes, complement activation, and migration of neutrophils. Antineural antibodies, directed against homogenate of human CNS, are frequently found in serum and cerebrospinal fluid of SLE patients with diffuse, nonfocal cerebral manifestations (Hanly et al. 1993). A subgroup of these group are lymphocytotoxic antibodies cross-reacting with brain tissue (Harten 1996).

It must also be taken into account that besides the ubiquitous vascular processes direct reaction of autoantibodies with brain structures can also trigger neuropsychiatric processes. Thus, in SLE patients, significantly elevated serum lymphocytotoxic antibody titres are found. More than 90% of the lymphocytotoxic antibodies in the serum of SLE patients react also with antigenic determinants present in homogenized human brain and on cultured human neuronal and glial cells (Butler et al. 1972; Bluestein and Zvaifler 1976; Utsinger 1976; Winfield et al. 1976). Moreover, SLE serum also contains some anti-CNS autoantibodies (Bluestein 1978, 1979). In the focus of the discussion concerning the pathogenesis of cerebral SLE are at present antibodies against ribosomal phosphoproteins (anti-P). Bonfa and coworkers (1987) established these autoantibodies in 18 of 20 patients in a group with completely different cerebral manifestations. No anti-P antibodies, however, were found in SLE patients without neuropsychiatric manifestations. The question remains whether this is a pathogenetic principle in itself or an epiphenomenon of the CNS damage.

Anti-P antibodies

Zvaifler and Woods (1985) consider, however, that the serum antibodies which are responsible for the CNS damage have to pass the blood-brain barrier, which normally prevents the contact of the serum proteins with the brain substance. Nevertheless, in about 90% of patients with CNS manifestations such as psychoses, organic brain syndrome, and generalized seizures, an increased titre of IgG anti-neuronal antibodies was found, whereas only 25% of SLE patients with localized vessel-related lesions had increased titres (Tourtellotte 1970).

Role of liquor barrier

In patients with SLE, a disturbance of the liquor barrier is thus assumed. Atkins and coworkers (1972) found immunoglobulins in the choroid plexi of two patients with CNS manifestations. They believe that the choroidal liquor barrier is disturbed by the deposition of immune complexes. On the other hand, it is apparent that choroidal deposition of immunoglobulin is a regular finding in SLE patients, regardless of whether CNS participation is involved. These deposits should also be found in other forms of immune complex-mediated vasculitis (Gershwin et al. 1974; Davis et al. 1978; Boyer et al. 1980).

The preferential fixation of immune complexes in the choroid plexus is perhaps explained by the fact that the choroidal capillaries are fenestrated in a similar way to the glomerular capillaries thus enabling passage of immune complexes from the circulation into the interstitium (Husby et al. 1979).

Two mechanisms of brain damage

Thus, it appears today that the complex picture of CNS disease in the context of SLE occurs by the combination of two different mechanisms:

1. By focal brain processes which are caused by immune complex lesions in small arteries
2. By diffuse anatomical, non-localizable brain cell damage due to autoantibodies with proof of LE cells

Peripheral nervous system

As vasculitis is a central pathogenetic mechanism in SLE, it is plausible that also peripheral nerves, being particularly well supplied with blood vessels, are involved. SLE results in damage to nerve fibres, rarely it leads to infarction with the surrounding connective tissue remaining intact. A neuropathy may then develop that is – typically for SLE – vasculitic in origin, progessive, and multi-focal (Schröder 1995a).

Cardiac manifestations

Clinical signs and symptoms of damage to the cardiovascular system are present in 50%–80% of SLE patients, and in the majority of lethal outcomes, heart involvement plays a role (Strauer et al. 1975). Whereas the SLE processes in the skin, kidney, myocard, endocard, and partly in the CNS are triggered by directly vessel-bound immune complex deposits, the manifestation in the pericardium, pleura, and synovial membrane is based on a completely different mechanism.

Affliction of mesodermal-mesothelial surfaces

All three surfaces belong to the mesodermal-mesothelial system. It concerns border tissues in which a capillary network is in close contact with a lacuna, separated only by a few fibres and a single layer of lining cells. This special anatomical situation facilitates, via physiological transudation, not only the formation of a liquid film at the surface, but in the context of multiple local or systemic processes (as also in SLE) is also disposed to plasma exudation with subsequent fibrin polymerization.
The exudated fibrin mobilizes macrophages, fibroblasts, and angioblasts from the pericardium and epicardium, as well as from the parietal and visceral pleura.
Thus, the connective tissue organization of the exudated fibrin begins, which then, in the course of time, switches to a persistent fibrotic scar tissue. This persistent scar tissue can, depending on the amount of exudation, be patchy or expansive. In extreme cases, both the pericardium and pleural sheets respectively can completely adhere to each other. It thus depends on the time-lapse between the fibrin exudation and the actual time of the pathological examination whether one finds fresh fibrin, loose adhesions or scarred fusions.

Pericardium

Exudative pericarditis is the most frequent heart complication in SLE with an incidence of about 25%. In contrast, scarred pericardial changes are found in 80% of autopsy cases (Rothfield 1985). The histological changes vary (with respect to what is said above) from small fresh fibrin coverages, accompanied by some lymphocytes in the surrounding submesothelial tissue, to widespread adhesions and total fibrotic scar plaques. The participation of the pericardium in SLE corresponds to that of a fibrinous pericarditis, as occurs also in the context of other immunologically orientated systemic diseases (e.g. RA and rheumatic fever, RF).

Myocardium

Myocardial participation in SLE is reported in up to 30% of SLE patients; Ropes (1976) detects it in 42% of autopsy cases. Pomerance (1975) describes myocarditis with perivascular fibrinoid necroses and fibroblast proliferation in 30% of all SLE patients.

Coronary arteritis

Coronary vessel arteritides are common in SLE patients, they are found in small arteries, arterioles, and venules, less frequently in extramural coronary arteries. A case of necrotizing coronary arteritis with lethal vessel blockage is thus described. Arteriosclerosis is, on the other hand, a common but uncharacteristic finding. Possibly, however, it is a late stage of a burnt-out arteritis. Whether old infarct scars of myocard can be correlated with the fundamental disease must, however, remain open.

Bulkley and Roberts (1975) see a connection between coronary sclerosis and corticoid therapy in SLE patients.

Endocardium

Libman-Sacks endocarditis is a non-bacterial, verrucous endocarditis and is a characteristic finding in 20–50% of SLE patients. Since the valve-margin vegetations do not or only minimally affect the valve mechanics, this valve process evades clinical observation. Its incidence in SLE patients can be estimated by larger autopsy series. Thus, in a review of 138 SLE cases, Harvey and coworkers (1954) reported that an endocarditis of the Libman-Sacks type was found in 1/3 of the autopsy cases. This was due to band-shaped vegetations at the commissure of the mitral and tricuspid valves, which consisted of a row of oval, whitish, tiny warts of 1–4 mm diameter which developed from small fibrin overgrowths and later grew like connective tissue into the valves. They may also be on the valve surface exposed to the forward flow of blood and may cover larger surfaces. Microscopically, these lesions can be seen to consist of fibrin, histiocytes, lymphocytes, plasma cells, and fibroblasts.

A sclerosing of the valves or a fusion at the valve margins as in rheumatic endocarditis does not belong to the picture of Libman-Sacks endocarditis. On the other hand, these valve changes can, in some cases, be secondarily colonized by bacteria which can lead to secondary valve destruction.

Pleuropulmonary manifestations

That which has already been said above is valid for the participation of the pleura. The pleura belongs to the system of mesodermal-mesothelial surfaces which, like in other systemic inflammatory diseases, caused by damage of the submesothelial capillary nets and plasma exudation, also take part in the systemic process.

The plasma exudation is followed by fibrin polymerization. The further progression corresponds to that in the pericardium (see above). Finally, fibrous adhesions and pleural fusions remain as witnesses of expired pleuritides.

"Silent" pleuritides

In SLE, as also in RA, a large proportion of the mild pleuritides progress clinically unrecognized. They are only discovered at post-mortem investigation. Thus, Ropes (1976) found in 24% of 58 and Haupt and coworkers (1981) in 18% of 120 autopsy cases of SLE patients different stages of pleural participation ranging from fibrinous exudation to total bilateral pleural fusion.

Lungs

In contrast to pleural participation, lung manifestations are clinically recognizable in 30%–70% of SLE patients and are more often diagnosed radiologically. The morphological picture is not specific and is frequently masked by infections or by complications of uraemic pneumonia. Thus, Matthay and coworkers (1974) observed an acute, mainly bilateral pneumonitis in 11.7%

of 102 hospitalized SLE patients. This, in general, wanes after the acute phase. It can also remain as a chronic infiltrate. Acute alveolar damage with interstitial oedema, hyaline membranes and, in some patients, an acute alveolitis is found at autopsy. A chronic interstitial pneumonitis with dyspnoe and pulmonary hypertonus can also develop in SLE patients (Perez and Kramer 1981).

Interstitial fibrosis

Haupt and coworkers (1981) found interstitial fibrosis in 5% of autopsy cases. Slight thickening of the alveolar walls via loosely fibrosing, sparse plasma cell infiltration in the interstitium, and occasional ulcerative necroses in the alveoles and bronchioles have been observed. In the case of the fibrosis taking a haemorrhagic course, arteriolitis with neutrophil infiltrates is found. Inflammatory changes predominate in the early stages, fibrosis in later phases.

Lymph nodes

Lymph node swelling can appear early at the onset of SLE. It can be generalized or can also be localized in one to two lymph node groups. Approximately 30% of patients suffer from lymphadenopathies, mainly in the neck region.

The histological picture conforms to follicular hyperplasia which may also be occasionally observed in RA: it is found in excessively enlarged follicles with extended, active germinal centres. The basic structure of the lymph organ is maintained. The fibrous capsule is not infiltrated. It is understandable that this giant follicle formation gives rise to misdiagnosis, in particular by confusion with follicle centre lymphoma (Brill-Symmers lymphoma). The lymph node process is, however, harmless and mostly disappears after the acute process has waned. It can, however, recur after re-activation.

Joints

The connecting link between this multisystemic immune complex disease and the group of rheumatic diseases is formed by arthralgias and arthritides. Even at the incipient stages of the disease, arthritides occur in 60–70% of SLE patients. Regarding symptomatology and pattern of the joints affected, these arthritides are similar to those in RA, to such an extent that one might mistake one for the other (Schneider and Specker 1996).

Clinical manifestations

The clinical picture brings RA to mind, to which belong, among other symptoms, morning stiffness, symmetrical attack of the proximal interphalangeal and metacarpal joints, and also of the knee and hand joints. In about 20% of SLE patients, the metatarsal joints and hips are also affected. Rothfield (1985) found movement pain and swellings in 78% of 365 SLE patients at the actual time of diagnosis. Ropes (1976) reported objective involvement of more than two joints in 74% of 142 SLE patients. The formation of typical swan neck deformities and ulnar deviation of the fingers is also identical with the pattern of the joint processes in RA.

No joint destruction

The essential difference to RA is that the deformations are not based on cartilage or bone destruction. The deformation in SLE is thus caused by changes in tendon and capsule tissue and not by joint destruction as in RA. Indeed, tenosynovitis is only rarely reported in SLE patients, but it must be assumed that exudative fibrinous processes occur in the tendon sheath which evade clinical observation and result in the typical tendon and capsule shrinkage. Since no joint destruction is present, stiffening and displacement can be successfully minimized by physiotherapy. Thus, there is also no indication for surgical intervention such as synovectomy or joint resection. Our knowledge of joint processes is based mainly on the analysis of only a limited number of synovial biopsies.

The observations of Labowitz and Schumacher (1971) in biopsies from 7 SLE patients agree essentially with our findings in 11 patients: we saw fibrin deposits in 4 patients, perivascular fibrosis and lymphocytic infiltration of the stroma with minimal formation of new blood vessels in 3 cases. Three times we saw a multi-staged lining cell layer and sparse lymphocyte infiltrates. We were impressed, moreover, by 5 cases with pronouncedly blunt synovial villi. In total, no changes which over-stepped the boundary of the uncharacteristic, exudatively distinguished synovitis were found in our own material or in that of other investigators. The histological picture indeed explains the pain, swelling, and morning stiffness, but offers no explanation for the impressive joint deformations in SLE. Therefore, we believe that there is not the slightest doubt about as yet unrecognized changes proceeding the collagenous tendon and in the capsular tissue, that are responsible for the shrinkage and shortening.

Synovitis

Exudative synovitis corresponds to the analogous changes which occur at other mesothelial surfaces (pericardium and pleura) and is understandably due to the capillary damage triggered by the immune complexes. Like other non-bacterial, purely exudative synovitides, it has no destructive character.

10 Systemic Sclerosis*

10.1 Definition

The definition of the Subcommittee for the Preliminary Diagnostic and Therapeutic Criteria for Systemic Sclerosis of the American Rheumatism Association (1980) is as follows: "Systemic sclerosis (SSC) is a disorder of connective tissue characterized by induration and thickening of the skin (scleroderma), Raynaud's phenomenon and other vascular abnormalities, musculoskeletal manifestations and visceral involvement, especially of the gastrointestinal tract, lungs, heart, and kidneys".

10.2 Epidemiology

The disease occurs world-wide in all races, predominantly in middle age, with an incidence of 1.2 cases per million and year, with a female predilection of 3:1 (Ruggieri and LeRoy 1986). According to Lawrence and coworkers (1998), the prevalence is 180 cases per 1 million inhabitants in Pennsylvania, but 400 cases per 1 million female inhabitants between 35 and 65 years of age. Within the group of patients aged from 35–44 years, the female-to-male ratio was 9:1, within the other age groups 3:1.

10.3 Clinical Manifestations

Heterogenous connective tissue disorder

The various types of clinical manifestations are evidence for the fact that SSC is a heterogeneous connective tissue disorder. A classification system for the different subsets of SSC was proposed by a panel under the chairmanship of Fine in 1996 as follows:

1. "Pre-scleroderma:" Raynaud's phenomenon plus nailfold capillary changes; disease specific circulating anti-nuclear au-

---

**Synonym:* Scleroderma

toantibodies [anti-topoisomerase-I, anti-centromere (ACA)]; and digital ischaemic changes.

2. Diffuse cutaneous SSC: onset of skin changes (puffy or hidebound) within 1 year of onset of Raynaud's phenomenon; truncal and acral skin involvement; presence of tendon friction rubs; early and significant incidence of interstitial lung disease, oliguric renal failure; diffuse gastrointestinal disease and myocardial involvement; nailfold capillary dilatation and drop-out; anti-topoisomerase-I (Scl 70) antibodies (30% of patients).
3. Limited cutaneous SSC: Raynaud's phenomenon for years (occasionally decades); skin involvement limited to hands, face, feet, and forearms (acral); a significant (10–15%) late incidence of pulmonary hypertension, with or without interstitial lung disease, skin calcification, telangiectasiae, and gastrointestinal involvement; high prevalence of ACA (70–80%); dilated nailfold capillary loops, usually without capillary drop-out.
4. Scleroderma sine scleroderma: Raynaud's phenomenon; no skin involvement; presentation with pulmonary fibrosis, scleroderma renal crisis, cardiac or gastrointestinal disease; antinuclear antibodies may be present (Scl 70, ACA).

The variable spectrum of SSC is determined by two basic mechanisms of the vascular changes and fibrosis. The predilection sites of the disease are particularly the lungs, heart, and kidneys, with involvement also of skin, gastrointestinal tract, skeletal muscles, and joints.

The skin changes start first at the finger tips and can in the course of time develop proximally and afflict the face and trunk.

Pulmonary involvement

The lung process in SSC is hallmarked by an interstitial fibrosis of the lung parenchyma and pleuritis. It is in the character of a fibrosis that the collagenous tissue becomes cell-poor and fibrerich and shrinks with disease duration. In the case of the lungs this means, on the one hand, that they lose their specific respiratory function, and on the other that an increasing constriction of the blood vessels and an increasing resistance to blood flow occurs. The thus resulting pulmonary hypertension progressively burdens the right heart and is an essential component of a lethal outcome.

Cardiac involvement

The heart disease is essentially caused by obstructive processes and by changes in the small myocardial vessels. These changes are not observed in coronary angiography and are not improved by by-pass operations (LeRoy 1985). Following diffuse cardio-angiopathy, a widespread myocardial fibrosis develops to which the systemic tendency to fibrosis contributes, too.

Renal involvement

The disease of the kidneys consists of a progressive sclerosing process of the interlobular arteries which is characterized by intimal proliferation, media atrophy, and adventitial fibrosis. The vascular kidney disease leads to an arterial hypertonia.

Thus, for the heart, which is already myocardially damaged, a fatal summation of myocardial fibrosis, pulmonary and arterial hypertonia develops; three factors which can lead to lethal heart failure.

Gastrointestinal involvement

Besides these main manifestations which, under certain circumstances, are lethal, the fibrosis in the region of the mucous membranes of the gastrointestinal tract, which affects approximately 90% of patients (Orringer et al. 1976), is important since it causes severe irritation, particularly via sclerotization of the oesophageal wall.

"Rheumatic" components

The "rheumatic" components, in the form of joint and muscle participation, constitute a less important sector of SSC in relation to the severe organ manifestations. The patients complain about arthralgia and stiffness of the joints, but at the same time a genuine arthritis cannot be detected. The joint problems result mainly from fibrous contractions of the tendons, tendon sheaths, and capsule tissue. In the synovial tissue, Schumacher (1973) found also a characteristic fibrosis, similar to that seen in other organs, alongside poorly reactive fibrin deposits and perivascular lympho-plasma cellular infiltrates. The picture of the synovial membrane thus appears to be very static. The dynamics of an arthritis, characterized by proliferation of the lining cells and synovial stroma cells, is absent. SSC patients often suffer from muscle weakness and atrophy. In these muscle sections, no inflammatory or fibrosing changes can be seen histologically. With histochemical methods, however, subtle changes in the form and composition of the fibres can be detected.

CREST syndrome

SSC can start suddenly and can make severe progress. In most cases, however, the disease begins insiduously. A slow-starting form hallmarks CREST syndrome which is characterized by a combination of calcinosis, Raynaud's phenomenon, oesophageal involvement, sclerodactylia, and telangiectasia.

Long-term observations have demonstrated, however, that the complete picture of SSC can develop even 50 years after these initial events (Ruggieri and LeRoy 1986).

10.4 Pathogenesis

The association of genes of the major histocompatibility complex (MHC) with systemic sclerosis in general, and with particular disease subsets, forms only part of the evidence for a strong role for the immune system in the pathogenesis of SSC. Long before advanced genetic studies were possible, familial associations of SSC with other rheumatological diseases, particularly those with striking autoimmune features, suggested the former (Korn 1996). The prominent inflammatory infiltrations, especially the T cells, in early skin lesions seem to imply immune mechanisms in the pathogenesis of SSC. Although the inflammatory cell infiltrate varies in intensity and distribution, its location around blood vessels and at sites of active connective tissue deposition suggests a pathogenetic role (Prescott et al. 1992). The increased DR expression of dermal T cell infiltrates suggests lymphocyte activation, which is also implied by raised circulating levels of lymphocyte and monocyte derived cytokines such as IL-1, IL-2, Il-4, and IL-6 (Needleman et al. 1992). Increased levels of circulating soluble forms of CD4 and IL-2R have also been observed. The resemblance of SSC to graft vs. host disease (GVHD) is further evidence of an immune cell-mediated process (Jaffee and Claman 1983). Several autoantibodies have been isolated, yet none of them has been proven to play a role in the pathogenesis of SSC (Korn 1996).

10.5 Pathology

The disease, the causes of which are still not plausible explained today (2000), is based on two different mechanisms which together shape the spectrum of SSC:

1. A disease of the small blood vessels, mainly of the small arteries and arterioles which was pointed out particularly by LeRoy (1985).
2. A diffuse heterotopic deposition and stratification of collagen fibres in organ structures. The fibrosis which thereby occurs, and the associated shrinkage process are perceived in the skin as being disturbing, whereas the analogous processes in the heart, lungs, and kidneys can, on the other hand, be life-threatening. We are indebted to LeRoy and his colleagues for a plausible concept which focusses on the repeated endothelial damage as the cause of the pathological fibrosis (Kahaleh et al. 1979).

Vascular lesions

Vascular injury and activation of monocytes and other cells lead to release of tissue factor and activation of the coagulation cascade. The resultant release of platelet-derived growth factor (PDGF) and transforming growth factor β (TGFβ) from platelets can activate fibroblasts (Korn 1996).

The question of Korn "why, in other disorders, such as rheumatoid arthritis (RA), where there is also immune cell activation and infiltration into sites of connective tissues, there is a preponderance of matrix degradation rather than matrix deposition" remains as yet unanswered.

The skin fibroblast is generally a quiescent cell that divides slowly. Normally, the production of extracellular matrix is regulated by stimulation and inhibition, and is adapted to demand at any given time.

With immune activation or inflammation secondary to tissue damage these signals are altered. The adhesion of lymphocytes, monocytes, and other inflammatory cells profoundly influences fibroblast properties, perhaps through direct cell contact but probably mainly through the elaboration and release of specific cytokines. These cytokines include IL-1 and IL-4, which stimulate both fibroblast proliferation and collagen biosynthesis, and IL-6, which stimulates the production of matrix metalloproteinases having variable effects on collagen synthesis (LeRoy 1994).

Platelet aggregation, myointimal cell proliferation and migration into the damaged region, and deposition of mucoid glycoproteins, collagen, and elastin fibrils occur in the small arteries. This material resists remodelling and resorption. As a consequence, restriction of the lumen and rigidity of the vessel wall occurs.

All this leads to the distinctive lesions of SSC. Platelet factors perhaps activate surrounding fibroblasts to secrete collagen in a cuff-shaped manner around the vessels. The processes in the intima and adventitia lead to atrophy of the media. Intimal proliferation with mucoid connective tissue deposition, media atrophy, and adventitial fibrosis, thus, characterize the vascular process in SSC.

The question of the initial endothelial damage is still, however, not satisfactorily solved, although a number of immune abnormalities and cytotoxic factors are described associated with SSC (Greenwald et al. 1978; Kahaleh and LeRoy 1983; Stuart et al. 1983).

Raynaud's phenomenon

Long-term observations have shown that the vascular process precedes fibrosis, thus alluding to the pathognomonic importance of Raynaud's phenomenon as a frequent precursor of SSC which may, under certain conditions, manifest itself many years later (LeRoy 1985). Raynaud's phenomenon occurs in 90% of patients with the classic skin changes of SSC (Rodnan 1972).

Intravital microscopic capillary findings

Intravital capillary microscopy at the finger-nail folds allows elucidation of the importance of the vascular components in SSC. Using this method, one sees in SSC patients an abnormal capillary pattern with dilated, distorted capillaries with irregularly spaced capillary drop-out (Maricq et al. 1976).

Pathologic fibrosis

Fibrosis in the skin of scleroderma patients is readily recognized by biopsy, and skin thickness has been correlated with the content of the major matrix component, collagen (Fig. 10.1). The generation of a fibrosis is normally a frequent and ubiquitous phenomenon in the general pathology. It arises following an inflammatory fibrin exudation which is followed by the development of granulation tissue which, after fading away, leaves behind a cell-free scar composed mainly of collagen type I. This involves a controlled, self-limiting process which also occurs in wound healing. Inflammatory or granulating precursors are, however, not observed in the widespread fibrosis which tends to occur in SSC. This points towards an uncontrolled pathological fibroblastic function. There are indications of cytotoxic factors not only damaging the endothelial cells but also stimulating the fibroblasts (Tan et al. 1981; LeRoy et al. 1983).

Moreover, other studies have shown that the thus induced proliferation selects a fibroblast population having a high collagen production which could perpetuate fibrosis. This was confirmed by investigations in which an increased accumulation of collagen was detected in cultures of dermal fibroblasts from patients with SSC (Perlish et al. 1976; Buckingham et al. 1978).

Pathogenetic concept

LeRoy and coworkers (1982) consider the following sequence as conceivable: endothelial injury – fibroblast proliferation (myointimal cell production) – high collagen synthesis – fibrosis. Lymphokines (Parrott et al. 1982), direct mononuclear leukocyte-fibroblast interaction (Hibbs et al. 1983), and glycosaminoglycans (Fox et al. 1982), among others, contribute to the factors which are in the position to stimulate fibroblast proliferation and collagen production. A disturbance of the feedback mechanism of collagen synthesis is also conceivable. In such a way, a pathological absolute or relative increase in collagen type III secretion could play a role (Fleischmajer et al. 1980).

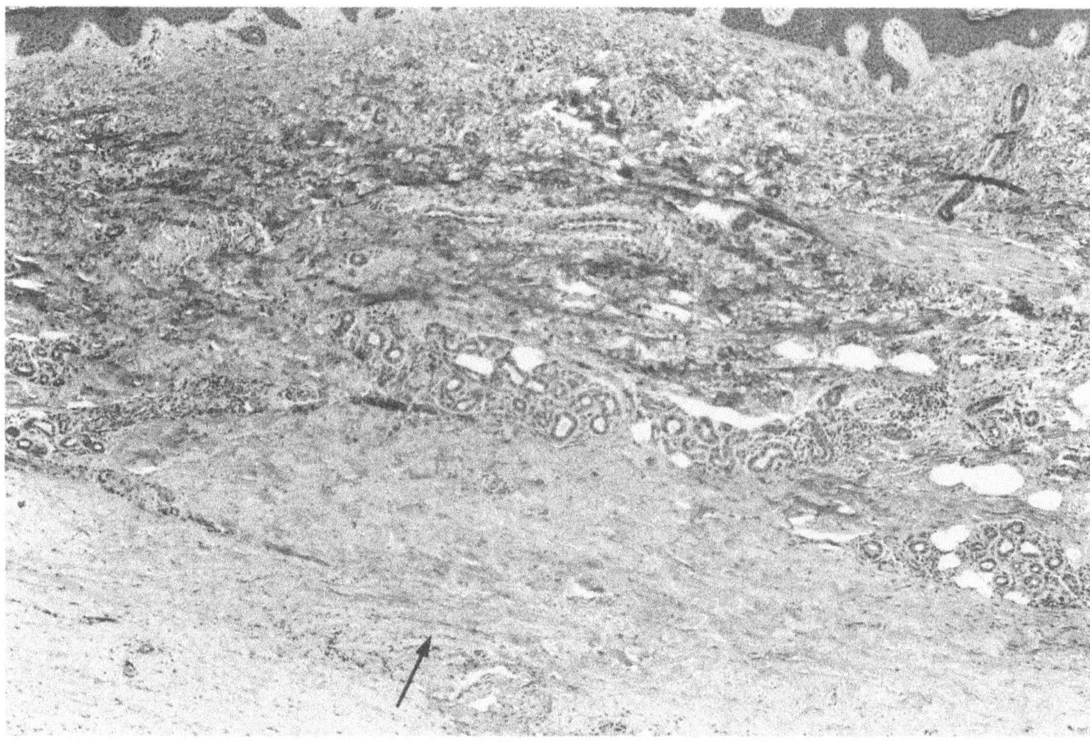

Fig. 10.1
Systemic sclerosis

Deposition of new, partly closely packed collagen (*arrow*) in the lower dermis and in the subcutaneous fatty tissue. Sparse lymphocytic infiltration in the upper dermis

LeRoy's (1972) original finding that dermal fibroblasts obtained from sclerodermatous skin maintain a higher level of matrix production in culture for several passages than do normal skin fibroblasts has been confirmed repeatedly (Vuorio et al. 1991). Related studies have indicated, however, that a subpopulation of fibroblasts may contribute disproportionately to the accumulation of extracellular matrix in SSC skin (Botstein et al. 1982). Indeed, subpopulations of fibroblasts responsible for increased collagen production in SSC have been identified by cloning and flow cytometry.
The investigations of Goldring et al. (1990) show even in fibroblast cultures from patients with normal dermis a heterogeneity concerning hormone responses, growth kinetics, and pattern of collagen synthesis.
The activation of increased synthesis and decreased degradation of collagen resulting in excessive deposition of extracellular matrix is, according to Gay et al. (1992), an effect of the vascular derived growth factors, e.g. PDGF.

11 Eosinophilic Fasciitis and Related Syndromes

11.1 Eosinophilic Fasciitis

Synonym: Shulman's disease.

11.1.1 Definition

In 1974, Shulman described for the first time a new disease profile, similar to scleroderma, which is characterized by a diffuse fasciitis with hypergammaglobulinaemia and blood eosinophilia which he later designated as eosinophilic fasciitis (EF) or diffuse EF.

As in scleroderma, the skin here is also "baked together" with the underlying structures, but, nevertheless, some differences exist which allow clear distinction of EF as an independent disease profile.

Scleroderma attacks preferentially the extremities whereas EF spreads more centrally and leaves the extremities free. Thus, it does not develop to Raynaud's phenomenon. Visceral participation does not occur in EF, in contrast to scleroderma. EF is distinguished from dermatomyositis (DM) by the absence of clinical, serological, and histological evidence of muscle involvement.

11.1.2 Clinical Manifestations and Morphological Findings

Stiffness and swelling

EF can occur stepwise, and also precipitously, mostly after intense physical exertion in unfit young men. In principle, however, it is observed in both sexes in all age groups. EF starts in one arm or leg with stiffness and swelling and can later systematically attack all four extremities. The skin and soft tissues of the extremities become ligneous and tensed. Contractures at the knees and elbows begin to develop. In extreme cases the stiffness can also encroach upon the foot and hand joints.

Morphological findings

The morphological substrate of this stiffening process is a hypertrophy of the collagen fibre bundles in the region of the fascia which are diffusely infiltrated by lymphocytes, plasma cells, histiocytes, and sparse eosinophils. Collagen hypertrophy and cell infiltration can spread to the septum of the neighbouring musculature and onto the connective tissue septa of the subcutis. Moreover, this tissue is oedematously drenched. The cutis itself is only in extreme cases involved in the process.

Collagen hypertrophy

Stiffness and tension result, thus, on the one hand, from the increased volume of the soft tissues of the extremities, on the other hand, however, they are also caused by the loss of the normal displacibility of the soft tissue layers which occurs via the trespassing infiltrating inflammatory process.

Bioptic findings

We are grateful to Barnes and coworkers (1979) for the painstaking pathological study on surgically removed biopsies in which skin, hypodermis, fascia, and muscle tissue were assessed. (The authors emphasize explicitly the uselessness of punch biopsies for the diagnosis of EF, since with these only skin and hypodermis can be obtained.) The analysis of 20 excisions from patients with clinically confirmed EF showed that EF is hallmarked more by its localisation than by the actual morphological picture. The disease target lies in all cases in the region of the fascia with variable extension into the subcutis and, in rare cases, also into the cutis itself. The inflammatory process extends in different amounts to the neighbouring musculature to which the fibrously thickened fascium is attached. The constituents of the inflammatory process are uncharacteristic: lymphocytes, plasma cells, histiocytes, and eosinophils. Barnes and coworkers demand at least three or more eosinophils per field of view at high magnification.

Eosinophilic infiltrates

Characteristic for EF are the consequences of the inflammation: the new collagen formation, which leads to fibrosis and to a 2–15 fold thickening of the fascia, is particularly pathognomonic for this disease. Inflammatory infiltration and fibrosis vary quantitatively depending on the duration and intensity of the process. The name-giving eosinophils can be sparsely present in the tissue and since they are moreover focally localized they can escape observation in a single sample excision. Furthermore, it should be considered that prior treatment with corticosteroids results, under certain circumstances, in their disappearance from the blood as well as from the tissue.

Thickening of fascia

Effect of corticosteroids

In two of the patients examined by Barnes and colleagues, a carpal tunnel syndrome (CTS) was identified (1979). Thereby, in both cases, synovial hyperplasia with lymphocytes and plasma cells as well as small and medium eosinophils, respectively, were found. Participation of the blood vessels is uncharacteristic. It consists of a perivascular deposition of lymphocytes and plasma cells which sporadically attack the vessel wall. Necrotizing vasculitides or thromboses were not found in the sample material. In immunohistologically studied tissue from eight patients, the authors of the study described deposits of IgG, IgM, and C3 in the fascia in five cases.

IgG, IgM, and C3

Treatment of EF

Corticosteroids have turned out to be effective in EF. With those a complete clinical remission of the disease is often successful, with normalisation of skin and subcutaneous tissue and retrogression of the flexure contractures. In most cases, however, relapses cannot be avoided. Only sporadically untreated spontaneous recovery is reported. There are also chronic cases which transform to scleroderma.

11.2 Toxic Oil Syndrome

New pathogenic aspects and also new puzzles were introduced in May 1981 by an explosive epidemic illness in Spain, the origin of which was ascertained to be the use of industrial grade denatured rapeseed oil marked as olive oil. Clinical signs and symptoms include fever, rashes, pneumonitis, myalgia, eosinophilia, neuropathy, pulmonary hypertension, and scleroderma-like skin changes (Berry 1993). By 1 June 1981, 315 of the 19,828 affected individuals had died (Shulman 1990). The primary cause of death had been pulmonary hypertension. The fundamental lesion was found to be an arterial vasculitis with some involvement of all vessel types.

Arterial vasculitis

It is noteworthy that those who fell ill with this toxic oil syndrome (TOS) had the following phenomena in common with EF: fasciitis, oedematous swellings, joint contractions as well as blood eosinophilia. However, in contrast to EF, which has no predilection for either sex, 90% of the severely affected TOS patients were female.

Mutuality with EF

11.3 Eosinophilia-Myalgia Syndrome

Myalgias with blood eosinophilia

A new facet arrived in October 1989 via a further syndrome associated with fascitis. It surfaced for the first time in New Mexico, USA: myalgias appeared accompanied by high-grade blood eosinophilia. In July 1990, already 1,531 cases were reported affected by the syndrome and 27 dead nationwide (USA; Swygert et al. 1990). Most of those affected were middle-aged females. Clinical findings include muscle weakness, arthralgia, peripheral oedemas, polyneuropathy, and rashes. In some cases, vasculitis and thromboembolism can be observed. The cause of this is today considered to be a contamination of L-tryptophan. It was used in products for treating premenstrual tension and insomnia, and it was a supplement in certain "health foods" included in dietary programmes. All these had almost exclusively been consumed by white women of the relevant age-group, which explains the gender- and age-related occurrence.

L-tryptophan

Morphological mutualities of EF, TOS, and EMS

The relationship of eosinophilia-myalgia syndrome (EMS) to EF and also to TOS exhibits itself not only in the common occurrence of blood eosinophilia and fasciitis but also in the fact that in numerous patients (in particular those with EMS and TOS) a myalgia also occurs. Oedematous swellings and contractures were also common phenomena. The histological picture in EMS was similar to EF and TOS, being described by collagen hypertrophy in the region of muscle interstitium and the fascia, rarely in the cutis. These tissue sections were infiltrated by lymphocytes, histiocytes, and less often by eosinophils (Bulpitt et al. 1990; Clauw et al. 1990; Fig. 11.1). Whereas in EF the sex ratio was equal, in EMS and TOS female patients predominated. Here also

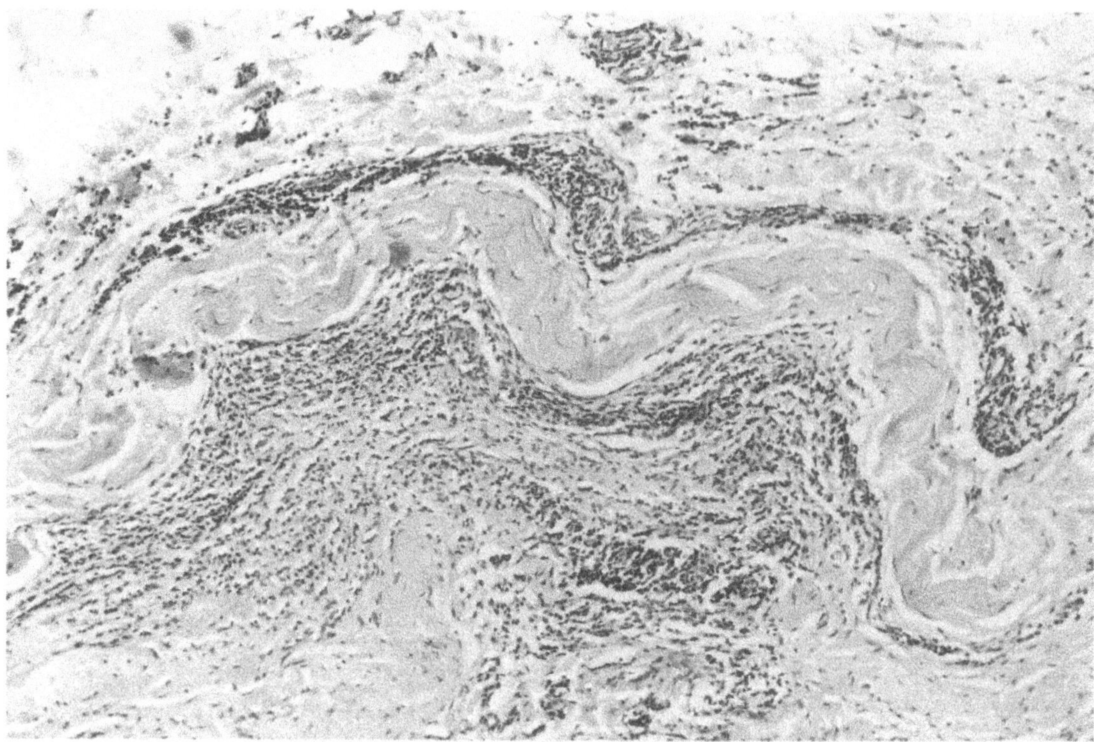

Fig. 11.1
Eosinophilic fasciitis

Arm. Fascia surrounded by lymphocytes, macrophages, and isolated eosinophils. Increase of collagen (15-year-old female)

previous bodily exertions were reported in several cases. Berry (1993) discusses the apparent similarity of TOS and EMS. He emphasizes aspects common to both entities: the involvement of the skin, fascia, muscles, lungs, and of the nervous system. Over time, these appear to evolve in a similar way in both conditions, with pulmonary hypertension being a severe to life-threatening sequel to the early systemic disorders. There are, however, significant differences: in TOS, lung involvement evolves at a later stage, and changes in blood lipid composition (elevated triglycerides) occur in TOS but not in EMS. In both conditions, vasculitis is the major pathological finding that may underlie many other findings. In general, the lesions of TOS are more severe than those of EMS.

Vasculitis – major pathological finding

11.4 Hypereosinophilic Syndrome

The fact that in the three diseases (EF, TOS, EMS) blood eosinophilia is the major common phenomenon directs attention towards hypereosinophilic syndrome (HES), which is hallmarked mainly by a high-grade eosinophilia (Fauci et al. 1982; Peters et al. 1988) but in which swellings, fasciitis and contractures are, however, absent. Therefore in future, the role of the eosinophils in the pathogenesis of these diseases has to be clarified.

12 Polymyalgia Rheumatica and Giant Cell Arteritis

Technical requirements for diagnosing muscle biopsies

If one expects an insight into the histological changes in muscle tissue, one should be aware of the fact that differentiated diagnoses are impossible to make using routinely prepared material, fixated in formalin. Material fixated with formalin and embedded in paraffin is advantageous only for detecting vasculitides and for ascertaining amyloid deposits. Variable degrees of shrinking of muscle fibres as well as fasciae do not allow to determine the diameters of muscle fibres such as is possible in biopsies prepared using a cryostat (Goebel 1999).
In order to be suitable for a differentiated light-microscopic diagnosis including enzyme-histochemical and immunomorphological procedures, the material must be frozen in isopentane in liquid nitrogen within less than 1 min after obtaining it. Semithin sections and electron-microscopic examinations require the material to be fixated in buffered glutaraldehyde (Goebel 1999).

12.1 Definition

The term polymyalgia rheumatica (PMR) designates an etiologically vague syndrome that affects older patients and is characterized by pain and stiffness in the shoulders and the pelvic girdle and by a highly elevated erythrocyte sedimentation rate (ESR).
Giant cell arteritis (GCA) affects medium and large muscular arteries with a well-developed internal and external elastic lamina. The affliction is segmental and multilocular, and it preferentially affects the temporal artery and other branches of the carotid artery. The special morphological sign of GCA is the formation of multinuclear giant cells.

Correlation between PMR and GCA

The connection between PMR and GCA seems to be close. There are varied clinical reports about the coincidence of both phenomena. But it has to be considered that they have progress curves which do not have to coincide with time. We ourselves have the impression that the burnt-out arterial process can escape observation if the minimal traces it leaves behind are overlooked and misinterpreted, respectively.

The question whether there is any association between PMR and GCA or not, must still remain open. The, in general, common manifestation of both, however, justifies their consideration in this chapter.

Nomenclature

The name "polymyalgia rheumatica" which was designated in 1957 by Barber is internationally accepted today. In contrast, the often synonymously used designation "polymyalgia arteritica" is still more puzzling since it leads to the assumption of a pathogenetic or even a causal connection between both phenomena.

Arteritis temporalis

GCA is a more general concept, whereas the frequently used designations "arteritis temporalis" and "arteritis cranialis" hide the fact that there is a vascular systemic disease which prefers only certain areas of the body and is characterized by the phenomenon of giant cell formation. It is therefore recommended to speak of a PMR-GCA syndrome in which a common origin of both components can be assumed.

12.2 Epidemiology

Prevalence of PMR

When considered as the primary process, the prevalence of PMR is estimated to be about 500 cases per 100,000 persons aged 50 years and older, with a yearly incidence of 53.7 per 100,000 persons aged 50 years and older (Chuang et al. 1982).

Prevalence of GCA

The prevalence of GCA is estimated to be 133 per 100,000 persons aged 50 years and older with a yearly incidence rate of 11.7 cases per 100,000 persons aged 50 years and older (Huston et al. 1978). Well-documented and arterial biopsy-certified PMR cases are rare in persons under 50 years.

Females are afflicted with the PMR-GCA syndrome twice as often as males. The reason for this is considered by Gerber (1989) to be the fact that more females are present in this age-group due to their higher life expectancy.

12.3 Etiology

The etiology and pathogenesis of PMR-GCA syndrome are still unclear today. Only a few facts support numerous estimations, thus frequent familial occurrence, including a pair of identical twins, and an apparent predilection of these conditions for Caucasians is reported, which indicate a genetic disposition (Liang et al. 1974a; Kemp 1977; Healey and Wilske 1978). Moreover, indications exist for an augmented association with HLA-DR4 (Calamia et al. 1981).

Genetic disposition

12.4 Polymyalgia Rheumatica

12.4.1 Clinical Features

Polymyalgia rheumatica (PMR) is a well-defined syndrome occurring in individuals older than 50 and most over 65 years and consisting of pain and morning stiffness in the proximal muscles. The very high ESR is a key to diagnosis, often being found to reach up to 100 mm/h (Westergren method). Bilateral pain and stiffness are noted in the neck and back as well as in the shoulder girdle and may radiate into the gluteal muscles and thighs. The dramatic response to corticosteroid therapy may be used as a diagnostic tool. The onset is acute, the disease then fully develops within approximately 2 weeks. It is frequently accompanied by depression and loss of weight.

Arthralgia

Arthralgia, joint swellings, and short-lived synovitides are no rarity. They can occur in every stage of the disease. The painful joint phenomena are oligoarticular, asymmetric, and can manifest themselves in large and small joints. Most often hand, finger, and knee joints are attacked. Occasionally, also sternoclavicular and shoulder joints are involved. PMR may begin before, appear simultaneously with, or develop after the symptoms related to the arteries.

12.4.2 Pathology

Mysterious disease

Particularly due to two reasons, PMR is still a mysterious disease:

1. The clinical symptoms, ESR, and successful therapy with cortisone undoubtedly indicate an inflammatory muscle disease. However, no plausible evidence is available for that.
2. The frequent mutual occurrence of the muscle symptoms with definitely detectable arterial changes logically suggests a vascular origin of the muscle disease. But there is no indication: stenosing vessel processes result in infarctions of the areas they supply. Changes of this kind cannot, however, be detected in the musculature in PMR.

We are thus confronted by two phenomena which indeed occur very often simultaneously but between which no mutuality and, in particular, no pathogenetic connection can be recognized.

Light-optical examinations

Light-optical examinations of biopsies which were taken from painful muscle segments progressed disappointingly. Neither in a defined study (Fassbender and Annefeld 1986) nor in longitudinal routine studies could we detect the slightest pathological changes, except for sporadic atrophy of type 2 fibres (age-related; Fig. 12.1). Some authors (Dubowitz and Brooke 1973; Schröder 1982; Engel and Franzini-Armstrong 1994) describe a distinct peri-capillary thickening of the basal membrane and a selective muscle fibre atrophy (type 2, in some cases type 2B only). In this regard, our data agree with those of other investigators. In particular, we could not find traces of acute or burnt-out inflammatory or necrotising processes.

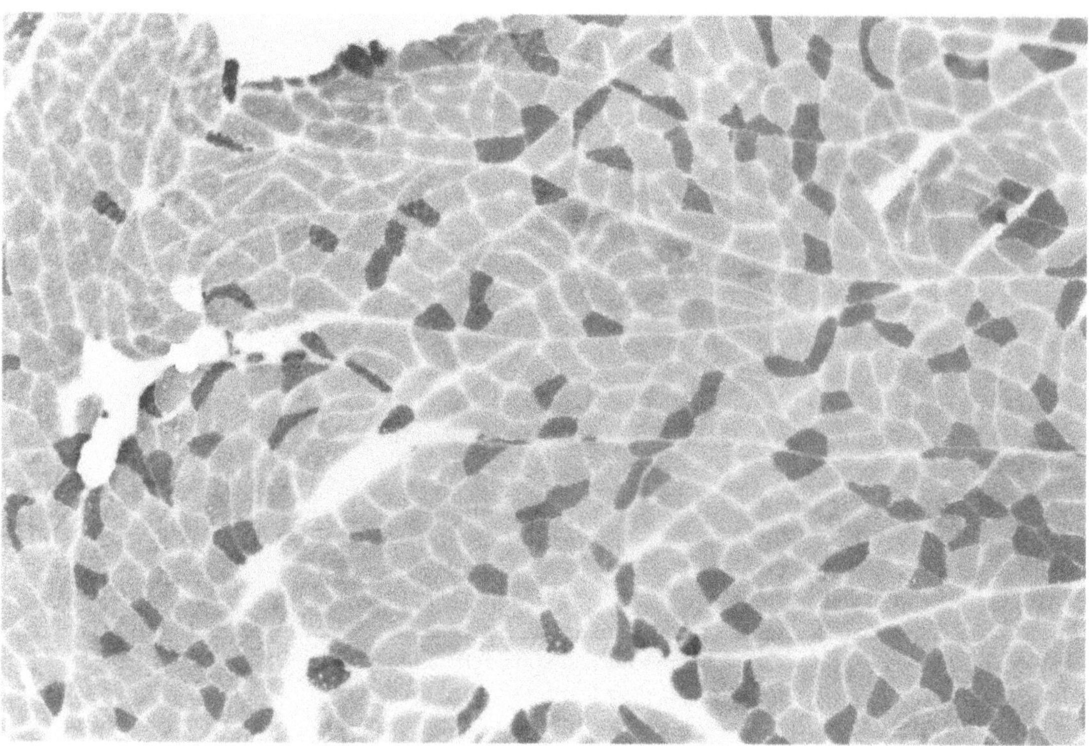

Fig. 12.1
Polymyalgia rheumatica

Excision from right m. trapezius. Slight changes in form of an atrophy of type 2 fibres. The dark type 2 fibres are atrophic, also isolated type 1 fibres. Myofibrillar ATpase after pre-incubation at pH 9.4 (66-year-old female)

Ultrastructural changes

Fassbender and Annefeld (1986) examined electron-microscopically the skeletal musculature of 21 patients with clinically confirmed PMR and classified the ultrastructural changes on the basis of 15 criteria (Table 12.1). These criteria include changes in nuclei, myofilaments, mitochondria, and in the T-system, furthermore glycogen depositions (Fig. 12.2) as well as lipid, lipofuscin, and myelin figures. The functionally most important ultrastructural change concerns the mitochondria (in the form of crystal depositions, deformations, new formation, accumulation; Figs. 12.3–12.5).

The changes found in muscles are focal, unspecific, and regressive in nature. The systemic assessment of all criteria results in a conspicuous accumulation of certain features: a constellation of characteristics, by which the ultrastructural picture of PMR obtains a specific profile. An additional comparative analysis of regressive skeletal changes and of processes in the region of the media of the muscular arteries demonstrates analogous morphological changes which point to a common harmful and overlying process in PMR and GCA. Changes in the ultrastructure of the kind and degree described cannot be explained by inflammatory or non-inflammatory arterial occlusions. Light-optical findings in muscle also correspond to this.

Synovial fluid and synovial tissue

Pathological findings in PMR are scarce. In synovial fluid, cell numbers of 1,000–8,000/µl with a neutrophil fraction of 40%–50% were observed (Hunder et al. 1969). Neutrophils in this

Table 12.1. Polymyalgia rheumatica. Analysis of changes in skeletal muscles

Case	Sarcoma	Nucleus	Filaments				Mitochondria				T-system	Cytoplasma			
	Wrinkling	Chain formation	Lysis	Dehiscence of the myo-filament	Smearing, "zig-zagging" of the Z-band	"Rod bodies"	Crystalline inclusion	Clumping	Bizarre forms	"Dense bodies"	Reduplication of the tubules	Lipofuscin accumulation	Lipid accumulation	Glycogen accumulation	Myelin figures
1	+	–	–	+	–	–	–	+	–	–	–	+	+	+	–
2	+	+	+	+	+	+	+	+	+	+	+	+	+	+	+
3	+	–	+	+	+	+	–	+	+	–	–	+	+	+	–
4	+	+	+	+	+	–	–	+	–	–	–	+	+	+	–
5	+	–	–	+	–	+	–	+	–	–	–	+	+	+	–
6	–	–	+	+	+	–	–	+	–	–	+	+	+	+	–
7	+	+	+	+	+	–	+	+	+	+	–	+	+	+	+
8	–	+	+	+	+	–	+	+	–	–	+	+	+	+	+
9	–	–	+	+	–	+	–	+	–	–	+	+	+	+	+
10	+	+	+	+	+	+	+	+	+	+	–	+	+	+	+
11	–	+	–	+	–	–	–	–	–	–	–	+	+	+	+
12	+	–	+	+	+	–	–	+	–	+	–	+	+	+	+
13	–	–	+	+	–	+	+	–	+	+	–	+	+	+	+
14	–	+	+	+	+	–	+	+	–	–	–	+	+	+	+
15	–	+	+	+	–	–	–	+	–	–	+	+	+	+	+
16	–	+	+	+	+	+	+	+	+	+	+	+	+	+	+
17	+	+	+	+	+	+	+	+	+	+	+	+	+	+	+
18	+	–	+	+	–	+	+	+	–	+	+	+	+	+	+
19	–	–	+	+	+	–	+	+	–	–	+	+	+	+	+
20	+	+	+	+	+	+	+	+	+	+	–	+	+	+	–
21	+	–	+	+	+	–	+	+	–	–	–	+	+	+	–

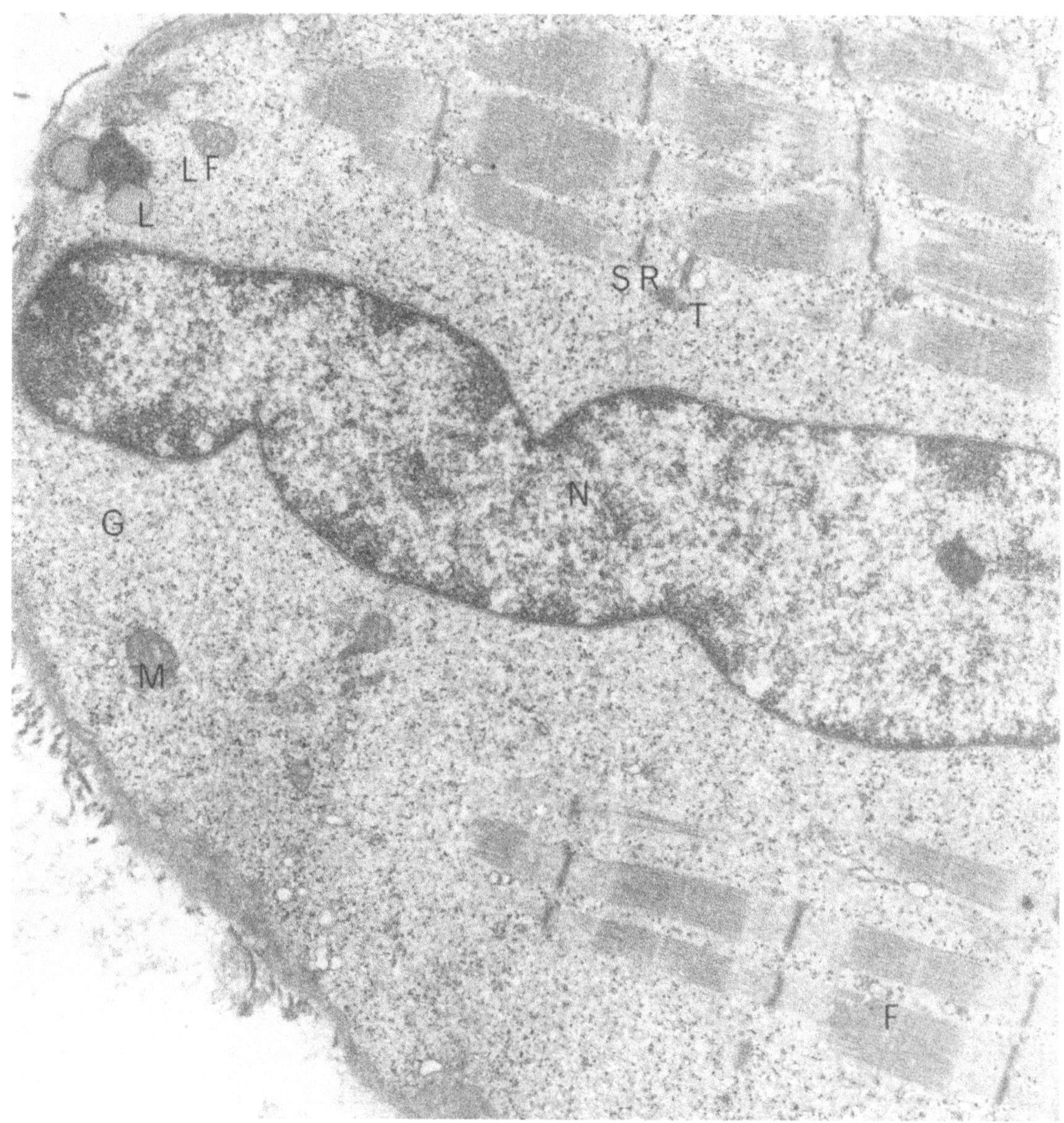

Fig. 12.2
Polymyalgia rheumatica

Excision from left m. deltoideus. Below the sarcolemma: cell nucleus (*N*), mitochondria (*M*), sarcoplasmic reticulum (*SR*), T-system (*T*), lipid (*L*), lipofuscin (*LF*); in the area of the destroyed filaments and between dehiscenced filaments (*F*), glycogen accumulation (*G*). (64-year-old female; 1:16,800)

order of magnitude do not endanger the joint cartilage since the amount of enzyme thereby released is far below the inhibitor level in synovial fluid. Synovial biopsies from knee, sternoclavicular, and shoulder joints revealed low-grade synovitides with lymphocyte infiltrations (Henderson et al. 1975). In a synovial biopsy from a knee joint of a patient with PMR, we saw a slight villi augmentation but, however, no fibrin exudation, no lining cell or stromal proliferation and no neutrophils, only some scattered lymphocytes. Thus it concerns the picture of a low-grade uncharacteristic synovitis, as we occasionally see it as an accompanying phenomenon also in degenerative processes.

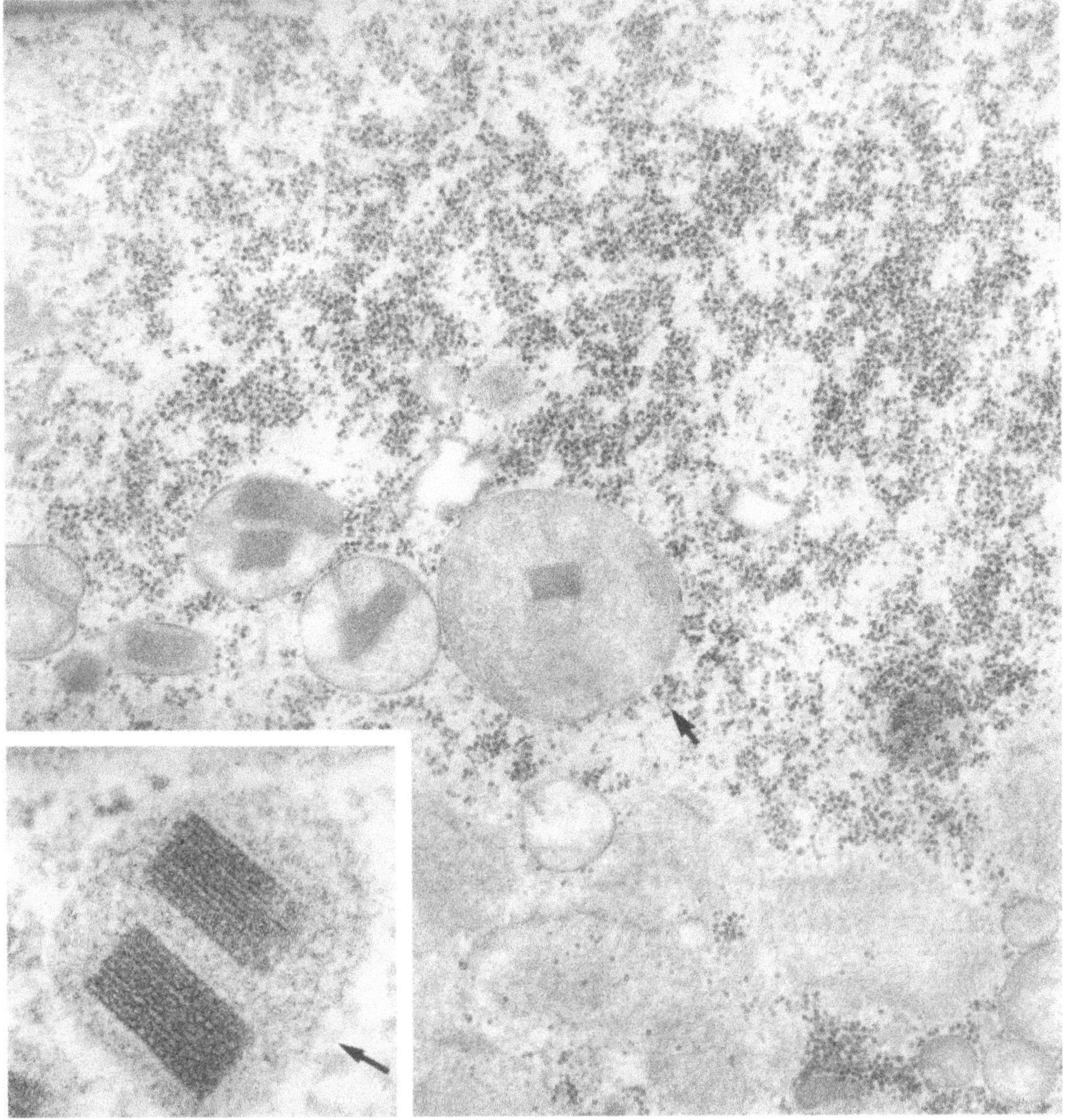

Excision from left m. trapezius. Paracrystalline inclusions (*arrow*) in mitochondria (62-year-old female; 1:28,500). *Insert:* excision from right m. trapezius. Crystalline inclusion (*arrow*) in mitochondria (63-year-old female; 1:186,000)

Fig. 12.3
Polymyalgia rheumatica

12.5 Giant Cell Arteritis

12.5.1 Clinical Features

The arterial process gives giant cell arteritis (GCA) its characteristic profile. The most common initial symptom is headache, visual symptoms are frequent and include diplopia, ptosis, and partial or complete blindness, which is mostly caused by ischemia of the optic nerve or tracts secondary to arteritis of the branches of the ophthalmic or posterior ciliary arteries. The ESR is elevated (>50 mm during the first hour). The pulsation of the temporal ar-

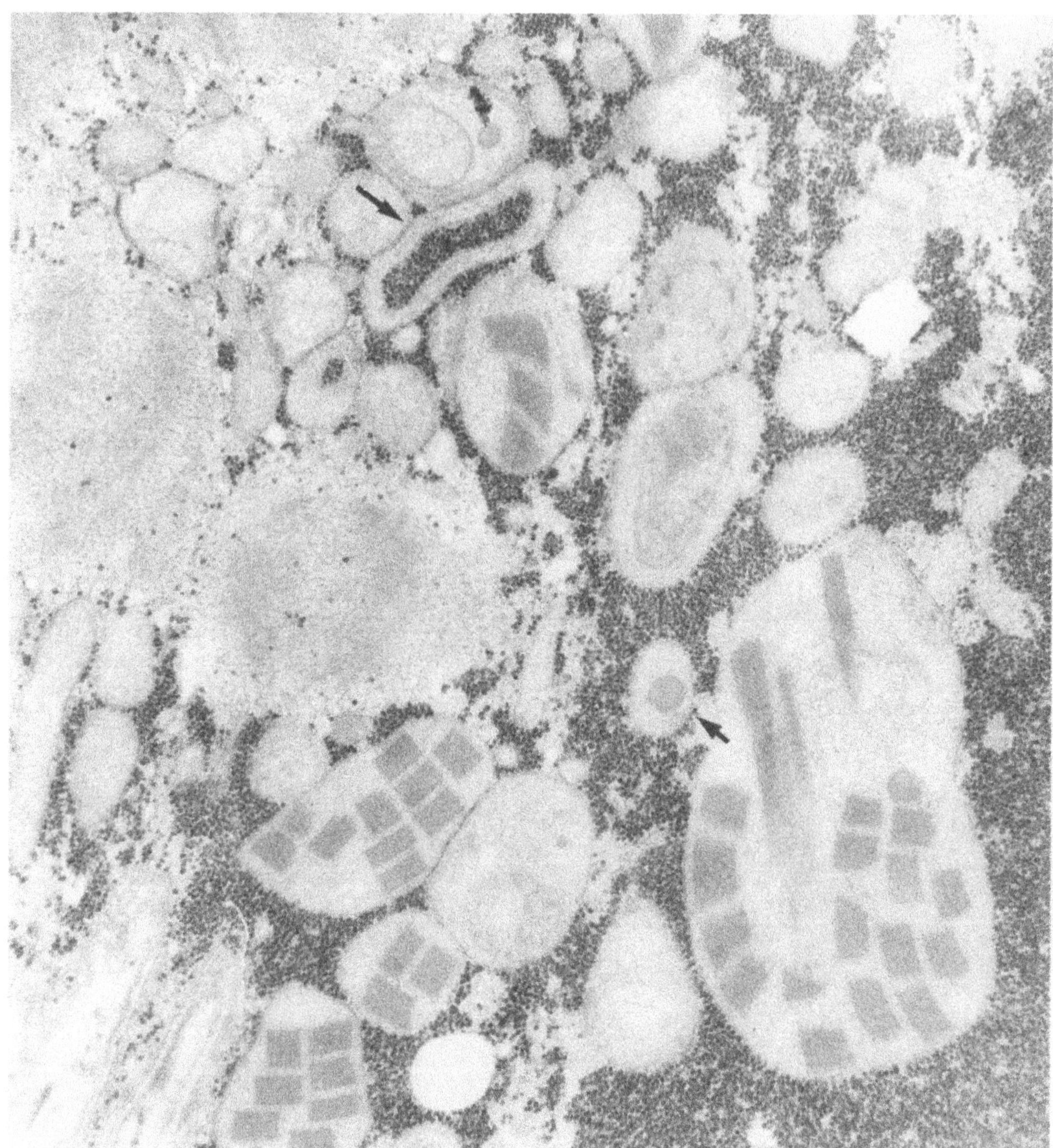

Fig. 12.4
Polymyalgia rheumatica

Biopsy from left m. trapezius. Accumulation of degenerated mitochondria, mitochondrium with "dense-body" without cristae (*long arrow*); sac-shaped widened mitochondrium with glycogen inclusions (*short arrow*); (70-year-old female; 1:28,500)

tery is diminished, patients often describe temporal artery tenderness. Classical complications include anterior ischaemic optic neuropathy leading to a loss of vision (Hayreh 1997).

12.5.2 Pathology

Only autopsy examinations can give guaranteed information about the spread of the vessel process. According to these, the arteria temporalis superficialis, the arteria vertebralis, the arteria ophthalmica, and the arteriae ciliare posteriores are preferred by

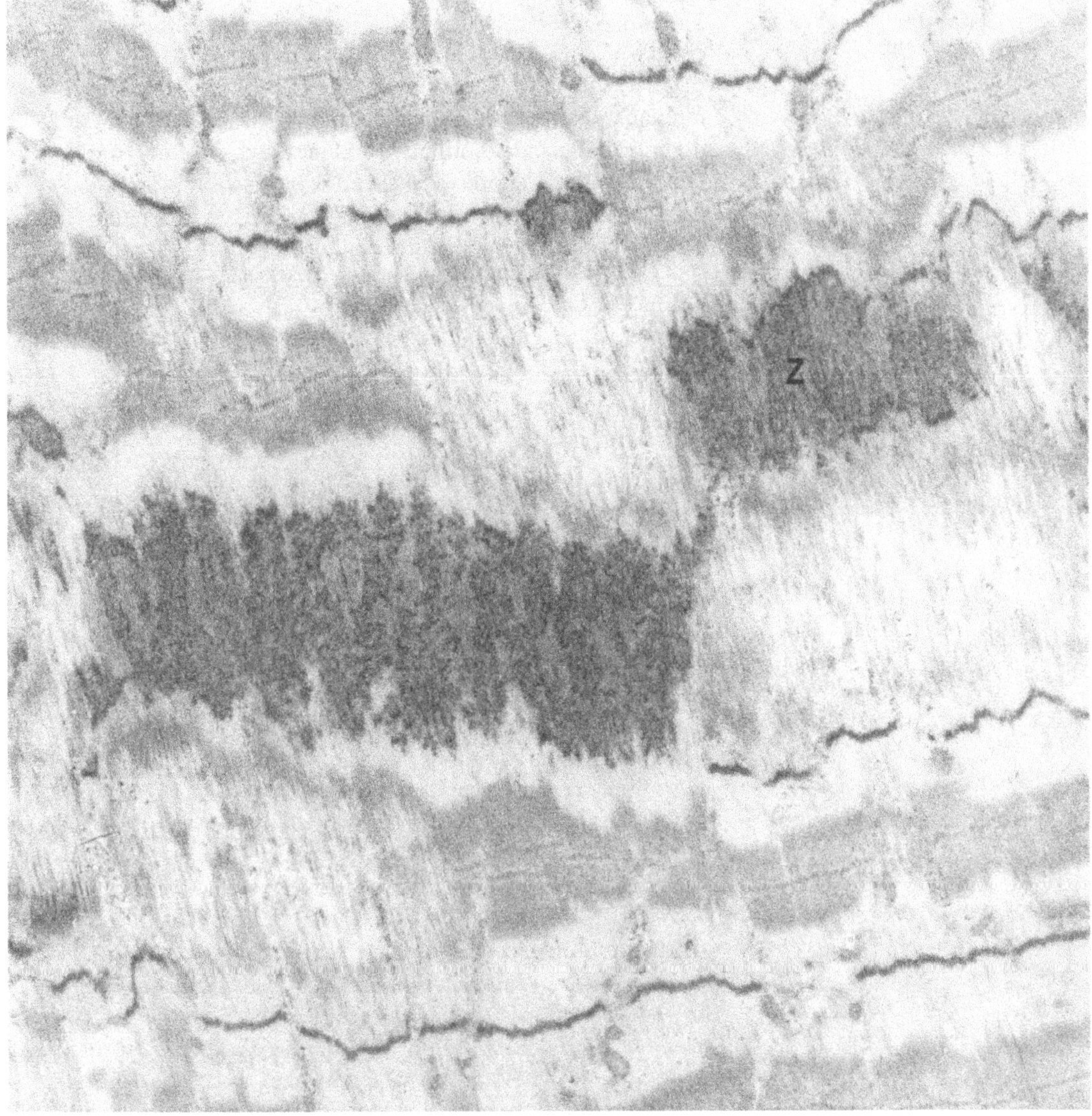

Excision from left m. trapezius. *Z*-band (*Z*) widened ("smearing"; 71-year-old female; 1:28,500)

Fig. 12.5
Polymyalgia rheumatica

the GCA. Moreover, the process can attack the proximal and distal aorta and internal and external carotid, subclavian, brachial, and abdominal arteries.

Two vessel areas

Thus, the GCA concentrates on two vessel areas: the head arteries or the branches of the carotid artery, respectively, and the branches of the proximal aorta. Already this attack pattern, particularly the predilection for the temporal arteries is highly characteristic for GCA. Involvement of large arteries, results in clinical symptoms in 10–15% of patients with GCA (Klein et al. 1975; Cid et al. 1998).

Morphological characteristics

The intrinsic specificity occurs, however:

1. In the primary destruction of the media without fibrinoid necrosis or the influence of neutrophils.
2. In the high consistency with which multinucleated giant cells are found in the destruction area.

Process dynamics

The morphological picture of the GCA is dominated by the process dynamics. It is hallmarked by the amount and duration of the arteritis. In the uncharacteristic early stage, small proliferating pads of the intima as well as small-focussed destructions of the internal elastic lamina with plaque-like swelling and degeneration of the smooth muscle cells can be found. The full range extends from a highly florid stage to an inapparent persistent residual scar in the media. The picture of the highly florid GCA can, in extreme cases, correspond to a panarteritis nodosa. It is labelled by two components:

Two components

1. The specific mostly segmentally limited destruction of the media and internal elastic lamina.
2. Unspecific, proliferative accompanying reactions of the intima and adventitia.

Media destruction

The specific nuclear process occurs after invasion of the elastica interna into the media. Here, in the florid stage, a fracture zone is set in which the connection to the muscle fibres is destroyed. They either disappear or lie distributed in small fragments irregularly between macrophages, sparse T lymphocytes, and eosinophils. B lymphocytes are extremely rare (Fig. 12.6). In this phase, single neutrophils are also found. We could never observe fibrinoid necroses or larger neutrophil accumulations. Striking is the splintering of the remaining muscle sections. The muscle fibre bundles are forced apart by macrophages and connective tissue cells.

Different types of giant cells

At this stage, giant cells of different origin and of different shape are found. Apart from histiocytic giant cells, that have phagocytized fragments of the elastica, giant cells of myogenic origin are observed. One sees rod-shaped cells in which the nuclei are aligned lengthwise, moreover round, oval and bizarre-shaped giant cells with pointed protrusions. In the cytoplasm, a regular, fine eosinophil granulation is recognizable, as well as inclusions which remind one of the fibrillation of muscle cells. In the florid stage, 50% of the giant cells which lie in close contact with the residual muscle contain oval, dark, and round vesicular cell nuclei with transparent karyoplasm (Fig. 12.7). In the region of the newly-formed, loose collagen fibrils without contact with the muscle fragments lie, in contrast, narrow oval giant cells with dark, peripheral nuclei which are similar to Langhans-type cells. Macrophages and giant cells localized in the media and along the elastic membranes, but not in the adventitia and intima, express metalloproteinases (Nikkari et al. 1996; Weyand et al. 1996), and thus have the potential to digest tissue components.

Spreading of destructive process

The destructive process can, on the one hand, be restricted to one or several wall segments (segmental involvement; Fig. 12.8) or it can also, in rare cases, surround the whole circumference of the vessel wall and destroy the media up to small muscle remains (Fig. 12.9). Between the residual muscle fragments lie the remains of the perished muscle fibres, in between which a loose avascular granulation tissue buds out of the intima. Sporadic neutrophils are found in the region of the dead muscle tissue. Eosinophils lie, in particular, at the outer circumference of the media. The adventitia is nearly always thickened by a concentric deposit of collagen fibres. Here also in the highly acute phase, we

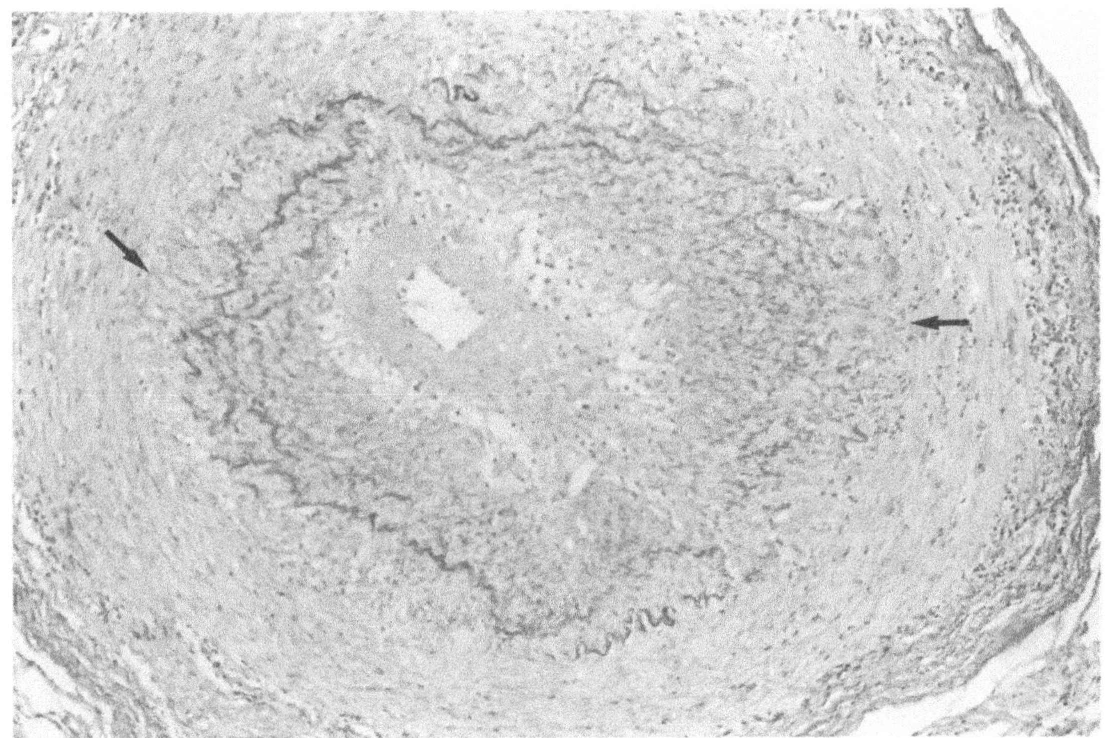

A. temporalis. Destruction of the muscularis with segmental splintering of the elastica interna (*arrows*). Thrombotic occlusion of the lumen with recanalisation. Concentric thickening of the outer media. Infiltrates of lymphocytes in the adventitia (76-year-old female)

Fig. 12.6
Giant cell arteritis

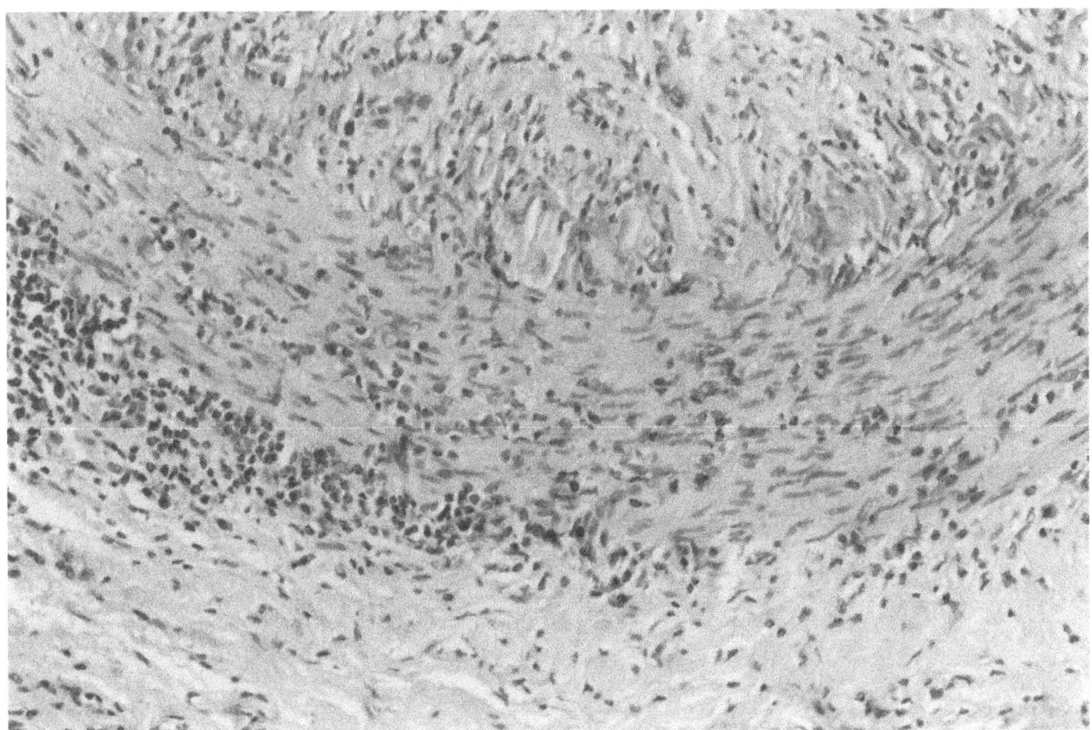

A. temporalis. Internal and external destruction of the muscularis through invading macrophages, giant cells, and neutrophils. Sparse cell infiltration in the adventitia (76-year-old female)

Fig. 12.7
Giant cell arteritis

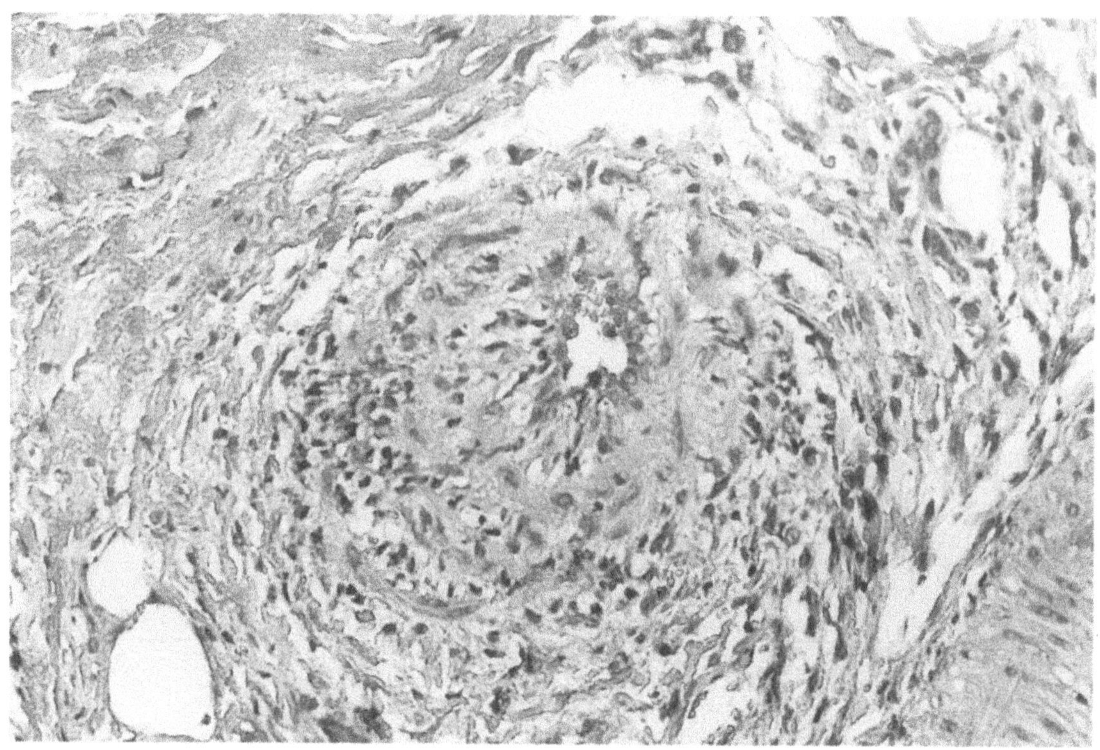

Fig. 12.8
Giant cell arteritis

Forearm muscularis. Predominantly segmental destruction of the artery wall through a granulation tissue containing macrophages, fibroblasts, and neutrophils with restriction of the lumen; at the bottom of the figure one giant cell (44-year-old female)

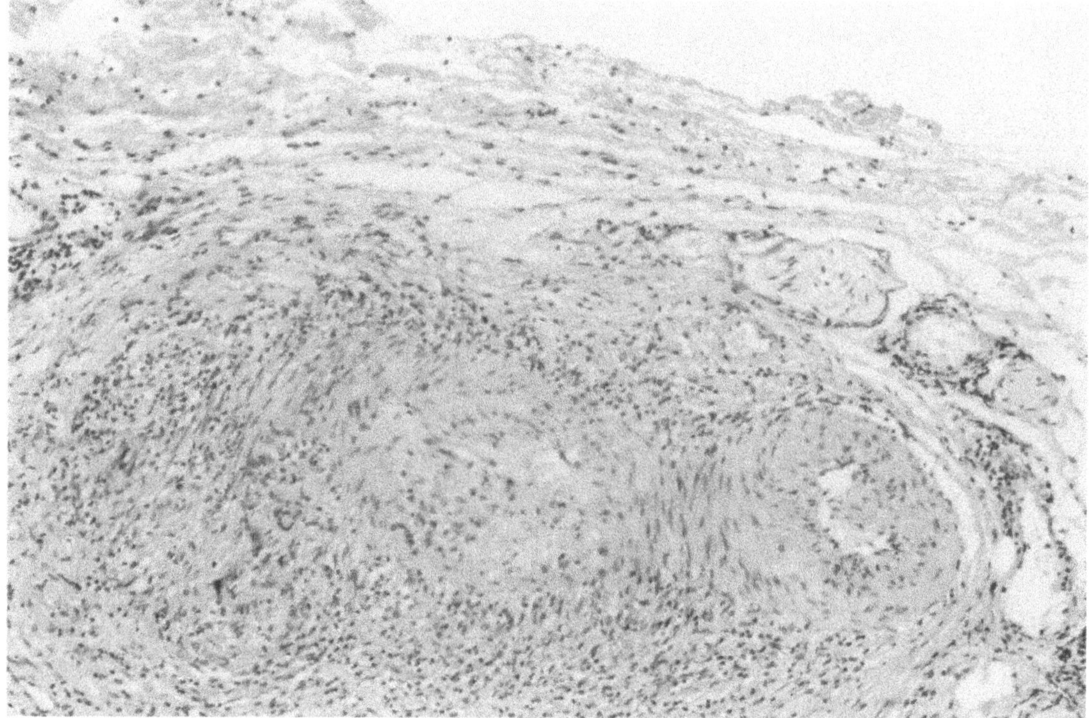

Fig. 12.9
Giant cell arteritis

A. temporalis. Destruction of all layers of the artery wall by macrophagocytically marked granulation tissue with isolated giant cells. High-grade restriction of the lumen (70-year-old female)

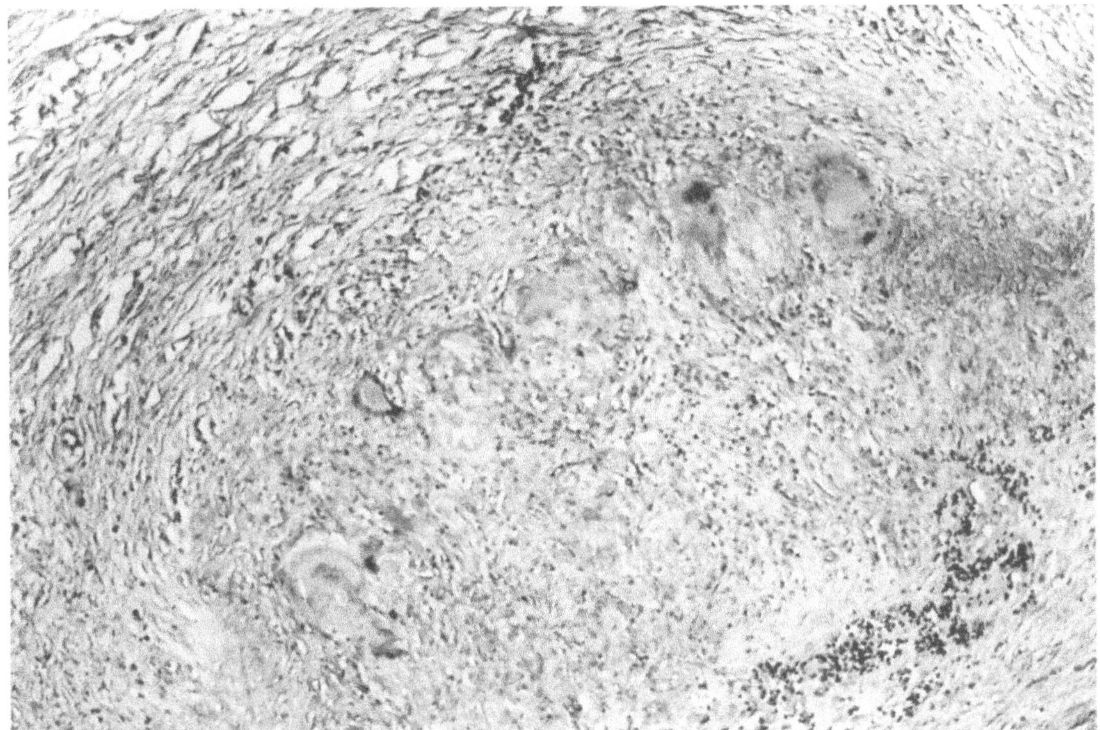

Total destruction of the A. temporalis. The perished blood vessel is replaced by scar tissue surrounded by giant cells, macrophages, neutrophils, and lymphocytes (84-year-old male)

Fig. 12.10
Giant cell arteritis

see sporadic eosinophils and lymphocytes but no neutrophils.

Secondary intimal fibrosis

The intima reacts to the primary media process with a high-grade fibroblast proliferation and collagen production whereby the clearing can be narrowed to total occlusion (Fig. 12.10). In the remaining space, a fibrin plug can deposit itself.

Subacute stage

In a later stage of the GCA, the cells in total are reduced and hallmarked by an increasing fibrosis which heals up the defects caused by the muscle destruction. In this phase, the giant cells are sparser but oval, dark-type cells with spindle-shaped peripheral nuclei persist.

Scar stage

After complete waning of the process hardly any traces are to be recognized. Intimal fibrosis alone is not uncommon in older people. One or more scarred invasions into the media are pathognomonic, however. The fibrosis thus progresses continuously from the intima into the muscle defect. Also in the adventitia, the burnt-out process has left behind traces in the form of a concentric fibrosis in which small lymphocytic foci are occasionally still to be found. Blood vessels branch from the adventitia into the destruction zone. At the outer edge of the media, occasional sporadic multinuclear giant cells can survive the process for a long time. Even if giant cells and lymphocytes are absent, a small residual scar-serration, protruding from the fibrosed intima into the media, can be an indication of a waned GCA. Frequently, the vasa vasorum of the artery affected are involved into the vasculitic process.

It has to be assumed that in a relatively large number of temporal artery biopsies, which in clinically confirmed PMR turned out to be negative, the findings described above are only slightly pronounced and were overlooked, and not assessed, respectively. Moreover, the question remains to what extent a small area within the biopsy is representative of the segmental vascular process. Interesting in this regard is an observation by Weyand, who deduced that temporal arteries from patients with the clinical diagnosis of PMR were found to contain gene-specific transcripts for IL-2, IL-1, and TGFβ, but not for IFNγ (Weyand et al. 1994; Weyand and Goronzy 1999). This would explain the discrepancies in different examination results.

Considerations of destruction mechanism

It is difficult to categorize the GCA under general pathological aspects since the progressing characteristic process is basically different from that of other arteritides. The media destruction precedes neither a neutrophil activity, as for example in polyarteritis nodosa, nor a fibrinoid necrosis, as for example in rheumatoid arthritis (RA). Even in relatively early stages in which the media destruction is "blooming", only sporadic neutrophils and no fibrinoid necroses are found. Striking, by contrast, in this stage is the excessive macrophage activity between and around small muscle fragments, intermingled with some fibroblasts, few lymphocytes, and scattered neutrophils. The ratio of macrophages to lymphocytes and neutrophils is estimated to be 20:5:1. Sparse eosinophils lie distributed outside the destruction foci near the adventitia. The significance of the giant cells which are known to belong to the inflammatory arsenal remains open.

Excessive macrophage activity

Immunoglobulin and complement deposits were detected intracellularly and on the lamina elastica interna in some temporal arteritides (Wilkinson and Russell 1972; Liang et al. 1974b). The specificity of the deposits and their correlation with the inflammatory changes have yet to be proven. Waaler and colleagues (1976) found anti-IgG activity in biopsies from patients with GCA. Higher levels of circulating immune complexes were detected in active phases of the disease (Papaioannou et al. 1980). The immune complex concentration is correlated with the height of the ESR and falls to normal levels after treatment or after waning of the inflammatory process.

Primary immunological muscle aggression

In total, the picture is vaguely reminiscent of a primary muscle destruction as we described in the myocardium for the special form of muscle aggression in rheumatic fever (RF). In both cases, destruction of the muscle fibres occurs without preceding inflammation. Observations of lymphocyte infiltrates in early stages support our assumption that a model case of autoaggression, directed against the muscle substrate, is present here. The molecular representation of T cell receptor molecules in the vascular lesions is highly suggestive of an antigen-driven immune response being the principal event (Weyand and Goronzy 1999).

Autoaggression

13 Vasculitides

13.1 Systemic Vasculitis

The relationship of the vasculitides to the rheumatic complex exists due to the fact that in the systemic inflammatory diseases, in which an immunological background is proven or assumed, the capillary system of the synovial membrane as well as the vascular system in other parts of the organism are reactive.

Role of vascular structures in inflammation

It is understandable that the "banks" of the blood network are primarily the substrate for an exudative inflammatory, systemic disorder. The wall construction and the flow rate determine the location, the kind, and the amount of damage.

The network of blood capillaries offers the largest contact surface to the flowing blood and thus also to the instigators, e.g. antigens and immune complexes. The capillaries which are surrounded only by a basal membrane and some pericytes can react by altering their endothelial tubules. Depending on the degree of damage, a disturbance of the permeability occurs which leads to leakage of serum, plasma, and formed blood constituents into the surrounding tissue, or to exudation into the neighbouring surfaces such as the synovial membrane, pericardium, pleura or peritoneum.

Endothelial cells

The activation of endothelial cells during exudation is brought about by various factors that may lead to changes in the cells' form and structure as well as to alterations in gene expression. Neutrophils are being recruited by interactions of adhesion molecules. The interaction of integrines and their receptors (e.g. ICAM-1 and VCAM-1) leads to an effective binding of neutrophils to the endothelium and, thus, paves their way to emerge via the next gap in the endothelial unit and then to infiltrate the area of inflammation.
An analogous situation exists also in small, medium, and large arteries and veins, with, however, three differences:

1. Due to the higher flow rate, the contact time is significantly shorter than in blood capillaries.
2. The contact surface between the blood-stream and the vessel wall is several fold smaller than that in the capillary network.
3. In contrast to the capillary network, the endothelial tubule is surrounded by a tight cuff consisting of multiple connective tissue and muscle layers which do not allow exudation into the surroundings but in such a case the vessel wall itself can become the substrate for the damaging substances which spreads over the blood stream.

The flow rate and size of the contact surface determine therefore that the exudations onto the mesothelial surfaces are more frequent than in vessel walls. Here also certainly lies a reason for the frequent occurrence of uncharacteristic, often minor synovitides as an accompanying reaction of different diseases. It also explains why, for example, in rheumatoid arthritis (RA) synovitides occur more often than vessel processes, although both endothelial surfaces have contact with the same circulating agents.
The flow velocity and contact area also explain the preferential attack of small blood vessels. Moreover, additional factors such as turbulences in the area of the vessel junction facilitate the local development of vessel processes.
In animal experiments, the frequency and amount of vascular damage can be increased by raising the arterial pressure. Nevertheless, there is still no explanation for the majority of localizations of the vascular processes which belong to the specific profile of defined systemic inflammatory diseases.

Pathogenic factors

Pathogenic factors in vascular processes which are not directly instigator-induced are mainly circulating immune complexes or immune complexes formed on the antigenic structure of the vessel wall. Thus, circulating immune complexes in high antigen excess tend, in particular, to deposit on the vessel walls. An impaired clearing function of the reticulo-endothelial system (RES) increases the pathological occurrence of circulating immune complexes. The studies of Gocke and coworkers (1970) have already shown that viral antigens participate in pathogenic immune complex formation. They showed this by the detection of hepatitis B surface antigen in the vessel wall of patients with polyarteritis nodosa (PAN).
The cytomegalovirus can also play a similar role at the onset of arteritis (Doherty and Bradfield 1981). Thus, in principle, an inciting role of viral antigen must therefore be taken into account

in immunological systemic diseases. The accompanying arteritides in malignant tumours indicate a possible role of tumour antigens.

Role of immune mechanisms

The role of cell-mediated immune mechanisms in the development of vasculitides is not yet adequately explained. It seems, however, probable that granulomatous reactions, as in Wegener's granulomatosis and in Churg-Strauss vasculitis, are the result of cell-mediated immune reactions whereby the sensitized lymphocytes react with local antigen and recruit macrophages.

Although the arsenal of pathogenic mechanisms of an immune-mediated vasculitis, which is known to date, is limited to circulating and locally-formed immune complexes and cell-mediated immune reactions, the profile of the various immune vasculitides is, nevertheless, very different. It thus concerns not only quantitatively but also qualitatively different processes.

Perivenous lymphocyte infiltrates

In skin biopsies of patients with different immunological systemic diseases, we see, with great regularity, lymphocyte mantles around small veins in the upper third of the corium. The density of these lymphocyte accumulations varies, but we never observed a close contact with the vessel wall and the lumen always remains unchanged, wide. We never found neutrophils amongst them. We have the impression, however, that a relationship exists between the density of the lymphocyte mantles and the intensity of the disease although we cannot interpret this phenomenon in which the vessel wall remains completely intact. We assume that the lymphocytes are recruited from the accompanying lymph vessels by circulating immune factors around the small veins.

Perivascular lymphocyte accumulations in OA

One often finds dense follicle-like lymphocyte accumulations without germinal centres in the "glass villi" in osteoarthritis (OA). On closer observation, small blood vessels in the centre of these sphere-shaped lymphocytic foci are recognizable. These often massive perivascular lymphocyte accumulations lie around intact blood vessels and have nothing in common with "vasculitis". They are an expression of local antigen reactivity and antibody formation, respectively.

Perivascular neutrophil infiltrates

In contrast, perivascular neutrophil infiltrates have a completely different significance. They penetrate the vessel wall and often occur sporadically in one of the three wall layers. They are always an expression of an unspecific vasculitis.

13.2 Different Types of Vasculitis

A classification that follows the suggestions agreed upon in the Chapel Hill Consensus Conference (Jenette et al. 1994) is oriented according to the vessels affected. It divides the vascular processes mainly under clinical aspects into vasculitides affecting small, medium, and large vessels. From the point of view of the pathology, a classification according to common pathogenetic mechanisms appears to be useful.

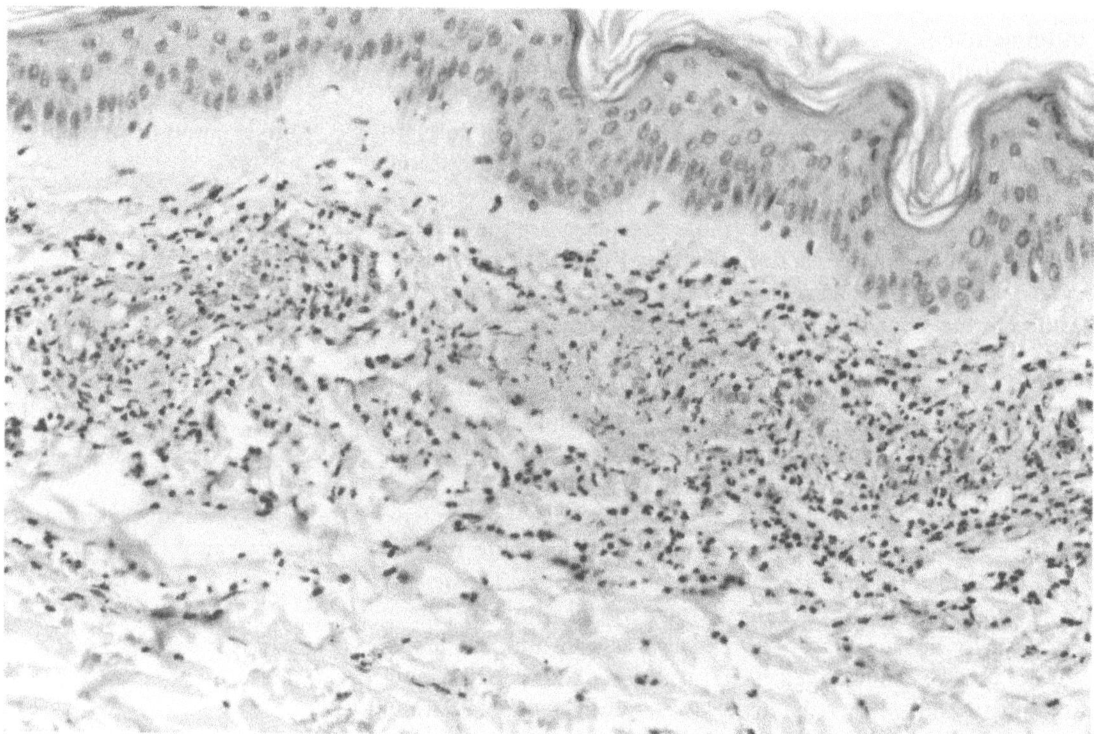

Fig. 13.1
Leucocytoclastic vasculitis

Small cutaneous blood vessels surrounded by neutrophils which also penetrate into the vessel wall. The process is surrounded by a border of lymphocytes (55-year-old female)

13.2.1 Leukocytoclastic Vasculitis

Synonyms: small vessel vasculitis, hypersensitivity vasculitis.

Zeek and coworkers described in 1948 the special form of leukocytoclastic vasculitis with primary skin involvement and a leukocytoclastic pathological profile. The wall of small cutaneous blood vessels is infiltrated by decayed neutrophils. According to the amount and duration of the infiltration, the vessel wall remains or is destroyed under the influence of the lysosomal neutrophil enzymes. Thereby the surrounding cutaneous tissue can be overlaid with leukocytic fragments (Fig. 13.1). Zeek and coworkers coined the designation "hypersensitivity vasculitis" for this disease. In their description, it occurs after some antigenic stimulus, such as the administration of horse serum.

Schoenlein-Henoch purpura

The specific vessel process in leukocytoclastic vasculitides is also encountered in other diseases in which the occurrence of circulating immune complexes has to be taken into account. Amongst these also is Schönlein-Henoch purpura, an anaphylactic phenomenon which occurs particularly in children often following an infection of the respiratory system, characterized by palpable purpura, joint swellings, in particular of the knee and ankle joints, as well as by abdominal cramps. According to the Chapel Hill Consensus Conference, Schönlein-Henoch purpura is a vasculitis with IgA-dominant immune deposits, affecting small vessels (i.e. capillaries, venules, or arterioles), typically involves skin, gut, and glomeruli and is associated with arthralgias or arthritis. The cause is assumed to be a hypersensitivity against bacteria and viruses. This is supported by the combined occurrence of synovial reactions and, under certain circumstances, life-threatening kidney involvement.

Hypocomplemententemic vasculitis

The type of leukocytoclastic vasculitis is also found in young adults (preferentially females) with hypocomplemententemic vasculitis with typical urticarial skin eruption and symmetrical involvement of small joints as described by McDuffie and coworkers in 1978.

Mixed cryoglobulinaemia

Also in mixed cryoglobulinaemia, leukocytoclastic vasculitides were reported by Lospalluto and coworkers in 1962 which proceeds with purpura and arthralgias. Moreover, the leukocytoclastic vasculitis is observed also in bacterial endocarditides, hypergammaglobulinaemic purpura, Sjögren's syndrome (SS), chronic active hepatitis, ulcerative colitis (UC), primary biliary cirrhosis, malign lymphoma, retroperitoneal fibrosis, and Goodpasture's syndrome.

Various diseases

13.2.1.1 Pathomechanism and Pathology

The morphological picture of leukocytoclastic vasculitis with flooding and infiltration of the vessel wall by neutrophils can be adequately explained by vessel contact with immune complexes and leucotaxis by complement components.

The common cause for vasculitides is an excessive production of immune complexes. Under normal circumstances, immune complexes react with complement, they are then – via complement receptors – bound to erythrocytes or macrophages and thus removed from the circulation. If this system is loaded beyond its limits or disturbed, immune complexes may gather on surfaces or – in the case of pathologically increased permeability – penetrate the endothelial tube and accumulate in tissue.

Neutrophils attracted by leucotactic complement factors (e.g. C3a, C5a) are activated and release tissue-damaging proteases and free radicals. Morphologically the leucocytoclastic vasculitis is characterized by a transmural inflammatory infiltration of neutrophils and cell debris, by endothelial oedema, fibrin deposits, and frequently by erythrocyte extravasations, too. At later stages, thrombosis may develop in the vessel affected.

Pathogenic considerations

The difficulty lies, however, in the comparison of leukocytoclastic vasculitis with other vasculitides, in which immune complexes and complement are also detected in the vessel wall but in which mostly no or only sparse neutrophils are present, as for example in RA vasculitis (see p. 130).

Noteworthy also is the fact that in hypersensitivity vasculitis debris is found but only rarely vital neutrophils. Since they only have a short life-span (half-life in the blood 6–7 h) whereas the debris can persist longer, the profile of leukocytoclastic vasculitis implies that here the leucotactic factors occur only in short episodes. The "mass burial place" of nuclear debris, impressing occasionally as "nuclear dust", is thus only explainable by multiple, but waned, immune complex contacts with complement activation. Probably the wall structure of the small vessels is not suitable for a longer-lasting deposition of immune complexes or the occurrence of circulating immune complexes is only short-lived and time-limited. We have never observed fibrinoid vessel wall necroses.

13.2.2 Polyarteritis Nodosa

Synonyms: periarteritis nodosa, panarteritis nodosa.

Using the designation polyarteritis nodosa (PAN), we agree with the suggestion of Conn and Hunder (1985) since the other two names do not always correspond with the local arterial process. PAN concerns a sharply defined, feverous disease profile, often with a fatal outcome, which was first described in 1866 by Kussmaul and Maier. Small and medium-sized arteries and veins are attacked. Males are afflicted with PAN twice as often as females, the preferred manifestation age lying between 40 and 60 years. It must be stressed that the diagnosis of PAN should only be made clinically or at autopsy. Skin or muscle biopsies can only support the clinical indication and may not by themselves be allowed, as is sometimes done, to serve as the basis of this diagnosis. On the other hand, very different arterial and vein processes can be observed in the course of this disease so that even with a negative biopsy result PAN cannot be excluded.

13.2.2.1 Clinical Features

The clinical picture is hallmarked by the actual localization of the vessel process. Of foremost importance is the participation of the kidneys. Infarction of the kidney tissue occurs via involvement of the arcuate and interlobular arteries. In most of the patients, affection of the small arteries in the region of the perineuriums or also of the larger arteries in the region of a nerve plexus causes peripheral nerve damage. Arthralgias are observed in about half of the PAN patients, in 20% asymmetric, episodic, non-destructive polyarthritides of the larger joints of the lower extremities occur at the beginning of the disease (Cohen et al. 1980). Leading symptoms of PAN are, moreover, abdominal ailments and general body weakness.

Autopsy results

Autopsy results explain the clinical symptoms of PAN. The vasculitic process can spread into the whole vessel system and thereby determine the disease profile. The autoptic finding often is already macroscopically highly characteristic and unmistakably: beneath the pericardium and under the serosa of the mesenterium, small, approximately glass pinhead-sized nodules are found which are occasionally aligned like a string of pearls along the adjacent arteries.

13.2.2.2 Pathology

Microscopically, these nodules which give their name to the disease turn out to be small, aneurismatic vessel protrusions (Fig. 13.2). These subserosal aneurysms are potentially in danger of rupturing. We have frequently observed such a fatal complication in PAN with pericardial blockage or bleeding into the abdominal space. It seems that the subserosal arteries are disposed, to a special extent, to aneurism formation because of the lack of opposing pressure from the surrounding tissue. The deeper lying arteries, however, play their fatal role mainly by occlusion of the vessel lumen, followed by infarction (Fig. 13.3).

Different vascular lesions

In the context of PAN diseases one can find microscopically very varied changes in the medium and small arteries and veins. It is thus concerned with variants which, on the one hand, are characterized by the extent, and on the other, by the duration of the local processes.

Specific vascular lesions in PAN

The specific picture of PAN is hallmarked by the complete affection of all wall layers and, above all, by necrosis of a larger vessel segment. The destruction of the wall layers is so complete such that it is never observed in any other vessel disease. It is therefore understandable that this dead tissue cannot sustain the arterial inner pressure and evaginates as far as the surrounding tissue pressure allows. Striking also is the wide zone of neutrophils, macrophages, fibroblasts, and lymphocytes which surround the attacked vessel area. Neutrophils are also frequently found in the necrotic wall segment. On the other hand, the destroyed vessel segment can also occasionally show the picture of a cell-free fibrinoid necrosis which is surrounded externally by macrophages, fibroblasts, and lymphocytes. In contrast to the leukocytoclastic vasculitis, the vessel walls in the florid stage of inflammation contain active neutrophils.

The acute vessel process can heal. It then leaves behind a markedly characteristic collagen media scar, surrounded by fibrosis of the adventitia and intima, mainly with vessel occlusion. In contrast to the wall musculature, the collagen scar is not able to compensate in long-term the chronic strain of the pulsating arterial inner pressure. Thus, in this area, typical aneurysms ("nodules") can develop which, in the course of time, can rupture.

Characteristic profile of PAN

Although here, as in many other vasculitides, immune complexes are present, PAN, nevertheless, shows a characteristic profile which differs from that of other forms:

1. Affection of small, but particularly medium arteries and veins in the whole organism
2. Total destruction of complete vessel wall segments
3. Strong perivascular infiltrative and proliferative reactions
4. Necrosis of wall segments by neutrophil infiltration
5. Focal affection of single arterial sections ("pearl necklace")
6. Predilection for subserosal arteries

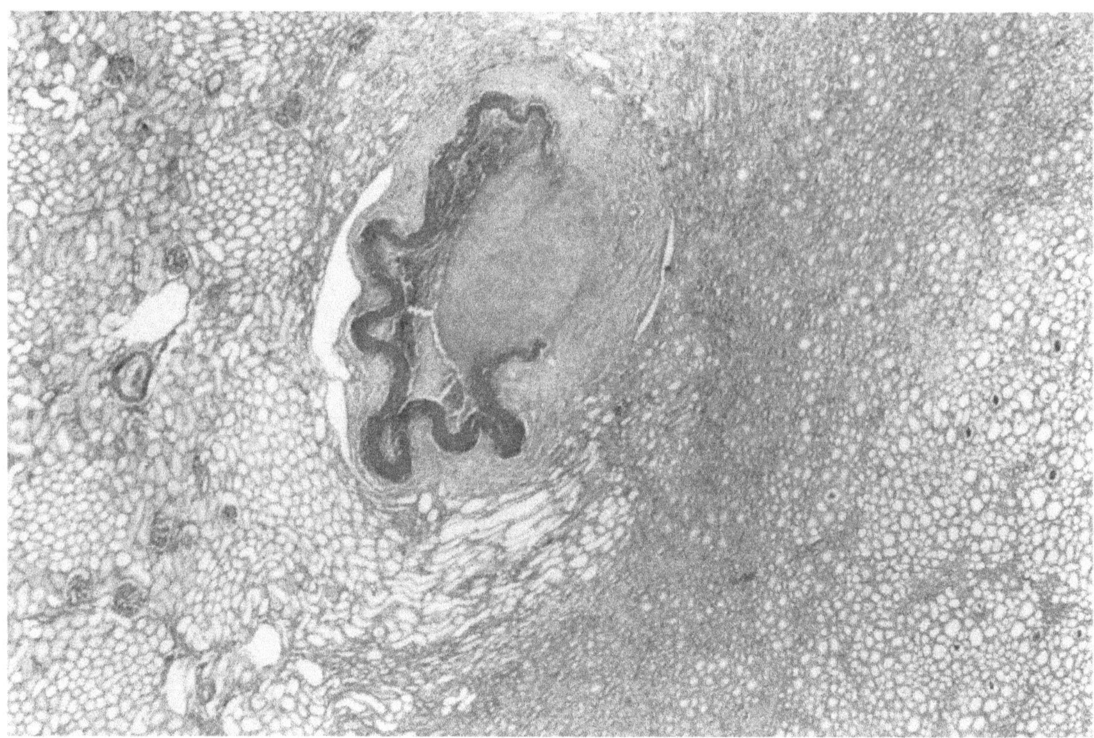

Fig. 13.2
Polyarteritis nodosa

Kidney. Segmental destruction of an artery wall with aneurysmatic protrusion. Vessel and aneurysm are thrombotically occluded. (Courtesy of J. Kriegsmann, Department of Pathology, University of Mainz)

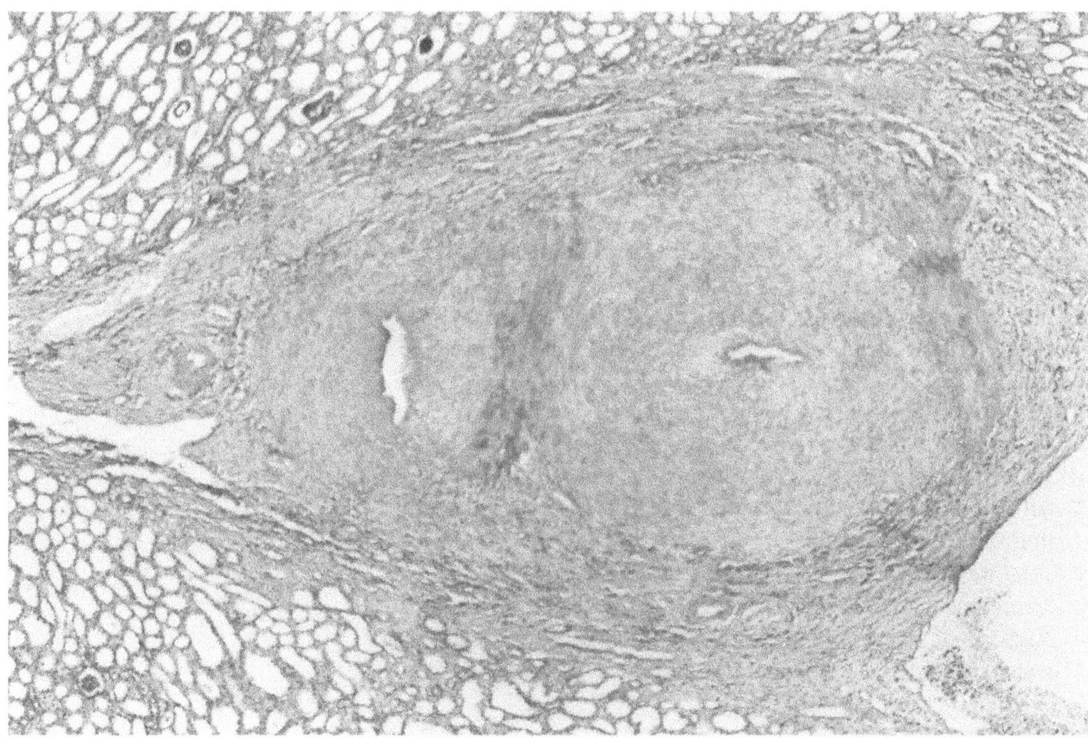

Fig. 13.3
Polyarteritis nodosa

Kidney. Scarred healing of the destroyed arterial tube with minor revascularisation. (Courtesy of J. Kriegsmann, Department of Pathology, University of Mainz)

13.2.2.3 Etiology

Also in PAN, there is no doubt about an immunological genesis. Thereby particularly the hepatitis B surface antigen triggers the vessel wall destruction by an immune complex mechanism (Gocke et al. 1970). This antigen was detected in 10%–54% of PAN patients in different studies (Trepo et al. 1974; Conn et al. 1976). The detection in individual sera was, however, only occasionally successful, so that the precise degree of correlation between hepatitis B surface antigen and PAN cannot finally be stated. A connection with the hepatitis C virus is also being discussed (Hunder 1996). The vessel damage in PAN is finally the work of immune complexe formation, cellular immune response, infectious agents (virus?), and antilysosomal antibodies (Sundy and Haynes 1995).

Hepatitis B surface antigen

Still today, no explanation is available for these specialities of the immune complex-dependent PAN. The search for anti-arterial wall antibodies was negative. Associations with HLA antigens are not found in PAN patients. Therefore additional factors must be involved which hallmark the specific disease profile. Hypothetically, an interference with the virus itself may be considered. Moreover, the permanent availability of the antigen could thereby play a role. The detection of active neutrophil infiltrates over a long period of time substantiates this.

13.2.3 Churg-Strauss Vasculitis

Synonym: allergic angiitis and granulomatosis.

In 1951, this vascular systemic disease was described by Churg and Strauss as an "allergic granulomatosis and angiitis". It is distinguished from PAN by an eosinophil-rich and granulomatous inflammation involving the respiratory tract and by necrotizing vasculitis affecting small to medium-sized vessels. Characteristic is also the intra- and perivascular localisation of the granulomata. Aneurysm formations with their often fatal complications do not belong to the picture of Churg-Strauss vasculitis. The disease is associated with asthma and eosinophilia.

13.2.3.1 Clinical Features and Etiology

The lung processes in the form of asthma, bronchitis, and occasionally also eosinophilic pneumonia precede the systemic vessel process by about 8 years. Bronchial asthma, atopia, and the pronounced eosinophilia have introduced the notation "allergic" to the disease profile. Churg-Strauss vasculitis, as most types of vasculitis, is rare and data of prevalence and incidence are limited. The disease usually affects adults.
The clinical picture is marked basically by the lung process and skin manifestations, especially subcutaneous nodules.
The causes of Churg-Strauss vasculitis are to date unknown. In four patients, Churg and Strauss found antibodies against Tri-

chinella but were unable to detect parasites in the tissue. The search for responsible agents continues without result, which is contributed to by the low incidence of the disease.

13.2.3.2 Pathology

Perivascular findings

The morphological picture of the vessel process is characteristic and clearly distinguished from PAN and other vasculitides. Striking is the spreading of the inflammatory process into a wide perivascular zone (Fig. 13.4). In the florid stage of the process, this region is infiltrated by an irregular mixture of eosinophils, macrophages, fibroblasts, and quite sporadic lymphocytes. Conspicuous is the high variability of cell nuclei: alongside narrow dark nuclei are found clumped, partly overlaid oval dark nuclei. These are probably macrophages. The cells lie loosely, net-like between small fragments of collagen fibres. From this, a granuloma-like cell mixture develops.

Vascular findings

The vessel process has a much lower destructive tendency than PAN. In the cases observed by us, the process was concentrated predominantly at the intima and adventitia (Fig. 13.5). The media lying in between remains unaffected for a long time. Finally, the intima process encroaches upon the bordering media structures. The external contour of the media is eroded also from the adventitia. In this phase, we found, however, no cell infiltration in the media. The intimal process reflects the proliferative destructive character of the disease. Whereas the intrinsic elements of the disease, such as neutrophils and lymphocytes, are absent except for very sporadic eosinophils, the picture is impressed by pathological cell elements. The cell nuclei show wide variation in form, size, and chromatin content. They are mainly macrophages and in between are also found some pathologically changed fibroblasts and sporadic cell forms which remind one of the Anitschkow's cells in the myocardium.

In one case, at the edge of the media, we saw a horse shoe-shaped cell chain with large dark nuclei varying in form and size. Thus, it was a question of a macrophage group. Some of these cells were tightly adjoined forming giant cells which, however, bore no similarity to those in giant cell arteritis. The cells surrounded a nucleus-free, homogeneous, weakly eosinophilic material which was suggestive of degenerated muscle fibres and the beginning of segmental media destruction.

We did not observe fibrinoid necroses. It can be concluded that the media destruction proceeds without the participation of neutrophils but is the work of activated macrophages which suggests an immune mechanism of some kind being responsible for this aggressive vessel process. Overall the impression arises that the media is destroyed in a pincer-like manner by the proliferation of intima and adventitia, without itself being the primary site of destruction, as is the case in other destructive vasculitides.

In one patient with active Churg-Strauss vasculitis, we also saw pronounced acute synovitis. The synovial villi were slightly augmented with fresh fibrin remnants on the surface. The lining cells were, in places, cuboid and multi-layered. In the loose, slightly

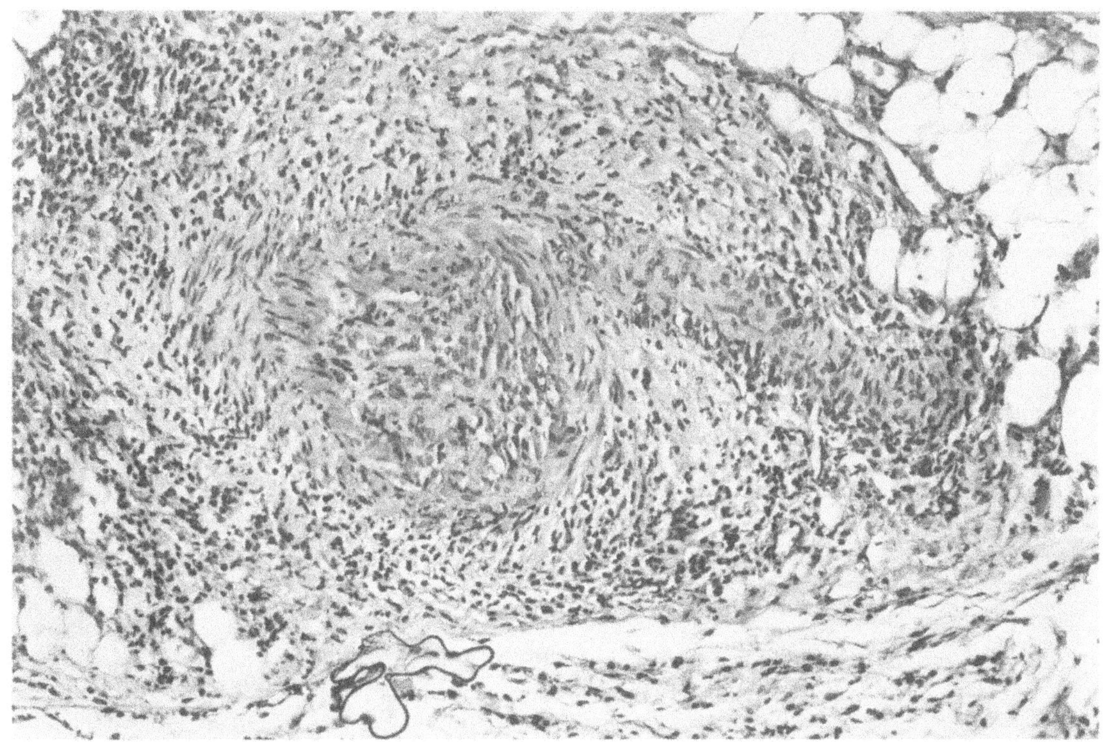

Lung. Artery surrounded by wide-spread formation of granulomata. Occlusion of the lumen by granulation and scar tissue (67-year-old male)

Fig. 13.4
Churg-Strauss vasculitis

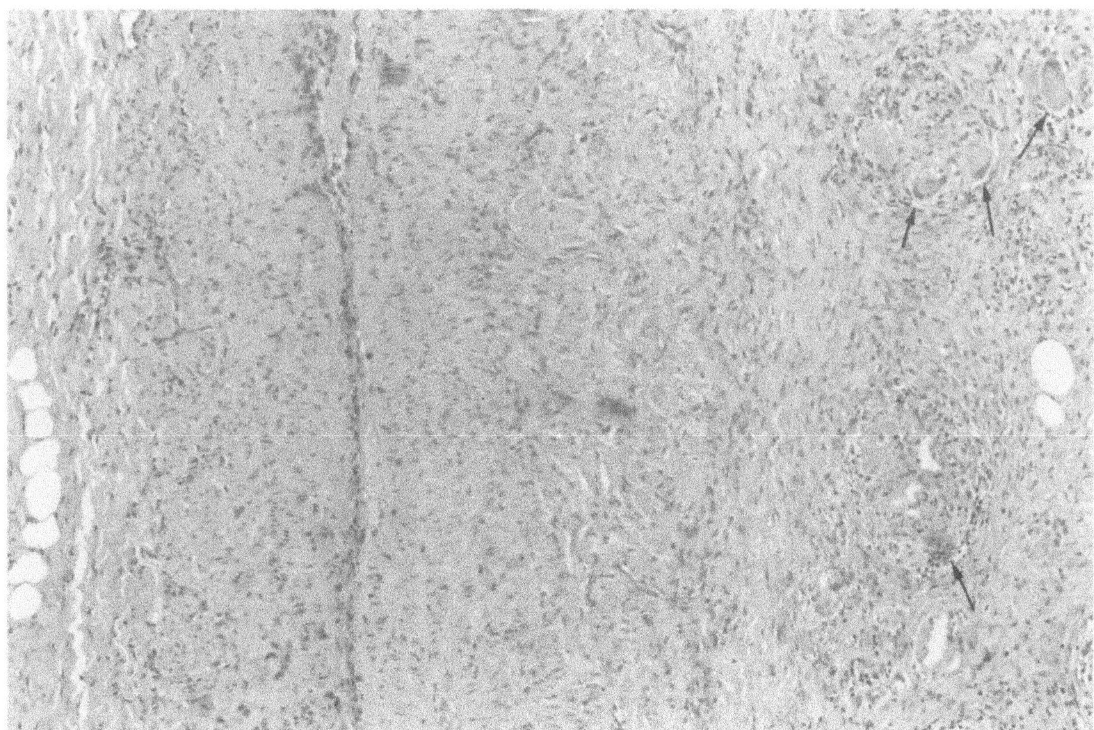

Elbow. Destruction of the vessel wall by a granulation tissue. Formation of granulomata in the surrounding of the vessel with giant cells (*arrows*; 30-year-old male)

Fig. 13.5
Churg-Strauss vasculitis

oedematous villi stroma, numerous newly formed, small diameter blood vessels were found. Densely packed lymphocyte mantles surrounded concentrically the small vessels. The close contact of the lymphocytes with the outer vessel wall was thereby striking. The vessel walls were, however, not infiltrated and the lumen remained free. We did not see eosinophils or neutrophils. Only the very dense lymphocyte infiltrates were unusual. We did not find granuloma formation in the synovial tissue. Thus, it concerns a picture of low-grade acute synovitis.

13.2.4 Wegener's Granulomatosis

Synonym: progressive necrotizing granulomatosis.

13.2.4.1 Clinical Features

The rarely occurring vasculitis first described by Wegener in 1939 belongs to the granulomatous type of vasculitis, for which the intrinsic substrate is a granulomatous process which can attack particularly the upper respiratory tract and also the lungs, kidneys, skin, and eyes. Kidneys are frequently affected in the form of a diffuse glomerulonephritis, respectively an interstitial nephritis. The necrotizing vasculitis affects capillaries, venules, arterioles, and arteries.

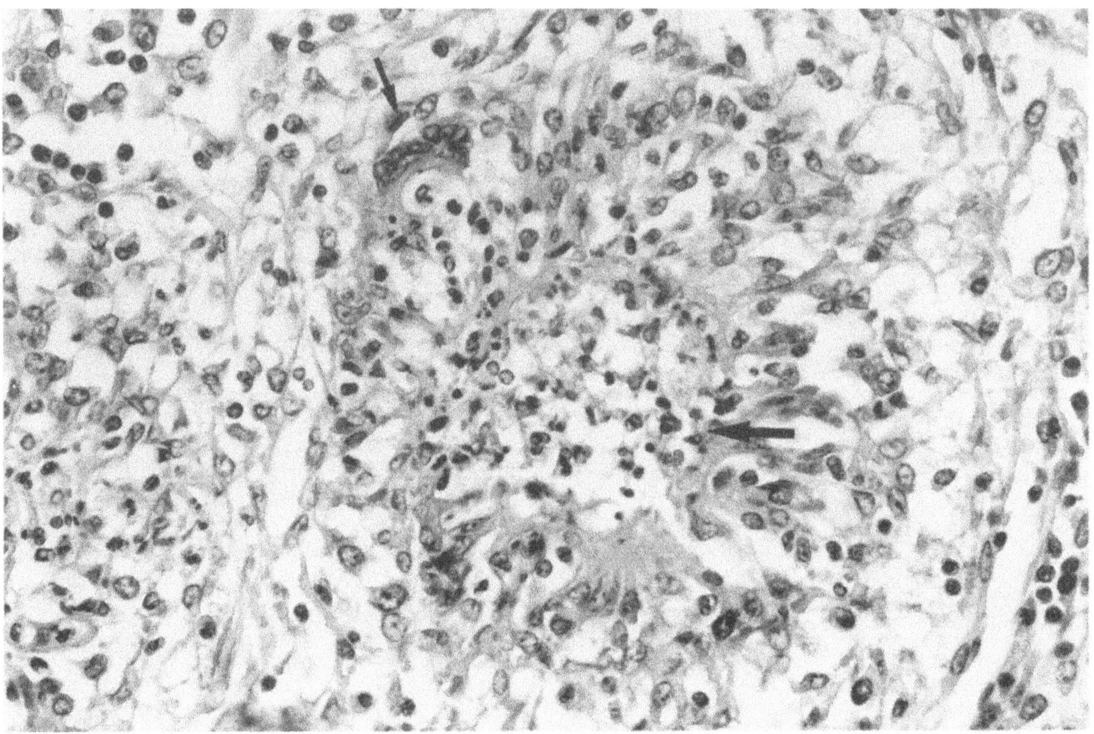

Fig. 13.6
Wegener's granulomatosis

Fresh granuloma in the lung. In the centre, remains of a vessel (*thick arrow*). Giant cells of foreign-body type (*thin arrow*; 43-year-old male)

Wegener's granulomatosis progresses biphasically: in the initial stage which can proceed for months or years as a local, restricted non-malignant disease, e.g. inflammation in ear, nose, and throat area and in the lung before the dangerous generalization stage with clinically recognizable systemic vasculitis occurs (Fig. 13.6). In more than two-thirds of the patients, in this phase, besides uncharacteristic arthalgia in about 30% of cases, arthritides without destructive tendency occur (Gross 1991).

13.2.4.2 Etiological Considerations

The etiology of Wegener's granulomatosis is still unclear. Rheumatoid factors are positive at low serum titres in over 50% of patients (Hunder and Lie 1986). ANAs are not present. The serum level of total complement and C3 is normal.

The understanding of the pathogenesis of Wegener's granulomatosis has been significantly broadened by the discovery of the anti-nucleophil cytoplasmic antibodies (ANCA). These are antibodies in the serum that are directed against parts of neutrophils and monocytes. Using immunofluorescence, two main patterns can be separated: a cytoplasmatic fluorescence (cANCA) and a perinuclear fluorescence (pANCA). cANCA are directed against proteinase 3 from neutrophils and are closely associated with Wegener's granulomatosis. pANCA are antibodies against myeloperoxidase and are mainly found in cases of microscopic polyangiitis (Hoffman and Specks 1998). Whereas in early, clinically inconspicuous stages of Wegener's granulomatosis cANCA is detected in about 50% of the patients, in the generalization phase it was found in about 98% of the patients examined (Reinhold-Keller et al. 1994). Since these cANCA are practically only found in the serum of patients with Wegener's granulomatosis and correlate in titre with the disease activity, they are valid as a marker for this disease.

ANCA

13.2.4.3 Pathology

The vasculitis, which attacks arteries as well as veins, is characterized by fibrinoid necroses with mononuclear infiltrates. The vessel walls are thickened, the vessel lumen is reduced and occluded, respectively. The elastica interna is destroyed (Fig. 13.7). The granulomata have a central necrosis, which is surrounded by fibroblasts. In between lie giant cells of foreign body type (Figs. 13.6 and 13.8).

Structural changes

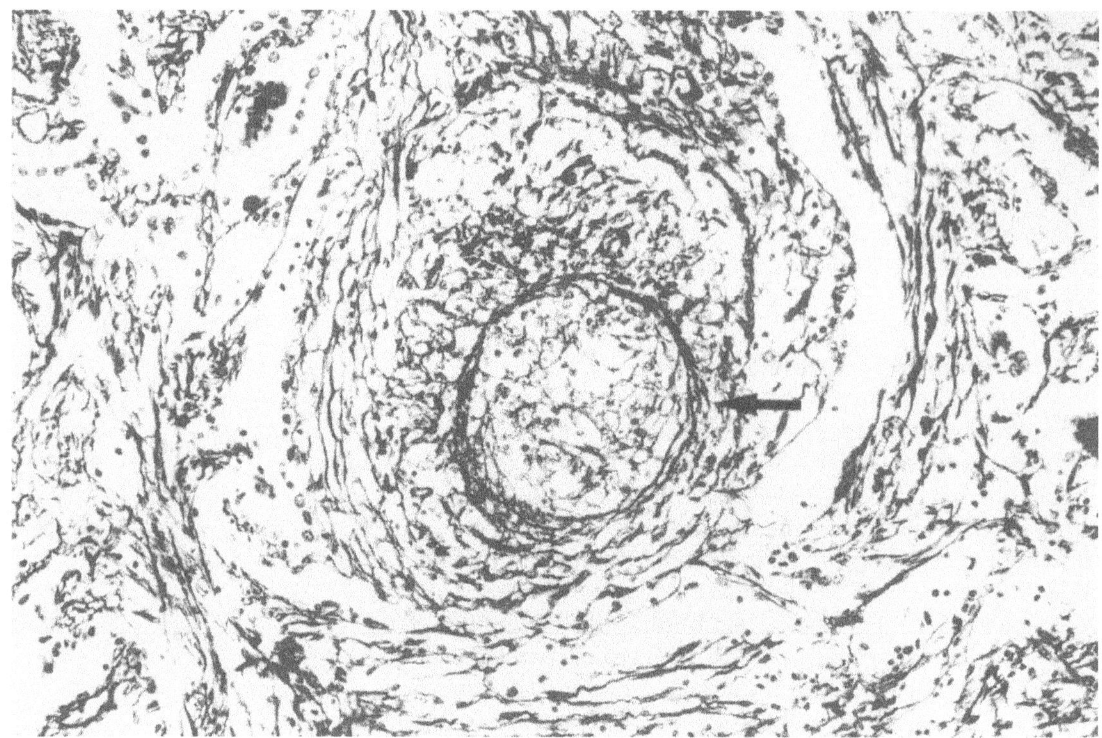

Fig. 13.7
Wegener's granulomatosis

Lung. Destroyed blood vessel (*arrow*) in the centre of a granuloma (43-year-old male)

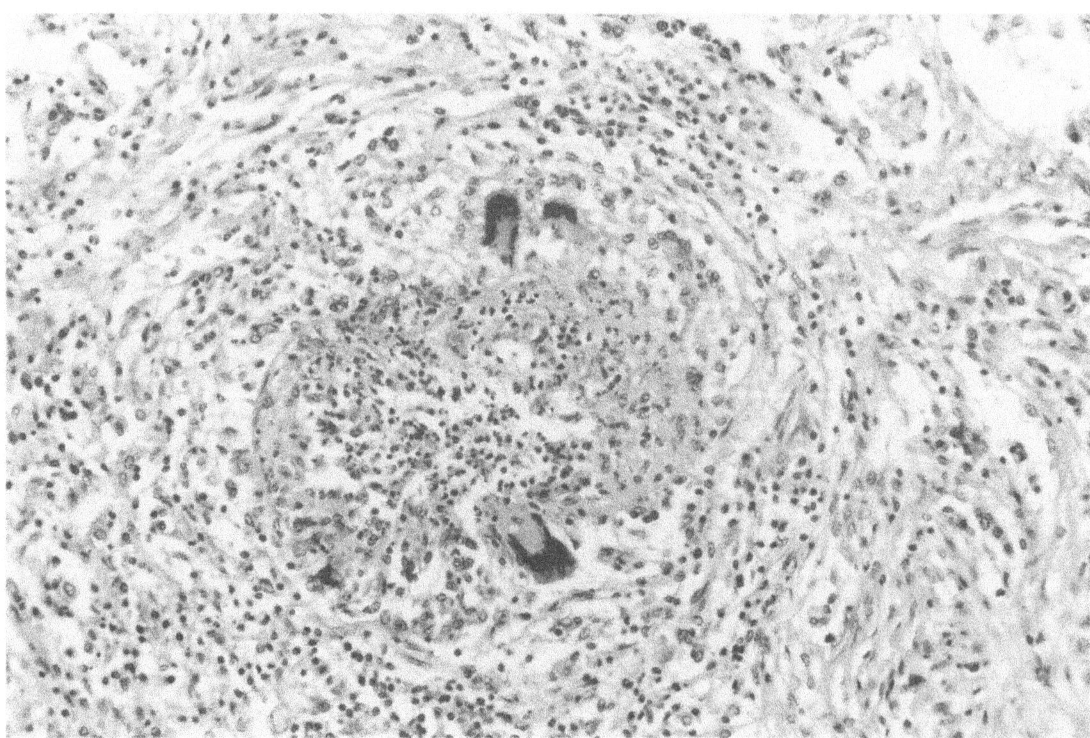

Fig. 13.8
Wegener's granulomatosis

Lung. Older granuloma with giant cells of foreign-body type. In the centre of the granuloma a necrotic artery (43-year-old male)

13.2.5 Kawasaki Disease

This disease which nearly exclusively attacks children was first described in Japan in 1967 by Kawasaki. It is defined by an arteritis involving large, medium-sized, and small arteries and is associated with mucocutaneous lymph node syndrome. Coronary arteries are frequently involved, sometimes also veins and the aorta are affected. The disease most often strikes Japanese or individuals of Asian descent. The rates of occurrence in Japan are highest in the age-groups 6–12 months and 2–3 years. The male-to-female ratio is 1.5:1.

HLA-Bs-22 was detected in most Japanese patients (Kato et al. 1978). In contrast, HLA-Bw-51 was frequently found in connection with an epidemic occurrence of this disease in the Boston area (USA; Krensky et al. 1981). A seasonal increment and the fact that the disease is sometimes occurring in epidemic form suggests that Kawasaki's disease is infectious in origin and that it strikes genetically predisposed individuals. Indications exist that house dust, either itself as an allergen or as a carrier for Rickettsia, is responsible for the disease (Fujimoto et al. 1982; Hamashima et al. 1982).

13.2.5.1 Clinical Features

Kawasaki disease begins very acutely with fever, coronary symptoms, conjunctivitis, "strawberry tongue", redness of the nose-throat area as well as diffuse swellings of hands and feet and development of erythema on hand and foot surfaces. The process is accompanied by swelling of the cervical lymph nodes. Arthralgias and non-destructive synovitides can frequently occur. After 7–12 days, this acute phase is followed by a subacute stage, characterized by irritability, anorexia, conjunctival injection, and myocardial dysfunction, approximately another 25 days later, convalescence begins. The elevated ESR, however, does not return to normal before approximately 70 days after the onset of the disease. In 25% of untreated patients, permanent myocardial damage may remain.

Epidemiological data and the clinical course suggest that Kawasaki disease is triggered by bacterial toxins and in that comparable to the "toxic shock syndrome", in which T cells can be activated by contact with superantigens. Bacterial toxins activate a great number of T cells without having to attach to the T cell specific HLA-II antigen complex (Leung et al. 1998).

13.2.5.2 Pathology

Structural changes

This relatively benign disease profile can, however, be complicated by necrotizing arteritides of the coronary arteries but also of the aorta and its main branches as well as the pulmonary arteries. Thus, it concerns a panarteritis in which the vessel wall is infiltrated by neutrophils and mononuclear cells whereby pictures arise which correspond to PAN in young individuals. The

wall destruction can lead to the formation of protrusions. The disease can progress fatally in 1%–2% of children by thrombosing of these aneurysms and occlusion of the coronary arteries (Conn and Hunder 1985).
In patients who have died from Kawasaki disease, vasculitis is found in small and medium-sized vessels, particularly in the coronary arteries. An activation of the endothelium can be proven and an infiltration consisting of macrophages and CD4+ and CD8+ T cells.

13.2.6 Takayasu Arteritis

Synonym: aortic arch arteritis.

13.2.6.1 Clinical and Immunological Features

Takayasu arteritis is a chronically progressive granulomatous disease of large vessels first described in Japan (Nasu 1975), but also frequently occurring in Mexico and India (Hunder and Lie 1986). Mainly girls and young females aged between 10 and 30 years are affected. The disease process has a predilection for the aortic arch and the branching vessels.
The etiology of Takayasu arteritis is still unknown today. Raised γ-globulin levels and the finding of anti-aorta antibodies in the serum of some patients (Ueda et al. 1971) suggest an autoimmune disease. The inflammatory process can attack the aorta and its branches either continuously or patchily, as well as infringe upon the coronary ostia and the aortic valve. Several months before arterial insufficiency caused by arterial narrowing develops, slight fever, arthralgias or mildly progressing arthritides frequently occur. Later, in most patients, weakened or sometimes absent pulses are confirmed in the extremities (pulseless phase).

13.2.6.2 Pathology

Structural changes

Granulating inflammation is found microscopically in the adventitia and media. The inflammatory process is characterized by an unusually dense infiltration of lymphocytes, plasma cells, and histiocytes (Fig. 13.9). In between only a few neutrophils and sporadic giant cells are found. This lympho-plasmacytic character differentiates the Takayasu arteritis from other systemic vasculitides, and suggests a cell-mediated immune mechanism for this disease. The immune process can destroy the musculo-elastic media of the large vessels and thus lead to aneurysmatic widening. After waning the process leaves behind a fibrotic scar on the vessel wall. In smaller vessels, a narrowing or even an obliteration of the vessel lumen can result.

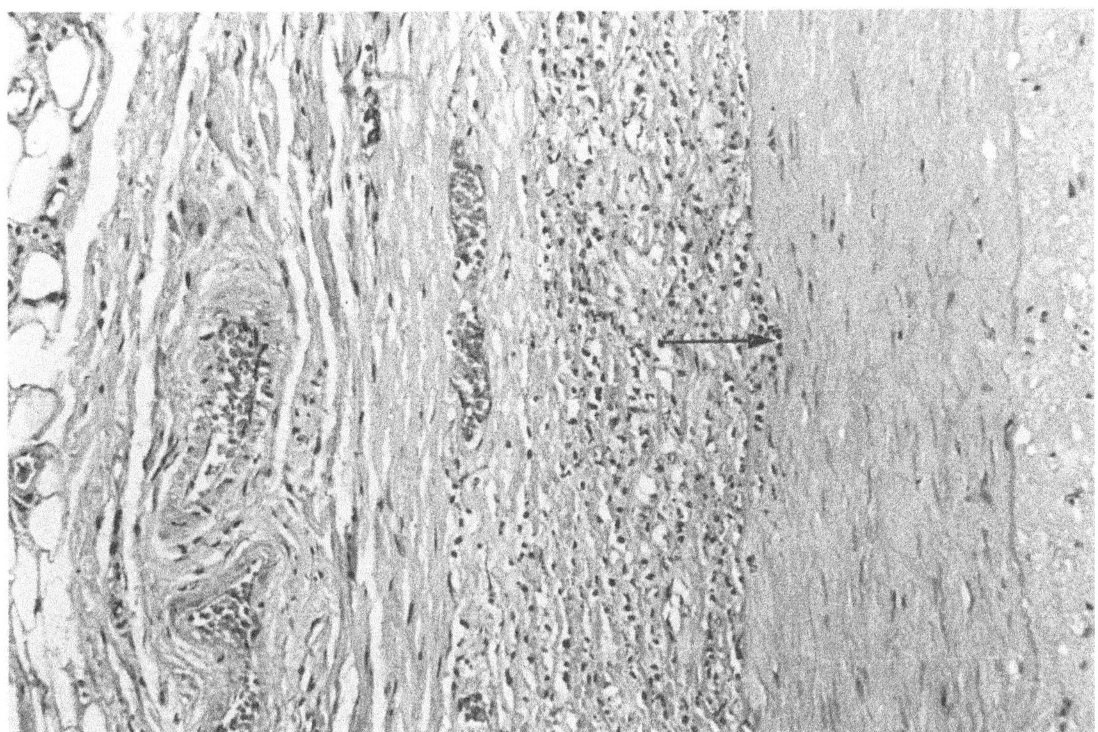

Carotid furca of the subclavian artery. Late alterations. Broad scar tissue with lymphocytes, plasma cells, and macrophages with spreading into the media (*arrow*). (Courtesy of J. Bohl, Department of Neuropathology, University of Mainz)

Fig. 13.9
Takayasu arteritis

14 Idiopathic Inflammatory Myopathies

14.1 Definition

We recognize today two main diseases of the skeletal musculature which have an autoimmune causation. Myasthenia gravis is characterized by a reversible fatigue of the musculature; its etiology is concerned with the formation of antibodies to acetylcholine receptors. This non-inflammatory process is in contrast to a heterogenous group of diseases which are included in the term "idiopathic inflammatory myopathies" (IIM). These are dermatomyositis (DM), polymyositis (PM), and inclusion body myositis (IBM). Clinically, they are all characterized by muscle weakness, histologically by inflammatory reactions in the muscle.

Leading clinical symptom: muscle weakness

14.2 Epidemiology

All three together have an incidence of 1:100,000 (Medsger et al. 1979; Banker and Engel 1986). DM is an illness of children as well as adults, and of women more frequently than men. PM develops mainly after the 20th year of age, IBM mainly after the 50th year of age, and of the latter, men are three times more frequently affected than women. All three forms are characterized by a predominantly proximal, often symmetrical muscle weakness (Dalakas 1991). A seasonal increment in frequency and the IIM's occurrence after infections indicate the significance of external factors influencing the development of myositides. The association of IIM with certain alleles of HLA-DRB1 and HLA-DQA1 as well as the familial occurrence suggest a genetic connection (Rider et al. 1998).

Genetic connection

14.3 Dermatomyositis

DM is well defined by a combination of characteristic skin rash and muscular weakness, the rash, however, sometimes may precede the muscle weakness. The skin changes affect face and upper body including the neck, chest, elbows, and the skin over the knuckle joints. Dilated capillary loops in the nail fold are characteristic and, particularly in children, the skin changes can calcify and ulcerate. In combination with progressive systemic sclerosis (PSS), DM can occur in the context of a "mixed connective tissue disease" (MCTD). Poisoning with impure tryptophan can give rise to a fasciitis with skin changes similar to DM. The muscle weakness may be accompanied by a considerable increase in serum creatine kinase (CK) as well as lactate dehydrogenase (LDH), aldolase, and glutamate oxalacetate transaminase (GOT).

Bioptic findings

A muscle biopsy is essential for the diagnosis. Sparse perivascular lymphocytes are found in the interfascicular septa of the perimysium (Fig. 14.1). Lymphocytes also occur rarely in the fasciculi themselves. Neutrophils are not observed! Endothelial hyperplasia of the intrafascicular blood vessels (Fig. 14.2) and fibrin thrombi cause microinfarcts marked by degeneration, necrosis, and regeneration of the muscle fibres, which lie in connected groups at the margin of the fascicles. This focal fascicular fibre degeneration was observed in 90% of children and 50% of adults with DM (Banker and Engel 1986; Carpenter 1988).

14.4 Polymyositis

PM develops within weeks and months. It occurs predominantly in adults and rarely in children. PM, previously rare, is today frequently seen in HIV-infected patients.

As PM lacks the impressive symptoms of DM, it must be differentiated from a range of diseases which may also present the somewhat non-characteristic symptom of "muscle weakness". Here, too, muscle biopsy plays a decisive role for the differential diagnosis against neuromuscular diseases. In contrast to DM, lymphocytes are found in the endomysium within the fascicle without recognizable relation to the scattered degenerated or necrotic muscle fibres (Figs. 14.3, 14.4). The blood vessels are unchanged.

14.5 Inclusion Body Myositis

The third myositic syndrome occurs three times more in men than in women. Muscle weakness is evident early in both distal and proximal regions of the extremities with possible involvement of the extensors of the foot and flexors of the fingers, and additionally the quadriceps, iliosopas, triceps, and biceps muscles. The diagnostic decision depends on biopsy findings: the histological picture resembles that of PM with a lymphocytic infiltration within the endomysium but above all the disease is characterized by the presence of the name giving inclusion bodies. These consist of basophilic granular inclusions distributed around the margins of slit-like vacuoles (rimmed vacuoles; Figs. 14.5, 14.6; Carpenter et al. 1978; Eisen et al. 1983; Lotz et al. 1989). With higher magnification, the vacuoles appear to contain granular material. Electron-microscopy shows membranous whirls in the granula.

Bioptic findings

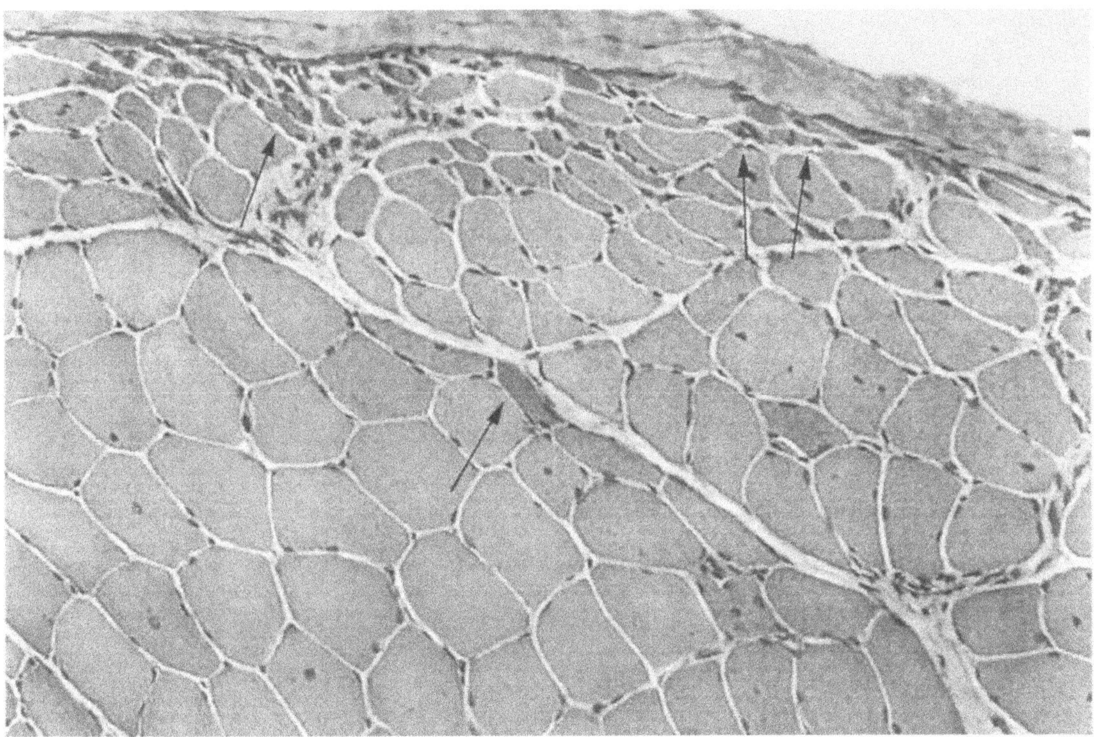

Perifascicular atrophy of muscle fibres (*arrows*), perivascular and endomysial lymphocytic infiltrates. (Electron micrograph, courtesy of J. Bohl, Department of Neuropathology, University of Mainz, Germany)

Fig. 14.1
Dermatomyositis

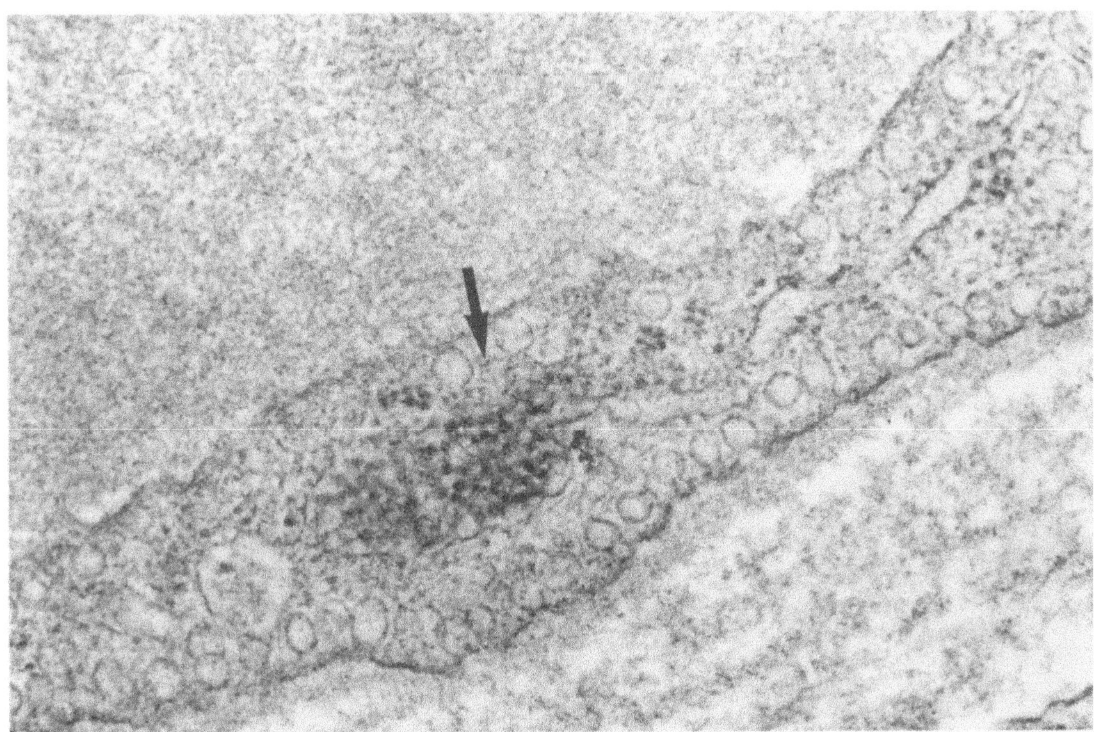

Endothelial cell containing undulating tubules (*arrow*, 1:60,500). (Electron micrograph, Courtesy of H.H. Goebel, Department of Neuropathology, University of Mainz, Germany)

Fig. 14.2
Dermatomyositis

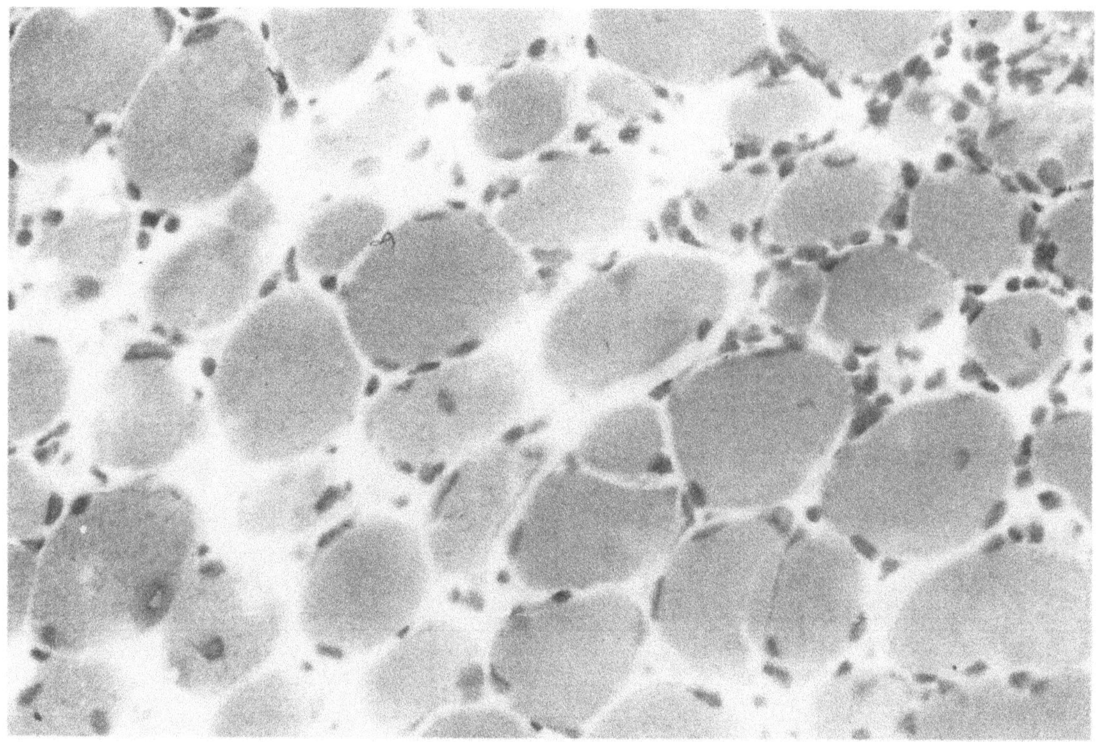

Fig. 14.3
Polymyositis

Interstitial lymphocytic infiltration amongst rounded muscle fibres (1:472). (Electron micrograph, courtesy of H.H. Goebel, Department of Neuropathology, University of Mainz, Germany)

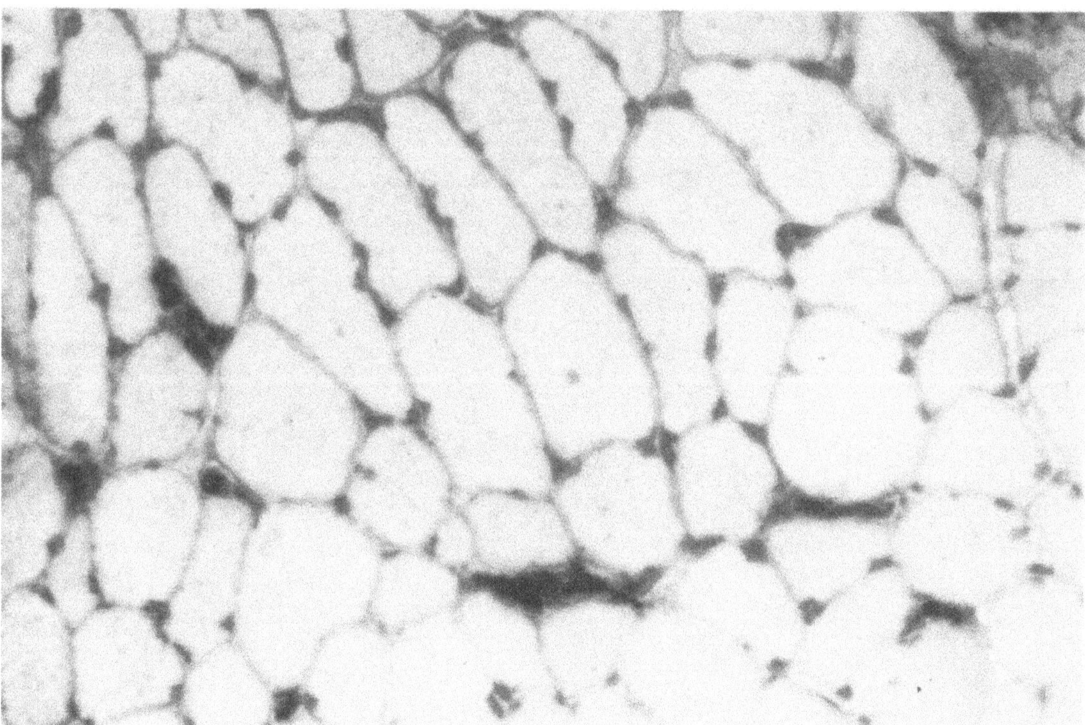

Fig. 14.4
Polymyositis

Expression of MHCI on the surface of muscle fibres (1:568). (Courtesy of H.H. Goebel, Department of Neuropathology, University of Mainz, Germany)

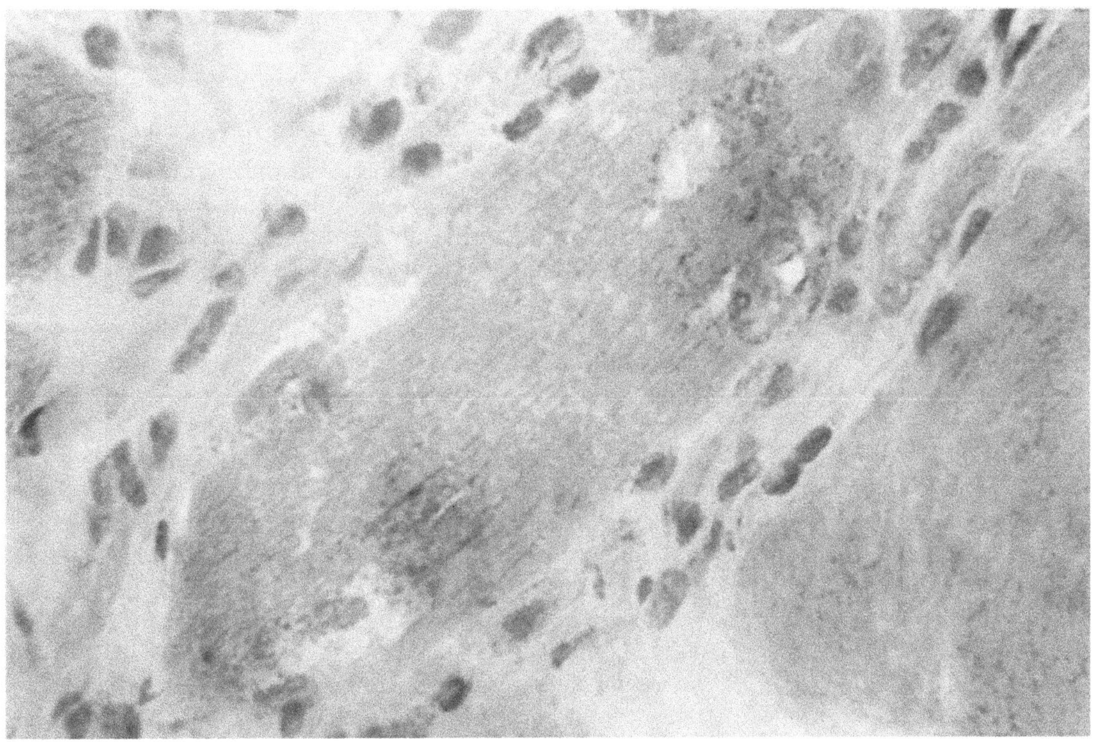

Partly "rimmed" vacuoles in muscle fibres (1:880). (Electron micrograph, courtesy of H.H. Goebel, Department of Neuropathology, University of Mainz, Germany)

Fig. 14.5
Inclusion body myositis

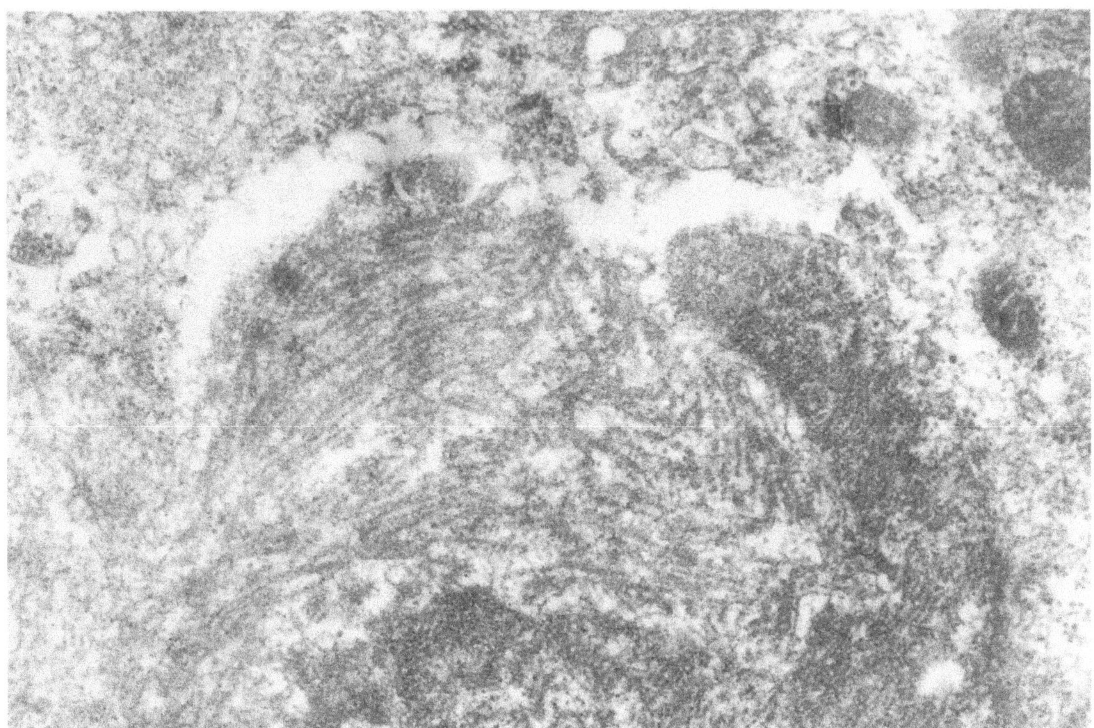

Inclusion body with aggregate of tubule filaments (1:54,000). (Electron micrograph, courtesy of H.H. Goebel, Department of Neuropathology, University of Mainz, Germany)

Fig. 14.6
Inclusion body myositis

Filamentous inclusions in the cytoplasm in the surrounding area of the rimmed vacuoles are pathognomonic for inclusion body myositis. The presence of several rimmed vacuoles and of more than one group of atrophic fibres as well as lymphocytic infiltrates in the endomysium denotes filamentous inclusions in the ultrastructure in more than 90% of cases (Lotz et al. 1989). It is, however, important to remember that paraffin embedding of the biopsy material releases the basophil granules so that an inclusion body myositis may be overlooked.

Pathogenetic considerations

If one considers the morphological changes of the musculature in the three IIM from the standpoint of the pathologist, it is difficult to classify these phenomena in the generally accepted concept of inflammation. Although elements of the complement cascade, i.e. the membranolytic attack complex C5b-9, can be identified, there are no indications of an inflammatory exudate, such as plasma exudation, fibrin polymerization or migration of neutrophils. Rather, the morphological substrate of IIM is limited to scanty lymphocyte infiltrates and muscle fibre degeneration. But lymphocyte infiltrates alone do not indicate an inflammation. They belong as is well known to the manifestations of the cellular immune process. This corresponds to the fact that the healthy non-necrotic muscle fibres are surrounded by CD8+ cells and macrophages which penetrate and, thus, destroy the fibres. As cytotoxic T cells can recognize antigens if these are presented together with the MHC-I antigen, it is possible that in PM and inclusion body myositis, the primary immunopathological mechanism is mediated by cytotoxic T cells and remains limited to cells, expressing the HLA-I antigen. In DM, however, the cell infiltrates contain a higher percentage of B cells and an increased ratio of T-helper cells (CD4+) to suppressor and cytotoxic T cells (CD8+). T-helper cells are found in the vicinity of B cells and macrophages. These findings are evidence for a humoral-immunologically mediated process, which in DM is directed primarily against the intramuscular vascular system (Arahata and Engel 1984; Banker and Engel 1986; Engel and Arahata 1986; Ringel et al. 1986; Engel and Emslie-Smith 1989). It is conceivable that antibodies that bind to components of the microvasculature trigger the complement cascade, which then induces lysis via the C5b-9 complex. Autoantibodies are produced in 60–80% of PM and DM cases. Some are myositis-specific antibodies directed against different aminoacyl-tRNA synthetases. These are immunologically diverse proteins differing in primary structure. The role of autoantibodies in the pathogenesis of the IIM is still largely unclear. In DM, immunoglobulins are found deposited in vessel walls, therefore, it seems most likely that autoantibodies are implicated in this disease (Plotz et al. 1995). The accepted immunopathogenesis of IIM corresponds also to the therapy with high dosage prednisone and immunosuppressives instead of a conventional antiphlogistic therapy which is suggested by the suffix "-itis".

15 Fibromyalgia Syndrome*

Among the rheumatic diseases, the painful conditions in the soft tissues are most frequent. They are of importance because of their chronicity and painful derangement of the general condition which can eventually restrict the working ability of the patients. The complaints about pain in the trunk or limbs do not, however, provide a physical or radiological diagnosis.

First description of "fibrositis"

In 1904, in a study of lumbago, Gowers introduced the term "fibrositis" for ailments of this type, making the obvious assumption that the inflammation occurring in the soft tissues is responsible for the painful phenomena. In 1920, Stockmann defined "fibrositis" as a state of chronic inflammation of the fascia, muscles, nerves, ligaments, tendons, periosteum, and subcutis which can affect all parts of the body, causing pain, tension, and stiffness.

Muscle conditions in rheumatic fever

In 1933, in his fundamental pathological studies of the rheumatic diseases, Klinge detected fibrinoid swellings and granulomata of the Aschoff type in skeletal musculature and in tendons which were interpreted as "soft-tissue rheumatism". These tissues were, however, removed post-mortem from patients who had died of rheumatic fever (RF). There was no correlation between the morphological findings and the clinical ailments. Thus, nowadays, these changes no longer belong in the category "soft-tissue rheumatism".

A more precise description of the vague term "soft-tissue rheumatism" was afforded by the designation fibromyalgia, whereby the disease is defined by the subjective syndrome ("algos" = pain).

ACR definition of fibromyalgia

In 1990, the American College of Rheumatology (ACR) defined fibromyalgia as a form of non-articular rheumatism characterized by widespread musculoskeletal aching and tenderness on palpation at characteristic sites called tender points (Wolfe et al. 1990). Characteristic for this pain syndrome is an increased sensitivity at certain points in the muscle or tendons. The focus of the pain is the musculature of the trunk. Fatigue, stiffness, and sleep disturbance often are accompanying symptoms. In connection with this, it is important to eliminate an underlying local pathological process such as bursitis or enthesopathy.

Unfortunately, the term "fibrositis" is still in use today and contributes towards preserving the historical error of Gowers and Stockmann. The description "fibrositis" still prejudges an inflammatory nature of the soft tissue conditions which, although phenomenologically plausible, is faulted by the lack of clinical signs of inflammation.

**Synonym:* fibrositis

Although fibromyalgia is no life-threatening syndrome and although it is open to debate whether it is to be classified as an actual disease, it is eminently relevant from an economic point of view. This is due to its high prevalence which is 0.8% in Finland, above 2.0% in the United States, and even 10.5% in Norway (Kennedy and Felson 1996). The fibromyalgia syndrome (FMS) predominantly affects women; the female-to-male ratio is 3.4% to 0.5% in the United States. Prevalence increases with age, in women between 60 and 79 years of age it increases to 7% (Wolfe et al. 1995). Especially in older patients, it is frequently difficult to differentiate FMS from rheumatoid arthritis (RA) or polymyalgia rheumatica (PMR). In these cases, muscle biopsies alone are of no certain diagnostic value, they can only help to rule out an inflammatory muscle disease (Urrows et al. 1994).

In blatant contrast to the enormous importance of fibromyalgia is the knowledge of its mechanisms and morphological changes.

Idiopathic pain phenomena

If looked at from today's viewpoint, fibromyalgia is, in the narrow sense, an idiopathic pain phenomenon with no connection to a superimposed basic disease, and without clinical and serological signs of inflammation.

The less than satisfying knowledge concerning pathogenesis and etiology makes the FMS an object of inter-disciplinary efforts of research by, among others, neurologists, psychologists, neuroendocrinologists, and virologists (Leventhal et al. 1991; Wortmann 1994; Pillemer et al. 1997; Wolfe et al. 1997; Martinez-Lavin et al. 1998; McBeth et al. 1999).

Tissue structures in fibromyalgia

In consideration of the pathomechanism of fibromyalgia it has to be taken into account that two completely different tissue structures are involved in this syndrome: the skeletal musculature and the collagenous tendon and capsule tissue. In the case of skeletal musculature it involves a parenchymatous assemblage of muscle cells. These muscle cells work actively and have a high oxygen requirement. The blood vessel network is therefore highly developed. On the other hand, the tendon and capsule tissue comprises a mature, rigid, bradytrophic network of collagen fibres with few fibrocytes. The low oxygen requirement of these sparse cells is in accordance with scanty vascularization. In contemplating these contrary anatomical structures, a completely different mechanism might be expected as the basis of fibromyalgia. Of greatest quantitative and qualitative importance are the pain phenomena in the region of the skeletal musculature. Hénriksson and coworkers (1982) as well as Bartels and Danneskiold-Samsoe (1986) attribute to their morphological findings a certain significance for diagnosing FMS. The most consistent and characteristic microscopic finding in the study of Hénriksson was the even distribution of moth-eaten fibres over the whole cross-section in muscles from painful tender areas. Electronmicroscopy of five specimens revealed mitochondrial abnormalities, myofibrillar *Z*-streaming, and cytoplasmic bodies. Adenosine triphosphate (ATP) and phosphocreatine were much reduced in the patients with fibromyalgia, lactate values were normal, but glycogen concentrations below normal.

Electron-microscopical examination of fibromyalgia muscle by Bartels and Danneskiold-Samsœ showed muscle fibres connected by a network of reticular or elastic fibres which are absent in normal muscle and which may be the cause of the disorder (1986).

In their light-microscopic studies of biopsies taken from the musculus trapezius of patients suffering from FMS, Bengtsson et al. (1986) found in 35 out of 41 biopsies moth-eaten fibres, these, however, were also found in the biopsies of 9 (out of 10) controls. Frequency of type I and type II fibres and the area of muscle fibres were the same in patients as in controls, capillary density too. Apart from degenerated and regenerated fibres, Bengtsson and coworkers also mention "inflammatory infiltrates". As this finding is unusual, and as it has been observed neither by other authors nor by us, it seems unlikely that they studied samples of patients suffering from ordinary FMS.

In order to elucidate the justification of the designation "fibrositis", we first attempted in 1973 to answer the question as to whether it has an inflammatory basis or whether it involves a purely functional, neurally-induced phenomenon. Using light- and electron-microscopical techniques, we studied numerous biopsies from patients who showed the clinical picture of fibromyalgia. The tissue was taken unequivocally from painful sites of the m. trapezius and m. deltoideus.

However, by light-microscopy we could never detect the slightest histological change which could provide an explanation for the painful symptoms. In particular, no traces of an acute or preexisting inflammation were found. Even in biopsies from focal, palpable, painful tender points we saw no pathological evidence by light-microscopy. These negative findings allowed us, however, to make the definite statement that in these patients the pain could not have been caused by any inflammatory muscle processes (Fassbender and Wegner 1973). This opinion was supported also by Yunus and coworkers (1981). We have therefore rejected the designation "fibrositis" since it can lead to false therapeutic consequences.

From 11 patients aged between 29 and 65 years with clinically defined FMS we studied electron-microscopically muscle biopsies taken from tender points in areas of the m. trapezius and m. deltoideus (and, as a control, from other non-painful muscle sections). Moreover, tissue was taken from four patients without FMS and studied in the same way (Fassbender and Wegner 1973). In all 11 cases, we found unequivocal ultrastructural changes in the tissue taken from the tender points. On the other hand, control biopsies from the non-painful muscle sections of the same patients and from the musculature of healthy individuals showed the regular ultrastructure of skeletal musculature.

EM findings

The electron-microscopical studies resulted in the following findings:

Whilst the skeletal musculature from the non-painful sections from patients with FMS and from healthy controls showed the regular structure of skeletal musculature with regular transverse striations, twinning arrangement of the mitochondria on either side of the *Z*-line, numerous triads, and normal glycogen content

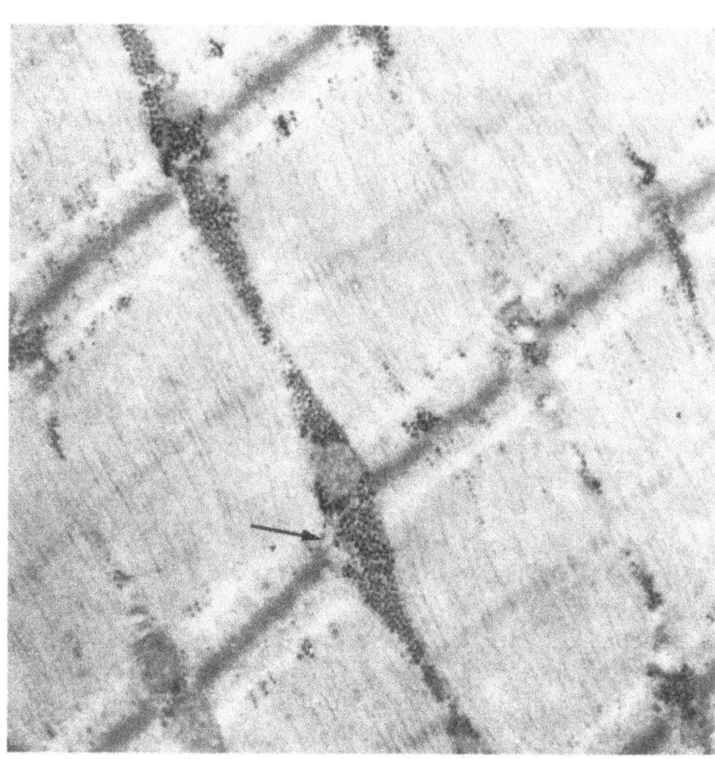

Fig. 15.1
Fibromyalgia syndrome

Normal muscle fibre in a state of contraction. Regular striations. Pairs of mitochondria are arranged along either side of the *Z*-line. Normal content of glycogen (*arrow*). Many triads. (Electron micrograph, 1:38,000)

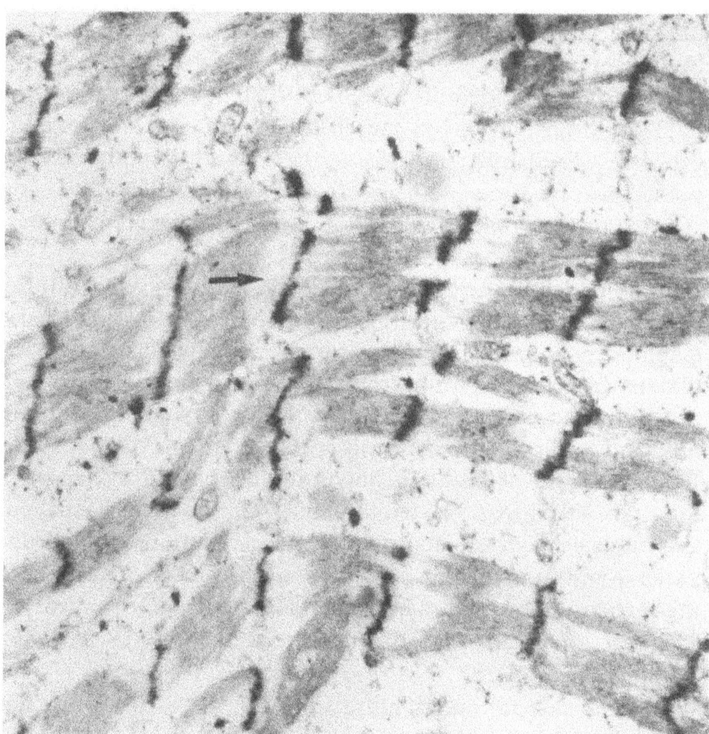

Fig. 15.2
Fibromyalgia syndrome

Segment of muscle fibre. "Moth-eaten" myofilaments in the *I*-band region (*arrow*). The intervening light zones correspond to myofibrils which have undergone dissolution (66-year-old female with "muscular rheumatism"). (Electron micrograph, 1:18,000)

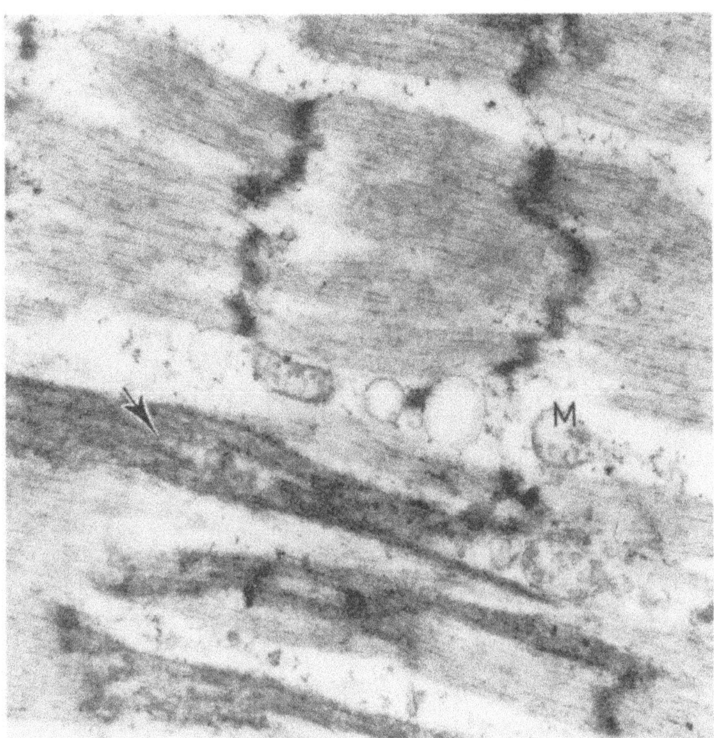

Fig. 15.3
Fibromyalgia syndrome

Segment of muscle fibre. Myofilaments in the *I*-band zone have been destroyed. The black lines (*arrow*) represent condensation of myofilaments. Some contractile material remains between the fibrils. Mitochondria (*M*) in various states of degeneration (66-year-old female with "muscular rheumatism"). (Electron micrograph, 1:38,000)

(Fig. 15.1), in the skeletal muscle which was taken from the tender points we saw all stages of parenchymal destruction. With respect to the level of destruction we defined the following stages:

Stage I

Swelling of the mitochondria and moth-eaten-like damage of the myofilaments in the region of *I*-band (Fig. 15.2).

Stage II

Myofilament destruction in the region of *I*-band and isolated myofilament condensation. The *Z*-bands still remain. One sees large areas in which the regular structure of the sarcomeres is completely abolished.

Stage III

Extensive condensation of the myofilaments and expansive clumping of the contractile elements (Fig. 15.3).

Stage IV

Complete disintegration of the contractile elements, particularly near the sarcolemma. Only finely granular material remains (Fig. 15.4). The fact that we found huge glycogen stores in the area of these muscle necroses suggests a disturbance in energy uti-

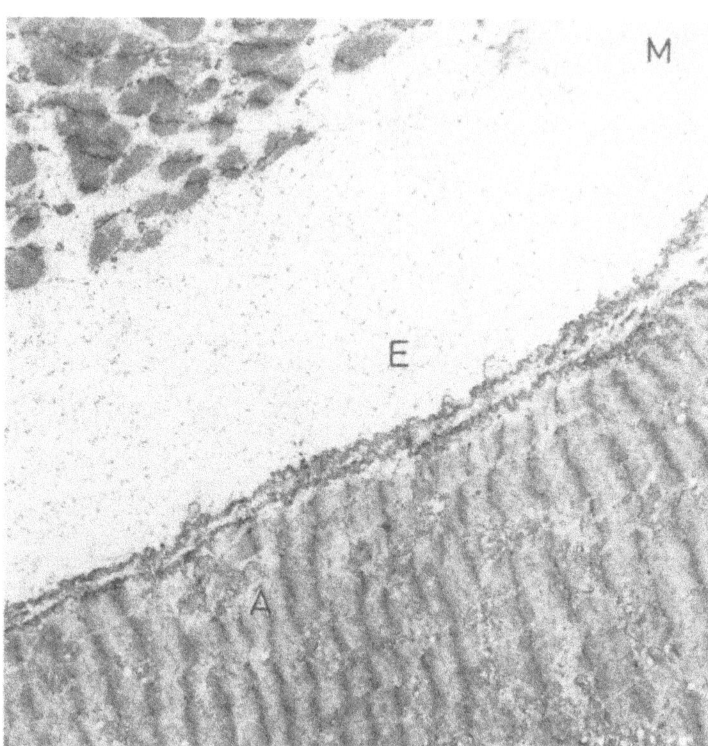

Fig. 15.4
Fibromyalgia syndrome

Segment of muscle fibre. The lower tangentially placed muscle cell only shows swelling of a few mitochondria. The upper cell shows a broad light border of fine granules. These represent remnants of necrotic myofilaments. At the *top* of the figure, there are partly intact myofibrils (47-year-old male with "muscular rheumatism"). (Electron micrograph, 1:7200)

lization. In 6 of 11 cases, we also saw striking changes in the muscle capillaries: the endothelial cells were swollen as a manifestation of acute damage. At the same time, secondary lysosomes appeared and, in single cases, the organelles were so increased that the capillary lumen was narrowed by the curvature of the endothelial cells.

The electron-microscopical findings correspond to various grades of degradation of the contractile elements of the skeletal musculature which, in certain cases, might be found together in the area of a single tender point. At the beginning, there is subtle destruction of single myofilaments and, at the end, complete disintegration of whole muscle fibres. The electron-microscopic picture also in no way shows any relation to an inflammatory process. An existing or pre-existing inflammatory mechanism can definitely be excluded by light- as well as by electron-microscopy. Much more in accordance with the observations are the moth-eaten-like disintegrations in the region of *I*-band as they can be produced in animal experiments by lack of oxygen (Büchner 1975). Subsequently, step-wise destruction occurs. Obviously, these electron-microscopical findings are not "specific" for fibromyalgia. They signal only a lack of oxygen within the scope of local hypoxia and are, thus, a signpost for an explanation of the pathogenesis.

Our hypothesis of local hypoxia as the cause of parenchymal destruction in the tender point foci has been confirmed by the studies of Brückle and coworkers (1990). In these studies, the partial pressure of oxygen (pO_2) in the lumbar musculature of 20 patients with tendomyopathy and 10 healthy subjects was measured with fine-needle polarographic probes. The mean pO_2 value of the healthy subjects was 34.6 mmHg. In the region of the tensed musculature of patients with FMS, the mean pO_2 value was increased to 44.4 mmHg. In the tender points, however, pO_2 was reduced down to 3 mmHg below the minimum for existence of the muscle fibres. This high-grade hypoxia probably also causes the local painfulness. Since the tonus of the muscle fibre in a tender point is increased several fold with respect to other musculature, it causes a higher oxygen consumption in these foci. A disparity thereby arises between the oxygen supply and demand. This „relative hypoxia“ (Fassbender and Wegner 1973) with a reduction of the oxygen partial pressure to one-tenth of normal is lethal for the highly active muscle cell. This gives an explanation for the decline of the myofilaments. The fact that pO_2 is increased in the other parts of the muscle that are not focally contracted but are rather wide-spreadly tensed, is explained by Brückle and coworkers (1990) as being due to an overcompensating active hyperaemia.

Local hypoxia

If one considers a muscle process within the scope of fibromyalgia under the aspect of the pathologically increased muscle tonus, the following consequences result:

Pathogenetical concept

1. The muscle tension means permanent and augmented work and therewith an increased oxygen requirement of the muscle cells.
2. In the region of the wide-spread muscle tension the organism responds to the increased requirement of oxygen with a reactive hyperaemia and hyperoxia.
3. In the case of tender points, in contrast, an excessive contraction in a focal muscle area takes place. The relative hypoxia which thus occurs leads to focal filament damage. The oxygen supply is further reduced via a disturbance of the microcirculation. The hypoxia, which can be detected with a fine-needle probe, lies below the minimum for survival of the parenchymatous muscle cells.

The observation that even under anaesthetisia no relaxation of these components occurs suggests that the process escapes neural control and has become independent. The cellular destruction causes further disturbance in the endothelial region, as observed by us. It is understandable that the painful tension experienced by the patients leads to a persisting vicious circle via a possible psychological fixation. Roy and Gutmann (1988) also viewed the reactive hypertonic hypoxia as the source of the muscle pain.
The minimal ultrastructural changes are unimportant for the function of the muscle.
The basic mechanism of the muscle process in the context of fibromyalgia is, thus, the pathological tension of certain muscle components. The reason for the pathological muscle tonus is, in

all cases, a neural disregulation. This can be triggered by various causes as, for example, cold or structural and functional misposture of the spinal column. Physical factors can also induce this mechanism, particularly in the region of the dorsal or neck musculature. Wolfe (1988) distinguishes between a "primary" form of fibrositis (fibromyalgia) and a "secondary" form which might be an accompanying phenomenon in RA and osteoarthritis (OA). This distinction is, however, dismissed by Smythe and Sheon (1990) as being unfounded since physiological examination failed to recognize any differences. The fact that only the surface muscle components are accessible for clinical and bioptical examination should not exclude the possibility that the deep autochthonous dorsal musculature between the spinal and transverse vertebral processes, as well as the deep neck musculature, might also participate in the myalgic pain symptoms. It would, of course, be difficult to understand if the pathological neural hypertonus was confined just to the surface muscle components.

Studies by Klein and coworkers (1992) indicate an association between FMS and disturbances of the serotonin metabolism. Accordingly, 74% of the patients with FMS have detectable antibodies against serotonin and gangliosides which are not observed in other rheumatic diseases. However, the pathogenetic significance of these antibodies remains to be established.

Tendon and capsule tissue

In contrast to the skeletal musculature, the pain phenomena in the insertion area of tendons and capsules has a substrate which can be observed by light-microscopy. In these tissue components, highly proliferative fibroblasts can sometimes be detected. The collagen fibres disappear (Fassbender and Wegner 1973) and, at the same time, no indication of inflammation is apparent. These changes are reactions of the tissue to mechanical or age-related degeneration processes in a practically cell-free, fibre-rich, primarily poorly vascularized bradytrophic tissue.

It thus has to be considered that the term "fibromyalgia", first, includes pain phenomena in completely different structures and, second, is functionally and neurally induced in the skeletal musculature, but arises under local influences in the tendon and capsule tissues, too.

Therapeutic consequences

The fact that morphological changes can be seen in fibromyalgia whereas inflammatory phenomena can be detected neither in the skeletal musculature nor in the tendon and capsule tissues, has the following consequences:

1. Further use of the term "fibrositis" is no longer justified since it could lead to non-indicated and unefficacious anti-phlogistic therapy. Unfortunately, however, this misleading designation has still not been expelled from common usage in current literature.
2. The described changes give a good starting point for physical and, possibly also, psychotherapeutic intervention.

16 Osteoarthritis*

16.1 Nomenclature

In 1913, the term "arthrosis" was coined by the German physician Friedrich von Müller based on observations of anatomical changes seen in cadaver joints. In doing so, he sought to distinguish primary degenerative processes of the joint, as they were regarded at that time, from primary inflammatory arthritides with secondary degenerative changes. The term "osteoarthrosis" takes into account the accompanying changes in the adjacent bone structure and currently is widely used in Europe.
"Osteoarthritis" (OA) is the term used in the Anglo-American literature, encompassing clinical symptoms by integrating the inflammatory episodes during the disease processes, which cause the patient with an arthritic joint to consult the physician. The term "osteoarthrosis" thus is based on morphological-pathogenetic findings, while the name "osteoarthritis" refers to the overall clinical-phenomenological features.

16.2 Definition

Contrary to rheumatoid arthritis (RA), which is a systemic disease with predilection for the joints, OA may run an asymptomatic course for many years and is exclusively characterized by the pathological changes at one or more joints. "It is a dynamic but slowly progressive, non-inflammatory degenerative disease of cartilages and other tissues of joints, primarily in older individuals with intermittent, inflammatory episodes" (Mankin et al. 1985). Sometimes the cartilage may be mechanically eroded down to the bone inducing pain which is not necessarily coupled with inflammation. It is only with the onset of a secondary synovitis that OA becomes apparent. To summarize: Synovitis transforms the arthrotic into an arthritic process.

Asymptomatic course

**Synonym:* osteoarthrosis

FDA and WHO definition

At an international workshop in 1994 in the United States, an interdisciplinary group of 75 leading clinicians and scientists [including representatives from the Food and Drug Administration (FDA) and the World Health Organization (WHO)] assembled to define the present knowledge on the etiopathogenesis of OA: "Osteoarthritis is a group of overlapping distinct diseases, which may have different etiologies but with similar biologic, morphologic, and clinical outcomes. The disease processes not only affect the articular cartilage, but involve the entire joint, including the subchondral bone, ligaments, capsule, synovial membrane, and periarticular muscles. Ultimately, the articular cartilage degenerates with fibrillation, fissures, ulceration, and full thickness loss of the joint surface" (Kuettner and Goldberg 1995).

16.3 Epidemiology

Large national studies

Epidemiological studies of Wagenhäuser (1969) form a good basis for the classification of OA. According to his studies of the Swiss population, 50% of those over 30 years have radiologically evidence of osteoarthrotic skeletal changes, which are, however, predominantly silent. In view of this high prevalence, it is inappropriate to designate "uncomplicated" OA as a disease, but more as biomechanical processes, which, over the course of time, may give rise to a painful, disabling illness. More information is provided from the results of three large studies based on interviews and clinical examinations conducted by the National Centre for Health Statistics, the Health Examination Survey HES I (Roberts and Burch 1966) and the National Health and Nutrition Examination Surveys I and II (NHANES I: Maurer 1979 and NHANES II: McDowell et al. 1981). The diagnosis of OA was based on radiological findings using the criteria of the "Atlas of Standard Radiographs". HES I was conducted on 6,672 US adults from 1960 to 1962 and indicated that estimated 37% had OA to some degree of the hands or feet. The rates ranged from 4% in individuals 18–24 years of age to 85% in those 75–79 years of age.

NHANES I was conducted between 1971 and 1975 and provides data on the prevalence of OA of the knee and hip. The overall prevalence rates ranged from zero in those 25–34 years of age to 13.8% in those 65–74 years of age. Rates of OA of the hip were 1.3% overall. The age specific rates ranged from 0.4% in men 25–34 years old to 3.1% in those 55–74 years old.

NHANES II was conducted between 1976 and 1980 and provides data on the prevalence of OA of the cervical and lumbar spine.

16.4 Pathophysiology and Pathogenesis

OA predominantly affecting the large, weight bearing joints of the lower extremities, needs to be distinguished from the Heberden-associated OA of the finger joints of different etiology and pathogenesis. Primary OA without local disposition has to be separated from the secondary form. To the latter group belong

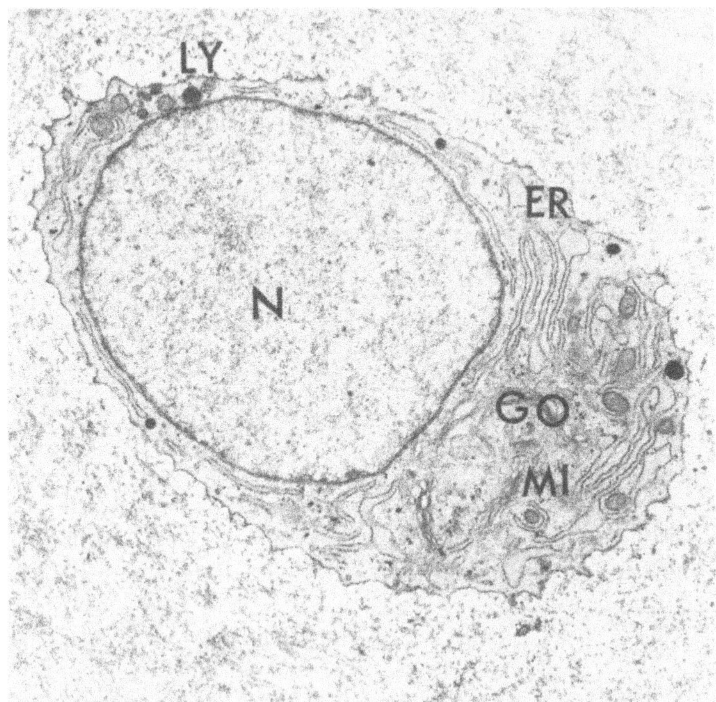

Fig. 16.1

Normal chondrocyte. *N*, nuclei; *ER*, endoplasmatic reticulum; *GO*, Golgi apparatus; *MI*, mitochondria; *LY*, lysosomes. (Electron micrograph: M. Annefeld)

osteoarthritic changes subsequent to pre-existing abnormalities as well as in the context of systemic diseases, e.g. RA.

Articular cartilage

The biomechanical characteristics of adult articular cartilage, which is only a few millimetres thick, and its surrounding connective tissue enable the joint to withstand the strain of large and complex mechanical forces over the course of decades. Implicit in this quality is the ability of the cartilage to bear loads many times that of body weight. This unique biomechanical property is due to the extreme swelling pressures generated by the hydrophilic nature of the aggrecan molecules within the matrix which is underhydrated, and the special architecture of the collagen network.

Articular cartilage contains remarkably few cells. The only living element, the chondrocyte, comprises only 2–5% of the adult tissue volume, depending on age and topographical location within the joint (Stockwell 1979).

The chondrocyte is a highly and terminally differentiated mesenchymal cell recognizable as early as the 6th week in the developing embryo. The advanced differentiation is reflected in the complex ultrastructure of the cartilage cell (Fig. 16.1).

The chondrocyte in the adult articular cartilage is distinct from all other cells of mesenchymal origin by the following characteristics:

1. The chondrocyte lives in a largely anoxic (anaerobic) milieu.
2. The chondrocyte lives in an avascular environment and receives its nutrients and eliminates its waste products by diffusion through the extracellular matrix.

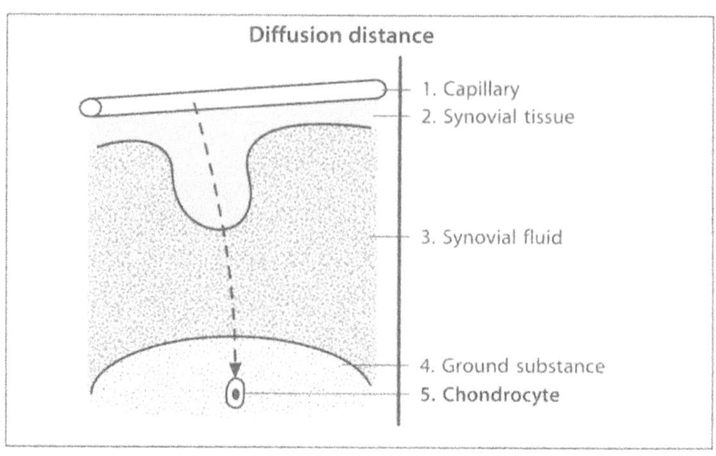

Fig. 16.2 Transit way between synovial capillary and chondrocyte

3. The adult chondrocyte is a post-mitotic cell and thus cannot be replaced if lost.
4. The chondrocyte lives without direct cell-to-cell contact.

With the completion of the growing phase, the articular cartilage loses contact with the blood vessels of the bone marrow through the zone of calcified cartilage. From this point on, the nutritional requirements for the synthetic and other metabolic processes of hyaline cartilage are provided by diffusion through synovial fluid and have to take the following route:

Transition route

- From the capillaries in the synovial membrane
- Through the synovial stroma and the lining cells
- Through the synovial fluid
- Through the cartilage matrix
- Ultimately to the chondrocyte (Fig. 16.2)

In comparison with the more direct blood supply of other tissues, the rather long supply line of cartilage is much more precarious and is vulnerable to interruption at any of the above stages. The removal of metabolic waste products of the chondrocytes also takes place by diffusion through the cartilage matrix the synovial fluid, the synovial stroma, finally to the lymphatic system. The chondrocyte lives suspended in its own matrix, which affords the cell a certain protection from environmental changes in pressure (Urban 1994). Chondrocytes in culture are able to synthesize and release predominantly the following molecules:

1. Predominantly collagen type II and up to 10% of minor collagens such as IX, X, XI, and small amounts of type VI
2. Populations of aggregating proteoglycans and non-aggregating (e.g. dermatan sulfate containing) proteoglycans
3. Cartilage matrix proteins
4. Proteases (e.g. metalloproteinases)
5. Metalloproteinase inhibitors [e.g. tissue inhibitor of metalloproteinases (TIMP)]

Proteins are synthesized in the rough endoplasmic reticulum (ER) and the polysaccharides added principally in the Golgi apparatus. The collagens are formed intracellularly as procollagens and polymerized extracellularly. In similar fashion, the intracellularly elaborated aggrecan monomers attain their final aggregated structure outside the cell.

Cellular heterogeneity

Adult articular cartilage can be divided, from the surface inwards, into three non-mineralized zones (I–III), which are sharply separated from a calcified zone (IV) by an interface, the tidemark (Aydelotte and Kuettner 1992).

Zone I

The tangential (superficial) layer shows the highest cell density. The most superficial chondrocytes are predominantly flattened, discoid, and lie parallel to the surface. They have fewer organelles than the deeper located chondrocytes of this layer, which show a less flattened shape. Consistent with their limited activity, the cell membrane of the upper tangential cells has only a few filopodia, in contrast to the deeper located chondrocytes and those found in the deeper zones.

Zone II

The typical functional active chondrocytes are found in the transitional (intermediate) layer, where they exhibit characteristic ultrastructures. The round to oval cells with more prominent cytoplasm than found in the cells of zone I are arranged singly or in small groups and are randomly distributed throughout the matrix. They have a round eccentric nucleus with a smooth membrane and frequently one nucleolus. The cell nucleus is surrounded by microfilament bundles arranged in parallel, which adjoin the nuclear membrane. Most of these perinuclear filaments may be intermediate filaments which are thought to resist stretch and play a role in bearing tension in the cell. The remaining cytoplasm contains numerous free ribosomes, abundant ER, and mitochondria. The Golgi apparatus is situated in a paranuclear position and consists of lamellar and vesicular structures.

The chondrocytes also contain paraplasmic inclusions, mainly consisting of glycogen and lipid droplets possibly representing stores for the predominantly anaerobic metabolic processes. The cell membrane of the active chondrocyte in the transitional zone shows a scalloped surface in the form of short finger-like processes which can become cut off from the cell to form vesicles. Further away from the chondrocyte, these matrix vesicles then lose their membranes.

Zone III

The chondrocytes found within their territorial matrix of the very deep layer of the radial (basal) cartilage zone are mainly ellipsoid and lie with their long axes vertical to the articular surface. They are grouped in an unit of radially-arranged columns of 2–6 cells which is called a chondron (Poole et al. 1988; Aydelotte et al. 1992).

Zone IV

Between non-mineralized and calcified cartilage, an interface (tidemark) is recognizable even after decalcification. Without decalcification, this tidemark is characterized by a narrow band of vertical striation. In the electron-micrograph, this corresponds to clusters of mineral that protrude 1–2 mm deep into the fibrillar space of zone III. After decalcification, the tidemark stains preferentially with a variety of dyes indicating the presence of a specialized extracellular matrix probably containing glycoproteins and lipids. The tidemark shares some staining properties with the cement-lines in bone (Schenk et al. 1986). In this zone, the chondrocytes are more sparsely distributed and most are apparently viable (Aydelotte et al. 1992).

Hunziker (1992) states that the chondrocytes in calcified articular cartilage are both structurally and functionally intact and surrounded by an envelope of non-mineralized pericellular and territorial matrices. These cells appear to be involved in the mineralization process, which may be reactivated along the tidemark at any stage in adult life in response to changes in loading patterns and trauma, leading to the hypothesis that this process may reactivate an "arrested growth plate" (Oegema and Thompson 1992).

Cellular activity

With advancing age, the chondrocytes in the tangential and also the transitional layers store increasing amounts of glycogen. The cell nucleus becomes darker with condensed chromatin as a sign of reduced cellular activity.

The early stages of "programmed cell death" can be recognized by the initial loss of cell volume. Loss of the nucleus is a definite sign of cell death. The dead chondrocytes leave behind lacunae filled with cell debris, myelin bodies, and frequently fat vacuoles. Collections of matrix vesicles are often found in the vicinity. This process means that an irreplaceable living unit responsible for the maintenance of the matrix is lost to the affected area of the tissue (Oegema and Thompson 1992).

Collagens

To date, different types of collagen have been identified in hyaline articular cartilage. Collagen type II is the predominant fibrous component and most minor (types VI, IX, and XI) collagens undoubtedly have important functions in determining the unique properties of the tissue (Eyre et al. 1987, 1992; Mayne 1989; Eyre 1991; Olsen 1992; Prockop and Kivirikko 1995).

It is known from the classic studies of Benninghoff (1939) that collagen fibres assume an arcade-like structure at the surface of articular cartilage. However, in the deeper layers, these fibres form a tissue-specific, three dimensional framework in which constituents, such as aggrecans or glycoproteins, are enmeshed or attached (Clark 1991). Such interactions reinforce the stability of this network. It is thought that two of the minor collagens are involved in the fibril formation process in the cartilage matrix (Nimni 1997).

Collagen type IX has been localized at intersection points between collagen fibrils. Since it is covalently bound to the collagen type II, it may function as a "connector" or "glue" molecule between type II fibrils (Eyre et al. 1987; Mayne and Burgeson 1987; Van der Rest and Mayne 1988; Vaughan et al. 1988). As a consequence, the collagen type II fibres become less extensible. Collagen type IX is assembled from three different peptide chains and to one of them a single chondroitin sulfate chain is covalently bound, making it thus a proteoglycan as well (Mayne and Burgeson 1987). It has been postulated that the collagen type II fibrous network becomes less rigid, if these "connector" molecules are altered or diminished. As a result, the tissue is able to swell and its biomechanical properties are altered. Collagen type IX is also closely associated with the type II collagen fibrils being localized within the fibres and may be involved in determining their diameters (Van der Rest and Mayne 1988; Mendler et al. 1989). Collagen type X (Schmid and Linsenmayer 1987) is synthesized only by hypertrophic chondrocytes and might play a role in the calcification process of the cartilage matrix (Von der Mark et al. 1992). Small amounts of collagen type VI have been identified in the pericellular matrix of articular chondrocytes, especially in osteoarthritic cartilage (Ronzière et al. 1990).

Aggrecan

The major proteoglycan within the articular cartilage matrix is termed aggrecan (Hardingham and Bayliss 1990; Hardingham et al. 1992). Aggrecan consists of a core protein (MW 220,000) to which anionic glycosaminoglycan chains (chondroitin sulfate and keratan sulfate) as well as *N*-linked and *O*-linked oligosaccharides are covalently bound. The molecular weight of aggrecan is dependent on the tissue and is between 2 to 3 million daltons. Aggrecan can interact specifically and non-covalently via its binding region with a small segment of a long polymer of hyaluronan. Up to 100 aggrecan monomers can interact with a single hyaluronan chain and thus form aggregates of more than 200 million daltons that, when reviewed by electron-microscopy, are more than 4 μm long (Rosenberg and Buckwalter 1986; Thonar and Kuettner 1987; Fig. 16.3). A third component of the aggrecan, the link-protein, binds to both the hyaluronan and the aggrecan core protein and stabilizes the attachment of each aggrecan monomer (Kimura and Kuettner 1986).

Several non-aggregating proteoglycans are also present in the cartilage matrix, including two smaller ones substituted with one or two dermatan sulfate side chains named "decorin" and "biglycan", respectively (Heinegard and Sommarin 1987; Rosenberg 1992).

Due to the high negative charge density, the aggrecan molecules are characterized by their tremendous capacity to bind water (Maroudas et al. 1992). The hydroelastic effect of hyaline articular cartilage operates through a pump effect which results in the dissipation of energy after dynamic or passive loading. Since in cartilage aggrecan molecules are present in an underhydrated form (only about 20% of its fully hydrated volume is occupied within the tissue), they attract water, providing a swelling pressure of several atmospheres within the tissue. The collagenous network restrains the mobility of the aggrecan molecules within the matrix and the pressure provides stiffness and shape of the tissue. When load is applied to the cartilage, water is extruded from the loaded region. However, the movement of this water is restricted by the aggrecan molecules which are already in an underhydrated state. Through this loading and the removal of the water from the aggrecan molecules, their highly charged side chains are also forced closer together, thereby increasing the ef-

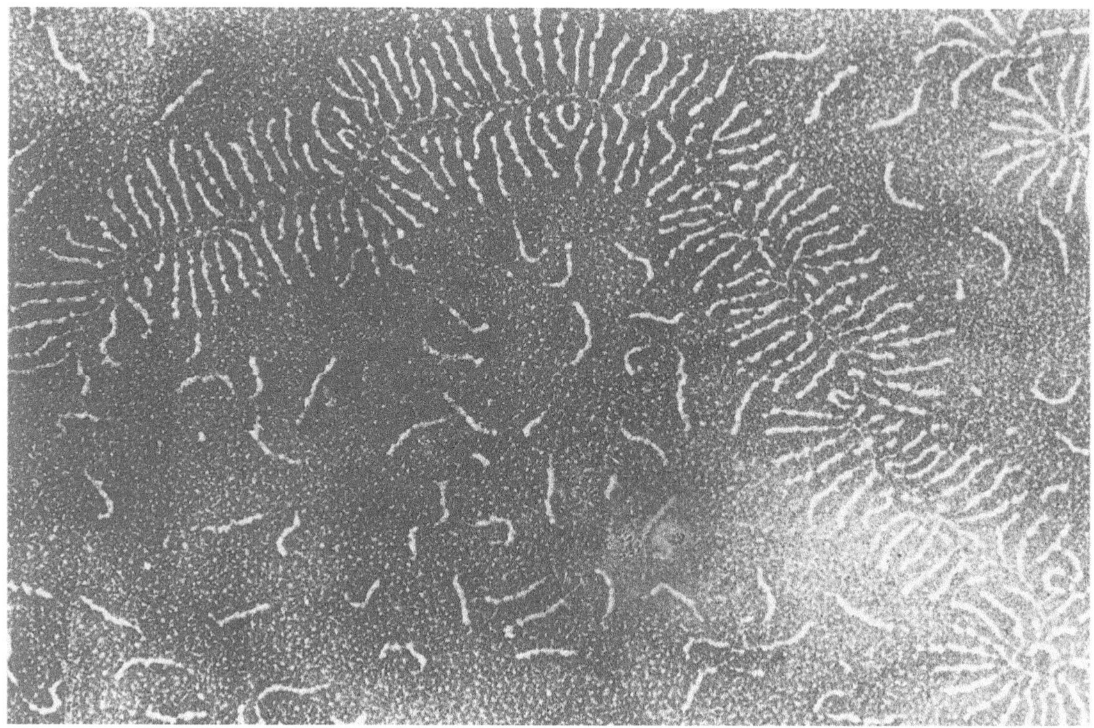

Fig. 16.3 Aggrecan macro-molecule. Proteoglycan molecules linked to hyaluronic acid filum. The binding is intensified by the link-protein

fective charge density. Ultimately, the deformation of the tissue reaches an equilibrium, when the load forces are counterbalanced by the swelling pressure of the aggrecan molecules (Urban 1990). When the load is removed, the compressed aggrecan molecules attract water mostly from the synovial fluid and the tissue regains its original form when the equilibrium between the restricting collagen fibres and the swelling pressure of the aggrecan molecules is reestablished (Maroudas and Grushko 1990; Sah et al. 1992).
This pump system facilitates the removal of cellular waste products during loading and an imbibing of nutrients for the chondrocytes during unloading. This process also represents a simple explanation for the shock absorption phenomenon of articular cartilage.

Shock absorption in the joint

However, it is hardly comprehensive that a few millimetres-thick layer of cartilage is able, over a long period of time, to sustain the load and pressure many times the body weight. An essential precondition of it is a corresponding nervous coordination of the surrounding muscular apparatus with the movement of the joint. As a result, the articular structure is increasingly endangered by an atrophy or a deterioration of the surrounding musculature. An additional important matter for shock absorption is a certain elasticity of the subchondral cancellous bone, which leads to adaption of the primary incongruent articular surfaces under load and, thus, allows for broader distribution of surface pressure.

Excessive loads cause microfractures of the subchondral trabeculae, which heal with callus formation and remodelling. The remodelled trabeculae may be stiffer than normal and less effective as shock absorbers (Brandt 1985a). Consequently, Todd et al. (1972) attach a certain importance to the effects of these microfractures in the development of OA. Radin (1972–1973) even sees in trabecular microfractures a primary cause for cartilage degeneration. In contrast, Mankin's experiments (1974) show that repeated impact loading leads to articular cartilage fibrillation and ultrastructural changes in the chondrocytes prior to changes in the mechanical properties of the subchondral plate.

Attempted repair processes

The potential of slow remodelling of the articular cartilage is retained throughout life (Von der Mark et al. 1992). Characteristic features of repair processes as response to tissue damage in OA are e.g. the formation of chondrocyte clusters (cell nests, pathological chondrons) and osteophytes as well as the remodelling of the zone of calcified cartilage.

Chondrocyte clusters

In the early phases of most forms of OA, the chondrocytes exhibit a state of hypermetabolism, upregulating biosynthetic processes to balance their increased catabolic activities. The chondrocytes appear to respond to the enhanced biomechanical stimuli by synthesizing different gene products which further lead to changes in matrix composition and a subsequent alteration in the biomechanical behaviour of the tissue (Bayliss 1990, 1992; Plaas and Sandy 1995).

Although the chondrocyte is regarded as a long-lived post-mitotic cell which lacks reproductive function, chondrocyte clusters are observed in the vicinity of fissures in osteoarthritic cartilage of the transitional and radial zones. The site of these cell clusters suggests that this increase of damage at the cartilage surface and the close contact with the synovial fluid may favour the proliferation of chondrocytes. However, these multicellular clusters are unable to synthesize normal matrix components (Aigner et al. 1992, 1993). Thus, these components do not contribute to a functionally intact matrix capable of bearing load. Therefore, in spite of the quite impressive cellular hyperplasia, little repair of the cartilaginous extracellular matrix occurs (Fig. 16.4).

Osteophytes

The formation of marginal new bone, which follows the original lines of the joint surface can be observed as part of the bone remodelling processes characteristic of OA (but also in RA following joint destruction). The centre of the osteophyte consists of crude compact bone and an abnormal spongiosa with irregular bone trabeculae of varying thickness. The osteophyte is covered by rapidly growing, newly synthesized fibrous cartilage (Fig. 16.5). Sweet and coworkers (1977) and Malemud and colleagues (1982) have shown in vitro that this cartilage forms sulfated proteoglycans rich in chondroitin 6-sulfate, but with a relative deficiency of keratan sulfate.

At first sight, it seems that the development of osteophytes at the marginal regions of the joint where lower pressure is applied, represents an attempt to restore the congruence of the joint surfaces after, at some other sites, the articular cartilage has undergone degenerative alterations.

Osteophyte formation in animal models

Gilbertson (1975) describes early osteophyte formation only 3 days after cruciate ligament trans-

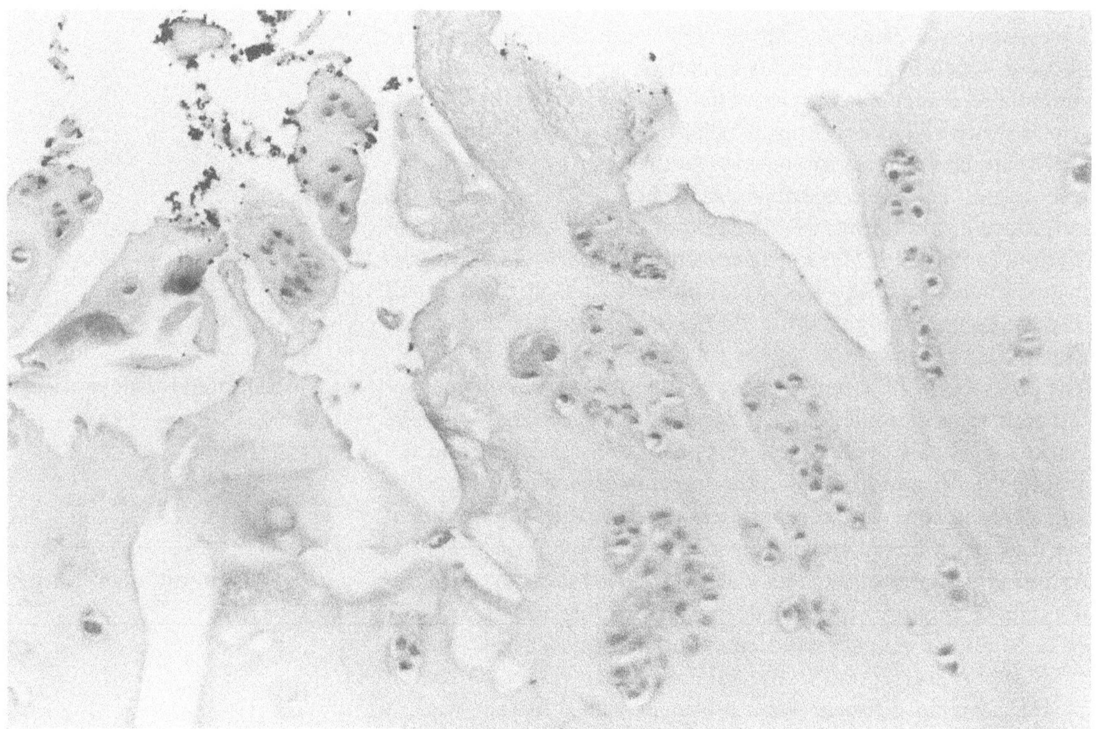

Fig. 16.4 Osteoarthritis

Knee-joint. Deep fissures and detachment of the articular cartilage. The developed spaces are surrounded by chondrocyte clusters

ection in the dog knee as a regular feature, and Williams and Thonar (1989) find prominent osteophyte formation after 3 weeks following injection of sodium iodoacetate into the guinea pig knee joint. Marshall and Olsson (1971), however, found that osteophytes developed in a dog knee joint although the articular cartilage did not show degenerative changes.

Thus, disturbed joint biomechanics fails to explain satisfactorily the development of osteophytes. Whether the proliferation of blood vessels plays a role, as suggested by Swanson and Freeman (1970), must remain open. However, the fact that biomechanical factors contribute to osteophyte formation has been indicated by studies of Palmosky and Brandt (1982): immobilisation of the joint following cruciate ligament transection in experimental OA in the dog prevents the development of osteophytes. Thus, the etiology of osteophytes still remains to be investigated.

Remodelling of calcified cartilage

Remodelling of the calcified cartilage is a continuous but very slow process in normal adult cartilage. According to Oegema and Thompson (1990) who were able to demonstrate progressive mineralization which resulted in an advancement of the tidemark following excessive load or impact loading on articular cartilage, biomechanical changes may stimulate such remodelling processes.

In OA, the non-calcified cartilage becomes thinner as a result of the advancing calcification zone. A characteristic feature is seen in the change of the tidemark: frequently, it duplicates or multiplies (Redler et al. 1975; Oegema and Thompson 1990,

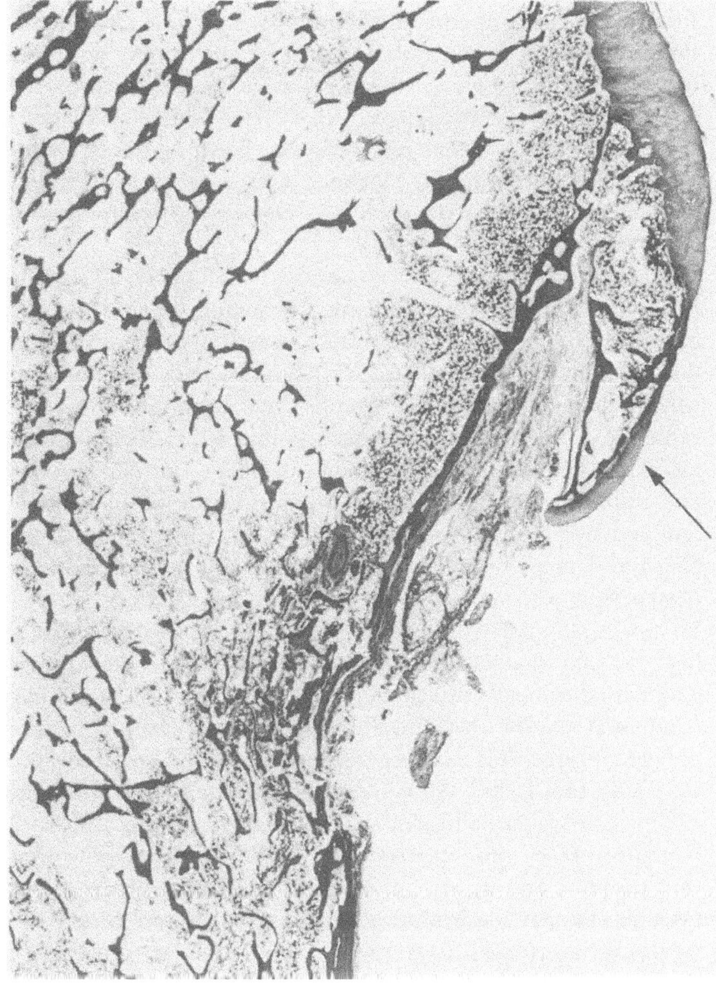

Marginal osteophyte (*arrow*) and considerable rarefaction of the spongiosa

Fig. 16.5
Osteoarthritis

1992). These processes represent other inadequate forms of articular cartilage repair.

Risks for the structural integrity

The structural integrity of the cartilage matrix, which is critical for the biomechanical function of the joint, may be compromised by the following external and internal factors:
The chondrocyte produces enzymes not only for matrix synthesis but also for its degradation. There is no danger to matrix integrity as long as these enzymes play their physiological role in the cycle of matrix turnover – a balanced anabolism and catabolism (Bayliss 1992; Plaas and Sandy 1995).
The maintenance of structural integrity of articular cartilage depends upon this balance between matrix synthesis and degradation. These processes are regulated not only by chondrocyte-derived enzymes (such as metalloproteinases; Murphy et al. 1981, 1990; Morales and Kuettner 1982; Woessner 1991) and enzyme inhibitors (such as TIMP; Hembry et al. 1985; Werb 1992; Murphy 1995) but, most probably, also by growth factors, hormones, and vitamins as suggested by in vitro and animal experiments. Experiments performed by Dingle and colleagues (1979) have

shown that inflammatory mediators such as IL-1 ("catabolin") released by synovial membrane act on bovine or porcine chondrocytes, leading to an increased release of proteolytic enzymes (Dingle and Tyler 1986; Tyler et al. 1992). On human cartilage explants, these mediators primarily downregulate aggrecan synthesis, thus disrupting the fine balance between anabolism and catabolism that ultimately results in chondrocytic chondrolysis (Aydelotte et al. 1986).

Cytokines

Cytokines, especially IL-1 beta and TNF-alpha (Martel-Pelletier et al. 1999), produced by inflamed synovium during the later phases of OA are most effective, even at low concentration, in downregulating the synthesis of aggrecan and may therefore contribute significantly to the progressive depletion of this molecule from the articular cartilage (Poole 1995). The aggrecan molecules remaining in the tissue can now occupy more space and imbibe water leading to a swelling of the tissue. This attempted but gradually failing repair results ultimately in mechanical damage to the extracellular matrix through continuous destruction of the collagen fibrous network.

Proteases

Proteases, singularly or in combination, can destroy the extracellular cartilage matrix components. Chondrocyte-derived collagenases do specifically attack collagen types II and IX in cartilage (Gadher et al. 1988). Enzymatic attack on the collagen network is only likely when it is exposed through loss of the protective proteoglycan coat (Scott 1990) secondary to extensive degradation of the proteoglycan and specifically the aggrecan molecules.

Hyaluronidase can theoretically degrade the hyaluronate (hyaluronan) and most of the other glycosaminoglycans, however, no endogenous hyaluronidase has been found in cartilage.

Aggrecan degradation is mostly attributed to metalloproteinases, among them stromelysin which cleaves the aggrecan core protein. The resulting fragments diffuse out of the matrix without being retained. It is noteworthy that stromelysin also can degrade the telopeptides of collagen type II and the associated collagen type IX, thereby loosening the collagenous network of the tissue. The decrease of aggrecan concentration and the loosening of the fibrillar structure lead to an increase in water content, and, thus, to a decrease of the biomechanical properties of the tissue.

The activation and regulation of these matrix metalloproteinases are carefully controlled via specific activation of the enzymes (or enzyme cascades) and controlled modulation by their inhibitor(s). Any disturbance of this balance results in either net proteinase activity or suppression of its activity via inhibition. In OA, for example, partially degraded fragments of aggrecan molecules can be detected in increased amounts: this appears to be due to the action of aggrecanase although other enzymes are involved (Lark et al. 1995). Aggrecanase is a recently discovered but not fully identified proteolytic enzyme which is highly specific for the degradation of aggrecan (Caterson et al. 1992). It may, thus, play a crucial role in the progression of OA.

Mechanical overloading

In contrast to this primarily biochemical viewpoint, Maroudas and colleagues (1986) consider that the primary event leading to the systematic degeneration of matrix components is unphysio-

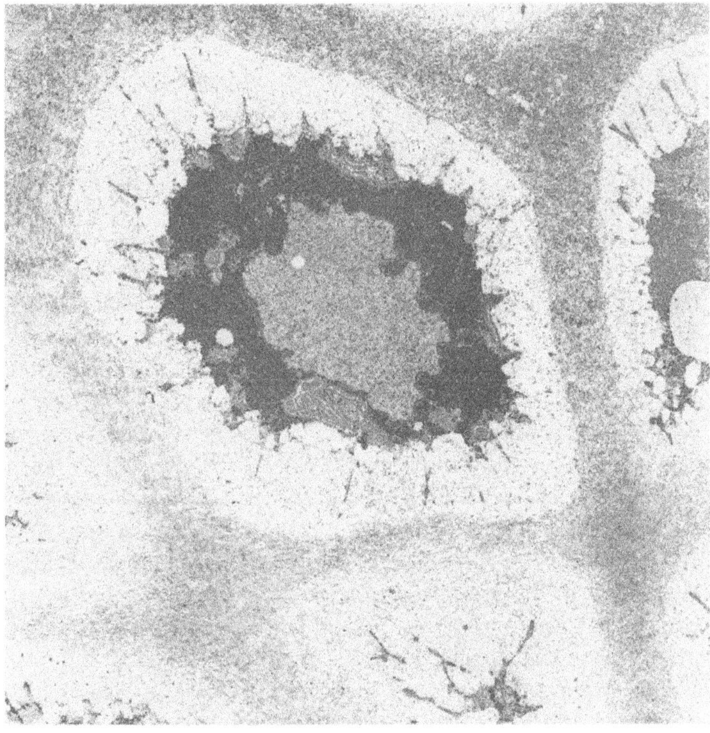

Fig. 16.6 Dead chondrocyte caused by Dexamethason. (Electron micrograph: M. Annefeld)

logical dynamic loading, leading to overstressing of the collagen fibre network. Rupture of the collagen network induces a release of aggrecan and causes an increased water influx with subsequent failure of the hydroelastic system.

A summary of the various factors that may compromise the integrity of hyaline articular cartilage includes:

1. Destruction of the collagen network secondary to mechanical overloading and physical trauma.
2. Loosening of the collagen network following enzymatic degradation of collagen type IX and/or type II through stromelysin.
3. Excessive release of chondrocyte proteases, mostly metalloproteinases, possibly induced by inflammatory mediators derived from the inflamed synovial tissue.
4. **Toxic damage** — Toxic damage risk to the chondrocytes by disease modifying agents, such as dexamethasone and some non-steroidal anti-inflammatory drugs (NSAIDs; Fig. 16.6).
5. **Nutritional insufficiency** — Damage to the chondrocytes due to inadequate nutrition secondary to interruption of the supply route between synovial capillaries and chondrocytes.
6. Alteration of specific, non-collagenous matrix proteins whose function is currently incompletely understood (Heinegard et al. 1995).

Singularly or in combination, these mechanisms ultimately lead to a qualitative deterioration of hyaline articular cartilage. This deterioration may be critical for loaded joints where an imbal-

ance can arise between the quality of the matrix and the mechanical load, leading to cartilage failure.
Although the etiology of OA is still not understood completely, it is unlikely that a single cause will be found to be responsible. More probably the different factors listed above may combine during the course of the OA disease process, with the predominance of nutritional, toxic, enzymatic or physical causes in individual cases (Hamerman 1989). This mosaic of factors responsible for the OA process is reflected in the clinical heterogeneity of OA and is a major impediment to the evaluation of therapy in this disease.

Mosaic of factors

Since there are no satisfactory diagnostic modalities (e.g. imaging) for the detection of the onset or early events of OA, new research focuses on disease markers, both in the synovial fluid and serum, by the use of mostly monoclonal antibodies which recognize specific epitopes on aggrecan and collagen fragments (Witter et al. 1987; Seibel et al. 1989; Lohmander 1990; Thonar et al. 1991). The development of such markers is based on the fact that alterations in the properties of joint cartilage and loss of matrix components are an integral part of the disease process. The degradation of the cartilage matrix may be a key event at the onset of OA. During this process, matrix molecules, or partially degraded macromolecules, are released into the joint fluid and eventually enter other body fluids. These molecules and fragments thus serve as valuable markers of cartilage matrix metabolism in the early stages of OA, before a diagnosis can be made by conventional methods (Lohmander 1992). One of these molecules in the synovial fluid, the cartilage oligomeric matrix protein (COMP), points towards a degradation of the cartilage matrix in OA but also to cartilage destruction in RA (Saxne and Heinegard 1985). According to investigations of Hummel and coworkers (1998), COMP can be secreted also by synovial stroma cells. The different origins of the protein can be differentiated with monoclonal antibodies.

The quality problem

As the quality of the matrix gradually deteriorates, a point is reached where the tolerance of the cartilage is exceeded and a stage comes where the aberrant composition of the matrix does not fulfill the biological requirements of the tissue. For each respective joint, a tolerance quotient can be defined through the formula:

$$\frac{\text{matrix quality}}{\text{physical stress}} = \text{tolerance quotient}$$

A negative quotient signifies that the tolerance limit for that particular joint has been exceeded (Fassbender 1988).
The atraumatic sliding of joint surfaces is dependent on their smoothness, which is guaranteed by embedding the aggrecan gel in the collagen framework. In addition, the cartilage surface is coated by a lubricating film of "pore water" and lubricin – a glycoprotein of about 250 kDa (Swann et al. 1981).
The work of Aydelotte and Kuettner (1988) has demonstrated that the chondrocytes in the upper 10% of the articular cartilage produce fewer aggrecan molecules than those in the deeper lay-

ers. This implies that the collagen fibres are less protected just at the point where loading- and sheer forces are directly applied. However, the small proteoglycans, decorin and fibromodulin, are more concentrated near the articular surface than in deeper tissue, and these are thought to influence collagen fibrillogenesis (Poole et al. 1993).

The first histochemical sign of reduced quality of the matrix, probably indicating the initial phase of the disease, is loss of staining with decreased avidity of Safranin-O and Alcian-blue reflecting the early loss of aggrecan.

Biochemical and biophysical deficiencies in the matrix predominantly affect the quality of the superficial structure of the hyaline cartilage. The earliest morphological sign of this structural insufficiency is an incipient denudation of the collagen fibre network, marking the first step towards mechanical damage (Figs. 16.7, 16.8). Small areas of roughness develop in the joint surface which, with increasing friction, expand in area. Subsequently, fissures develop, increasing in number and depth over the course of time. Based on the arcade-like structure of the collagen fibres, these fissures initially run parallel to the surface and then orient vertically in the deeper layer above the tidemark. Meachim and Brooke (1984) describe small horizontal fissures arising secondary to loading between the calcified and non-calcified zones.

Fissures

Complete denudation of the collagen fibres leads to a progressive phase. The joint surface becomes roughened with fissures and cartilage separation and may advance to complete abrasion of the cartilage substance. In this way, the smooth joint surface becomes fibrillated, and, during this process, flakes of cartilage which are partially free are moved by joint activity (Figs. 16.9, 16.10). Such fragments become strangulated and detached from their origin and are freely floating in the synovial fluid. This event may be responsible for the onset of pain in an OA patient who is getting up and starts to walk. Further joint movement will tend to cause some smoothing over of the initial foci of surface injury. In the vicinity of cartilage tears, there are nests of chondrocytes consisting of many cells in the form of dense and irregular clusters (see Fig. 16.4). It appears, however, that such cells are not capable of forming sufficient amounts of a new functional matrix and that the cartilage defects are thus not repaired (see p. 329).

The ability of viscous joint fluid to act as a lubricant compensates to some extent for the superficial roughening of cartilage; in the absence of this, erosions would proceed more rapidly. Synovial fluid alterations, as they may occur in the course of an accompanying synovitis, may therefore be of serious consequence for the fate of the surviving cartilage.

Destruction and removal of articular cartilage are usually accompanied by a compensatory formation of new subchondral bone. Thus, eventually a focus of complete cartilage erosion is matched by sclerotic eburnated bone (Fig. 16.11). Removal of cartilage from the zone of maximal loading reveals a bare smooth surface of bone which through the abrasive effects of movement, takes on the polished appearance of ivory. The loss of articular cartilage may, however, be accompanied by so few symptoms that the joint may retain adequate mobility.

Eburnisation

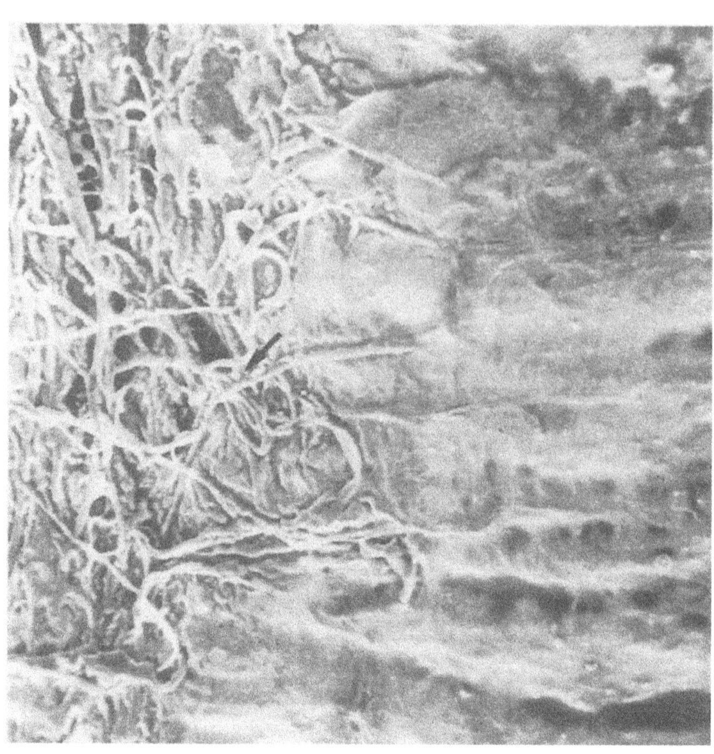

Fig. 16.7
Osteoarthritis

Fifty-six-year-old female. Articular cartilage of the knee with beginning denudation of the collagen fibre net (*arrow*). *Right*, collagen bundles covered with proteoglycan matrix. (Scanning Electron micrograph)

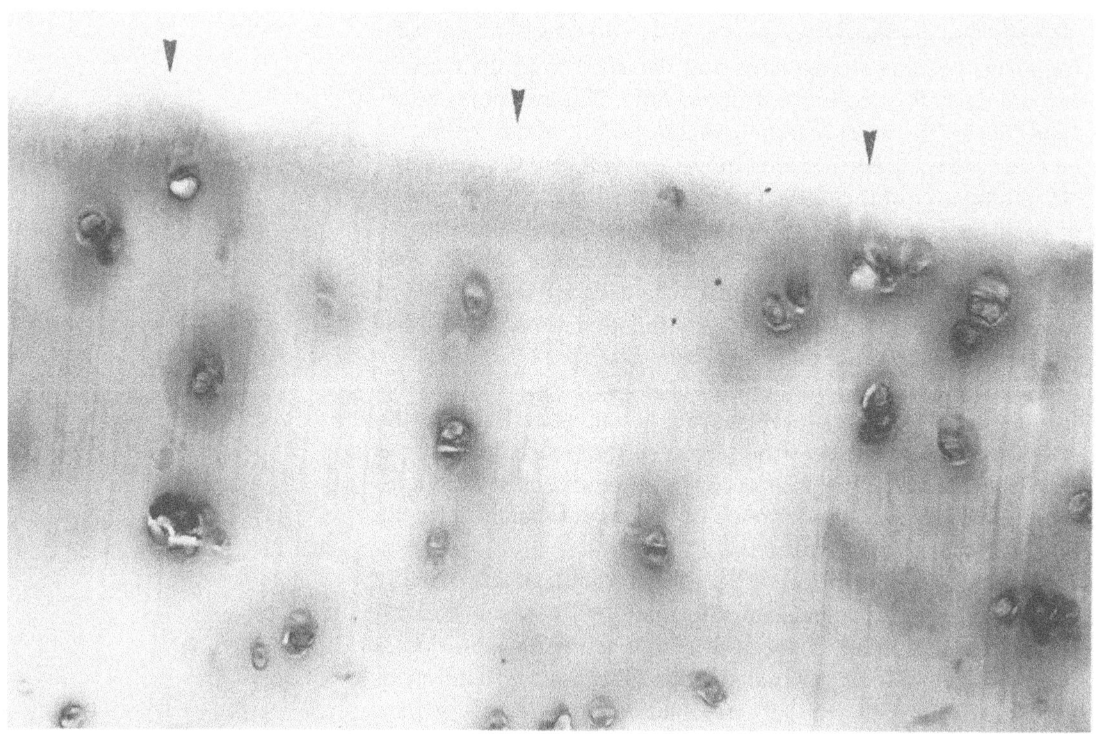

Fig. 16.8
Osteoarthritis

Knee-joint. Discrete unmasking of collagen fibres at the surface of the articular cartilage (*arrows*). Sustained chondrocytes up to the surface (semi-thin section)

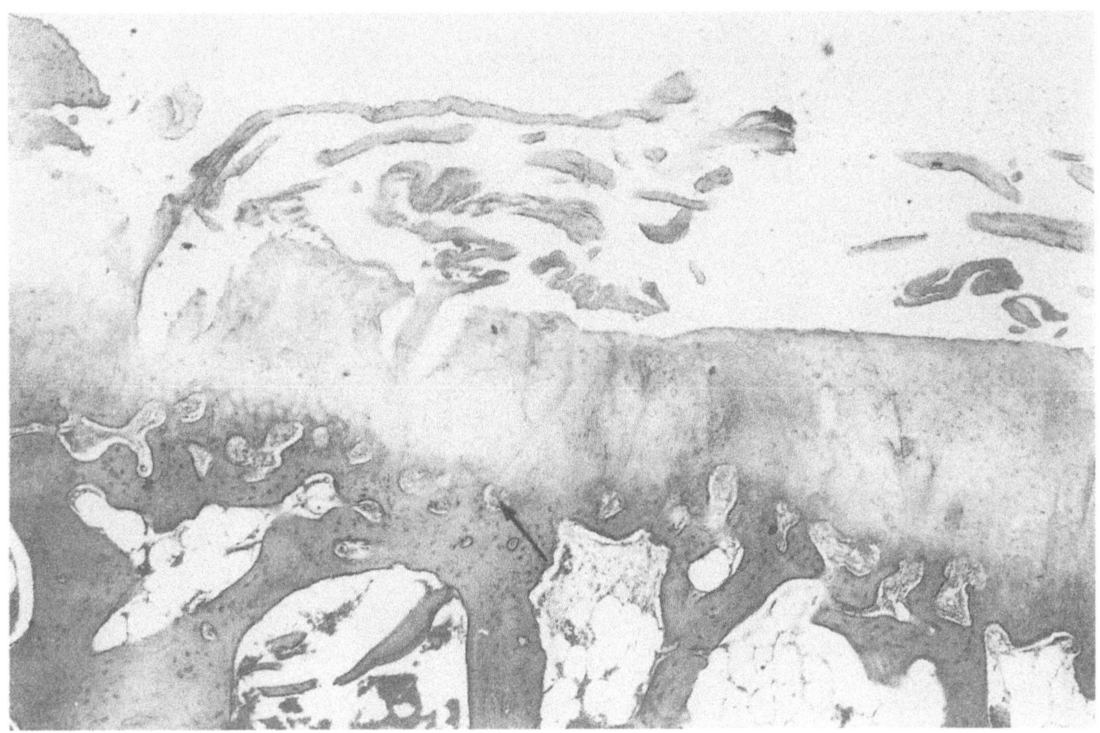

Knee-joint. Detachment of fragments from the articular cartilage. Subchondral osseous lamella partially perished. Early sclerosis (*arrow*)

Fig. 16.9
Osteoarthritis

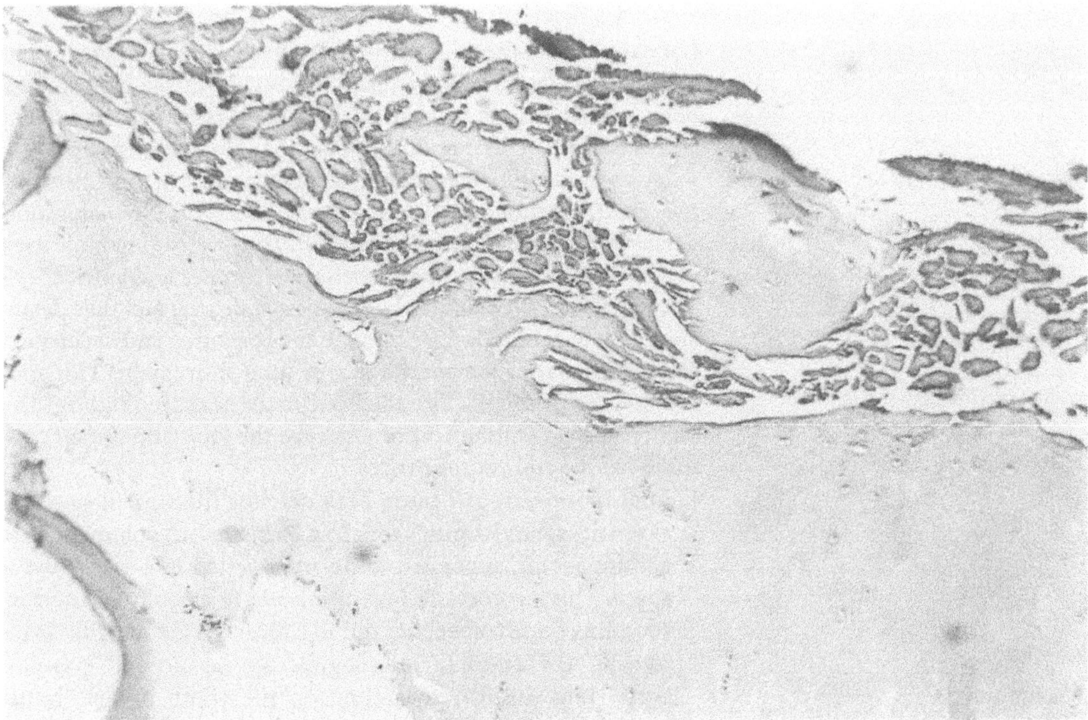

Knee-joint. Crumb-like grinding of the cartilaginous tissue

Fig. 16.10
Osteoarthritis

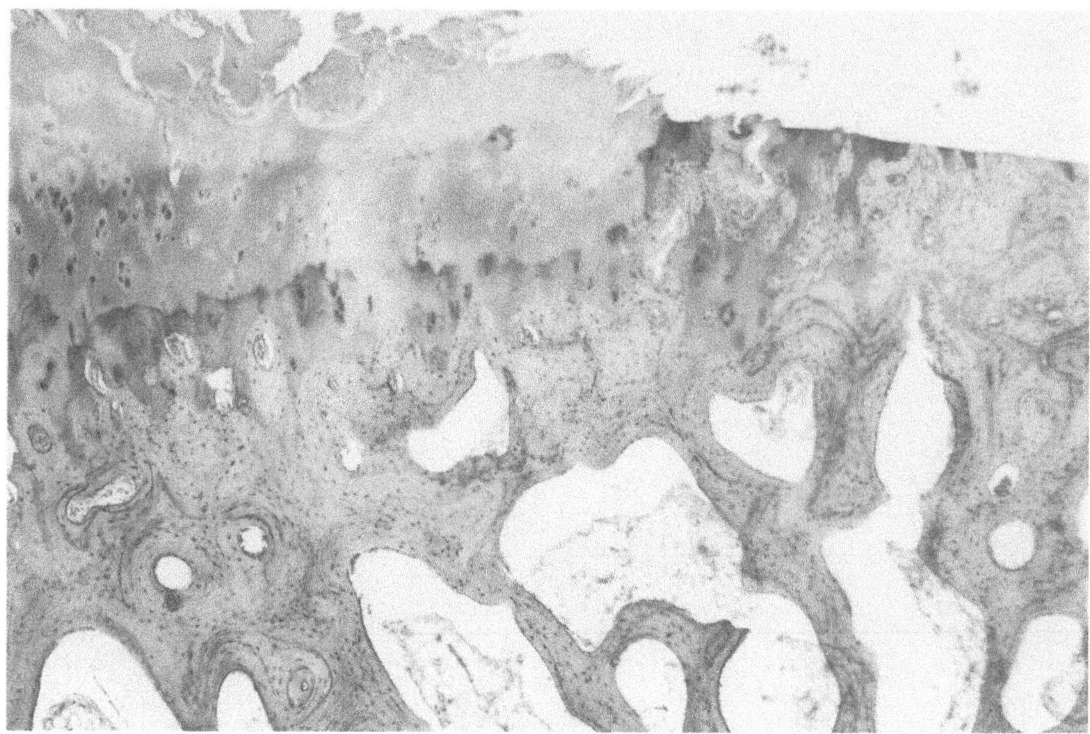

Fig. 16.11
Osteoarthritis

Knee-joint. *Right*, abrasion of the sclerosed (eburnated) subchondral bone. *Left*, remnants of cartilage. New osteones reveal adaptation of subchondral bone to the changed mechanic situation

Concurrent with the decrease in hydroelastic quality of the hyaline articular cartilage, bone remodelling occurs in the subchondral bone with the disordered formation of densely packed osteons (eburnisation). This remodelling leads to an extensive plate-like sclerosis of the initially small bone lamellae. It is highly likely that this rigid subchondral lamellar bone constitutes an additional danger for the remaining cartilage, which with loading finds itself in a position analogous to that between hammer and anvil.
The rigidity of the sclerosed bone plate hides the fact that the inelastic bone can no longer tolerate the pressures and sheer forces resulting from the mechanics of joint movement. This may lead to breakthroughs into the bone marrow space (Fig. 16.12).
The resulting communication between the joint and the marrow space has several consequences:

"Pseudo-cysts"

1. Joint movement can cause both detritus from cartilage abrasion and synovial fluid, which is increased in volume due to accompanying synovitis, to be transmitted into the marrow space. This hydrostatic pressure leads to atrophy of the surrounding bone trabeculae and to a recess of the marrow space causing the familiar radiological appearance of "pseudo-cysts" (Fig. 16.13). Depending on the width of the "bottle neck", these pseudo-cysts may contain fragments of bone and cartilage. A foreign body reaction may ensue with the appearance of foreign body giant cells, neutrophils, and fibrin deposition.

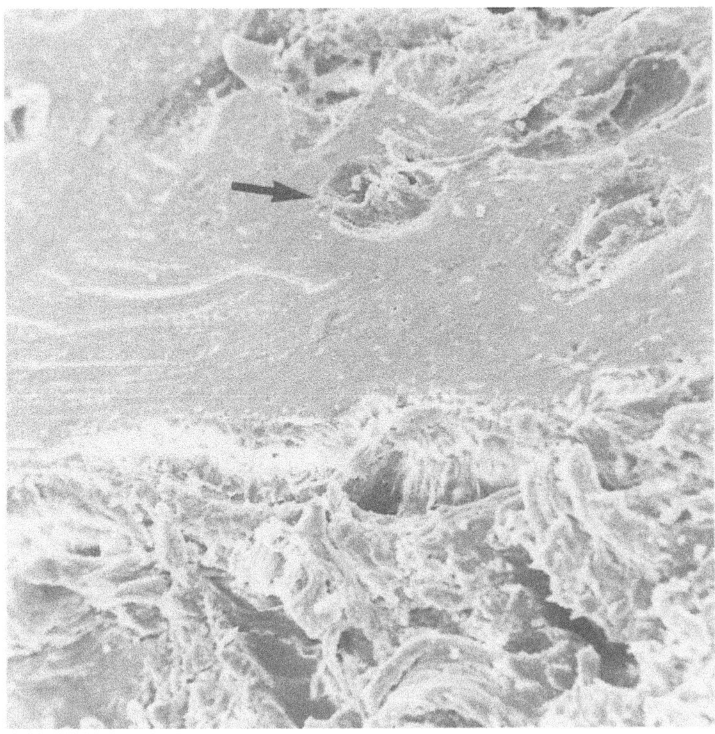

Fig. 16.12 Osteoarthritis

Knee-joint. The lower part of the picture shows lacerated collagenous fibres. Sclerosed (eburnated) subchondral bone plate is evident in the upper part. Several marrow spaces are abraded and opened. Connective tissue protruding out of the marrow space to the articular surface (*arrow*). (Scanning electron micrograph)

2. The products of degradation in these cysts may trigger or maintain an accompanying synovitis.
   Over the course of time, the pseudo-cysts in response are walled-off by a gradually developing thicker layer of bone which clearly separates them from the surrounding marrow space.
   Initially, marked osteoblastic and osteoclastic activity is seen. The detritus within the cysts is gradually organized into a fibrous scar tissue.

Fibrous repair

3. Connective tissue and blood vessels may spread from breaks in the marrow space into the avascular joint space and, thus, form a layer of fibrous cartilaginous tissue that may bridge the cartilage defect and lead to repair (albeit qualitatively inadequate) of the joint surface (Figs. 16.14, 16.15).

Synovial processes

During the attrition of cartilage in the degradative phase, fragments of collagen fibres, proteoglycans, and calcium hydroxyapatite crystals may be found in the synovial fluid. Inflammation may then develop in the synovial tissue and through the action of mediators phagocytic degradative enzymes are released.

Characteristic villous formation

Synovitis found secondary to OA or in trauma develops from an irritation of the lining cells which undergo mild proliferation. Thereby, club-shaped villi form which are initially delicate, then become solid with the development of a sparse stroma with oc-

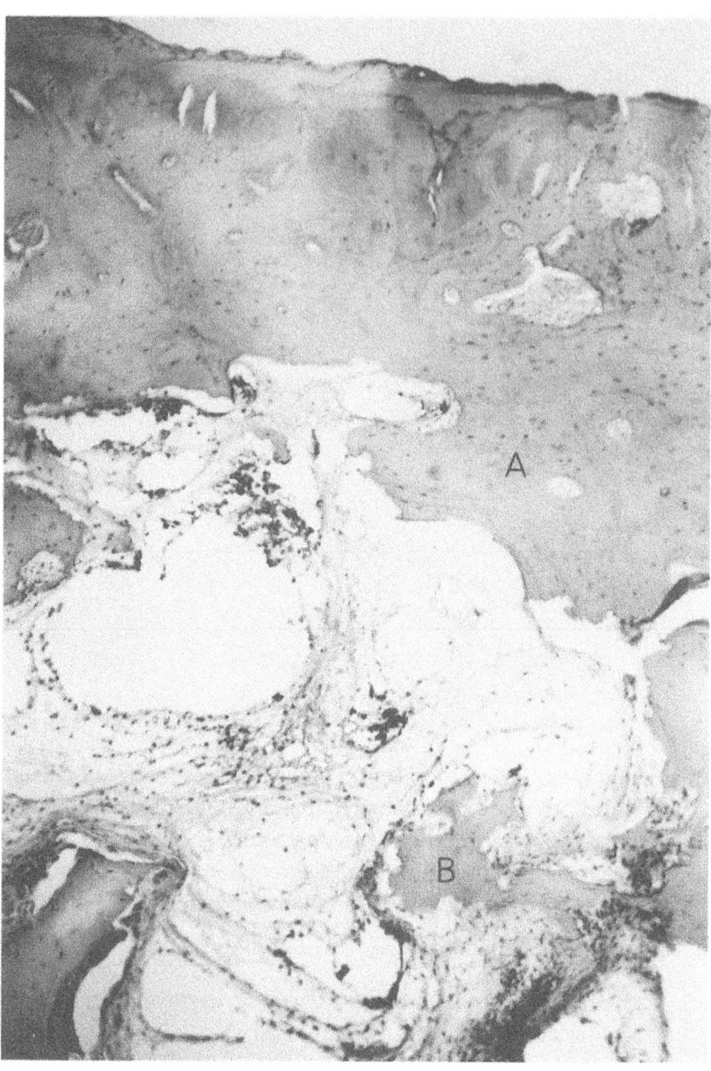

Fig. 16.13
Osteoarthritis

Knee-joint. Bone cyst comprises loose scar tissue. The sclerosed (eburnated) subchondral bone (*A*) is perforated (*B*, newly formed bone)

casional blood vessels. These dainty villi are often found in large numbers in OA and synovitis following intra-articular injuries. Lining cell proliferation with following villous formation leads to an increase of the synovial surface, which hereby is available for the absorption of the substances resulting from cartilage abrasion. The height of the lining cell layer mirrors the stage of the inflammatory process at any given time. In contrast to the "villi" seen in systemic synovitis (see p. 66), we call these villi "proliferative villi" (Fig. 16.16). With the course of time, the villi increase in volume; they become distended and can be recognized by their loose, transparent stroma containing relatively few blood vessels. We have termed this type of villus distinctive for OA and traumatic synovitis, "vitreous (glass) villus" (Fig. 16.17).

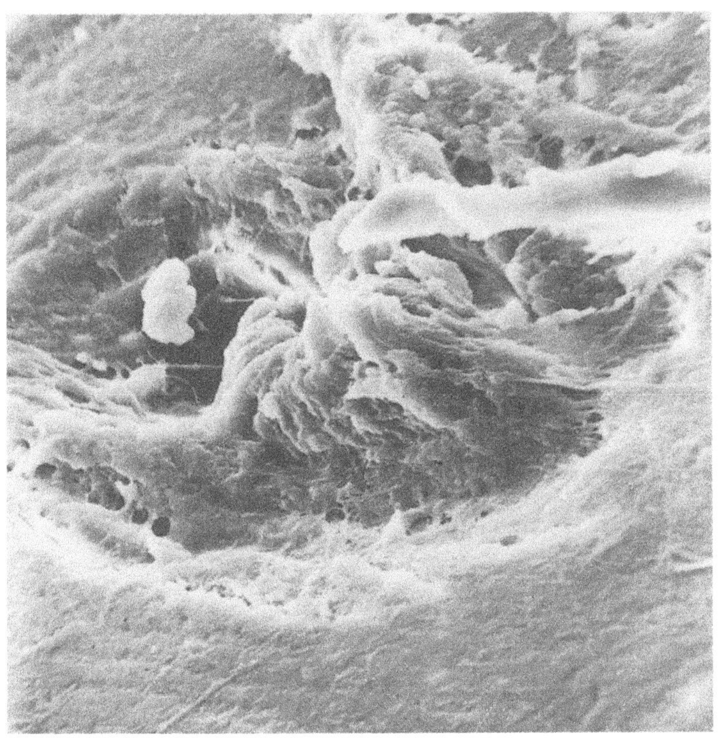

Knee-joint. Connective tissue of marrow protruding through an erosion of bone into the articular cavity (segment from Fig. 16.12; scanning electron micrograph)

Fig. 16.14
Osteoarthritis

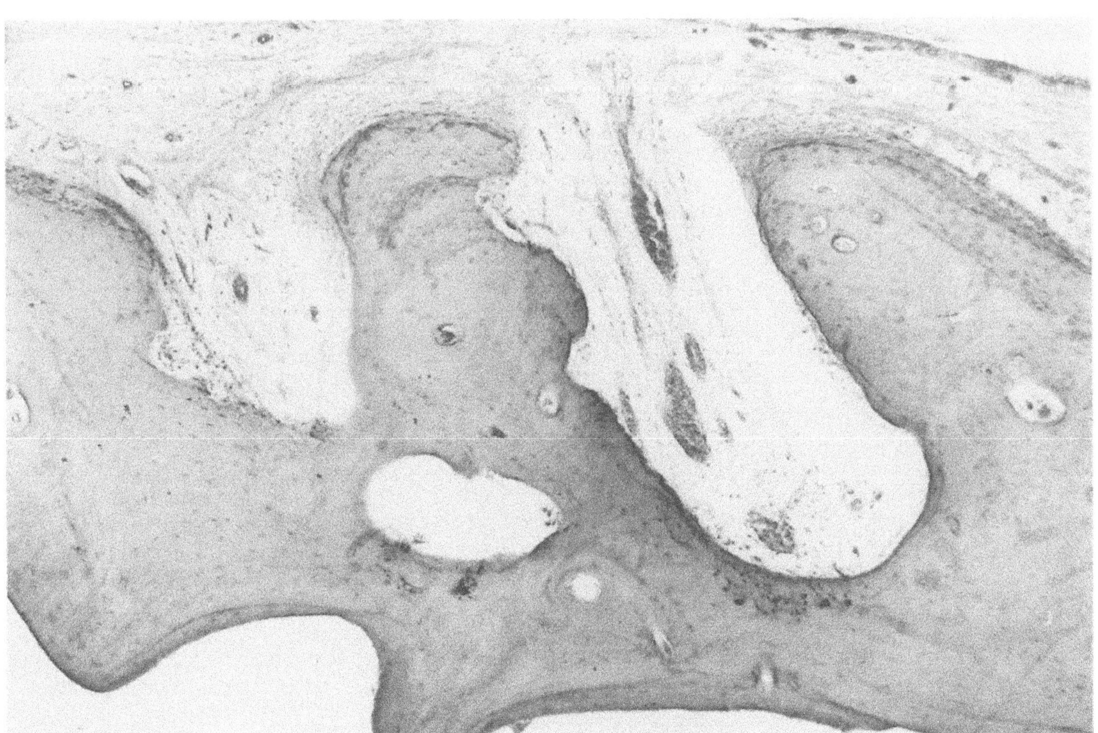

Knee-joint. "Repair" of a cartilaginous defect through a scar plate consisting of myelogenic connective tissue

Fig. 16.15
Osteoarthritis

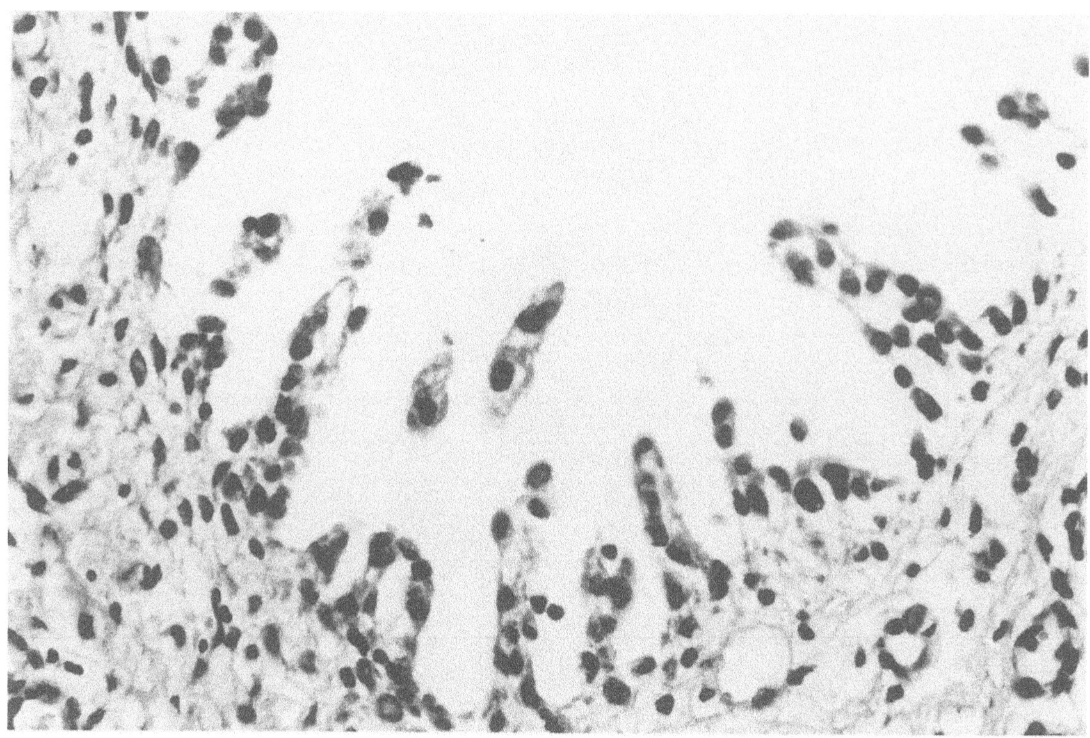

Fig. 16.16
Osteoarthritis

Accompanying synovitis with beginning villous formation in form of delicate solid lining cell sprouts ("proliferation villi")

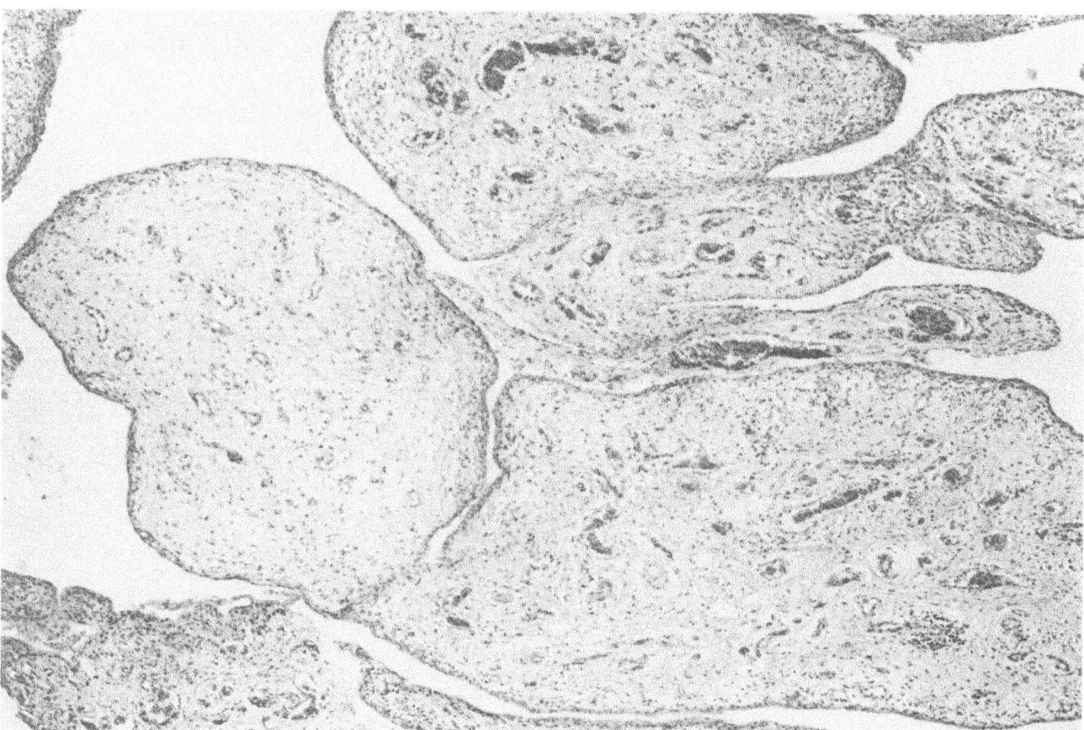

Fig. 16.17
Osteoarthritis

High-grade synovial hyperplasia as remnant of repeated accompanying synovitides. Subsided inflammatory process. The lining cell layer is single-layered, flat. Several persistent lymphocytic foci. Paltry formation of new blood vessels ("vitreous villi")

Apart from the persistent marked villous formation, the acute inflammation found in OA and traumatic synovitis can also be recognized by the discrete deposition of fibrinous exudate, lining cell hyperplasia, and diffuse lymphocytic infiltration (Figs. 16.18, 16.19). Larger collections of fibrin leading to villous remodelling as seen in RA are not a feature of OA and traumatic synovitis. As the secondary synovitis subsides, lymphocytic infiltrates may persist for months and years in the stroma of the villi in the form of small round follicles with a central small blood vessel, sometimes with real germinal centres (Figs. 16.20).

Lymph follicles

In how far diffuse or focal lymphocytic infiltrations in the synovial membrane in OA not only in the phenotype are identical with those in RA must remain open. Immunology and molecular biology have to show whether the findings of Johnell and coworkers (1985) are lasting, according to which the content of T cells, macrophages, and cell presenting HLA-DR antigens in the synovial membrane in OA differs from RA only quantitatively keep valid with time.

Degeneration of synovial tissue

These lymphocytic foci are no sign of actual inflammation, but suggest the processes of antigen presentation and antibody formation and may bear witness to the triggering of immunological mechanisms within the context of OA.

The equipment of the synovial membrane in OA with immunocompetent cells is an expression for an immunological reaction with cartilaginous antigens occurring in the course of cartilage and bone destruction (collagen fibres type II, proteoglycanes, and chondrocytes) from which one may draw conclusion to the further progress of OA (Johnell et al. 1985; Fassbender and Zwick 1995).

Secondary chondrocalcinosis

The episodic periods of synovitis occurring during the course of OA lead to increasing formation of clumsy villi. With the gradual loss of joint congruency, the hypertrophic-thickened synovial membrane is subjected to increasing trauma causing an increase in hyalinisation of the villous stroma, disappearance of blood vessels, and atrophy or loss of the lining cell layer. After the blood vessels have perished, a chondroid metaplasia can be observed within a ragged hyalinized synovial tissue with flattened, fibrinoid-swollen, irregular borders totally unrecognizable as synovial membrane. This „burnt-out“ tissue is structureless and not able to initiate an inflammatory reaction (Figs. 16.21, 16.22).

The chondroid metaplastic transformation of synovial tissue provides the pathobiological conditions for the deposition of pyrophosphate crystals. This secondary chondrocalcinosis which establishes at the end stage of synovial scarring is clinically insignificant.

Fibrosis and hyalinisation of the synovial tissue occurring in OA lasting over several decades lead to a decline of the supporting capillary network. As a result, the supply of nutrients to the remaining articular cartilage is decreased and the destruction of the articular surface is accelerated.

Extrinsic and intrinsic synovitis

Thus, the synovitis secondary to OA or to trauma is induced by cartilage-derived fragments in the synovial fluid, i.e. "extrinsic", while the inflammatory reaction in systemic synovitis (e.g. in RA) arises via the synovial capillary network, i.e. "intrinsic". Accordingly, the morphological appearances of synovitides in OA or traumatic synovitides are fundamentally different from those seen in systemic synovitis.

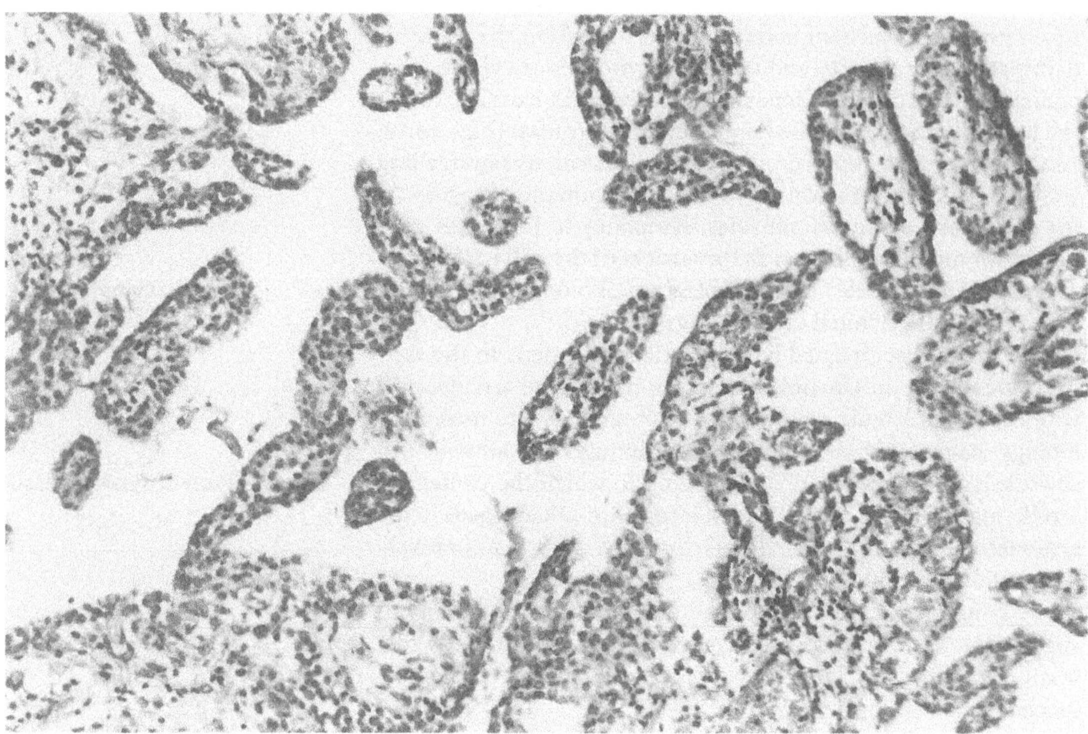

Fig. 16.18
Osteoarthritis

Hyperplastic accompanying synovitis. The lining cell layer is single- or double-layered, cuboid. Paltry, diffuse lymphocytic infiltration in the loose stroma

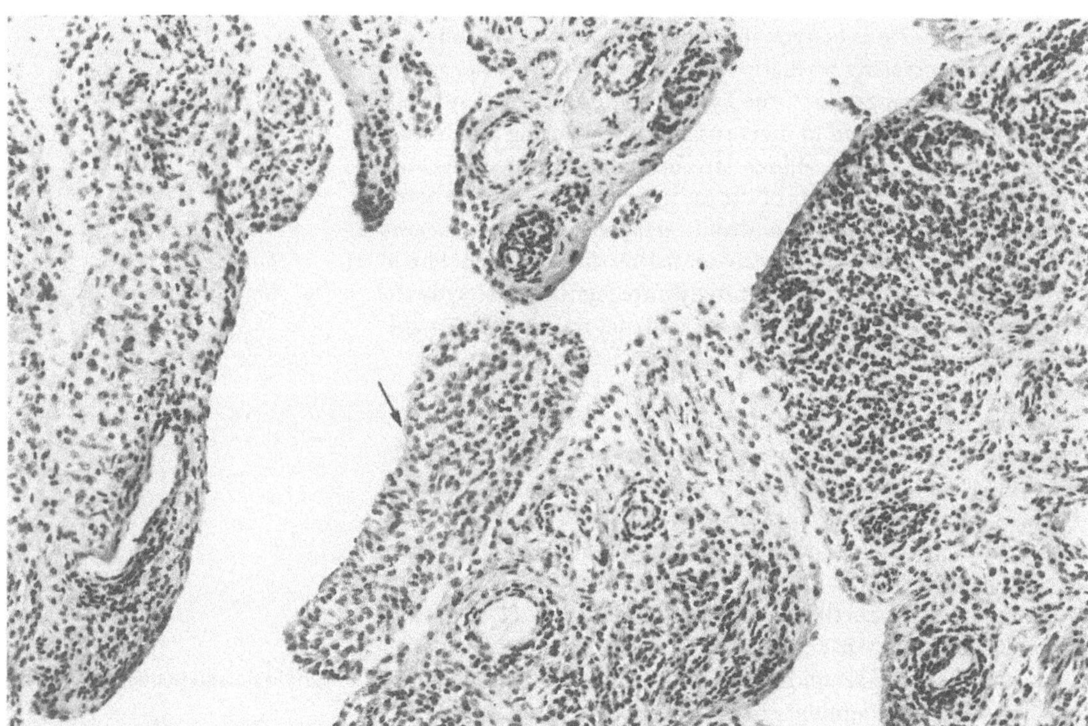

Fig. 16.19
Osteoarthritis

Marked hyperplastic accompanying synovitis. The lining cell layer is single- or multi-layered, cuboid (*arrow*). Considerable lymphocytic infiltration. Paltry formation of new blood vessels

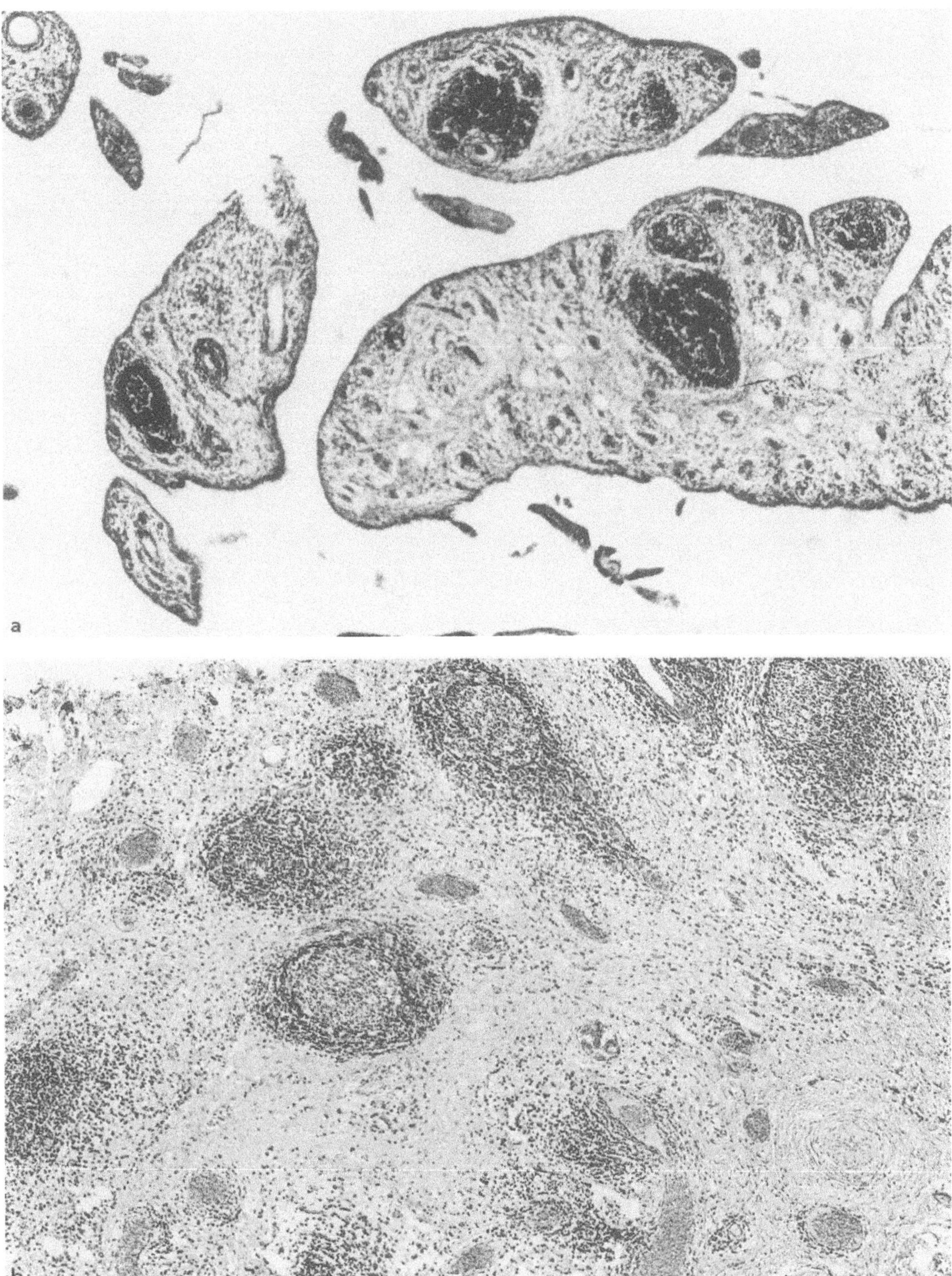

a Persisting lymph follicles in an old synovial villus with fibrotic stroma and flat lining cell layer. The inflammatory process is burnt-out. **b** Knee-joint. Lymph follicles with extensive germinal centres within the fibrotic stroma of synovial villi

Fig. 16.20 a,b
Osteoarthritis

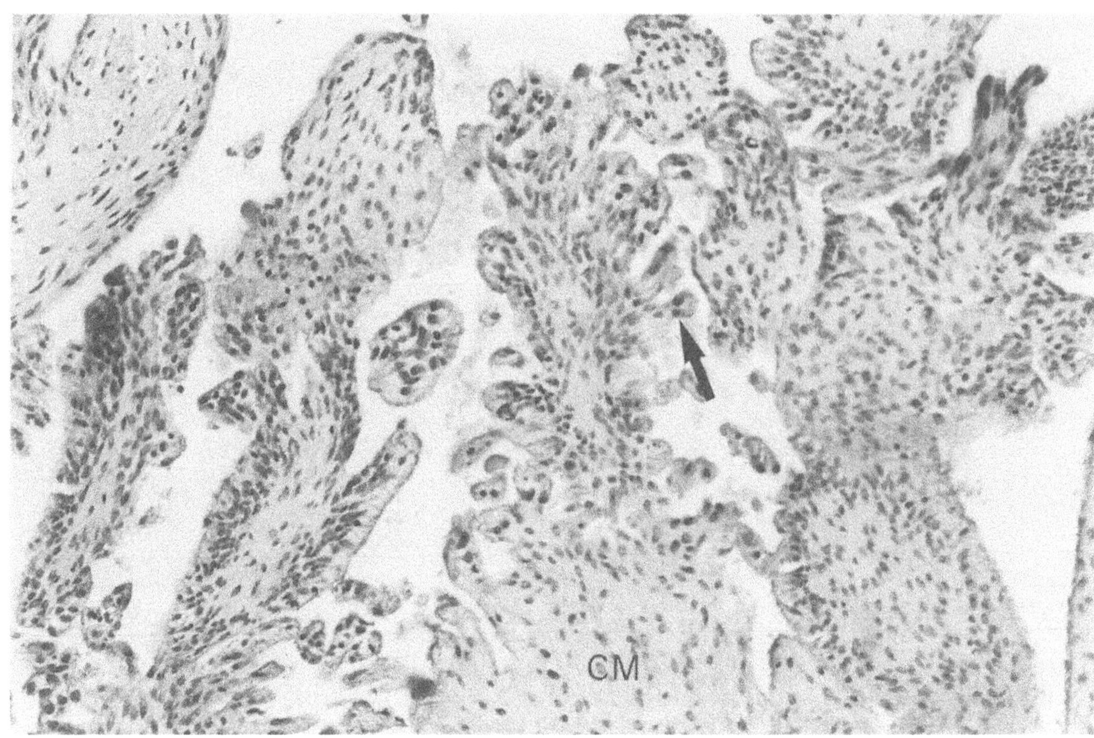

Fig. 16.21
Osteoarthritis

Hip-joint. Synovitic recidivation with buds of delicate proliferation villi (*arrow*) at the bottom of an old scarred synovial membrane with hyalinisation and chondroid metaplasia (*CM*)

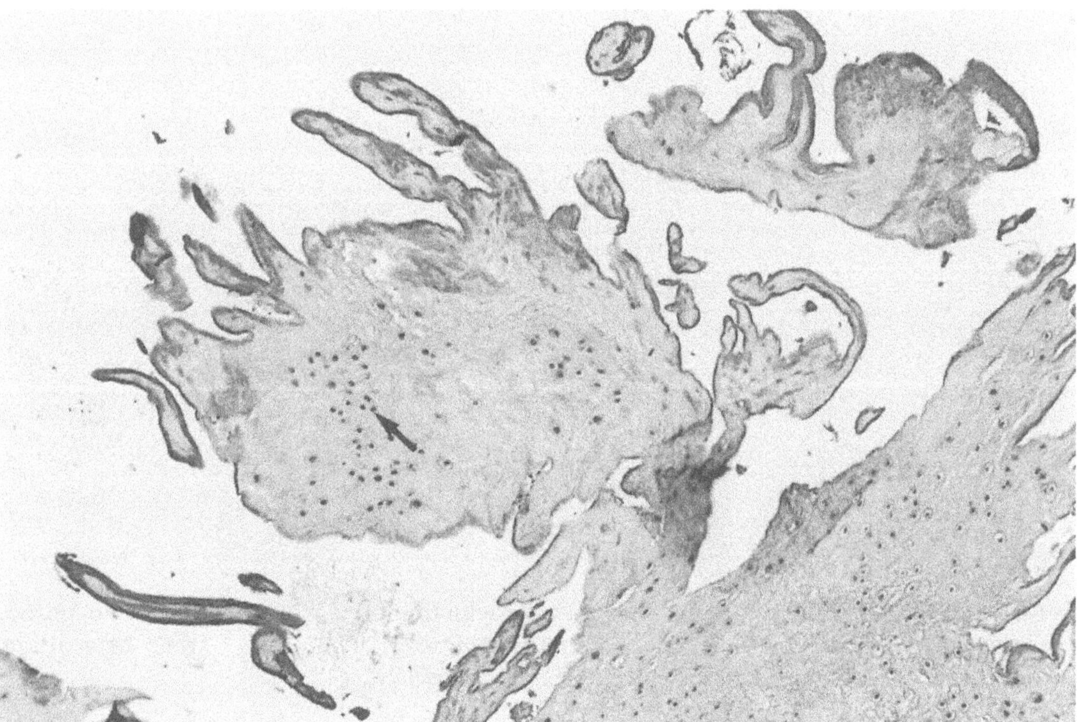

Fig. 16.22
Osteoarthritis

Knee-joint. Scarred residual state after accompanying synovitides coursed over years. Fibrotic and hyalinized synovial membrane. Large areas show chondroid metaplasia (*arrow*). The surface is mechanically lacerated

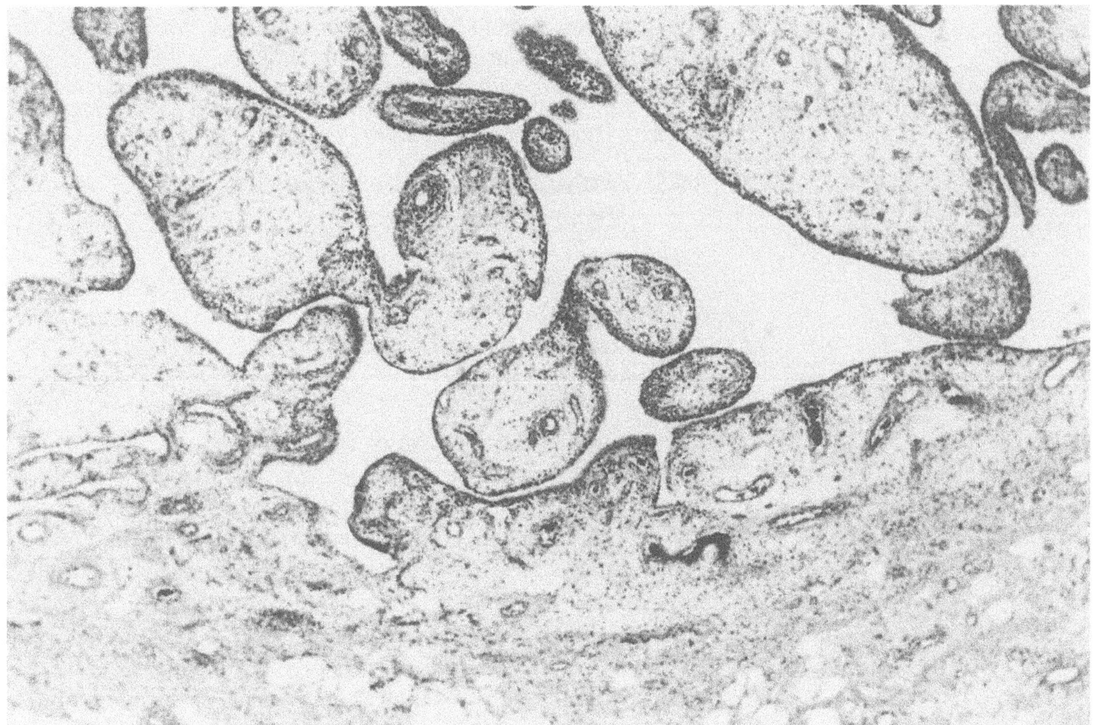

Hip-joint. Persistent villous hyperplasia after chronically recurrent accompanying synovitis and formation of plump villi

Fig. 16.23
Osteoarthritis

Changes occurring secondary to destructive mechanical forces are most often seen with OA of the hip.

Peculiarities of coxarthrosis

In coxarthrosis, further predisposing components can be added to the general factors being responsible for the genesis and development of OA. Solomon (1976) and Murray (1965) estimate that up to 80% of hip OA are secondarily based congenitally on developmental defects. X-ray studies of the hip joint have suggested to some investigators that acetabular dysplasia is the basis of most of the OA cases of the hip.

Legg-Calvé-Perthes disease

Legg-Calvé-Perthes disease is an avascular necrosis of the proximal capital femoral epiphysis. Its peak incidence occurs between 4 and 8 years of age. The condition is more common in boys than in girls. The softened femoral head is distorted and the surface incongruities lead to development of OA (Brandt 1985b).

The changes of the synovial membrane in OA of the hip differ quantitatively from those of other joints: the villi are generally more numerous, shorter, and plumper. The height of the lining cell layer varies depending on the state of irritation of the local process. The stroma of the villi is distinctly more fibrotic. The newly formed blood vessels are wider and show thicker walls than during OA in other joints (Fig. 16.23). The infiltration of lymphocytes and plasma cells is focal. In contrast, siderophages are often found in the fibrous stroma next to small bone fragments. They give evidence of numerous traumas which occur over the years in the joints of patients suffering from OA.

Frequently, fragments of bone and cartilage can be seen within the fibrous scar tissue as well as in hyalinized fibrous parts of tissue. The joint capsule tissue which undergoes hyalinisation and chondroid metaplasia is not infrequently the site of focal deposits of calcium pyrophosphate crystals (see p. 343).

16.5 Polyarthrosis of the Fingers (Heberden's Arthrosis)

The classification of primary OA currently defines three categories:
1. Idiopathic OA
2. Generalized OA
3. Erosive OA

These categories include OA of small finger joints.
Based upon the structural changes and the different biomechanical environment, we would like to classify on etiological, pathological, and morphological grounds the non-erosive and erosive OA processes of the finger joints as distinct from OA affecting the large joints.
OA of the finger joints predominantly occurs in women around the time of menopause. The distal interphalangeal joints are most commonly affected, but in a few cases, the proximal interphalangeal joints also may be involved (the lack of involvement of the metacarpophalangeal joints helps to diagnostically distinguish OA from RA). In finger OA, small nodules appear over affected joints. In 1802, Heberden gave the following description of these phenomena characterized by their location as well as their relationship to the sex and age of the patients:

Heberden's node

> "What are these small hard nodes, the size of a pea which are frequently seen on fingers, slightly proximal to the finger tips and close to a joint? They are not the nodules of gout since they occur in patients who have never suffered from this disease. They remain for the rest of the patient's life and are never painful. They never become inflamed. They are disfiguring rather than disturbing, but they may interfere somewhat with finger movements."

Heberden's nodes develop over the marginal osteophytes of the interphalangeal joint. They arise in the overlying skin secondary to degeneration of the collagenous subcutaneous tissue. In this way, small cystic swellings are formed which may become reddened and, in contrast to Heberden's description, can be moderately painful. The content of the cysts tends to mucilaginisation.
The joint changes themselves, which only develop later, were not described by Heberden, although they are known as "Heberden arthrosis" in the European continental literature. The OA is progressive and may often affect all terminal interphalangeal joints symmetrically. The process commences with cartilage degeneration, reactive osteosclerosis, osteophyte formation, and metaplasia of cartilage.
Similar changes as seen in finger OA can also occur in the toe joints. The radiographic appearances of this form of polyarthrosis demonstrate loss of joint space of the terminal and interpha-

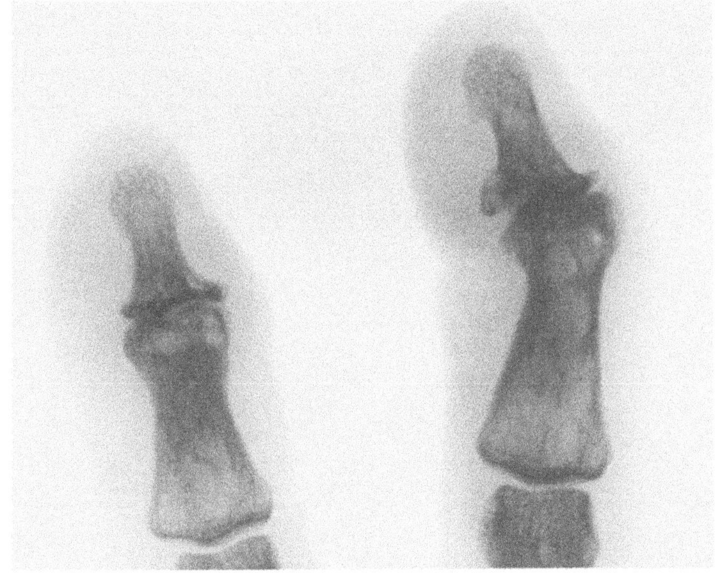

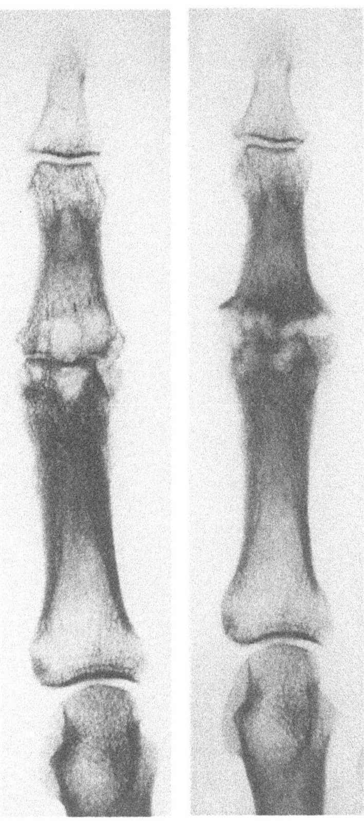

Left: Fifty-three-year-old female. Partial subluxation of distal interphalangeal joints
Right: Fifty-six-year-old female. Subchondral cysts affecting the proximal interphalangeal joints

Figs. 16.24 and 16.25 Polyarthrosis

langeal joints with maintenance of the contour and bone structures and subluxation (Fig. 16.24). The appearance of small capsular ossifications is an important diagnostic distinction from RA (Müller and Schilling 1982).

About 4%–5% of patients with finger OA have evidence of destructive changes, most frequently in the interphalangeal joints. In this destructive form, the joint surface is underminded by formation of cysts and destruction of articular bone (Fig. 16.25). There is also a tendency to repair with formation of new smooth contours or bony ankylosis. As with other forms of OA, the primary degenerative process may later be associated with secondary inflammation. The radiographic destructive appearances may lead to confusion with RA. Characteristically, however, erosive OA is associated with a particularly painful OA of the first carpometacarpal joint (termed "rhizarthrosis" in the European literature). Similar involvement is also seen in the toes where the first metatarsophalangeal joint is predominantly involved.

Synovitis

Communication with marrow spaces following tissue destruction may be a major factor in this. In cases of this destructive form, we have observed the histological features of chronic synovitis. Small fragments of bone were seen in the tissue (Fig. 16.26). The fibrous tissue capsule also contained bony frag-

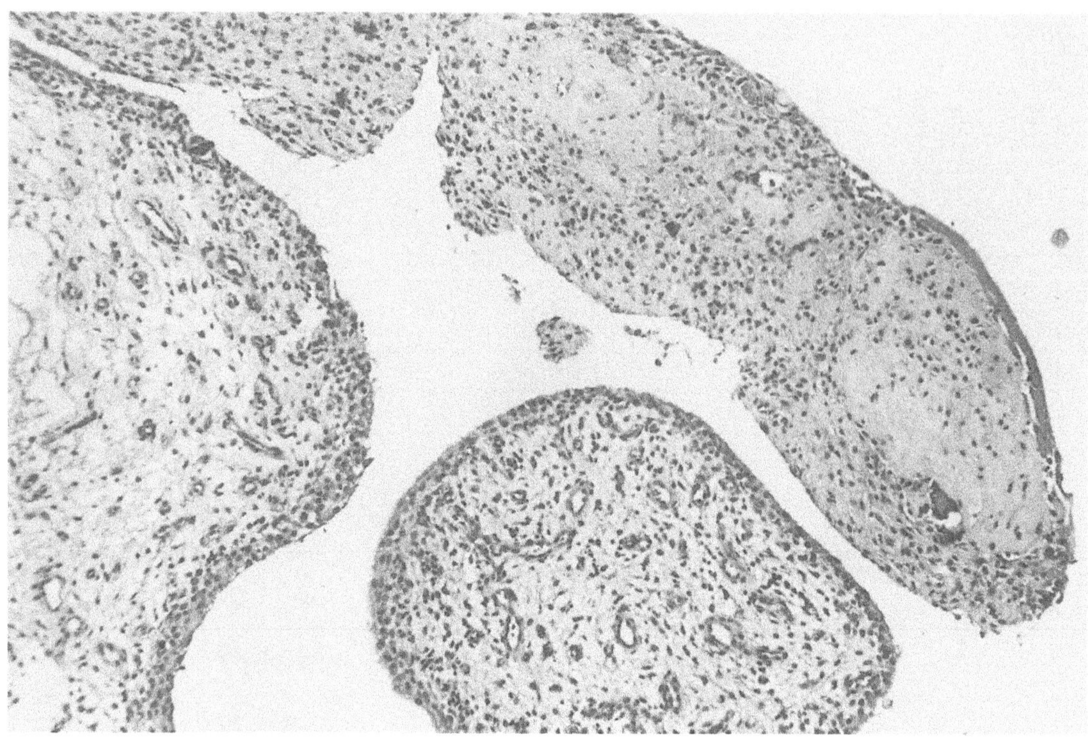

Fig. 16.26
Polyarthrosis

Proximal interphalangeal joint. Synovitis showing lining cell hyperplasia with adherent fibrin. Villus on right of picture shows bone and cartilage fragments

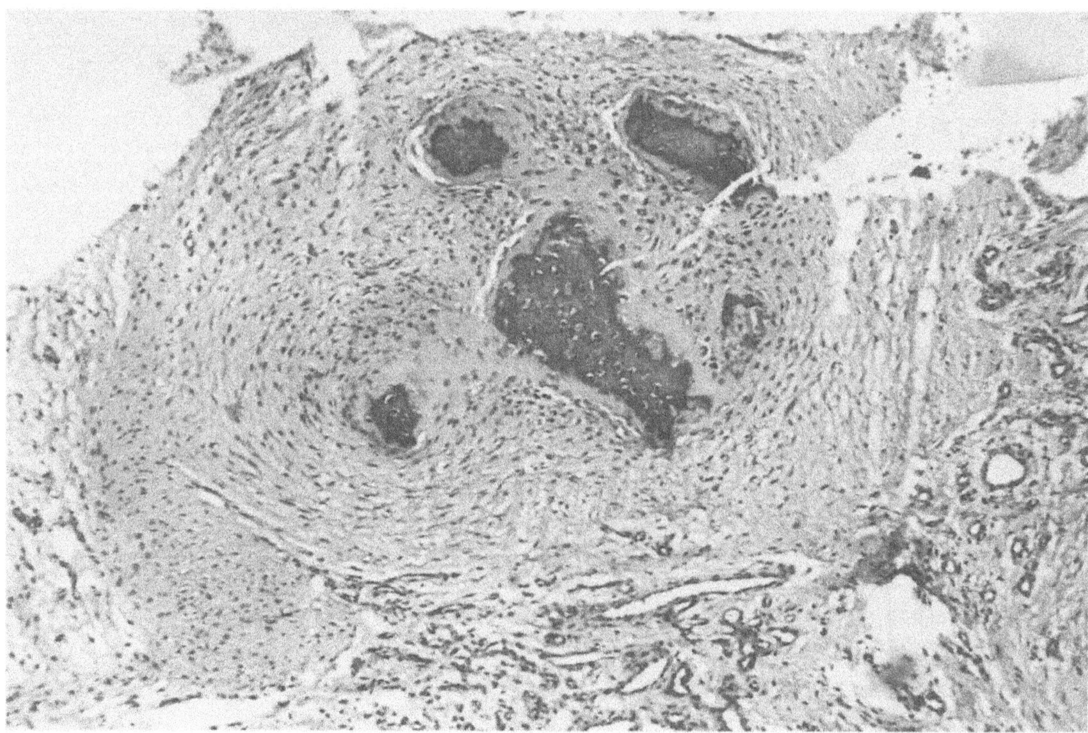

Fig. 16.27
Polyarthrosis

Distal interphalangeal joint. Bone fragments in scarred synovial tissue

ments surrounded by seams of osteoid and a fibrous capsule as witnesses of the destructive process (Fig. 16.27). In a few cases, the synovial tissue contained remarkable foamy structures surrounded by fibroblasts while in the fibrous capsular layer there were lymphocyte collections around small vessels.
Involvement of the proximal interphalangeal joints is regarded as an equivalent of Heberden's nodes and is often falsely associated with the name Bouchard (1837–1915). The changes described by Bouchard affected younger patients with flexion deformities of their fingers and these patients were said to have had gastric dilatation as an associated feature (Crain 1961).
While OA of the large joints essentially is the result of mechanical stress, the process of finger polyarthrosis is in this way not explainable. We consider that neuro-vascular influences may here play a significant role. The survival of joint cartilage in the adult is in any case based on a critical metabolic supply situation. This may explain why neuro-hormonal disturbances of the climacteric may be of special significance and introduce a systemic factor affecting joint cartilage, especially that of terminal finger and toe joints. Such disturbances may lead to cartilage loss and bone erosion and re-formation. Thus, it is understandable that especially the end-phalanges, which in the climacteric are poorly supplied with blood, suffer under trophic disturbances. We consider these structural changes in finger polyarthrosis (Heberden's nodes) as collapse of cartilaginous as well as osseous tissue as a consequence of vascular insufficiency. Inflammatory or proliferative processes, which possibly could play a role in the joint destruction, have never been observed in our material from patients with finger polyarthrosis.

Neuro-vascular influences

16.6 Generalized OA

Heberben's nodes are frequently associated with OA of the hip, knee, and cervical spine. This has given rise to the concept of "generalized OA" occurring as part of a systemic process (Kellgren and Moore 1952). This syndrome mainly affects women in the 5th to 7th decade. Since Heberden's nodes are found in 60% of women over the age of 55 years, the co-existence of OA of the large joints is extremely likely (Lawrence 1969).
OA of the cervical spine affects all of the major spinal articulations including the intervertebral disks, the apophyseal joints, the ligamentous connections between the vertebrae, and the vertebral bodies themselves.
Osteophyte spur formation on the vertebral bodies is prominent, most frequently seen at the anterior aspect of the vertebrae. Apophyseal joint involvement characteristically exhibits joint space narrowing, bony sclerosis, and spur formation.

OA of the cervical spine

16.7 Pathological Remarks

Although the involvement of various joints simultaneously can be attributed to the aging process, the results of recent cartilage research give insight into the fate of the articular cartilage. They reveal that the matrix components are part of a complex system whose integrity guarantees the quality of hyaline cartilage. The chondrocytes are responsible for the synthesis of the elements of the matrix as well as for the production of degradative enzymes. It thus is likely that synthesis and degradation form part of a very highly regulated process adapted to the biological environment. It also is possible that genetic defects may give rise to impaired chondrocyte function. In both events, a systemic failure of the entire chondrocyte system may be possible.

17 Crystal-Associated Arthropathies

Metabolic diseases

The crystal-associated arthropathies are a group of metabolic diseases in which crystals (especially monosodium urate, calcium pyrophosphate dihydrate, and calcium hydroxyapatite) are deposited in and around joints. One can differentiate three crystal-induced arthropathies: gout, calcium pyrophosphate dihydrate crystal deposition disease, and hydroxyapatite crystal deposition disease.

17.1 Gout

Synonym: monosodium urate arthropathy.

17.1.1 Definition

It seems likely that the word "gout" takes its origin from the Latin "gutta" denoting a drop, in which form the putative toxin was supposed to be deposited in an affected joint.

Hereditary disposition

Löffler and Koller (1955) decided that the origin of the word "gout" was derived from an old German term for "speaking", since it was a matter for much discussion. Gout is a disease resting on a hereditary disposition and showing a familial aggregation. It is characterized by hyperuricaemia associated with a complex disturbance of the metabolism of purines; the classical picture is one of recurring attacks of particularly painful acute arthritis and the deposition of monosodium urate crystals in the articular, periarticular, and subcutaneous tissue.

17.1.2 Historical Background

Already Hippocrates entitled the "podagra" ("gouty foot") as the most painful of all joint diseases.

Sydenham's description

A more differentiated description of the acute gout we owe to Sydenham (1683; Fig. 17.1). He attributed gouty arthritis quite rightly to "be caused by gluttonous feast of the night before. The patient goes to sleep in apparently good health and is awakened by sudden onset of pain about 2 h after midnight, usually affecting the great toe but occasionally also the heel, sole or ankle. The pain resembles that of a subluxation of these bones. This is quickly followed by shivering and fever in proportion to the pain which is mild at first but grows gradually more violent every hour" (from Sydenham quoted in Copeman 1964).

The caricatures of the 18th and 19th century illustrate the pain as well as the corpulence and social stature of those suffering from acute gouty attack (Fig. 17.2).

Political and social components

A political component was added to the social significance of urate gout as it used to be a disease that afflicted the wealthy and those belonging to leading classes. That Alexander the Great (356–323 B.C.) and Charlemagne (768–814 A.D.) were vexed by the disease was significant enough for the historians to pass it on to posterity. The lives of several English kings were affected by the symptoms of urate gout. The wedding of Henry VII (1457–1509) with Lady Margaret, for example, had to be postponed due to an attack of gout. One therefore understands Sydenham, being a victim of the disease himself, lamenting: "For humble beings like me there is only one, pathetic comfort: unlike any other disease, gout kills more of the wealthy than of the poor, more of the educated than of the simple minds, famous emperors, kings, generals, naval officers, and philosophers fell victim to it. It is here that nature proves its impartiality: those who are being favoured in one respect, are being punished in another" (Mertz 1990).

17.1.3 Epidemiology

Gout is uncommon before the third decade of life. It occurs with increasing frequency from the second to the sixth decade, showing some preference for the fourth decade. The prevalence varies worldwide. It is similar in Europe (0.3%) and North America (0.27%; Lawrence 1960; Wyngaarden 1960). Among 4,663 Parisian men aged 20–44 years, the prevalence was 1.1% in the age group 35–39 years, and 2% in the group 40–44 years of age (Zalokar et al. 1981). The prevalence of gout is related to the serum urate levels. Over 90% of patients with gout are men. The age of peak incidence in men is earlier than that of women, who rarely

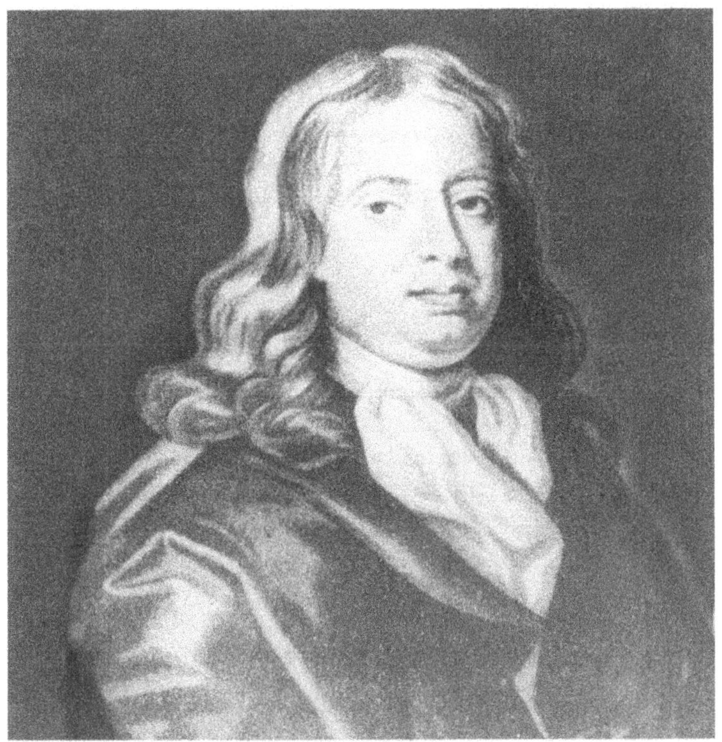

Thomas Sydenham, 1624–1689, physician in London

Fig. 17.1

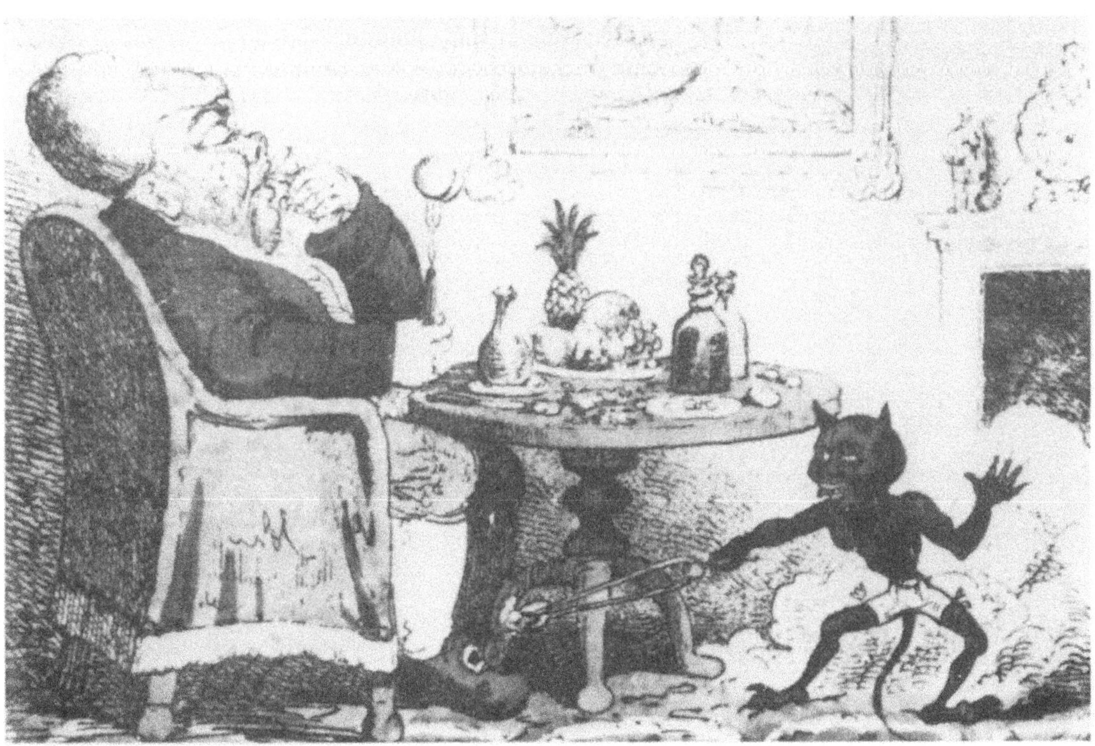

Onset of gout. Engraving (chalkography) by George Cruikshank (1792–1878), published April 9, 1818 by S.W. Forbes. British Museum, London (Mertz 1990)

Fig. 17.2

develop the disorder before menopause (Turner et al. 1960; Harth and Robinson 1962).

Significance of nourishment

The significance of nourishment for the development of gout show the disappearance of gout during the war and the enormously increased incidence of the disease in the 1950s and subsequent years in West Germany rising from a few cases per 1,000 to the present incidence of 2% amongst males (Schilling 1967).

17.1.4 Clinical Manifestations

Metatarsophalangeal joint

Non-articular tissue

Mechanical factors and micro-trauma of tissues may play a part in the articular involvement of gout. In 70% of cases, the first joint to be affected is the metatarsophalangeal joint of the big toe (Fig. 17.3). The severe local disease, which is associated with systemic signs of inflammation, gives the false impression of septic arthritis. Urate may, however, also be deposited in non-articular tissues such as bursae, tendons, and tendon sheaths. Tissue deposition is favoured by local factors such as low turn-over and pH of tissue fluid. Uric-acid precipitation shows some association with the occurrence of sulphated mucopolysaccharides in connective tissue.

The characteristic course of gout is marked by three phases: an acute gouty attack, an intercritical phase, and a chronic tophaceous phase.

Acute gouty arthritis

The symptoms and signs of acute gouty arthritis are preceded by hyperuricaemia of some duration. Classic site of initial attack is the base of the great toe. Other common initial sites of involvement include instep, ankle, heel, knee, wrist, fingers, and elbows (olecranon bursa).

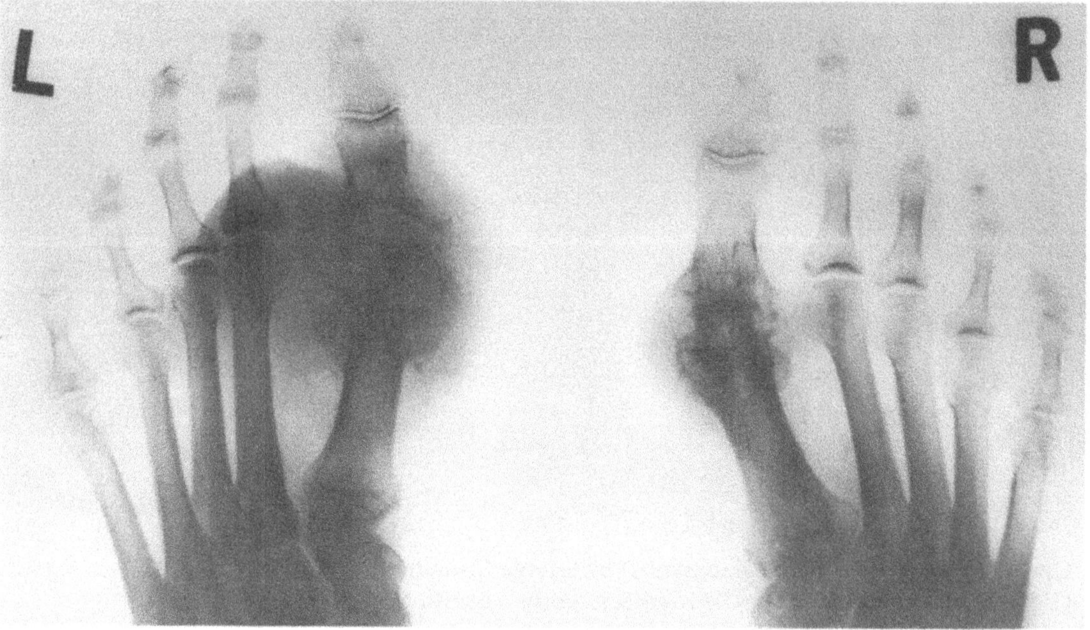

Fig. 17.3
Gout

Destruction of metatarsophalangeal joints of both big toes with tophi in soft tissues. Male aged 56 years with advanced gout

About 80% of initial attacks are monarticular. Polyarticular attacks are more common in elderly women and in patients with gout accompanying myeloproliferative disorders or the use of cyclosporine. Initial attacks may subside in several hours or may persist for only a few days. Severe attacks may last many days to several weeks. The acute relapsing gout is marked by attacks which, if untreated, last from several days to several weeks with intervals of complete clinical remission. An asymptomatic phase, termed intercritical period, in which the patient is once again well, can follow. This freedom from symptoms period is an important feature in the diagnosis of gouty arthritis. This intercritical period can be interrupted by further attacks.

Relapsing gout

Intercritical period

It is only in the later phase of disease that chronic gouty arthritis becomes established, usually involving several joints together with the multifocal appearance of gouty tophi. This chronic tophaceous phase is characterized by the identifiable deposition of solid urate (tophi) in connective tissues.

Chronic tophaceous phase

The clinical significance of an urate granuloma depends on its location. Tophi situated in the subcutaneous tissue, which tend to undergo calcification, may ulcerate and become secondarily infected. In this phase of the manifested gout, the serum urate concentration ranges in general between 9 and 11 mg/dl. Tophaceous gout is often associated with an early age of onset, a long duration of active but untreated disease, frequent attacks, high serum urate values, and a predilection for upper extremities and polyarticular episodes (Nakayama 1984).

Clinical significance

Typical locations for tophaceous depositions are the helix of the ear, the olecranon, the prepatellar bursa, ulnar surfaces of the forearm, and achilles tendons. Virtually all parenchymal organs except the brain have been sites of tophus formation in one or another report (Lichtenstein et al. 1956; Stark and Hirokawa 1982).

Typical locations

Patients with urate gout frequently suffer also from diabetes mellitus (10%–25%), overweight (up to 70%), adiposis hepatica (>60%), and hyperlipoproteinaemia (>40%).

17.1.5 Etiology

Other than the rare, primary, genetically determined hyperuricaemia, the etiology of which is still unknown, secondary hyperuricaemia is the decisive factor in the pathogenesis of gout. This secondary form may originate in two ways: by increased uric acid production from endogenous as well as exogenous purines in the presence of normal renal function, or by impaired uric acid excretion (in the presence of a normal rate of production). The increased production of uric acid may have several origins, in which enzyme defects play an important role. Apart from a primary, genetically determined disposition or reasons to develop secondary hyperuricaemia, some exogeneous factors must be involved which are dietary in nature.

Hyperuricaemia originating in 2 ways

17.1.6 Pathology

Crystals of urate are deposited in the form of clusters of big needles in form of a chalky-white precipitate on the surface of articular cartilage or in connective tissue as so called tophi (Figs. 17.4–17.6).

The material penetrates through surface lesions more deeply into the cartilage substance and this is followed by further destruction (Fig. 17.7). Such erosions may coalesce into large lesions (Fig. 17.8). Tissue destruction is mediated by granulomata called forth by urate crystals. These act as foreign bodies in the connective tissue and attract histiocytes. This progresses into layers of uni- and multi-nuclear macrophages surrounding a necrotic centre (Fig. 17.9).

Granulomata

The necrotic centre of the urate granuloma contains bundles of urate needles (Figs. 17.10, 17.11). Since they are water-soluble, they are usually lost in formalin-fixed material. After fixation in alcohol, however, the crystals show impressive polarising microscopial phenomena. The monosodium-urate crystal is negatively bifringent and when viewed in a plane parallel to the axis of the compensator it is yellow, while at right angles to this it appears blue. In this way, a differentiation from calcium-pyrophosphate crystals of pseudo-gout is obtainable. These show positive bifringence and therefore a reversed colour pattern.

Monosodium-urate crystals

The clinically recognizable deposition of urate tophi in soft tissues and above all in articular structures characterizes the chronic phase of gout. In addition, the destructive gouty arthropathy is often complicated by secondary degenerative changes. In this way, grotesque tumescences at hand and feet can develop.

Chronic phase

In the course of time, the granulomata become surrounded by a vascular fibrous capsule and the gouty tophus is macroscopically visible (Fig. 17.12). Urate deposition in a joint is usually associated with synovitis which in course of months as a chronic inflammation leads to further joint damage by means of pannus and fibrosis.

Synovitis

The pathological diagnosis of gouty synovitis depends on the microscopical finding of typical urate depositions in the specimen. The accompanying synovitis itself is entirely unspecific. It shows a villous hyperplasia, the extent of which depends on the duration of the local process. Proliferation of lining cells hinges on the degree of the actual irritation. We could never observe proliferation of synovial stroma cells, but, opposed to that, we see lymphocytic infiltrates. Neutrophils, however, only found sporadically.

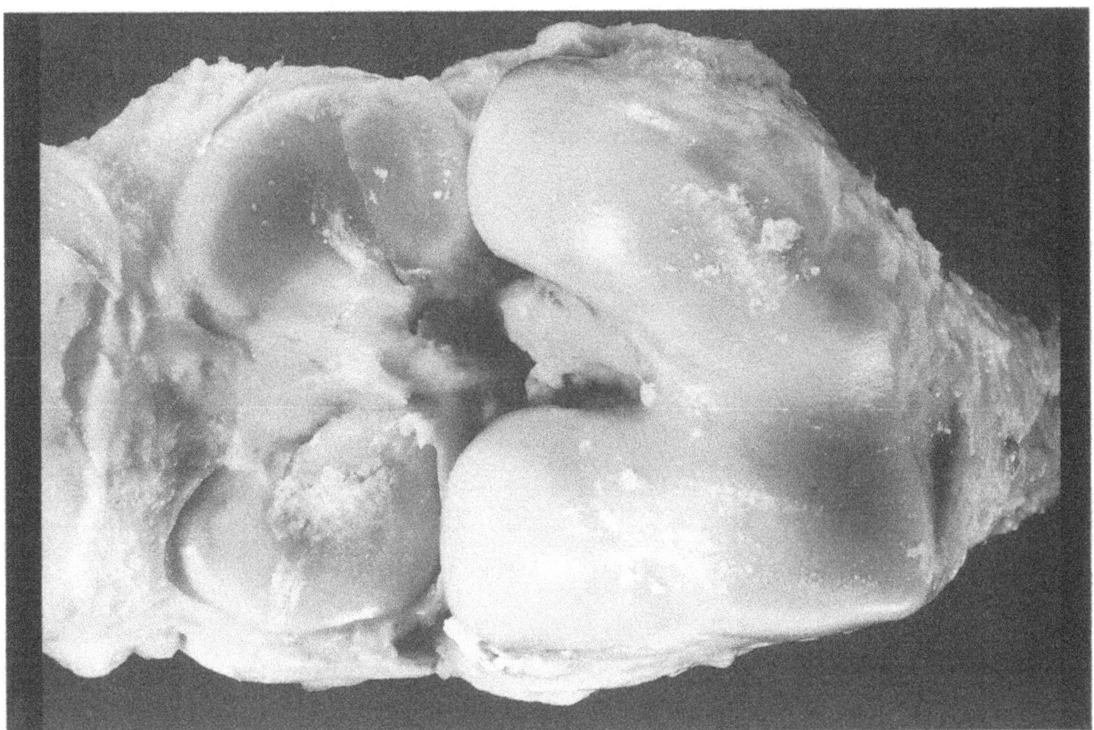

Urate deposit on cartilage of gouty knee joint. (Photograph by E. Uehlinger, University Department of Pathology, Zurich)

Fig. 17.4
Gout

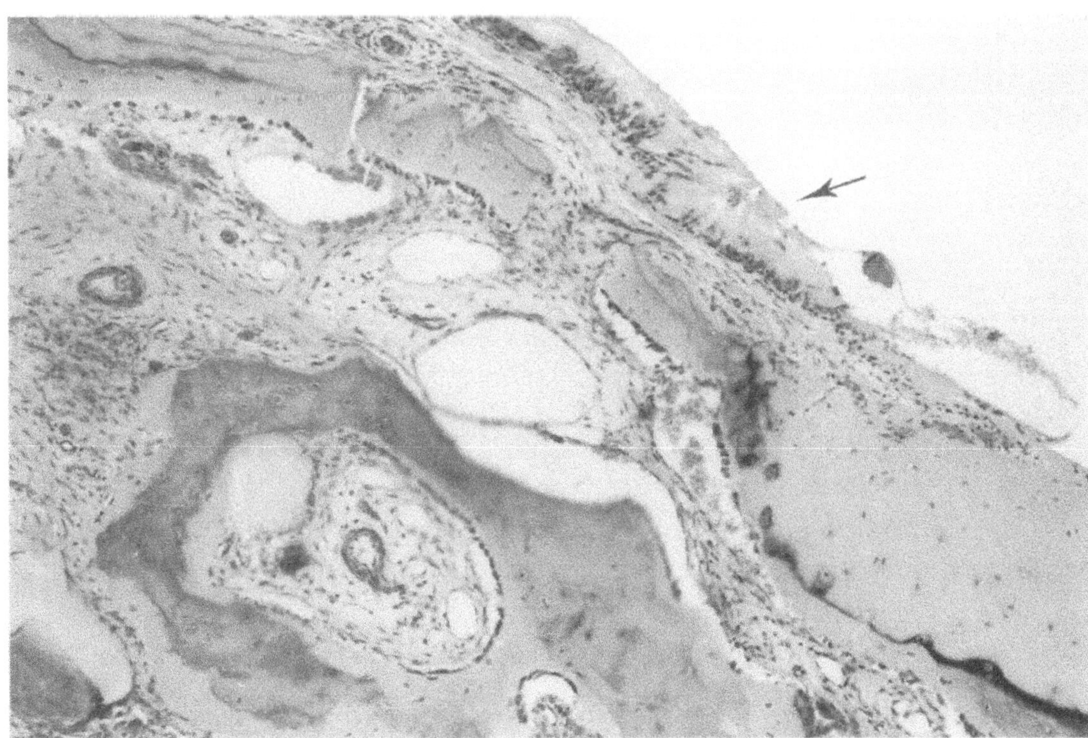

Finger joint. Cartilage destruction in a zone of urate crystal deposition on the joint surface (*arrow*). The darker outlines of macrophages are recognizable

Fig. 17.5
Gout

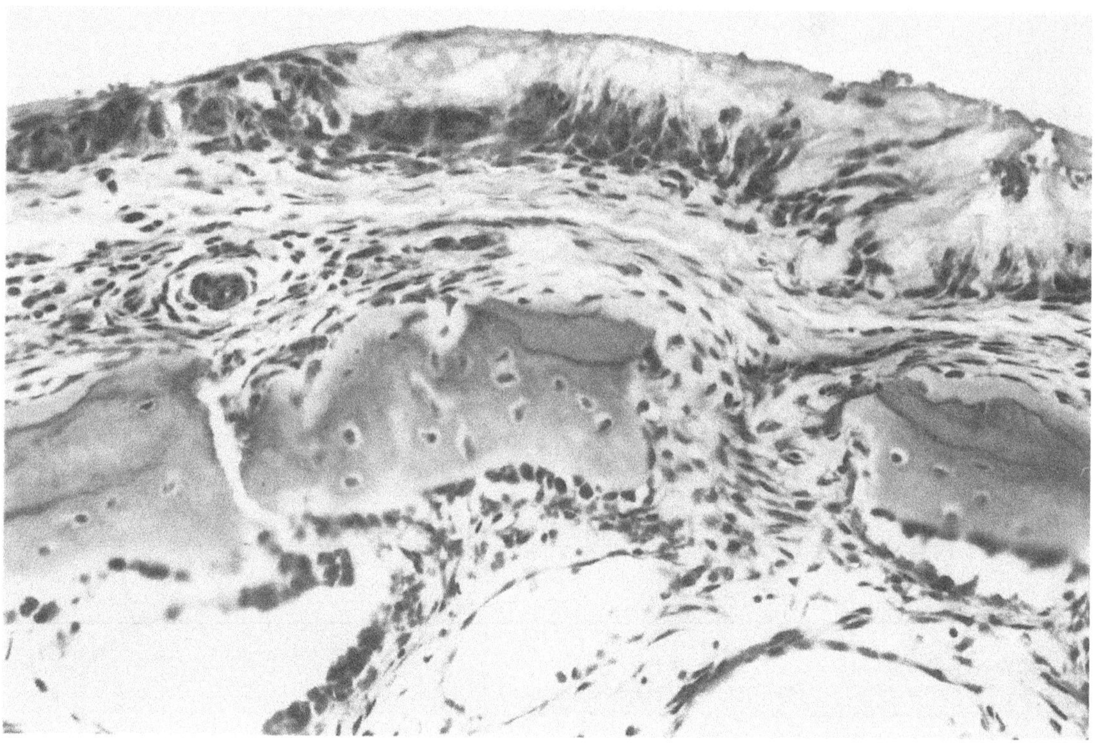

Fig. 17.6
Gout

Segment taken from Fig. 17.5. Urate deposits, surrounded by macrophages at joint surface. Local destruction of cartilage and subchondral bone

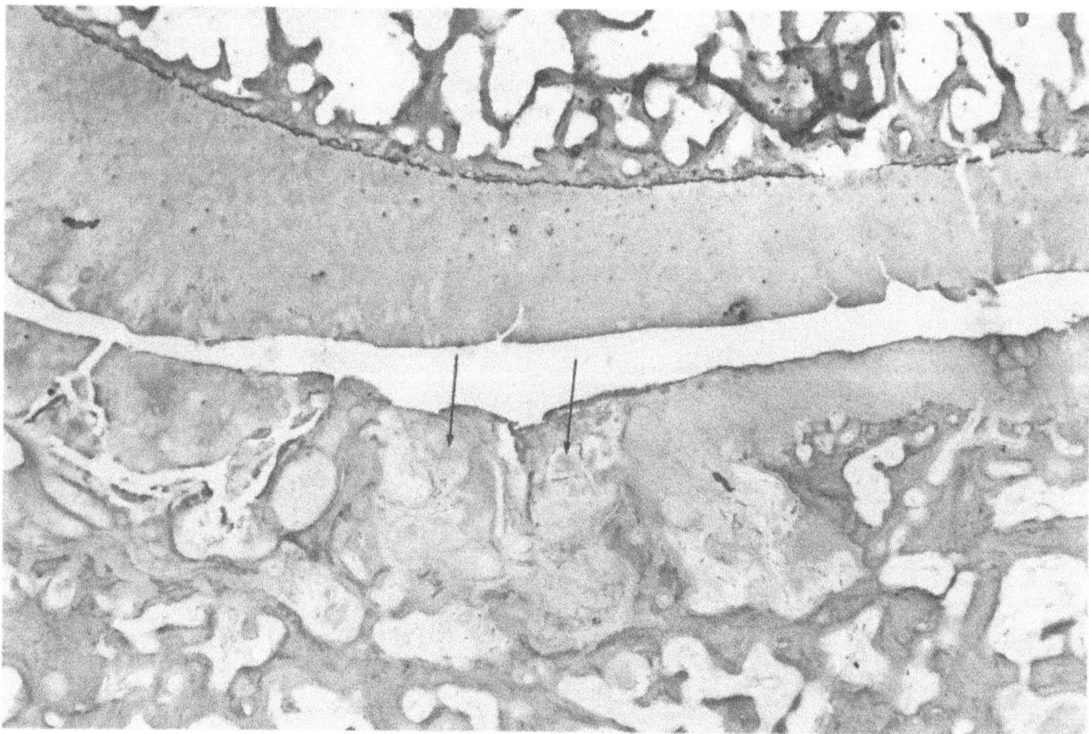

Fig. 17.7
Gout

Finger joint. Superficial urate granulomata (*arrows*) with destruction of neighbouring cartilage and bone

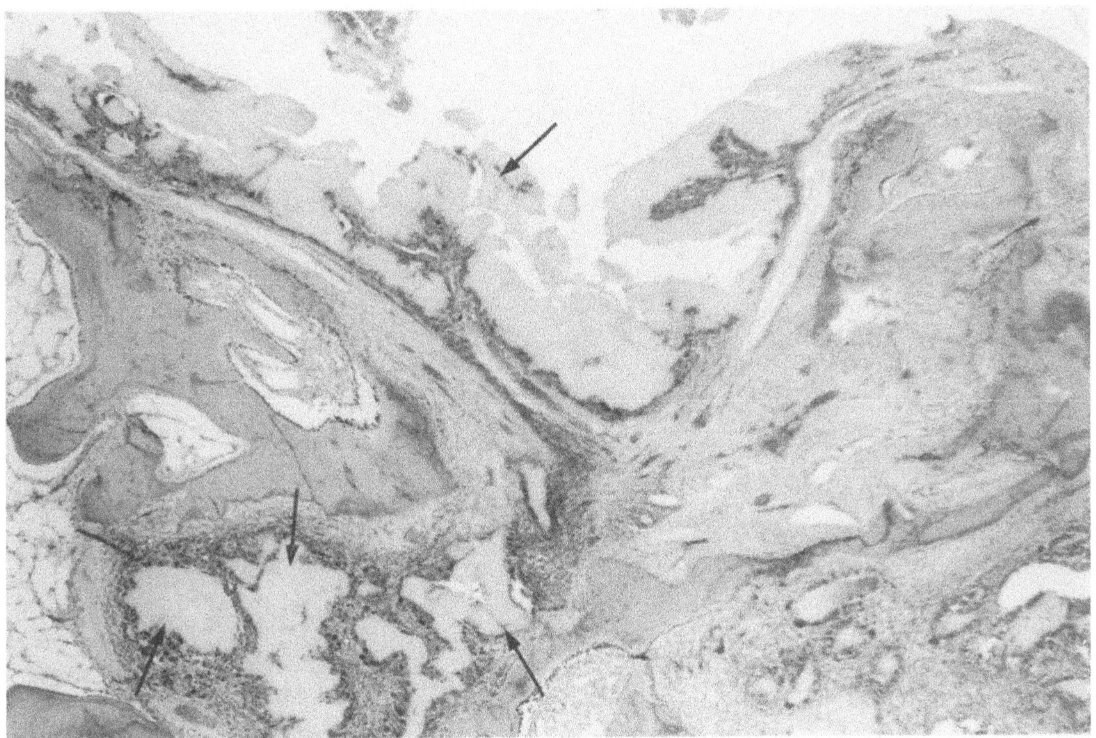

Widespread urate deposits (*arrows*) with macrophageal reaction replacing articular cartilage in a big-toe joint

Fig. 17.8
Gout

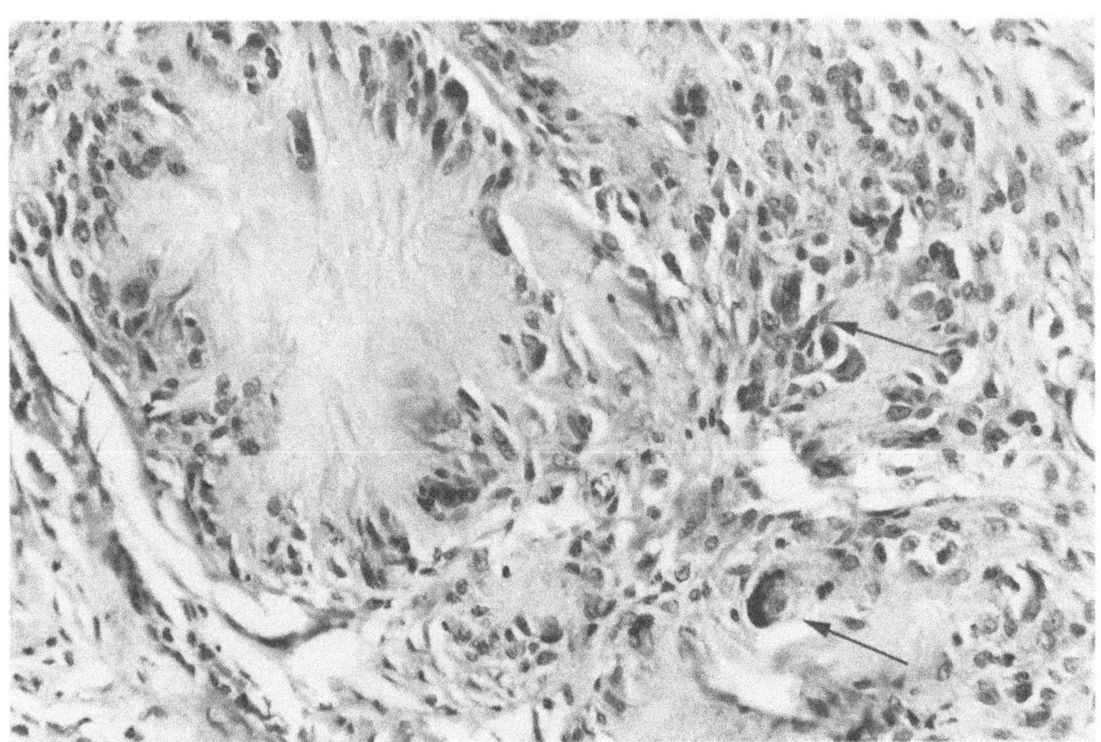

Finger joint. Recent urate granulomata, surrounded by macrophages and foreign-body giant cells (*arrows*)

Fig. 17.9
Gout

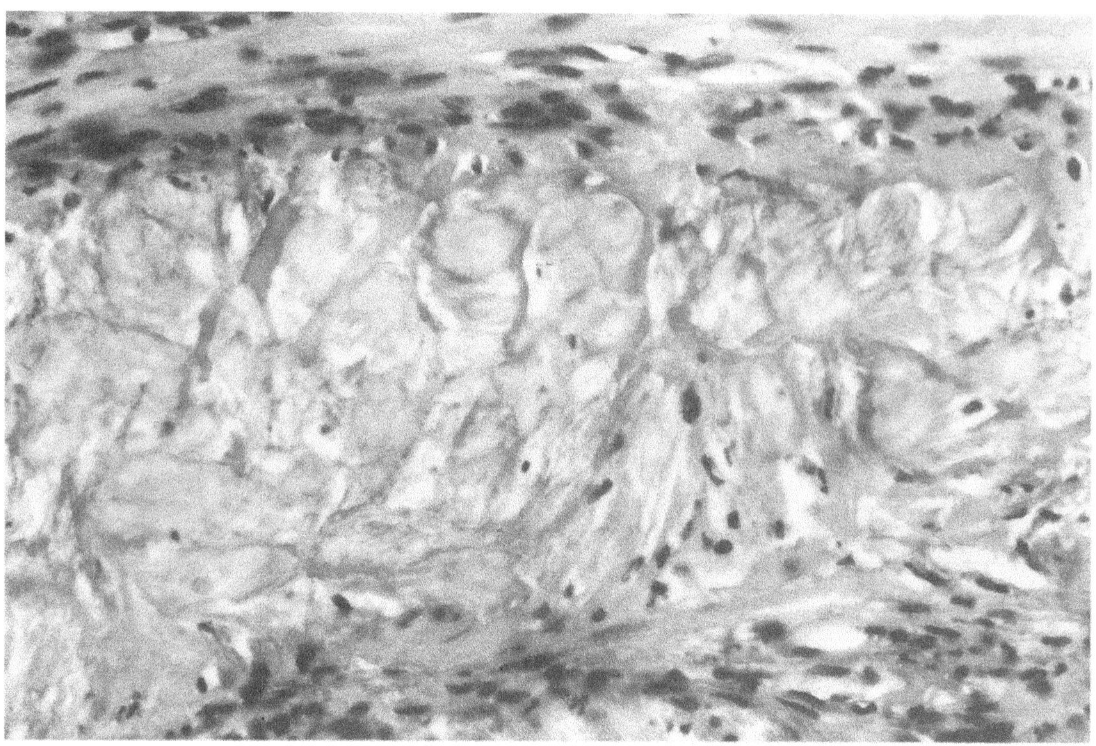

Fig. 17.10
Gout

Big toe. Collections of urate crytals in a tophus

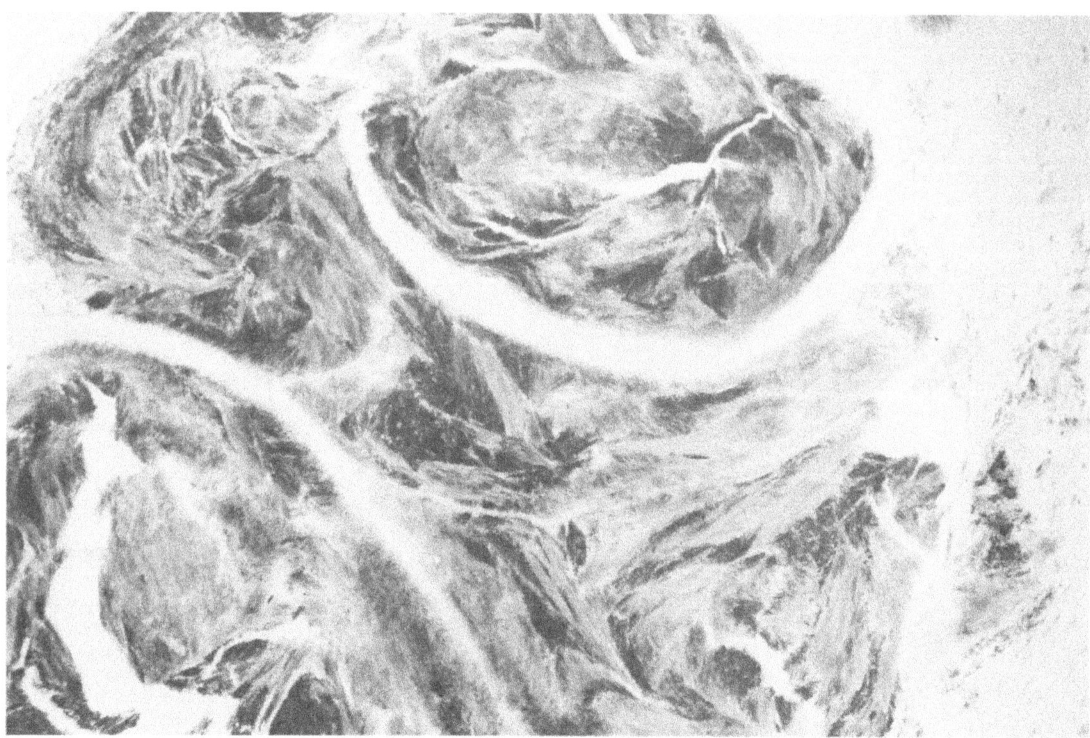

Fig. 17.11
Gout

Sheaves of urate crystals in an ear tophus

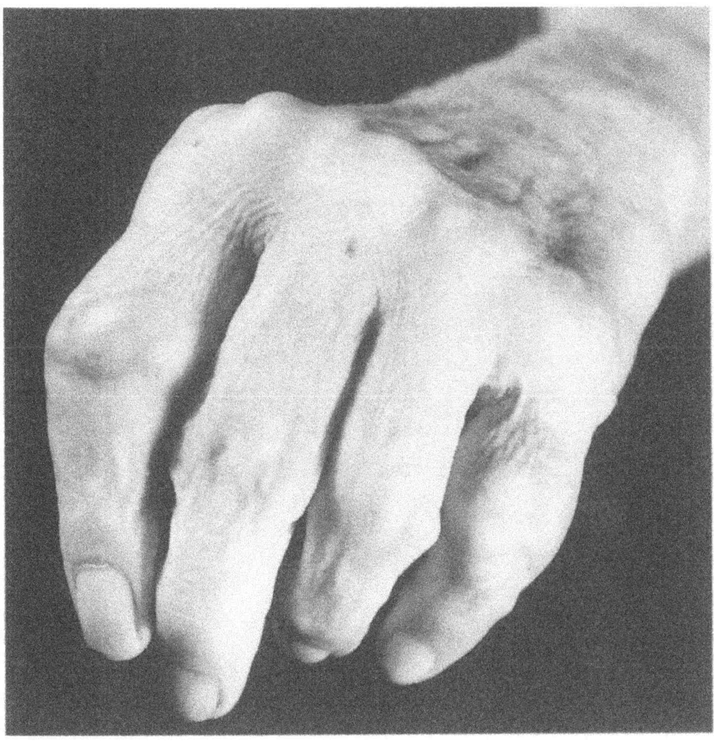

Subcutaneous tophi in the soft tissue of the dorsal aspect of the fingers of male aged 67 years with advanced gout. (Photograph by E. Uehlinger, University Department of Pathology, Zurich)

Fig. 17.12
Gout

Granulomata in bone

Following loss of articular cartilage and break-through into adjacent bone, the granuloma does not confine itself to the marrow spaces, but involves the surrounding spongiosa of bone (Fig. 17.13). This process accounts for the extensive destruction of the gouty arthritis (Figs. 17.14, 17.15). Remarkable presentations may arise when tophus material covers the eroded contours of bone seams (Fig. 17.16). Deposits of urate in the periosteum and adjoining tissue may induce to the formation of new bone (Fig. 17.17). This leads to the kind of structure which radiologists have termed "tophus prickles" or "bays". Urate granulomata may affect any joint but show a distinct preference for the lower extremities.

"Tophus prickles"

Electron-microscopy

In her fundamental electron-microscopical investigations in 1969, Gieseking demonstrated that the organic material surrounding the crystals in the centre of a gout nodule is entirely unstructured. Her studies give an insight into the mechanisms of tissue destruction by urate crystals (Fig. 17.18).

No collagen fibre remnants are recognizable. It appears that the fibrils have disintegrated as far as their molecular components. The collagen fibres which have been split into protofibrils are impregnated with amorphous material, apparently dissolved uric acid (Fig. 17.19). This has led to the conclusion that the dissolution of the collagen fibres is not produced by the crystalline material but precedes crystal formation. Gieseking considers the fibre disintegration to be due to a pH change resulting from the presence of uric acid. A small alteration of pH in the surround-

Dissolution of collagen fibres

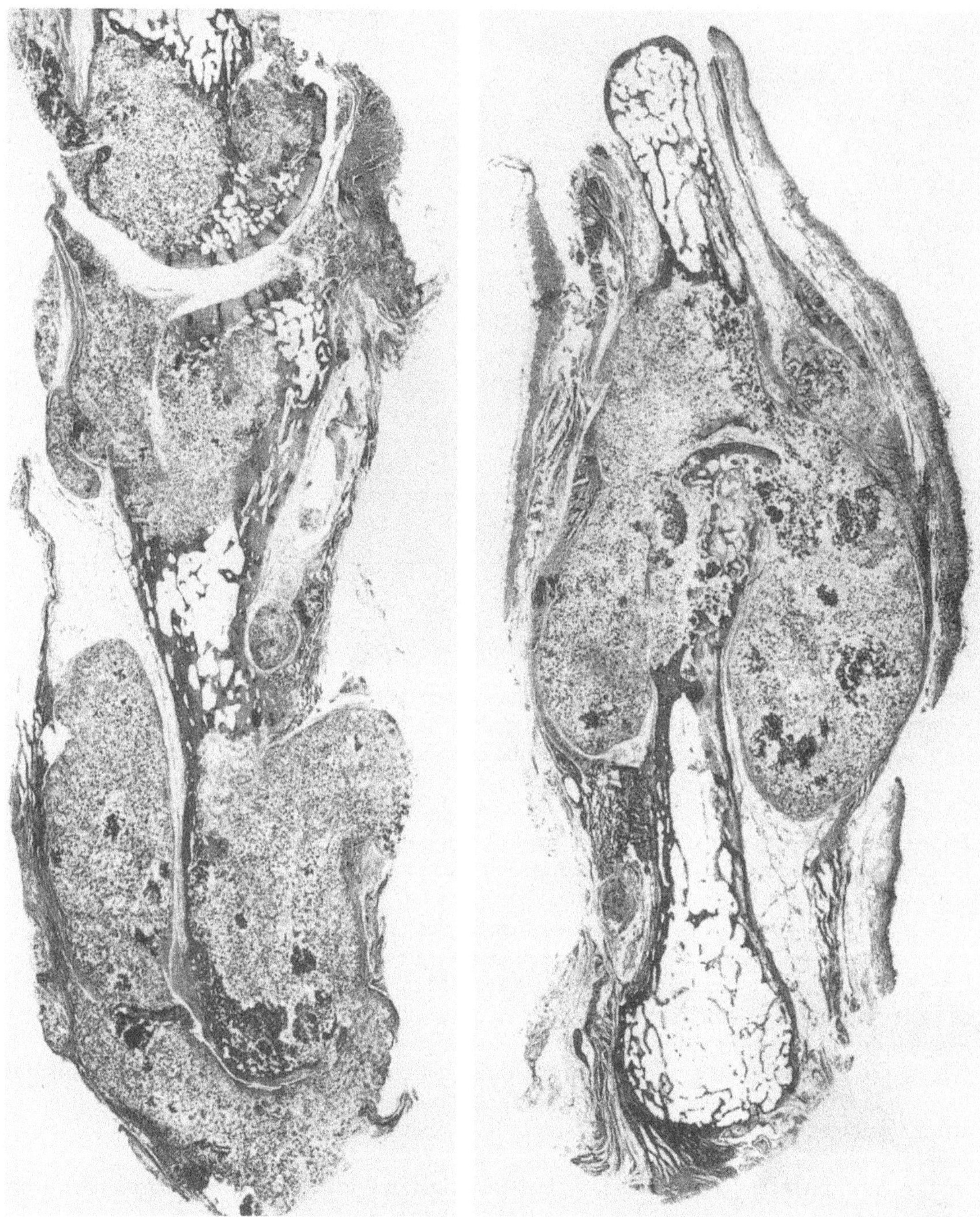

Fig. 17.13
Gout

Extensive tophi involving phalanges. They have spread into the synovial tissue and show subchondral break into bone (big toe). (Photograph by E. Uehlinger, University Department of Pathology, Zurich)

ing milieu is capable of disrupting the lateral bonds between the molecular chains of collagen. The tissue reactions are, however, caused by precipitates of uric acid. Gieseking studying the cells surrounding a gouty tophus, found that they have the characteristic submicroscopic structural features of histiocytes, at the surface of which there is an unusually large number of cytoplasmic

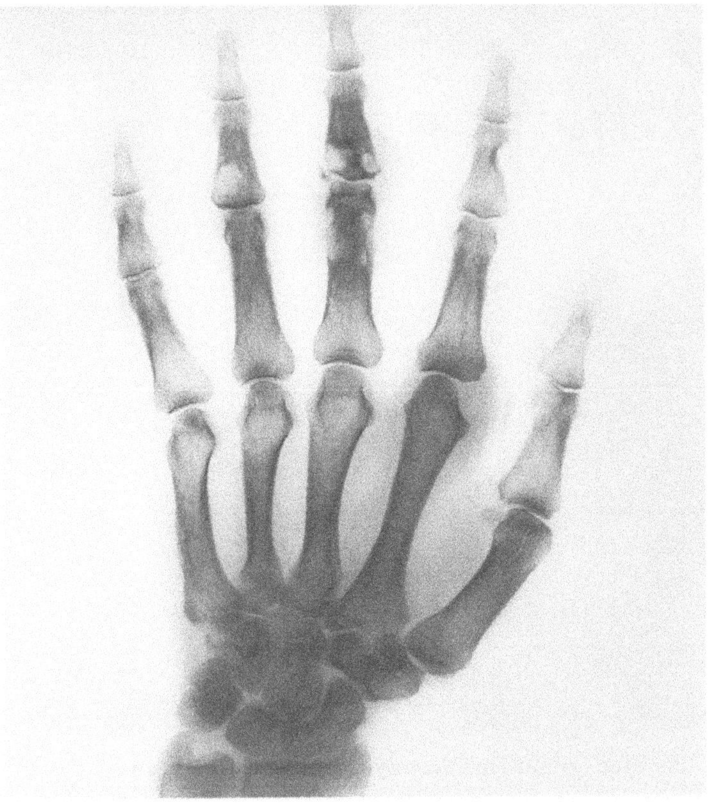

Juxta-articular bone destruction and soft tissue tophi in advanced gouty arthritis

Fig. 17.14
Gout

fringes. These are interspersed among the urate deposits in the centre of the nodule. Near these cell surfaces, the crystals appear to be fragmented. The cytoplasmic processes enclose these fragments and together with the surrounding separated cell membrane they are interiorized within the histiocyte cytoplasm. The cytoplasm contains many such resorptive vacuoles with crystal fragments of varying size. These are further split into fine, electron-dense granules which occur diffusely in the cytoplasm following disruption of the vacuoles. Gieseking draws attention to the similarity of these end-products of intracellular crystal decomposition within histiocytes to the small granular inclusions which occur in the capillary endothelial cells when uric acid enters these during its passage into the tissues. The granular form which the bound uric acid takes in the cytoplasm is quite different from the extracellular macro-crystalline needles which are deposited in the tissues.

Crystal fragments

The lack of formed cells in the central zone of a gouty tophus is a sign of the cytotoxic effect of urate crystals. Although the surrounding histiocytes have processes which project into this zone between the crystals, the cells themselves do not appear to migrate into this zone. The first row of histiocytes to come into contact with crystalline material and which phagocytoses some of the more coarse particles, shows typical changes of necrobiosis, while histiocytes at the periphery show no such features.

Cytotoxic effect

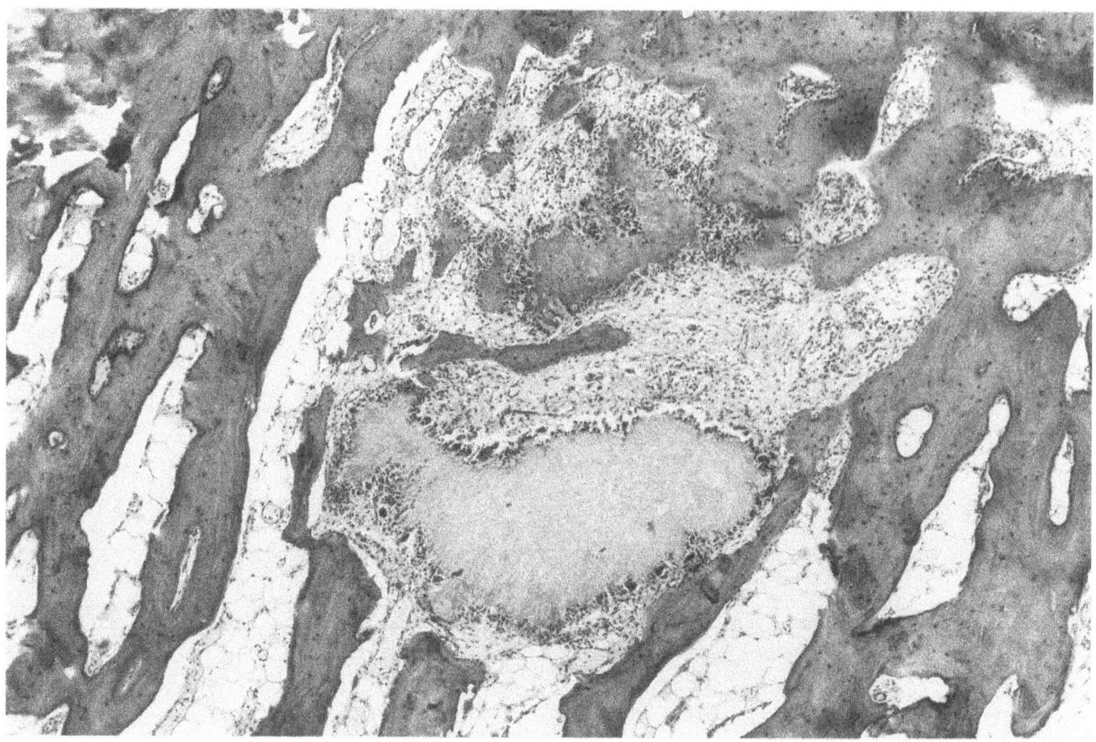

Fig. 17.15
Gout

Toe. Urate granuloma destroying spongiosa of bone

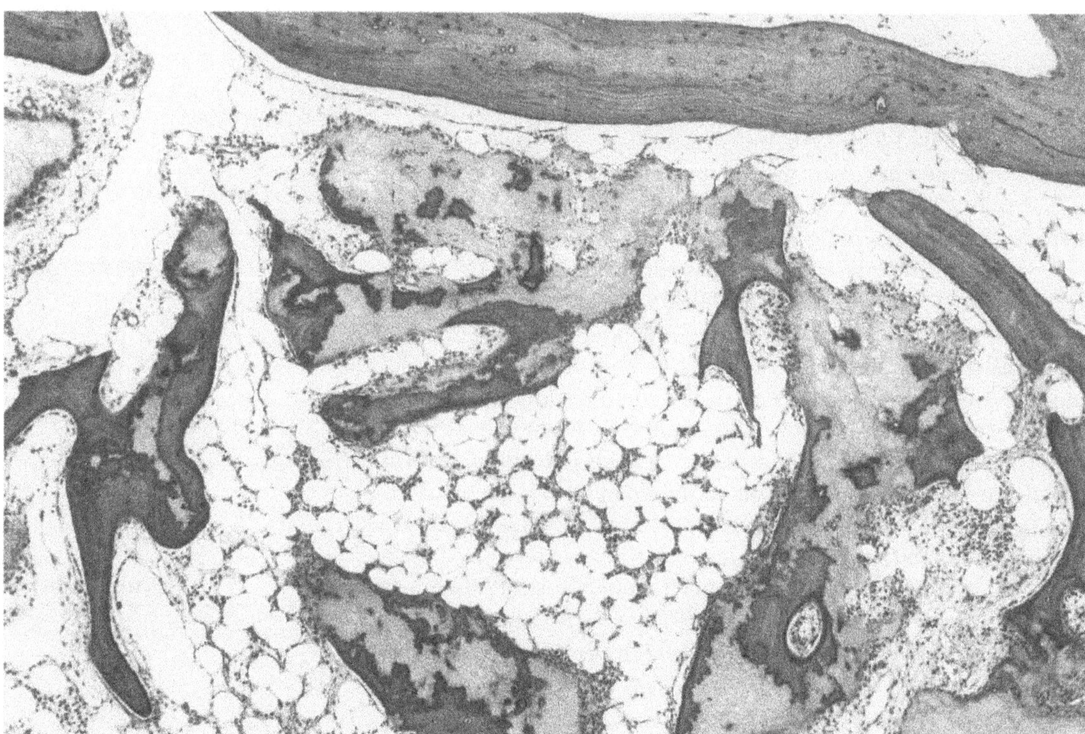

Fig. 17.16
Gout

Toe. Fragments of destroyed bone lamellae, surrounded by urate granulomata (light grey material)

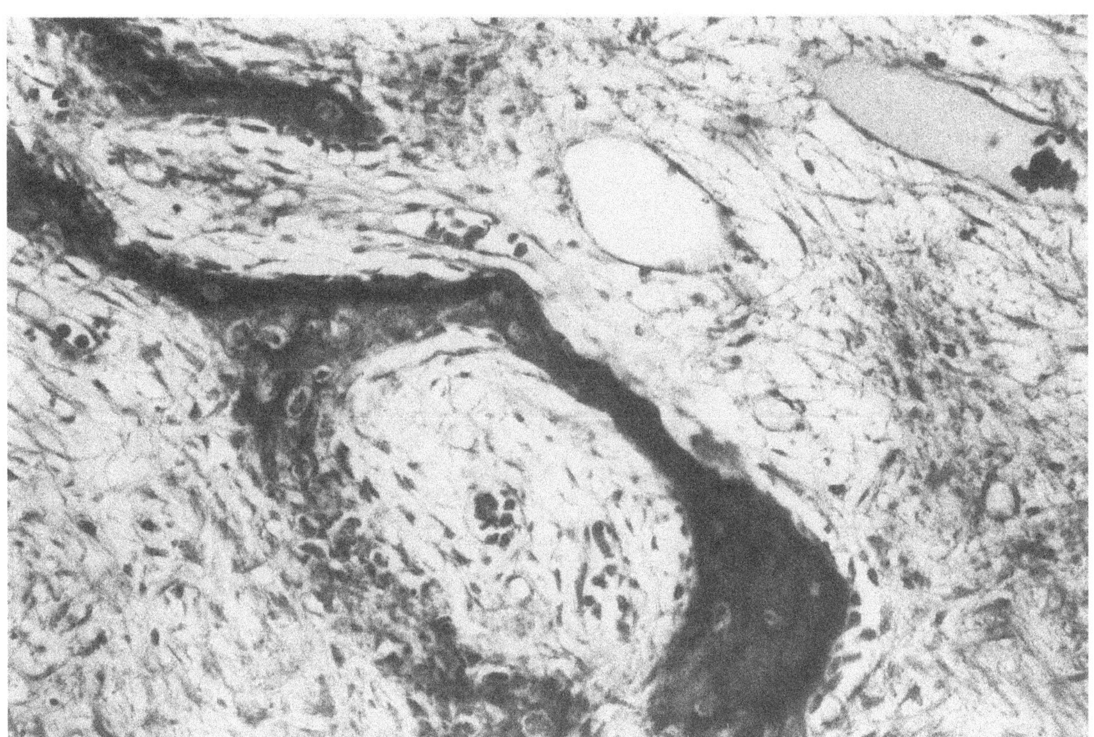

Toe. New formation of fibrous bone in connection with urate granuloma close to periosteum

Fig. 17.17
Gout

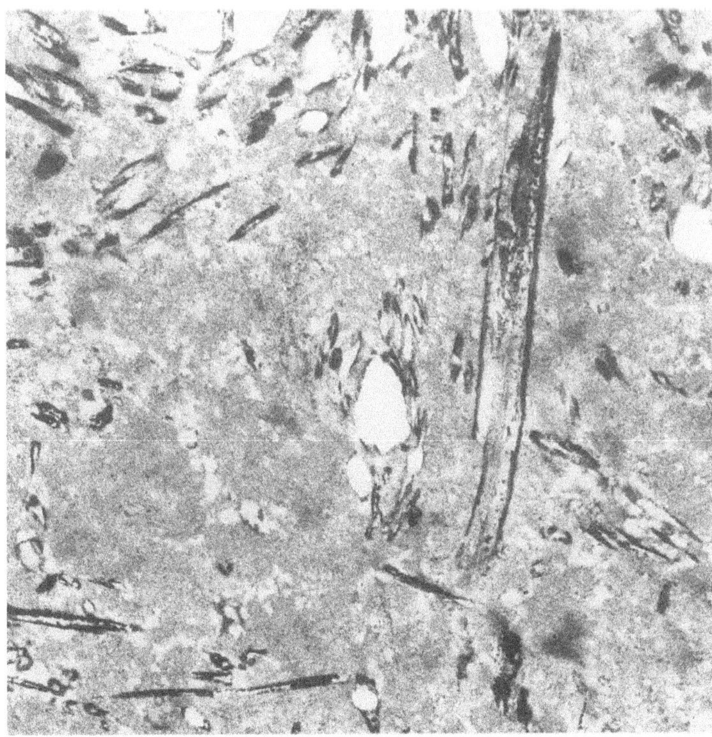

Dissolution of amorphous-appearing matrix containing crystals in centre of gout nodule. (Electron micrograph, 1:18,000). (Photograph by R. Gieseking, University Department of Pathology, Munster)

Fig. 17.18
Gout

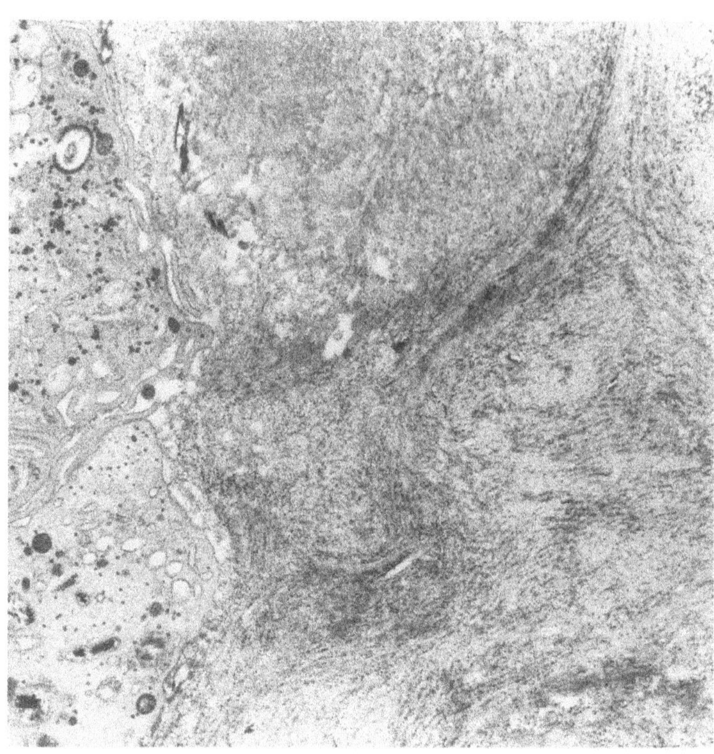

Fig. 17.19
Gout

Lysis of collagen fibres at the periphery of a gout nodule. The fibrillar elements of collagen fibres have been broken down to protofibrils and impregnated with an amorphous refractile material, probably uric acid. (Electron micrograph, 1:10,000). (Photograph by R. Gieseking, University Department of Pathology, Munster)

Synovial fluid

Although neutrophils are plentiful in synovial fluid, especially in acute attacks of gout, they do not form part of the tissue reaction proper. The synovial fluid neutrophils contain phagocytosed crystals of urate with smooth straight facets which do not project beyond the cell. In contrast to the urate crystals, the calcium-pyrophosphate crystals of chondrocalcinosis are more rounded and tend to project beyond the confines of the cell.

17.1.7 Kidneys

Lethal complication

While erosive and destructive arthritis dominate the clinical features of gout, renal involvement constitutes a potentially lethal complication. In 60% of patients suffering from gout, pathological changes in the kidneys are observed, approximately 37% of the latter are pathognomonic.

Renal damage may, in fact, occur by means of a clinically non-apparent hyperuricaemia preceding the articular manifestations of gout. Hyperuricaemia may lead to the formation of small tophi in the interstitium referred to as urate nephropathy. Deposition of

Urolithiasis

uric acid crystals in the collecting tubules, an entity referred to as uric acid nephropathy (up to 50%), as consequence leads to uric acid urolithiasis (up to 20%; Fig. 17.20). Urate nephropathy is not

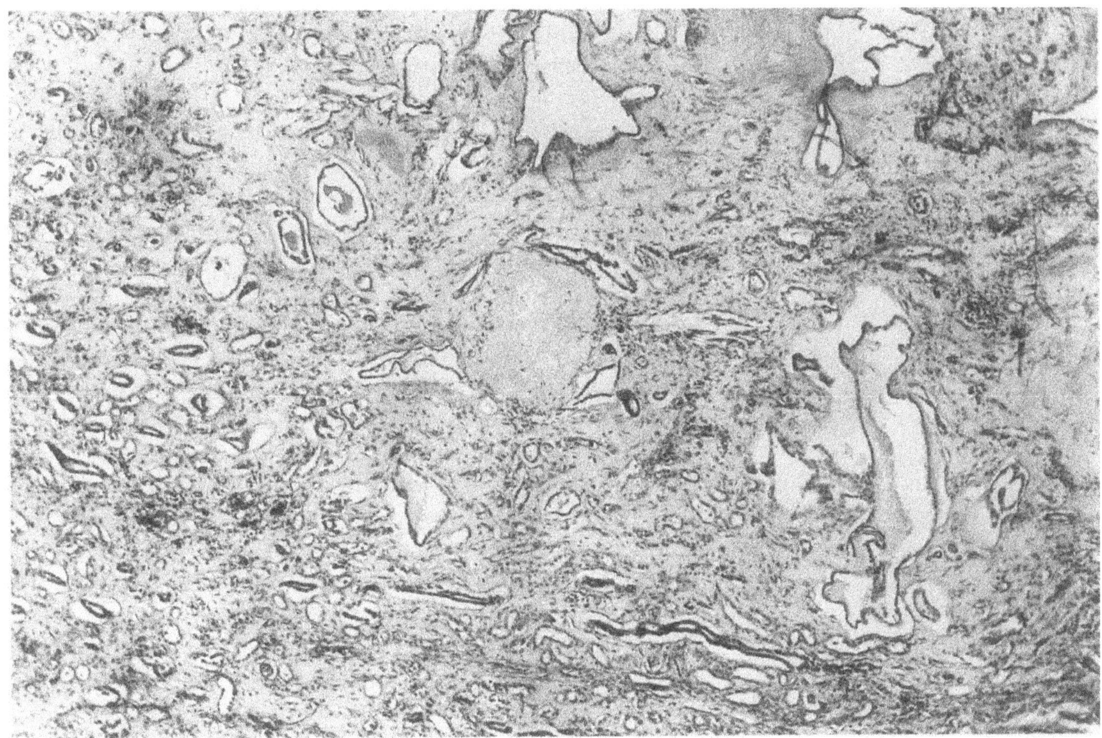

A small urate granuloma in the renal medulla with hydronephrosis

Fig. 17.20
Gout

uncommon, by pathological criteria at least, in patients with gout, regardless of the accompanying excretion of uric acid. In contrast, both uric acid nephropathy and urolithiasis are more common in patients with excessive uric acid production and excretion. Urate nephropathy is only slowly progressive and does not materially reduce life expectancy of the treated patient (Fessel 1979; Reif et al. 1981). Urine retention as well as leucotactic activity of urate favour the development of interstitial nephritis.

Glomerular sclerosis

Apart from these mechanisms, a few cases show glomerular sclerosis, which may cause hypertension. This affects the renal arterioles with development of arteriosclerosis, leading in turn to the loss of further glomeruli. Thus, a vicious circle is established. Hypertension leads to left ventricular hypertrophy, and this in turn raises the danger of relative coronary insufficiency.

Coronary sclerosis

Coronary artery sclerosis is in any case not uncommonly found in hyperuricaemic patients. It is not clear whether we are dealing here with the coincident several components of a constitutionally conditioned syndrome, or whether hyperuricaemia per se is the cause of vascular disease.

Deposition in connective tissue

It is in principle possible for urate to be deposited in the connective tissue of any structure and there result in a foreign-body reaction; in advanced cases, aorta, myocardium, aortic and mitral valve, epiglottis, vocal cords, and vertebral bodies may occasionally be affected in this way. The necrotic centre of a tophus shows a tendency to undergo calcification and sequestration.

Secondary infection

Secondary infection and chronically infected fistulae may occur and may dominate the final stages of the disease.

17.2 Calcium Pyrophosphate Dihydrate Crystal Deposition Disease

Synonyms: calcium pyrophosphate arthropathy, chondrocalcinosis, pseudogout.

17.2.1 Definition and History

Intrasynovial crystal deposition of calcium pyrophosphate dihydrate (CPPD) was discovered by McCarty and Hollander (1961) and Kohn et al. (1962) in the course of a study of patients with acute arthritic episodes which were presumed to be gout.

"Pseudogout"

McCarty et al. (1962) named the newly found crystal associated disease "pseudogout". Since that time, crystal deposits have gained increasing interest as pathogenetic factors of acute arthritides.

Chondrocalcinosis

The deposition of CPPD crystals in joint structures proceeds asymptomatically in most cases, even when crystals are detectable radiologically. But, similar to monosodium urate crystals in gout, they could trigger a crystal-induced synovitis with phenomena which have already been described by Zitnan and Sitaj (1958) as chondrocalcinosis. The term chondrocalcinosis refers to the detection of calcium mineral salts in the articular fibrous or hyaline cartilage.

17.2.2 Epidemiology

Prevalence

The disease is endemic to certain areas of Slowakia, Chile, and The Netherlands; a high incidence of the hereditary form is observed. In general, CPPD deposits in joints are fairly common. Prevalence increases with age. Findings from autopsies indicate an increasing prevalence in the knee joint from 16.6% in patients from 50 to 90 years of age to 50% in patients older than 90 years (Mitrovic et al. 1988). Except in destructive pyrophosphate arthropathy, no major sex differences have been reported.

17.2.3 Clinical Manifestations

Three forms

Usually polyarticular

The disease may be present in three different forms: hereditary, sporadic-idiopathic, and secondary (in patients with hyperparathyroidism, haemochromatosis, hypothyroidism, amyloidosis, hypomagnesiaemia, or hypophosphataemia). Trauma may also precipitate calcium pyrophosphate dihydrate crystal deposition disease (CPDD). Calcium pyrophosphate dihydrate (CPPD) crystal deposits are usually polyarticular, symmetric and related to concurrent or subsequent cartilage degeneration. According to McCarty (1986), the extent to which these crystals initiate an inflammatory reaction depends on the "dose". McCarty classifies the disease into six types under phenomenological aspects, i.e. depending on the clinical picture which partly may mimic other types of arthritis:

Type A

Pseudogout

Pseudogout: the type A pattern is marked by inflammatory episodes lasting approximately 1 day to 4 weeks. Such episodes are self-limiting and usually involve only one or few peripheral joints. In extreme cases, the attacks may be as severe as those of urate gout. But the average attack takes longer to reach peak intensity and is usually less painful and disabling. About 25% of patients observed by McCarty show this gout-like type A pattern. Men predominate.

Type B

Pseudorheumatoid arthritis

Pseudorheumatoid arthritis: approximately 5% of his patients have multiple joint involvement with subacute attacks lasting for weeks or even months. At these patients, McCarty describes symptoms of nonspecific joint inflammation. About 10% of patients with CPPD-related arthritis have positive tests for rheumatoid factors, usually in low titre.

Types C and D

Pseudo-osteoarthritis

Pseudo-osteoarthritis: the clinical picture of these patients is marked by progressive joint degeneration. McCarty attaches half of his patients to these types. Women predominate. McCarty differentiates between patients with inflammatory components (type C) and patients without inflammatory components (type D).

Type E

Asymptomatic CPPD crystal deposition

Asymptomatic CPPD crystal deposition: this type is even so a common form of CPDD. Most joints with CPPD crystal deposits visible on X-ray films are not symptomatic, even in patients with acute or chronic symtpoms in other joints.

Type F

Pseudoneurotrophic joints

Pseudoneurotrophic joints: McCarty postulates that neurotrophic joints actually develop in that 5% of the tabetic population that happens to have underlying CPPD crystal deposition.

Common to all these types are occasional histological CPPD deposits in joint tissues, frequently only be detected by radiographic means. To what extent the chondrocalcinosis influences the manifestation of the respective type, McCarty leaves undecided. Bjelle (1979) suggests a classification comprising five types and designating the respective clinical picture: acute, chronic, familial, destructive, and asymptomatic.

17.2.4 Etiology and Pathogenesis

To date, there is no conclusive explanation for the pathogenesis of CPDD. Hyperparathyroidism, haemochromatosis, and hypomagnesiaemia are assumed to facilitate the deposition of CPPD crystals via increased concentrations of inorganic pyrophosphates (PPi) in the synovial fluid (Doherty et al. 1991). But also in patients not suffering from any metabolic disturbances, the synovial fluid concentration of PPi may be elevated. Howell et al. (1984) conclude (from their research) that the ectoenzyme nucleoside-triphosphate-pyrophosphohydrolase degrades the nucleotides excreted from damaged chondrocytes into the extracelluar space to PPi. This is then deposited around the chondrocytes. Their explanation is based upon results of their earlier studies performed to analyse the production of PPi in cartilage from patients with osteoarthritis (OA) and chondrocalcinosis. Immediately after removal, the cartilage specimens were incubated in synthetic media. Human ulcerated osteoarthritic cartilage as well as cartilage from patients with chondrocalcinosis extruded PPi into the medium. This is in contrast to normal synovial membrane and articular cartilage, as well as that from patients with avascular necrosis, rheumatoid arthritis (RA), and femoral neck fractures.

Role of chondrocytes

It is not yet clear, whether cartilage destruction is the prerequisite for the formation of CPPD deposits, or whether the deposits promote OA. Mohr (1991) examined the cartilage of hip joints from patients who had femur fractures; he found CPPD deposits even in those parts of the hyaline cartilage that were not affected by OA. On the basis of their studies on surgically resected joints, Sokoloff and Varma (1988) claim that determining the potential connection between OA and crystalline deposits is not possible.

Age and CPPD deposition

The fact that CPPD crystal deposits are observed more frequently with increasing age suggests that the degenerative changes in joint structures are of pathogenic significance. The observations of Pritzker et al. (1983) from a well-defined population of free-ranging Rhesus monkeys with age-associated CPPD deposition also point in this direction. The crystal-bearing matrix in these animals showed morphological features identical to those in humans.

In contrast to gout, in which raised levels of serum uric acid are responsible for localized deposition, no systemic elevation of pyrophosphate levels are found in plasma of patients with CPDD.

17.2.5 Pathology

In contrast to gout, which is a systemic, metabolic disorder, CPPD deposition is a localized metabolic abnormality. The pathogenic substrate consists of small, irregularly shaped crystals (Fig. 17.21), which, when viewed with a polarisation microscope, appear positively bifringent. Electron-microscopically, they appear plump, electron-dense, and centrally vacuolated (Mohr 1984). Mohr (1991) describes that in the early stages, CPPD deposits are found in the superficial and middle layers of the cartilage; in severe cases, multiple deposits permeate the entire cartilage.

Importance of cartilage structure

Topographically, these deposits are confined to hyaline cartilage and fibrocartilage in the meniscus of the knee (Fig. 17.22), in the symphysis pubis or in the annulus fibrosus of the disc. The specific importance of the cartilage structure for the CPPD crystal

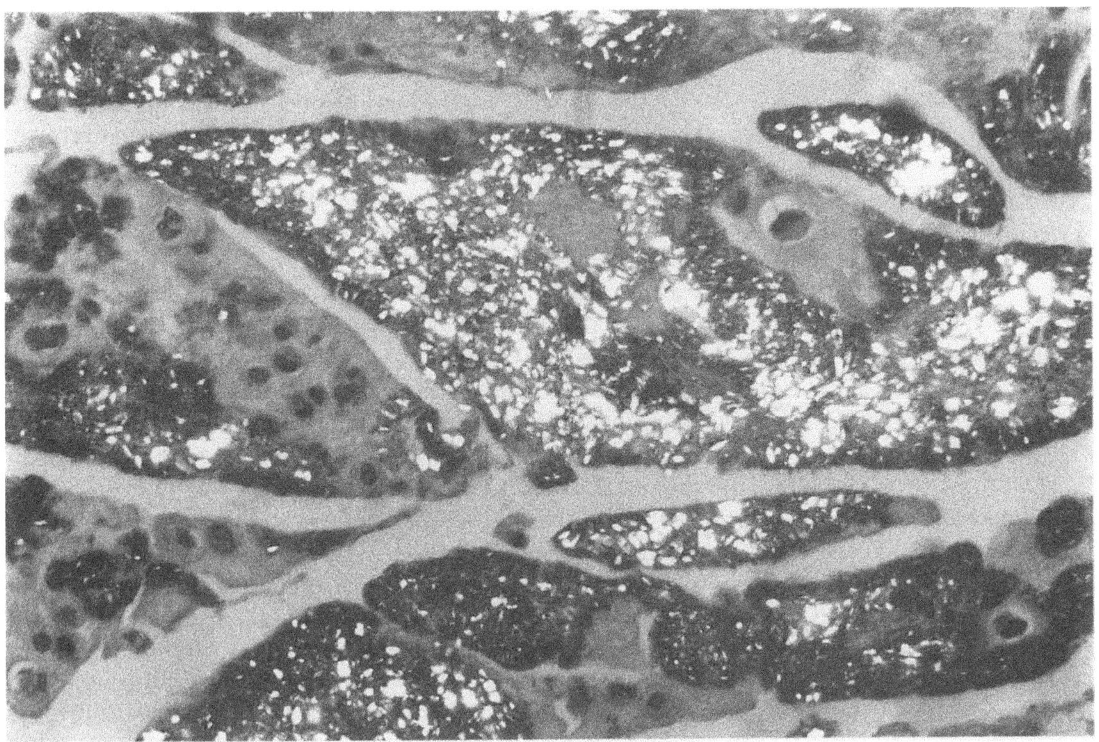

Knee joint. Deposits of pyrophosphate under polarized light: the hyaline cartilage is almost completely splintered

Fig. 17.21
Chondrocalcinosis

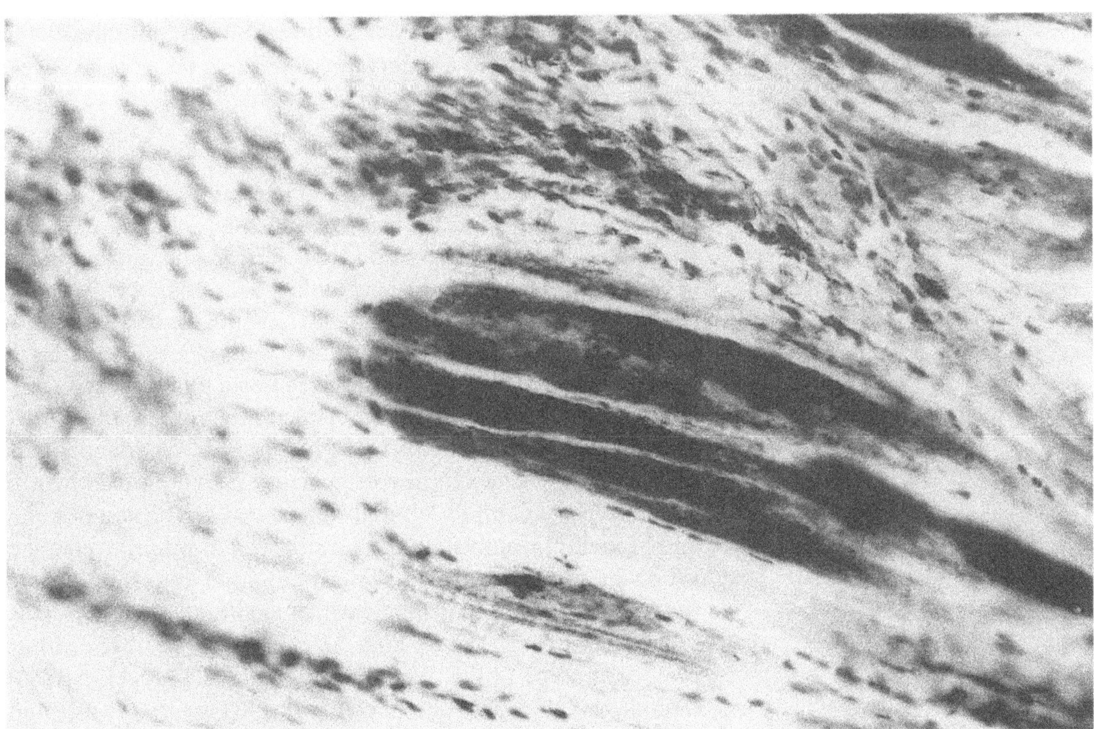

Knee joint. Pyrophosphate impregnating collagen fibres of a meniscus

Fig. 17.22
Chondrocalcinosis

deposition manifests itself by the fact that their deposition in the articular capsule tissue, tendons, and ligaments presupposes chondroid metaplasia of these tissues. Chondroid metaplasia is the last stage of connective tissue degeneration, which starts with fibrosis and then leads to hyalinization and loss of vascularisation. In this avascular tissue, the fibroblasts either die or transform into cells with the phenotype of cartilage cells. Around these cells we can detect ultrastructurally a coating of collagen type II.

Chondroid metaplasia

Granular matrix

The CPPD crystal deposits are located around the lacunae in large tophus-like masses in the vicinity of clefts in degenerated cartilage. This granular matrix stains more densely than its surroundings with alcian blue, colloidal iron, and PAS and consists predominantly of aggrecans. An abnormally high content of aggrecans is a constant finding in this area.

Initial deposits of PPi

The initial deposits of PPi, according to McCarty (1986), appear in rims around chondrocytes, larger deposits are associated with cell necrosis in the periphery. The PPi diffusing from chondrocytes may precipitate as a very sparingly soluble calcium salt. The crystals are deposited extracellularly in a glycosaminoglycan-rich perichondral matrix. These deposits coalesce to form nodules within the articular tissue (Pritzker et al. 1980). CPPD crystals are extremely insoluble and an experimental clinical attempt at crystal dissolution has failed. The primary changes responsible for crystal deposition may occur in the ground substance, the "soil", that permits nucleation and growth of the crystals. This speculation may also apply to gout in which hyperuricaemia is a frequent but not sufficient antecedent factor leading to the formation of monosodium urate crystals. In vitro studies of McCarty (1986) point to a reduction of ambient Ca2+ as a cause of the increased solubility of CPPD crystals. This leads to "crystal shedding" which acts as a source of a local acute or a systemic arthritis.

"Crystal shedding"

After the CPPD crystals reach the joint cavity, they are coated with various polypeptides, some of which have biological activity. A chemotactic glycopeptide [cell-derived chemotactic factor (CCF)] is released from the neutrophils after phagocytosis of the CPPD crystals. Animal experiments and in vitro studies show that injection of monosodium urate crystals or CPPD crystals into human and animal joints is followed by a phagocytosis which triggers again an acute inflammatory reaction (Mandel 1976; Mandel and Mandel 1982). This process is dose dependent and reversible. In vitro experiments explain this mechanism by activation of Hagemann Factor and subsequent generation of kinins and bradykinin, activation of plasminogen to plasmin, and activation of complement pathways. Yet another requisite factor is the recruitment of neutrophils which again release a non-dialysable chemotactic factor after phagocytosis of monosodium urate crystals or CPPD crystals (Spilberg et al. 1977, 1979, 1980).

Phagocytosis of crystals

Acute inflammatory reaction

Phlogistic potency

Overall, the phlogistic potency of the CPPD crystals is distinctly smaller than that of the monosodium urate crystals. An explanation for this is offered by the experiments of Schumacher and coworkers (1975) who showed that in the presence of neutrophils synthetic CPPD is phagocytozed noticeably more slowly than monosodium urate crystals. The CPPD crystals seemed less reactive than urates as hydrogen-binding agents. Moreover, monosodium urate crystals have a stronger membranolytic effect on the lysosomes than CPPD crystals. The majority of CPPD deposits remain asymptomatic even if they are X-ray detectable. The clinical manifestation occurs via attacks due to rupture of preformed clusters of CPPD crystals from local avascular cartilage into the adjacent synovial cavity.

Synovial process

The synovial process of the CPDD as described above is not very impressive. Only in the acute phase can one find a fibrin film on the synovial surface and in single cases neutrophils and lymphocytes in the stroma. In the inflammatory response not only neutrophils but also mononuclear cells take part in the phagocytosis of crystals (Fig. 17.23).

Ultrastructural studies

In ultrastructural studies of synovium, Schumacher (1976) found deposits of CPPD crystals only at sites of surface phagocytic cells and adjacent interstitium.

Histological detection

The low water solubility of the CPPD crystals, in contrast to the monosodium urate crystals, enables their histological detection, even in formaldehyde-fixed tissue.

Crystal identification

The clinical diagnosis of CPDD requires the direct identification of crystals in joint puncture fluid. Phagocytozed CPPD crystals have blunt ends and in general lie strictly intracellularly, whereas the needle-shaped monosodium urate crystals protrude from the cell (Fig. 17.24).

Polarisation: CPPD – monosodium urate crystals

The crystals show different polarisation patterns: the CPPD crystals show a blue (positive double fringence) parallel to the compensatory axis, the monosodium urate crystals a yellow colour (negative double refraction).

Low-grade inflammation

Since the acute phase is brief, resting conditions predominate in biopsy material, which are characterized by traces of pre-existing, low-grade inflammation, as in villous hyperplasia, which is distinguished by the number and intensity of preceding attacks. The lining cell layer is, moreover, flat and single-layered. No cell proliferation and no fibrosis is found in the stroma, it remains mainly transparent. Lymphocyte infiltration of varying density may still be present in the region of small blood vessels a long time after the last attack. Plasma cells and neutrophils are rare. The synovial picture corresponds, thus, to that of a synovial hyperplasia with arthrosis and internal joint damage, respectively. It is obvious that no direct danger for the joint cartilage results from this modest synovial process, even in an acute state. However, as in all synovial processes and also in the scope of OA, the question as to what extent cytokines are produced in the synovial membrane and cause the release of proteases from the chondrocytes, must remain open.

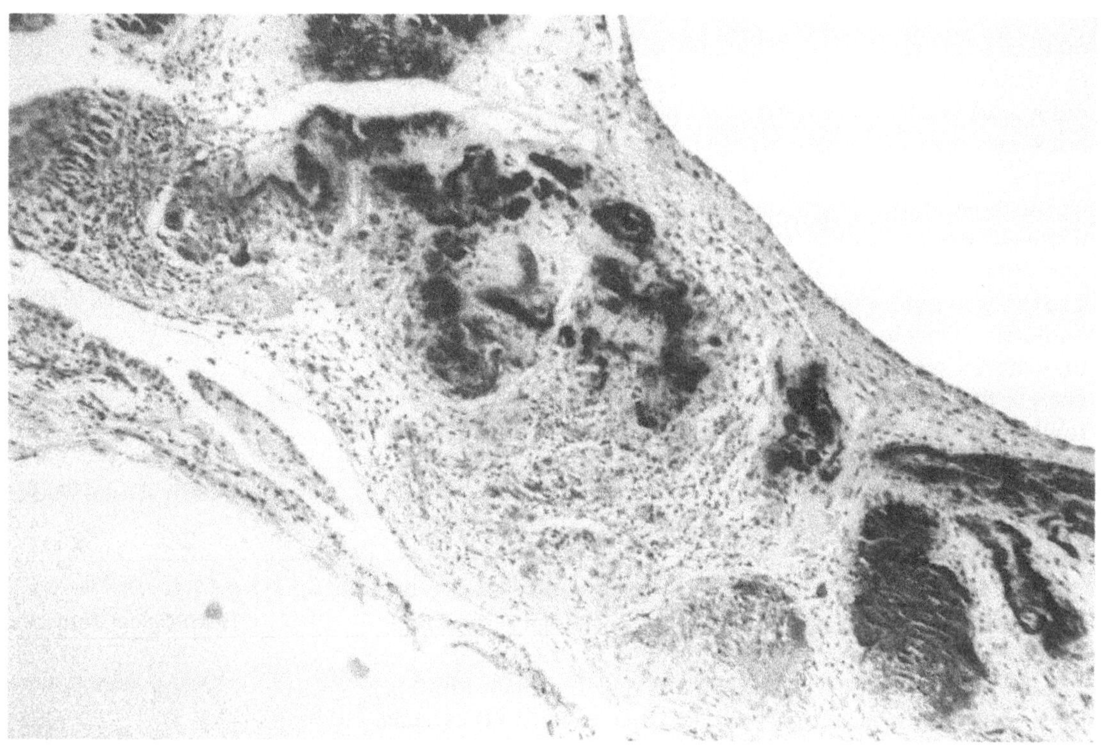

Fig. 17.23
Chondrocalcinosis

Knee joint. Pyrophosphate with foreign-body reaction in chondroid metaplastic synovial tissue

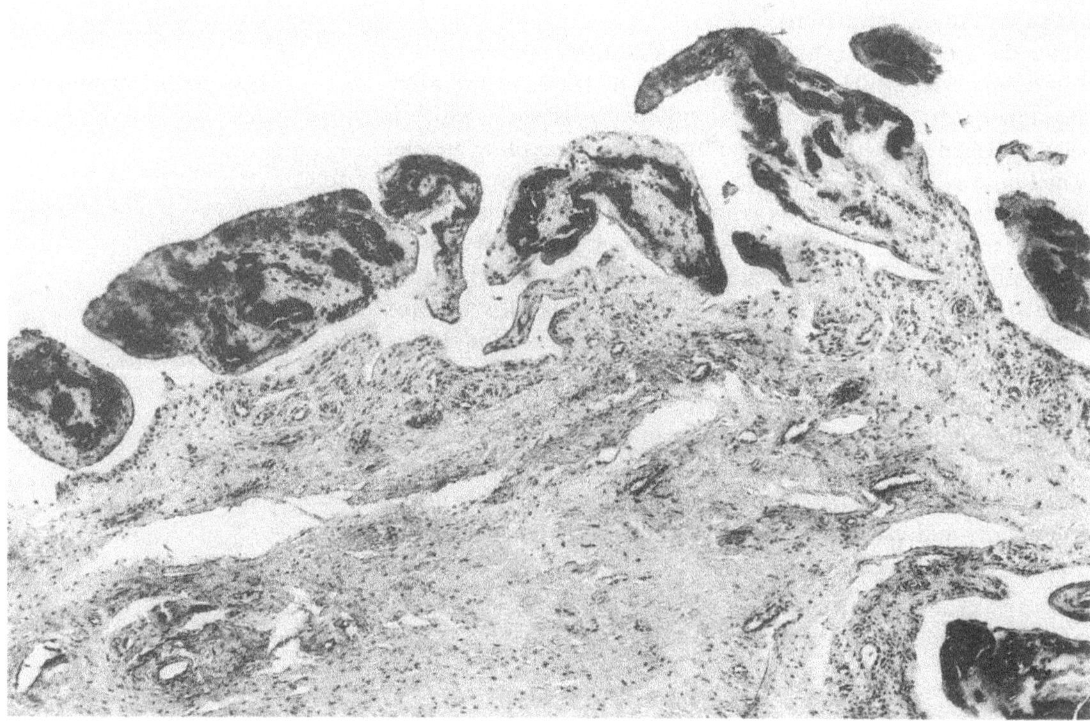

Fig. 17.24
Chondrocalcinosis

Knee joint. Pyrophosphate deposits in chondroid metaplastic synovial villi

17.3 Hydroxyapatite Crystal Deposition Disease

17.3.1 Definition

A further common crystal-associated arthropathy is caused by deposition of basic calcium phosphate as hydroxyapatite. Since the hydroxyapatite crystals in humans measure only 200×30–70 Å, they can only be recognized as aggregates by electron-microscopy. It seems that aggregate formation is also a prerequisite for the phlogistic effect of the hydroxyapatite crystals.

17.3.2 Clinical Manifestations

The occasional detection of these crystals in synovial fluid in acute and subacute synovitides as in OA (Dieppe et al. 1976) and in neutrophils of synovial effusions (Schumacher et al. 1976) would merely have remained a pathogenetically interesting phenomenon had it not been shown that a clinically well-defined disease state, the so-called Milwaukee shoulder, exists. The Milwaukee shoulder correlates strictly with the detectability of hydroxyapatite crystals in both the synovial fluid and the joint capsule with the periarticular structures. In contrast to that, the CPPD crystal deposits which occur in CPDD are confined to the joint cartilage or chondroid metaplastic tissue.

"Milwaukee shoulder"

The Milwaukee shoulder syndrome (synonymous with "apatite-associated large joint lysis" or "cuff-tear arthropathy") resembles in clinical features the arthropathy with chondrocalcinosis (CPDD). It predominantly affects elderly females (McCarty et al. 1981). They suffer as a result of damage to the rotator cuff of the shoulder. Although the dominant side is predisposed, the other side may also be affected to a lesser extent. The syndrome may also develop in males following trauma. The knee joints, particularly the synovial tissue, from patients with Milwaukee shoulder syndrome often show degenerative changes as seen in the shoulder. McCarty (1986) assumes, moreover, that the other large joints are affected in a similar way. Numerous other sites of deposition are also reported (e.g. elbow, wrist, hand, foot, ankle, hip, neck).

"Cuff-tear arthropathy"

Other sites of deposition

17.3.3 Pathology

The structural process is characterized by glenohumeral joint degeneration and calcification of the collagenous capsule tissue which, in many cases, is recognizable by X-ray (Fig. 17.25). In such cases, the synovial fluid is essentially acellular. McCarty (1986) attributes the residual haemorrhage to microtrauma due to the instability of the joint. Intense effusions can cause disintegration of the joint capsule facilitating entry into the subcutaneous tissue. By light-microscopy small non-descript masses can be seen in the synovial fluid. These seem to be aggregates of hydroxyapatite which look like snowball-like structures under the scanning electron-microscope.

Aggregates of hydroxyapatite

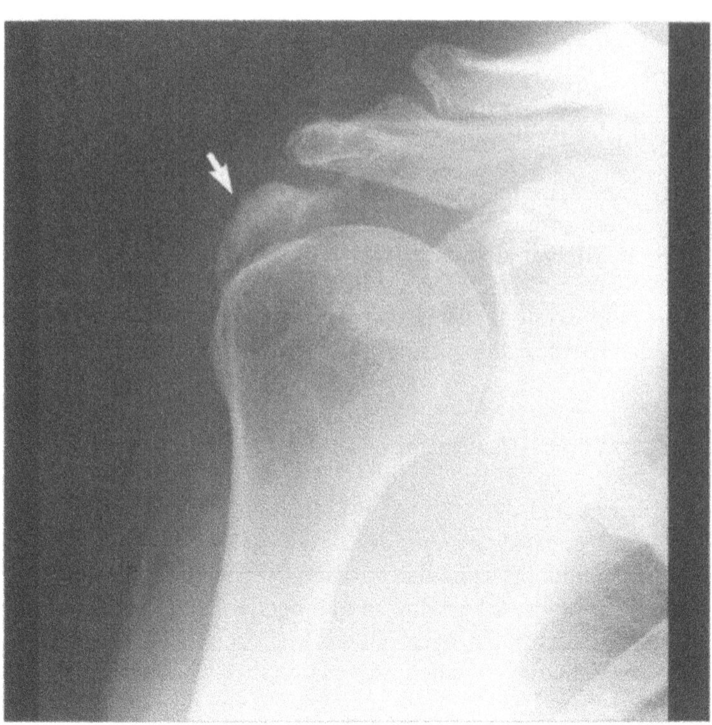

Fig. 17.25
Hydroxyapatite periarthropathy

Hydroxyapatite deposition in the aponeurosis of the rotatory cuff (*arrow*) of the shoulder ("Milwaukee shoulder"). Female aged 66 years. (Courtesy of G.M. Lingg, Radiological Institute of Rheuma-Heilbad AG, Bad Kreuznach, Germany)

Destructive nature

Electron-microscopy

The fact that active synovial collagenases and neutral proteases, and also components of collagen types I, II, and III can be detected in synovial fluid indicates the destructive nature of the disease. At the same time, the affinity of the hydroxyapatite crystals for collagenous tissue plays an essential role. With the aid of transmission electron-microscopy they can be visualized in the tendons and typically in the rotator cuffs of the shoulder, 1–2 cm from the insertion at the greater trochanter in the region of the fibrocartilaginous metaplasia of the tissue (McCarty 1986). The importance of the preceding chondroid metaplasia for the deposition of crystals bears resemblance to the corresponding process of chondrocalcinosis (see p. 374).
Schumacher and colleagues (1976) demonstrated the phlogistic potency of hydroxyapatite crystals using dogs by injecting them intra-articularly with a solution of synthetic CaP mineral of the apatite class. These dogs subsequently developed a marked synovitis with swelling and heat in the injected joint.

Uncharacteristic inflammatory reaction

In humans, the synovial membrane exhibits an uncharacteristic inflammatory reaction with exudation of sparse fibrin, focal synovial cell hyperplasia, and infiltration of a few lymphocytes. Occasionally, cartilage fragments can also be found. However, only the findings of intra- or extracellular crystal aggregates are pathognomonic. The detection of these crystals for routine histological diagnosis fails because the tissue fixation methods customarily used prevent the detection and identification of the crystals. This necessitates the aid of transmission electron-microscopy, employing the corresponding fixation and embedding techniques. Exact crystal analysis is successful with electron diffraction and Fourier transform infrared spectroscopy (Mandel and Mandel 1982). Thus, the pathologist often has to disappoint the referring physician who seeks confirmation of his suspicion of a case of hydroxyapatite crystal deposition disease with a synovial biopsy.

From the impression given by the findings of Schumacher and colleagues (1983) that synovial fluid samples from 60% of patients with OA contain predominantly hydroxyapatite and also CPPD crystals, Howell (1985) raises the question of whether OA may instead precede hydroxyapatite deposition disease or chondrocalcinosis, and that the mineral formation is a consequence of disarrayed cartilage metabolism as a spin-off or secondary effect of OA.

18 Ochronosis

18.1 Definition

Ochronosis is characterized by a bluish black pigmentation of connective tissue in patients with alkaptonuria, usually apparent clinically in the cartilage of the ear, in the skin, and in the sclera (Schumacher 1993).

18.2 History

The earliest clinical observation, that of a boy who passed dark urine, was made by Scribonius in 1584. Boedeker, in 1859, isolated homogentisic acid from the urine of a patient with alkaptonuria. Urine from affected patients becomes dark on standing due to alkalisation under the consumption of oxygen. LaDu and his collaborators in 1958 demonstrated the absence of enzyme homogentisic acid oxidase in the liver of a patient with alkaptonuria, ochronotic spondylosis, and peripheral arthropathy.

18.3 Clinical Features

Alkaptonuria

Alkaptonuria is felt to be transmitted by a single recessive autosomal gene (Schumacher 1993). The present concept of the mode of transmission of alkaptonuria has been substantiated by several careful family studies in which complete pedigrees were available (Knox 1958). One family had HLA-B27 in eight of ten members with alkaptonuria (Gaucher et al. 1977). Typical is a dark-blue discoloration of the auricular cartilage, especially of concha and anthelix. Also the sclera and the skin over the malar areas, nose, axilla, and groin are often pigmented. Alkaptonuria results in a generalized degeneration of joints similar to osteoarthritis (OA). But the external remodelling is less prominent than in idiopathic OA (Lagier 1980).

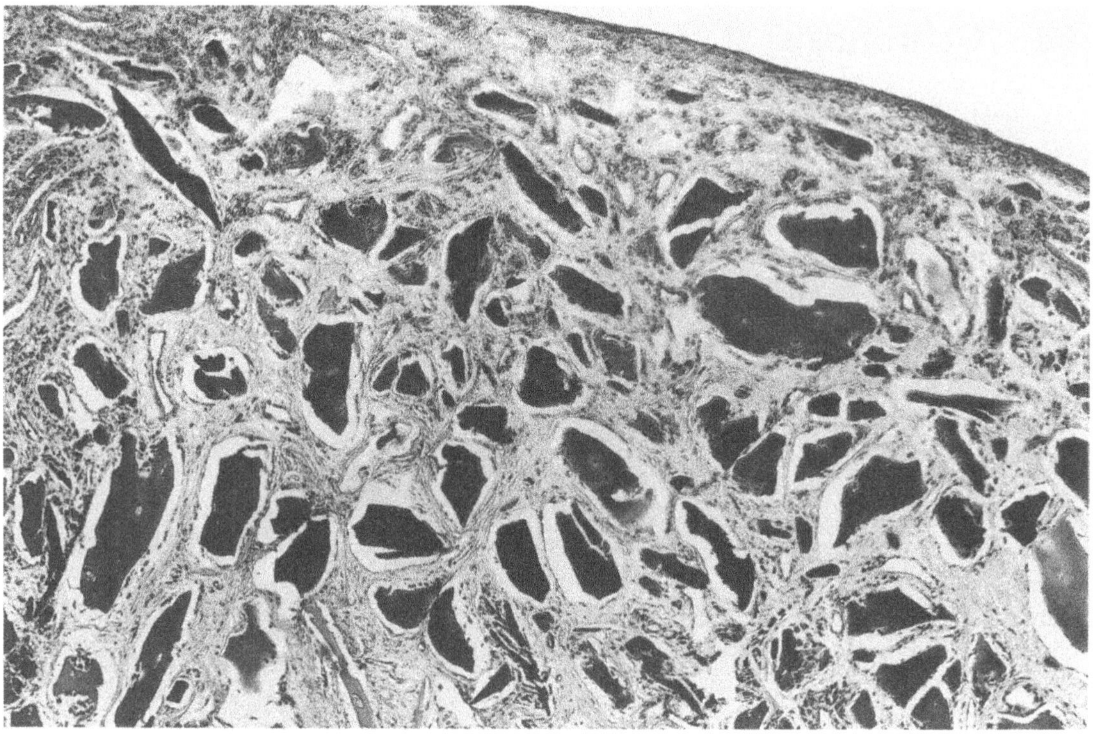

Fig. 18.1
Ochronosis

Deposition of pigmented cartilaginous fragments in the fibrotic synovial membrane

18.4 Pathology

Ochronosis has a special predilection for cartilage. Intra- and/or intercellular deposition of pigment, i.e. the accumulation of an unknown polymer of homogentisic acid, leads to the characteristic discoloration (Fig. 18.1).

Destructive changes

The pigmented cartilage is extremely brittle. The decrease in cartilage quality has its effects mainly within structures that are under mechanical strain. It is, therefore, understandable that degenerative and destructive changes of the spinal column are the most impressive manifestation of the disease. The majority of patients with ochronosis past the age of 30 years develop spondylosis. This includes a calcification or ossification of the nucleus pulposus of the intervertebral discs and breakdown of the vertebral endplates. Spondylosis starts in the lumbar spine; years later, the dorsal and finally the cervical spine become involved. Stiffness of the lower back slowly progresses to rigidity, and lumbar kyphosis may develop.

Peripheral joints

Degenerative changes in peripheral joints are less frequent and develop later than spondylosis. The joints most commonly affected are the knees, but also shoulder and hips can be involved. Pain, stiffness, flexion contractures and limitation of motion are the most common features. Effusion occurs in about half of the cases. The cartilage surface is eroded, chondrocytes and the intracellular matrix contain pigment. Degenerated chondrocytes are observed as well as pigmented calcified or uncalcified microshards, and granulation tissue with macrophages. The changes in bone are less severe than those in cartilage. Pigment is present in the calcified matrix. Diffuse or granular pigmentation is found in a few osteocytes, while several of them are condensed or reduced to cellular fragments. Pigment is also found in osteoclasts but not in osteoblasts (Di Franco et al. 2000). In the synovial fluid, homogentisic acid can be demonstrated, its concentration is much lower than in the urine. Occasionally, black specks of ochronotic cartilage are seen floating in the fluid (Reginato et al. 1973; Hunter et al. 1974; Stiehl and Kluger 1994). Leukocyte counts in a large series by Hüttl ranged below 1,000/µl with predominantly mononuclear cells (1970). Cells containing ochronotic pigment can be observed. In the synovial membrane calcium pyrophosphate crystals can be proved without signs of inflammation (Schumacher and Holdsworth 1977; Table 18.1).

Table 18.1. Diagnostic features of alkaptonuria, ochronosis, ochronotic spondylitis, and peripheral arthropathy (Schumacher 1993)

Alkaptonuria
- Urine turns black
  - On alkalinization
  - On standing
  - When tested for sugar by Benedict's reagent: in addition, yellow-orange precipitate forms
- Positive family history

Ochronosis
- Pigmentation of cartilage and skin
  - Pinna of ear, eardrum, and cerumen
  - Sclera
  - Skin over malar area, nose, axilla, groin
- Prostatic calculi

Ochronotic spondylosis
- Calcification and ossification of intervertebral discs
- Disproportionately little osteophytosis
- Sacroiliac joints not fused and no "bamboo" spine
- Loss of lumbar lordosis
- Spine rigid and stooped, knees flexed, stance typical

Ochronotic peripheral arthropathy
- Knees, shoulders, and hips most commonly affected
- Synovial fluid contains small amounts of homogentisic acid and is noninflammatory, except with occasional calcium pyrophosphate crystal-associated inflammation
- Brittle cartilage fragments and pigmented "chards" in the synovium
- Osteochondral joint bodies common
- Small joints of hands and feet usually not affected

19 Bacterial Arthritis*

19.1 Definition

The term "septic arthritis" is often used as a synonym for bacterial arthritis (BA), but this usage is not only inaccurate semantically, it is according to our observations actually misleading. The term suggests that the clinical symptoms of BA represent at least some evidence of sepsis, and at most the full clinical manifestation.

The clinical picture of bacterial-pyogenic arthritis is unmistakably characterized by pus, consisting of extensive fibrin exudates and masses of neutrophils. Classically, the causative organisms are gram-positive staphylococci, gonococci, and, less frequently, streptococci.

Whether this qualitatively thoroughly defined process becomes clinically manifest as septic, as merely arthritis, or as a clinically latent arthritis depends on the number of causative organisms and on the extent of the purulent inflammation. The morphological appearance is so specific, that a BA can clearly be differentiated from the basic immune process and/or from the basic non-bacterial process.

19.2 Clinical Features

The bacterially infected joint is one of the possible sites of origin for the development of a sepsis. The term "sepsis" (Greek: "decay") in its generally accepted word usage is associated with a range of classical symptoms, the most notable being chills, intermittent fever, and polynuclear leucocytosis which occur as a result of bacteraemia. It is, thus, concerned with symptoms which are medically unmistakable. Clearly this type of characteristic septic arthritis should be treated as a clinical emergency with the intervention of antibiotics.

Septic arthritis

In clinically diagnosed BA, however, the complete picture of sepsis is not usually present, and, thus, has led to a critical examination of the term "septic arthritis". Deesmochok and Tumrasvin (1990) observed chills in only one-third of their patients with BA.

Bacterial arthritis

---

* *Synonym:* septic arthritis

Fever may also be absent, as is shown by the observations of Kelly et al. (1970), Rosenthal et al. (1980), and Goldenberg and Reed (1985). The incidence of leukocytosis is equally unreliable; Rosenthal and colleagues (1980) found it in only 39 out of 63 patients with BA.

In other words, the predominant clinical symptoms of sepsis are not constant in BA. It is therefore not correct to equate a local BA with a generalized bacterial process giving rise to the clinical picture of a sepsis, and for the doctor it is a misleading conception.

Bioptic findings

Until now, diseases classified as "BA" have been diagnosed either by clinical or bacteriological criteria, but we have been led by our bioptic material to a completely different approach.

The pathological diagnosis "BA" is based on the presence of the following clear morphological features in the joint tissue:

1. Lamellated fibrin masses, which are permeated predominantly with a lot of neutrophils.
2. Infiltration of the synovial membrane by bacterial toxins and the proteases of the neutrophils, enzymatic degradation of the synovial structure, and the subsequent formation of granulation- and scar tissue. In addition, there are some further characteristics which develop as a consequence of the bacterial process (see p. 390).

In comparing these clear morphological findings with the clinical symptomatology and the subsequent diagnosis, provided by arthroscopic biopsy, there seemed to us to be a major discrepancy between morphological processes and clinical symptomatology.

Thus, we found in the period from the beginning of 1990 to the end of 1992 in 7,210 joint biopsies from patients with unspecific arthritides 375 cases with morphological features of a clear active or regressing BA. However, only in 34 of these patients (9.1%) had the possibility of a BA been considered by the referring clinic. In none of the remaining 341 cases was a BA suggested; many were merely diagnosed "unspecific rheumatic pain" as an indication for an arthroscopic biopsy. None of the 375 patients had been treated with antibiotics. This bacterial infections are quite evenly spread throughout all age groups, with only a slight increment at old age. En detail, age-related distribution in our material is as follows: 0–10 years, 7.3%; 11–20 years, 10.3%; 21–30 years, 13.7%; 31–40 years, 12%; 41–50 years, 17%; 51–60 years, 18.8%; over 60 years, 20.8%.

"Clinically latent bacterial arthritis"

We have called this clinically undetected disease process "clinically latent bacterial arthritis" (CLBA). This CLBA largely corresponds to what clinicians have pragmatically termed "low-grade infection".

The fact that a majority of these cases of CLBA observed by us were already regressed at the time of biopsy is evidence for the self-limiting character of the process.

To summarize:

- Without biopsy examination, this CLBA would not have been detected.
- The fact that CLBA made up approximately 5% of the cases in our unselected biopsy material shows that this disease process is by no means rare!

Self-limiting course

It might be concluded from this clinically undramatic self-limiting course of CLBA that it is harmless. Our examinations show, however, the opposite, as we find severe damage of the joint cartilage and synovial membrane depending on the age and type of the process (see below).

Because of the term "septic arthritis" there is a danger for patients that if the full picture of a sepsis is not present the physician may await a clinically distinctive symptomatology to indicate the bacterial character of the joint disease process. In other words, if the doctor makes his antibiotic intervention dependent on clear symptoms of a bacterial joint process, he may overlook CLBA with the risk of considerable joint damage.

Three different types of BA

Thus, three different types of BA must be distinguished:

1. The "true" septic arthritis with the systemic indications of a bacteraemia, which is treated as a clinical emergency.
2. The clinically manifested BA, but without systemic "septic" signs; nevertheless, the local process needs antibiotic intervention.
3. The relatively frequent CLBA we observed, with no typical symptoms, which is self-limiting also without antibiotics.

Clinical significance and prognosis

Clinical significance and prognosis of the three types are different:

In type 1, there is the danger of systemic metastases of the infecting agent principally in lungs and brain, in some cases with a fatal outcome. In type 2 (clinically "low-grade infection"), the purulent bacterial process is limited to the joint and leads to considerable damage. In type 3, it remains similarly limited to the joint. The difference from type 2 is purely quantitative, i.e. according to our observations only a part of the synovial membrane is involved in the purulent bacterial process. This is the explanation for the relatively discrete, uncharacteristic symptomatology and its self-limiting nature. However, this process may also damage the joint.

Infective agent

The fact that in this CLBA a bacterial infection is not suspected explains why in general the physician in charge does not order a bacterial examination. In those cases, however, in which a bacterial culture is routinely done at each biopsy, it is found that as with "classical" BA, mostly *Staphylococcus aureus* or *Staphylococcus epidermidis* are identified.

Staphylococcus

Path of infection

The obvious idea that CLBA could be induced in the joint by a previous injection or other operative manipulation, is refuted by the fact that in none of the 375 cases we examined had any manipulation of the joint been undertaken. We have therefore no doubt that CLBA originates haematogenically. Evidence for this is the observation that in 30.9% of these cases joint involvement was oligoarticular. According to our present state of knowledge, silent bacteraemiae are not infrequent. They can occur following a minor treatment, endoscopy, and unnoticed trauma or skin infections and are, in general, without effects. In particular, there appears to be no preference of the infective agent to colonize the region of the joint (Goldenberg and Reed 1985; Esterhai and Gelb 1991). One may rather suspect that bacteraemia may lead to infection in other tissues of the organism, there also being silent, self-limiting, and showing no characteristic symptoms and sequelae. By contrast, the synovial membrane, due to its irritability and anatomical location, reacts with an exudative inflammation and pain. In some of our CLBA cases, skin infections were found but in most cases there was no evidence of the source of the silent bacteraemia.

Pattern of joint disease

As in "classical" BA, we also find in the above-mentioned 341 cases of CLBA that in the majority, i.e. 235 cases (68.9%), the knee joint was involved and, in descending order of frequency, the joints of the hand, ankle, finger, elbow, hip, shoulder, toe, and the sternoclavicular joint.

Symptomatology of CLBA

In the 341 patients with CLBA ("low-grade infection"), which had not been considered by the clinic to be BA, we have determined additionally the following symptoms: low pain on loading and on movement of the joint involved in 67.4%, effusion in 45.7%, low swelling in 46.3%, and low pain at rest in 31.6%. Only in 5.5% is redness and in 2.9% heat apparent. In the majority of patients, only one of the classical phenomena of inflammation may be present.

It is interesting to compare these 341 cases with the 34 patients in which BA was provisionally diagnosed. In the latter, the symptomatology also had no clear definition; it depended more on whether or not the physician associated the case with a scanty symptomatology possibly being BA. In this type of BA, parameters indicative of inflammation are frequently not helpful. ESR can be between 6 and 140 mm per h. Due to the relatively small numbers of causative agents, their detection is only possible during a short period of time. The provisional clinical diagnosis of the 341 patients with CLBA was "unspecific monarthritis" in 48.3% of cases, "rheumatoid arthritis" (RA) in 17.6%, and "unspecific oligoarthritis" in 8.8%. In the remaining 25.3% of cases, "osteoarthritis" (OA), "psoriatic arthritis" (PSA), "juvenile chronic arthritis" (JCA), "villo-nodular synovitis" (VNS), "reactive arthritis" (REA), "urate gout", and "Lyme arthritis" were suggested. There were no suspicions of a bacterial infection: in other words, the diagnosis "BA" depended in these cases on the objective morphological signs of bacterial processes.

19.3 Pathology

The histological differences among the non-bacterial arthritides are discrete and often only quantitative, but the morphological picture of BA is basically distinctive and unmistakable. The details involve all the components of the synovial "scene".

The fibrin exuded in the non-bacterial arthritides forms a thin film over the whole synovial surface and only in occasional cases extends further. The fibrin exudation in all types of BA, however, is much more impressive. Large fibrin masses are often found which have become detached from their synovial place of contact and lie free in the synovial cavity (Fig. 19.1). In contrast to the homogeneous fibrin of the non-bacterial arthritides, the fibrin of BA contains masses of neutrophils. The enzymatic action

Lamellated fibrin

and disappearance of these neutrophils result in the striking la-

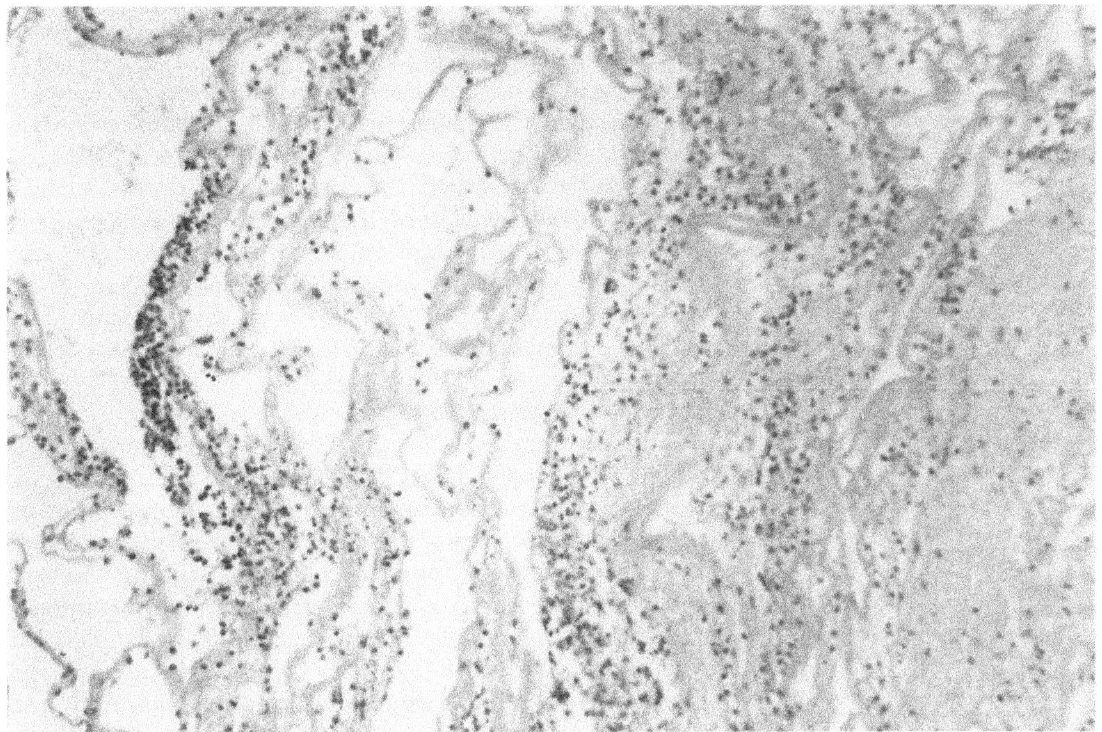

Fresh lamellated fibrin masses (pus). Numerous neutrophils in fibrin gaps

Fig. 19.1
Bacterial arthritis

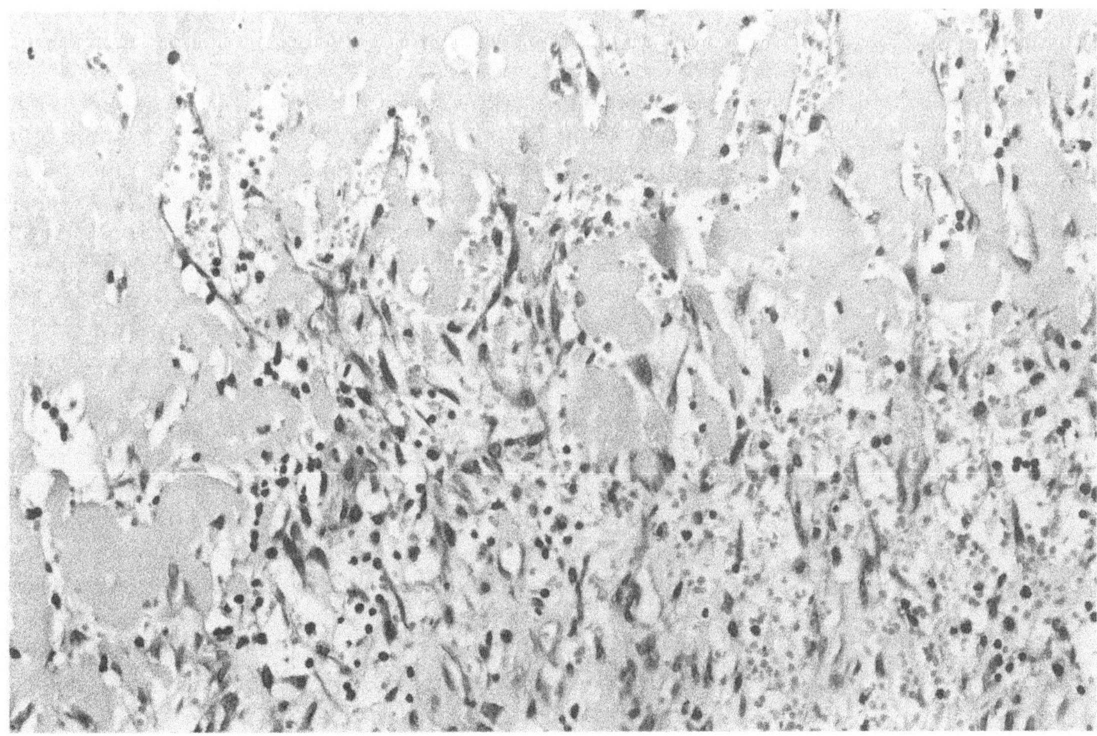

Fresh fibrin masses at the surface of the synovial membrane. Synovial tissue is transformed into a cell-rich granulation tissue, from there macrophages, fibroblasts, and angioblasts invade into the fibrin. Neutrophils in the gaps of the fibrin as well as in the granulation tissue

Fig. 19.2
Bacterial arthritis

mellated structure of the fibrin, which forms the clearly characteristic and unmistakable picture of BA.

Synovial membrane

Under the influence of bacterial toxins and neutrophil enzymes, the synovial membrane sustains a variable degree of severe damage with loss of structure. The synovial villi are destroyed and a smooth surface is formed. The damage usually goes even deeper and leads to the formation of the loose synovial stroma in a granulation tissue rich in cells and blood vessels (Fig. 19.2). This contains a great number of neutrophils as well as lymphocytes and macrophages. As pointed out already by Bywaters and Ansell (1965), neutrophil infiltrations of the synovial membrane are not part of the morphological picture of RA. This also applies to the other non-bacterial arthritides.

Articular cartilage

In contrast to the non-bacterial arthritides, the neutrophil-containing joint exudate reacts highly aggressive with the articular cartilage. The proteases liberated by the disintegration of the neutrophil masses degrade the matrix of the cartilage. In addition, there is the damaging effect of the bacterial toxin. The damage to the joint surface is considerable and not to be confused with that of RA: multiple crater-shaped depressions in the cartilage surface which also destroy the bone and can extend to the medulla are often visible containing fibrin remnants mostly mingled with neutrophils. The evidence for the acute cartilage damage in BA is the presence of variably sized sequestra of cartilage in the lamellated fibrin mass (Fig. 19.3). Their form is mainly oval and their edges are smoothed under the influence of the degrading neutrophil enzymes, in contrast to detached fragments of cartilage in OA and cartilage particles which are inclusions in the scar tissue in RA.

Sequestra of cartilage

Regressing BA

The changes described characterize the florid stage of BA, but the picture of the fibrin exudate differs during the regression of the bacterial inflammation process: the neutrophils die and leave behind nuclear debris, in the spaces between the fibrin lamellae. A few neutrophils may survive intact. Weeks or months after a fully regressed BA, the debris has also disappeared, the characteristic lamellation of the fibrin, however, remains (Fig. 19.4). The spaces between the lamellae of the old fibrin are empty.

Remodelling of synovial membrane

The synovial membrane also begins to recover. At first, a thin single layer of covering cells appears over the scar plate and, then, the first delicate short synovial villi are formed. But it is only many months later that the synovial membrane has fully recovered from the BA damage, and the remodelling has progressed to the stage that one can speak of an intact synovial membrane (Fig. 19.5).

Traces of BA

BA leaves its traces, however, which can still be perceived many years later. The fibrosing of the normally loose synovial stroma depends on the intensity and the duration of the process. Vessels that have developed during the bacterial process also remain behind. In areas of major destruction of the synovial surface, shrub-like, densely-layered, small blood vessels remain situated radially to the surface. With time, the number of vessels decreases while the calibre of those remaining increases.

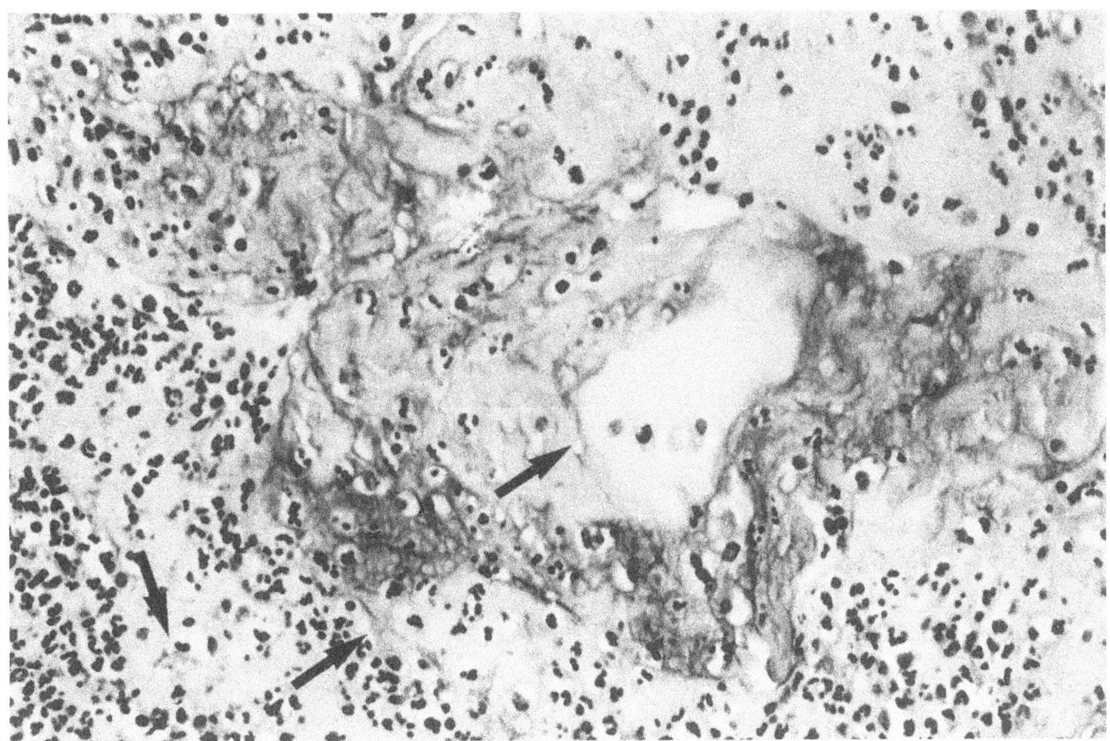

Fresh fibrin masses, interspersed with numerous neutrophils (pus). In the centre, enzymatically degraded sequestra of cartilage (*arrows*)

Fig. 19.3
Bacterial arthritis

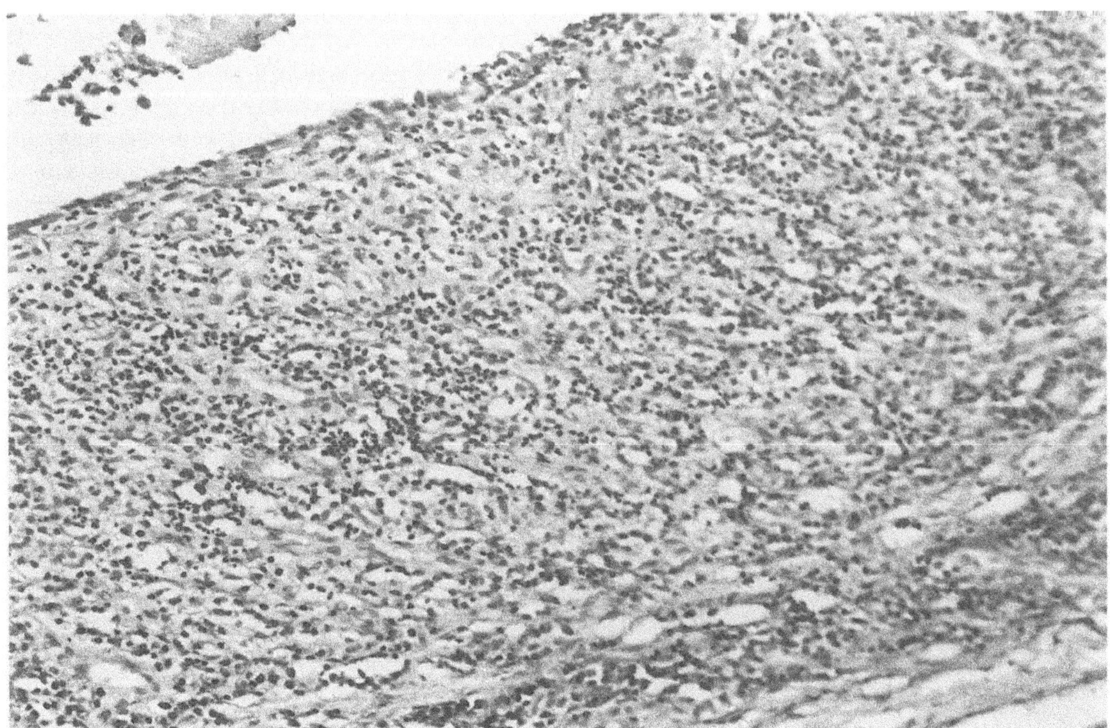

The synovial membrane is destroyed and transformed into a young, cell-rich scar tissue. Still some sporadic foci with neutrophils

Fig. 19.4
Subsiding bacterial arthritis

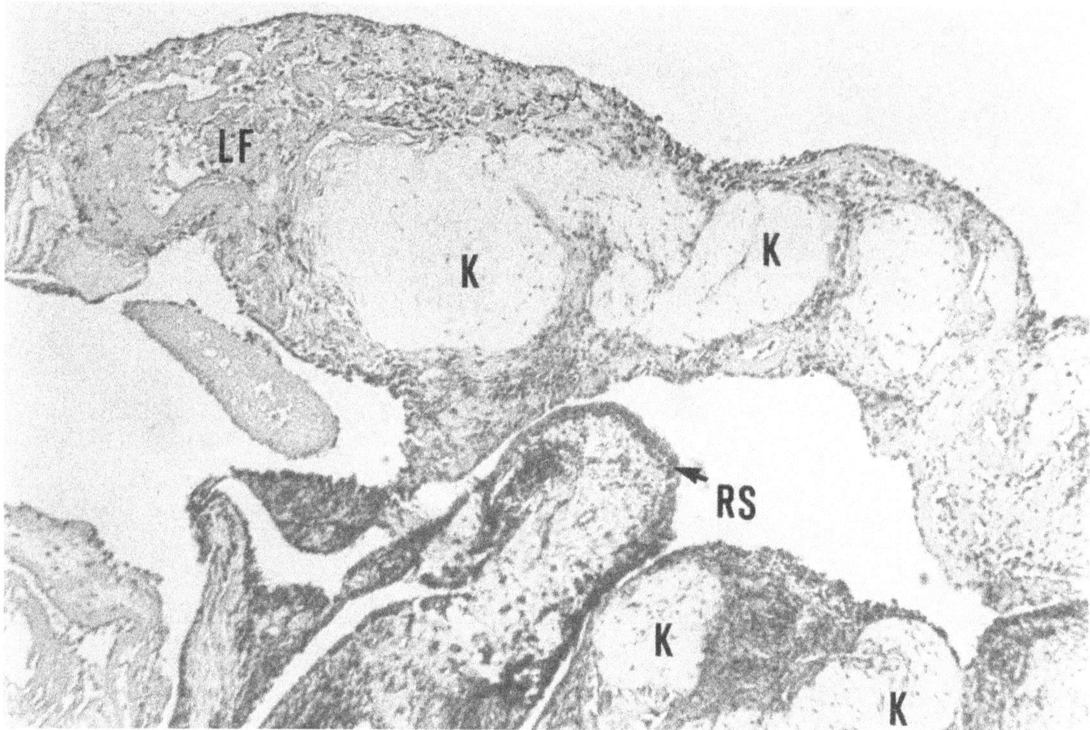

Fig. 19.5 Remnants of a bacterial arthritis, passed off weeks ago. Numerous enzymatically degraded sequestra of cartilage (*K*) in old, lamellated fibrin masses (*LF*). At one site, a regenerated lining cell layer (*RS*)

Other traces bearing witness to the destruction brought about by BA are the round and oval sequestra of cartilage enclosed in scar tissue. Immunological and other non-bacterial processes do not leave such a picture. Thus, a former bacterial synovitis can be diagnosed many months or even years later, especially if previous surgery and trauma are excluded (Fig. 19.6).

The reason why the purulent bacterial process manifests itself clinically in one case and in another remains clinically latent, is provided by the extent of the pathological process. We see that in CLBA it is often only one sector of the synovial membrane that is affected and the remaining areas are completely intact. In other cases, by contrast, the joint area is largely or fully involved in the bacterial-purulent process.

As CLBA mostly affects only parts of the synovial membrane and is self-limiting, the question arises as to the significance of these processes for the patient: the presence of degraded cartilage sequestra partly derived from larger fragments also found in CLBA is evidence of the damaging effect of the bacterial toxin and neutrophil enzyme on the articular cartilage. A regeneration of the hyaline cartilage of the same quality is not possible, so the remaining defect must be corrected with connective tissue and later with fibrous cartilage. It can only be speculated as to how far such scars on the surface of the hyaline articular cartilage predispose to later OA.

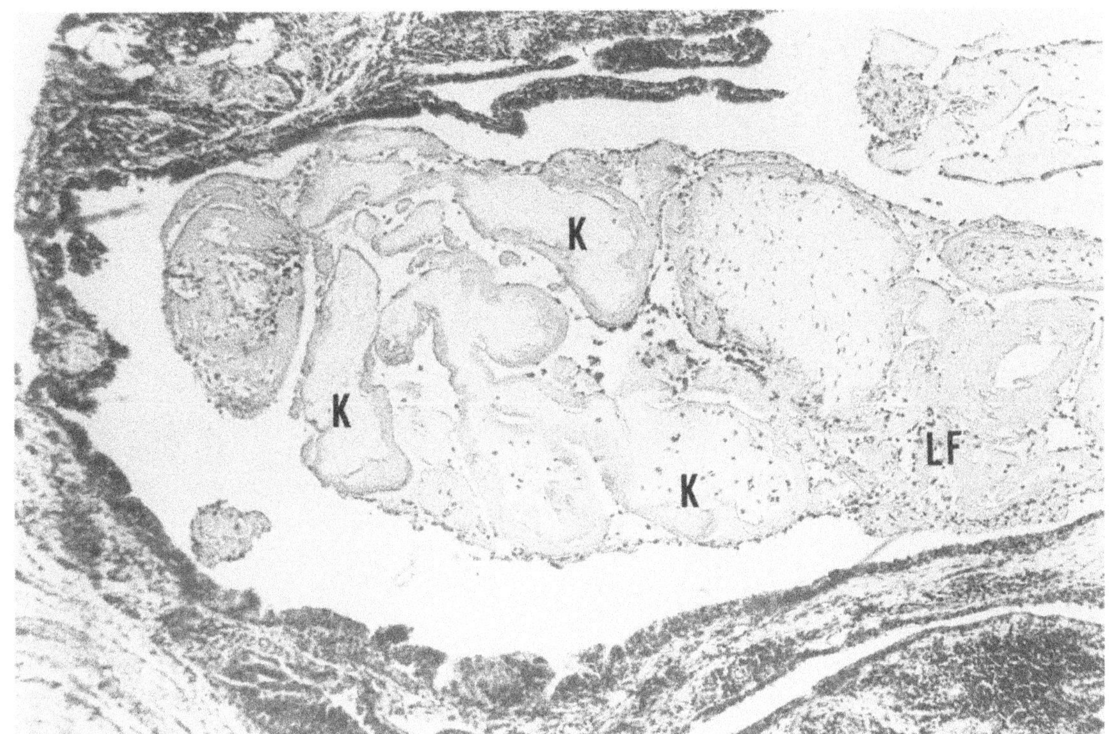

Remnants of a bacterial arthritis, passed off months ago. Synovial membrane is partly regenerated. First steps to new villous formation (*arrows*). In one synovial lacuna, old, lamellated fibrin masses (*LF*). Fibrin is free of cells (*K*, old enzymatically degraded sequestra of cartilage). In the regenerated synovial membrane, dense, focal infiltrates of lymphocytes

Fig. 19.6

20 Bacterial Superinfection

20.1 Definition

Septic bacterial superinfection

Kellgren and colleagues (1958) have described the susceptibility of the rheumatoid joint to superimposed bacterial infections. These present clinically as septic diseases needing appropriate therapy. We have not had any biopsies from patients with a current real septic superinfection, because in these cases intensive antibiotic therapy is required and biopsy is not indicated.

Clinically latent bacterial superinfection

We discovered, however, in our own biopsy material from patients with rheumatoid arthritis (RA), osteoarthritis (OA), and other rheumatic diseases bacterial superinfections (CLBS) as an incidental finding. They had developed in a clinically latent manner and had been hitherto unsuspected.

In a study (1989 1990) of 2,355 unselected consecutive joint biopsies (Hebert et al. 1990), we found a CLBS present in 149 (13.5%) of the 1,106 cases of RA, in 19 (8.8%) of the 216 cases of OA, and in 92 (8.9%) of 1,033 cases with various other rheumatic diseases. The most frequently superinfected joints were the knees. These processes had remained clinically undetected because the bacterial infection often affects only a segment of the synovial membrane and the number of infective agents and their virulence are relatively low in relation to the cellular defence (neutrophils). The process is therefore self-limiting and does not develop into a sepsis. The presenting symptoms were attributed in these patients to the underlying non-bacterial systemic arthritis.

20.2 Pathology

Primary bacterial infections (BA; see p. 385) and bacterial superinfections are basically identical processes. The clinically latent superinfection that we observe is also characterized by the same morphological features, such as fibrin masses and numerous neutrophils, the latter of which, depending on the duration of the process, exist only in the form of cell debris or have left their traces as lamellated fibrin. While the immunological and other non-bacterial synovitides do not destroy the fundamental structures of the synovial membrane, but on the contrary over-emphasize the tendency to develop villi in the form of a villous hyperplasia, a bacterial purulent superinfection destroys the syn-

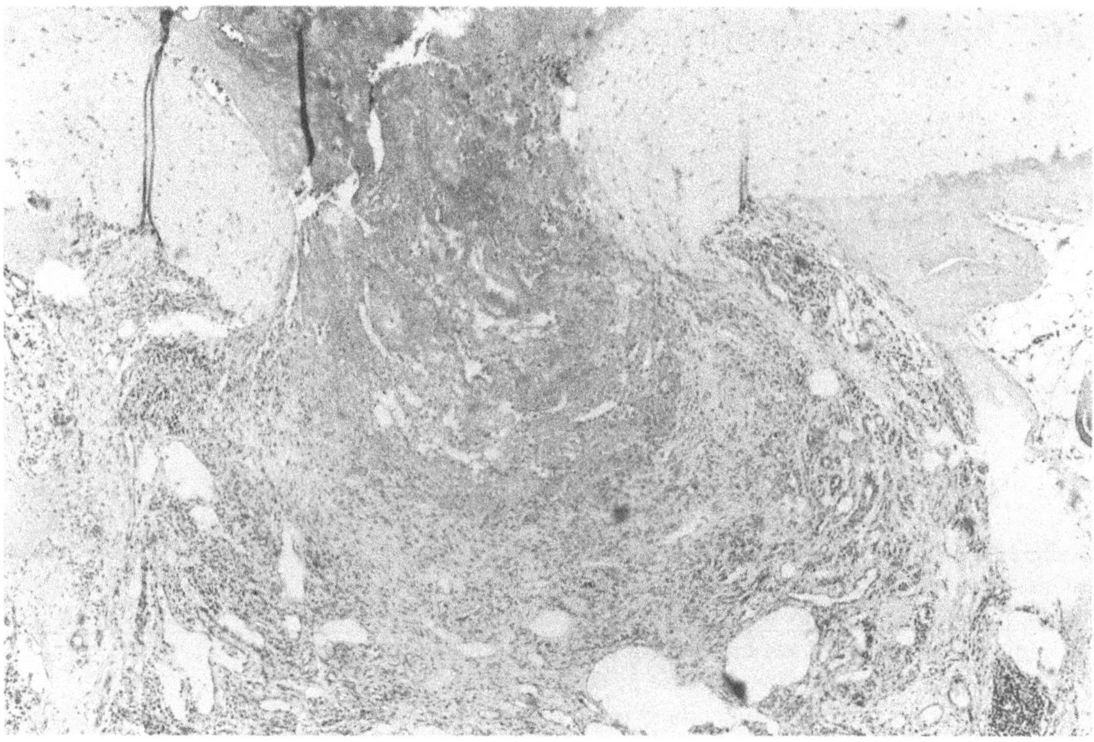

Fig. 20.1
Bacterial superinfection

Ankle joint. Funnel-shaped destruction of articular cartilage by bacterial superinfection in RA. The defect is filled with fibrin and neutrophils. Beginning scarred encapsulation in the medullary space (54-year-old female)

ovial architecture. In this area, the villi have perished. The smooth surface is covered by granulation tissue and fibrin. These "bald" patches are evidence of a bacterial devastation. As such they can unmistakably be distinguished by changes caused by RA or other non-bacterial synovitides. Different than in primary BA, the parts destroyed by neutrophil proteases lie within conserved villous structures. While the surface of the synovial membrane may regenerate, scars and numerous newly formed vessels will always remain within the synovial stroma to bear witness to the bacterial episodes.

In bacterial superinfections, also as in BA, the typical, funnel-shaped destructions of the articular surface up to the medullary space can be seen (see p. 390; Figs. 20.1, 20.2).

The neutrophil proteases degrade the fibrin into the lamellar structure characteristic of bacterial infection. In the fibrin, numerous variably sized, mainly oval, smooth edged enzymatically degraded cartilage sequestra are found.

Resolving bacterial infection

Bacterial superinfection is resolved by the action of the local neutrophil defence mechanism on the relatively low concentrations of markedly leukotactic bacteria. In this way, the infection is overcome in a short time without therapeutic intervention. After cessation of bacterial leukotaxis, the numbers of neutrophils are reduced. Between the fibrin lamellae there remain dead cells and, after a time, only nuclear debris which later also disappears. The bacterial infection is thus terminated.

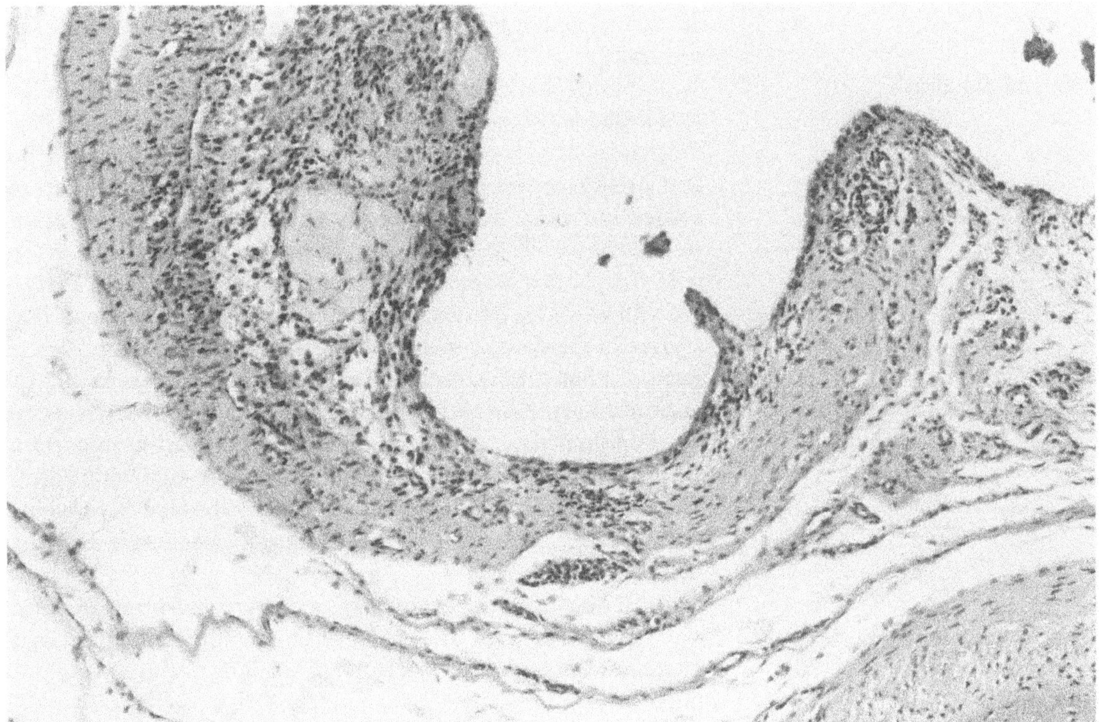

Wrist joint. Older, funnel-shaped fracture in old scar pannus. In the granulation tissue old fibrin remnants and enzymatically degraded cartilaginous sequestra (60-year-old female)

Fig. 20.2
Bacterial superinfection in RA

Scarring and reconstitution of synovial membrane

In the bacterial superinfected area of the synovial membrane, not only is the lining cell layer destroyed but also the deeper layers of the synovial stroma. The original synovial architecture is replaced by a cell-rich granulation tissue and later by a highly vascular scar tissue. The granulation tissue contains lymphocytes together with neutrophils grouped at the contact place of the fibrin covering. The self-limiting process can involve greater or smaller sections of the synovial membrane. After several months, the traces of a resolved bacterial superinfection can still be recognized by the lamellation of the fibrin masses (even when there is no more evidence of nuclear debris), but above all in the scarring destructuring of the synovial membrane followed many months later by its restructuring, and finally by the rebuilding of the characteristic synovial villi.

20.3 Etiology

Staphylococcus aureus or Staphylococcus epidermidis

As CLBS has a limited course, there is only evidence of bacteria in the acute phase and before the sterilizing action of the neutrophil enzymes takes place. They are mainly discovered in routine synovial fluid investigations undertaken before a bacterial infection has been suspected. In these, evidence of *Staphylococcus aureus* or *Staphylococcus epidermidis* is regularly found. In the acute phase, the ESR is clearly raised (between

40–80 in 1 h) but this is related to the activity of the arthritis in general.

Path of infection

We cannot subscribe to the opinion that this latent superinfection is due to previous joint injections as we found these as a factor in only 24% of our RA patients with superinfection. It is true that in 40% of the cases previous joint injections had been recorded but since in the majority of patients no manipulations were done we feel that as in the primary bacterial arthritides (see p. 387), the haematogenous path of infection is the most likely.

We believe that in patients with arthritides, two components have a share in the development of bacterial superinfections:

Promotion due to therapeutic agents

Asymptomatic bacteraemias are not unknown even in the healthy. In arthritis patients, bacteraemias are possibly favoured by antiphlogistic, steroid, and non-steroid drugs, but in particular through the use of immunosuppressive and cytostatic agents. The haematogenous origin is supported by the fact that we quite often find a CLBS in two or more joint biopsies in the same patients.

Promotion due to synovial structures

As in all non-bacterial arthritides, a villous hyperplasia develops over a period of time. The crypts of this multiply folded synovial membrane surface are very suitable sites for bacterial colonization.

The bacterial superinfection, although self-limiting and clinically not ostentatious, is, nevertheless, highly significant for the affected joint. This is shown by the fact that even after several months, the lamellated fibrin masses contain cartilage sequestra which have been dislodged from the joint surface and under the action of the neutrophil proteases have been partly or wholly degraded (see above); months later, only weak basophil shadows remain in the fibrin. How far the bacterial toxins damage the matrix of the cartilage and the chondrocytes cannot be estimated from our biopsy material.

Augmention of joint destruction

It must be taken into account, nevertheless, that bacterial superinfections, as discovered incidentally in our biopsies, are not rare in the course of non-bacterial (immunological) arthritides and are a feature of the recurrent episodes which augment the destruction of the joint.

We have the impression that the great number of bacterial superinfections in our tissue specimens from RA patients can be at least partly explained by the actualisation of the disease process through this inflammation which leads to operative or bioptical interventions.

Arising from these findings, we conclude that recurrent, limited, clinically latent episodes of bacterial superinfection influence the course of many non-bacterial arthritides (especially in RA) and play a part in the basic clinical manifestation, the symptomatology, and progress of the disease. Perhaps these bacterial episodes also reinforce the false notion that higher neutrophil counts in the synovial membrane or fibrin are part of the morphological picture of RA. This was shown not to be the case already by Bywaters and Ansell (1965).

21 AIDS and Rheumatism

In human immunodeficiency virus (HIV) infections, the expectation is met that opportunistic joint infections occur. Thereby unusual infective agents are observed. Acquired immunodeficiency syndrome (AIDS) is of special interest with regard to its interaction with rheumatic diseases, the basis of which, according to our current knowledge, lies in an immunological mechanism, the role of which in the pathogenesis, however, is not entirely explained. From this point of view, the appearance of AIDS in which there is a defined disturbance of the immune system, namely damage to the CD4+ helper lymphocytes, provides the role of a nosological experiment. It gives the possibility of studying the role of the helper cells in the pathogenesis of these rheumatic diseases. The consequences for systemic diseases of immunological disturbance are difficult to define accurately because of the complexity of the involved immunological mechanisms. If one reviews the reports available up-to-date, there appear to be two kinds of effect that HIV infection has on systemic "rheumatic" diseases: on the one side, there are Reiter's syndrome (RS), psoriatic arthritis (PSA), Sjögren's syndrome (SS), polymyositis (PM), and vasculitis, and, on the other side, rheumatoid arthritis (RA) and systemic lupus erythematosus (SLE).

Immunological disturbance

21.1 HIV Infection and Reiter's Syndrome

Two different forms of RS

In HIV-infected patients, two different forms of RS are observed, namely a severe, cumulative form and a mild, intermittent form, which can also occur in HIV-negative patients. Data of the prevalence of RS in HIV-infected individuals range from 1.7% (Calabrese et al. 1991) to 9.9% (Berman et al. 1988) and are thus clearly higher than in the normal population. The classical triad, arthritis, urethritis, conjunctivitis, is not always marked, in particular, conjunctivitis rarely occurs. The changes are especially striking in the feet, giving rise to the term "AIDS foot". Marked muscular wasting along with enthesopathy and plantar fasciitis are dominant characteristics in both forms of HIV-associated RS. These changes can precede the onset of AIDS. It is under-

"AIDS foot"

standable that in these cases immunosuppressive therapy would have catastrophic effects.
In 79%, HLA-B27 is present in HIV patients with RS (Winchester 1990) and, thus, does not differ significantly from HIV-negative patients with RS. The same applies for direct preceding infections. Immunopathologically, mainly CD8+ lymphocytes together with the HIV p24 antigen is reported. As a microbial persistence in RS is highly probable, this might explain its higher prevalence in HIV-infected patients who have a dysfunction of the normal clearance mechanism.

21.2 HIV Infection and Psoriatic-Like Arthritis

From an investigation by Duvic and coworkers (1987), the prevalence of psoriasis in HIV-infected patients of 1%–2% was similar to that in the normal population. The course of the disease in AIDS patients, however, is considerably more severe. The musculoskeletal involvement resembles that in RS, but includes patients whose distal interphalangeal joints are affected. How far AIDS-associated psoriasis is identical with the idiopathic form is not yet fully elucidated. At least, the frequencies of specific HLA alleles deviate from each other. As in RS, a mild, intermittent form, in contrast to an aggressive cumulative form, can be differentiated.

21.3 HIV Infection and Sjögren's Syndrome

DILS

In patients with HIV- or HTLV 1 infection, there is a peculiar phenomenon which is probably a variant of SS. This disease entity described as DILS (diffuse infiltrative lymphocytosis syndrome) is characterized by an enlargement of the parotid gland and xerostomia. Histologically, there is a diffuse infiltration of glandular and also extraglandular tissue by CD8+ and CD29+ lymphocytes. DILS is differentiated from conventional SS by the lack of autoantibodies.

21.4 HIV Infection and Polymyositis

CD4+ lymphocytes bearing HIV-antigens

In HIV infections, all stages of PM are observed. The onset is usually insidious, the pathological mechanism as yet unknown. Histologically, there is a diffuse infiltration with CD4+ lymphocytes bearing HIV-antigens on their surface, CD8+ lymphocytes, and monocytes.

21.5 HIV Infection and Vasculitis

In the context of the AIDS disease, various forms of vasculitides are observed, namely:

- Associated with cytomegalovirus infection
- Associated with eosinophilia

- Manifested as necrotizing vasculitis resembling the pattern of periarteritis nodosa with involvement of the central nervous system
- Manifested as leucocytoclastic vasculitis in mononeuritis multiplex

In addition, granulomatous vasculitides are observed.

21.6 HIV Infection and RA and SLE

The concept that attributes an obligatory role to CD4+ helper-cells in the pathogenesis of RA was tested in an unplanned experiment.

Unplanned experiment

The elimination of the CD4+ T cells in HIV infections could theoretically give an insight into the mechanisms of these diseases, in which this cell system is ascribed a leading pathogenetic role. There are indeed individual observations in which symptomatic improvement of RA and SLE in AIDS patients does occur (Bijlsma et al. 1988; Furie et al. 1988). In the course of time, however, more and more observations hinted at a possible co-existence of both diseases. According to these, the destruction of CD4+ cells by the virus did not influence the activity of RA (Ornstein et al. 1995). Müller-Ladner and colleagues (1995) reported on the histological and immunohistological findings in a patient with both HIV-disease and RA, in whom ongoing joint destruction was documented on autopsy, without the presence of T cells. Thus, recent scientific data appear to show that active RA may occur independent of the presence of CD4+ lymphocytes in both the peripheral blood and the joint.

Co-existence of both diseases

The destructive process in RA is the product of highly proliferated, synovial cell elements (tumour-like proliferation, tlp) and not that of inflammatory cells and their metabolites (see p. 89), this accounts for the corresponding independence of this RA-typical process from CD4+ lymphocytes.

In contrast to that, the mutual exclusion of HIV and SLE has been documented by Fox and Isenberg (1997). They used stored serum, the precise timing of HIV seroconversion was determined and the early effects of HIV infection on SLE examined. This infection resulted in clinical improvement and the disappearance of autoantibody production. The observations submitted so far seem to indicate that CD4+ lymphocytes do play a role in the pathogenetic chain of events in SLE but not in that of RA.

Mutual exclusion of HIV and SLE

22 Tuberculosis

Manifestation in skeletal system

In about 1% of patients with tuberculosis of the lung, the *Mycobacterium tuberculosis* invades the skeletal system in the form of a haematogeneous dispersion (Davidson and Horowitz 1970). It occurs chiefly in adolescent patients and preferentially in the vertebrae of the thoraco-lumbar region and the weight bearing surfaces of hip, knee, and ankles.

In over 80% of these cases, spinal tuberculosis begins in the anterior part of the vertebral body (Partridge 1986). The disease process can then shift to the neighbouring vertebra via the intervertebral disc and also break through into the paraspinal tissue as a "cold abscess". In untreated cases, the vertebral bodies are destroyed and collapse. This can result in kyphosis and also eventually compression of the spinal cord.

Synovial tuberculosis

In cases in which we could detect bioptically a clear synovial tuberculosis, it clinically was presented as "unclear" monarthritis of the hip, knee, wrist, and ankle joints. In none of these cases was there a suspicion of tuberculous disease.

22.1 Pathology

Tuberculosis can manifest itself in the synovial tissue in two forms:

1. Proliferative granulomatous type:
   The morphological picture of tuberculous synovitis is variable: the typical tuberculous granulomata are round and consist of densely layered epithelioid cells with weakly eosinophil cytoplasm and light, oval cell nuclei which on aging of the granuloma become oblong and darker. Giant cells of the Langhans type with numerous peripheral nuclei are certainly typical for the epithelioid cell granuloma, but they can also be absent. Depending on its age, the tuberculous granuloma is progressively encircled by collagen fibres with lymphocytes lying in between and surrounding it in an annular form. This lymphocytic infiltration is, however, usually less well defined than with sarcoidosis granuloma. The most important constituents of the tuberculous granuloma are, however, the epithelioid cells. Here, we are dealing with a special macrophagocytic reaction of the phosphatide fraction of the *Mycobacterium tuberculosis*. Impressive as these granulomata are, they, nevertheless, do not permit the pathologist to make an uneqivocal diagnosis since the picture presented does not

Diagnostic difficulties

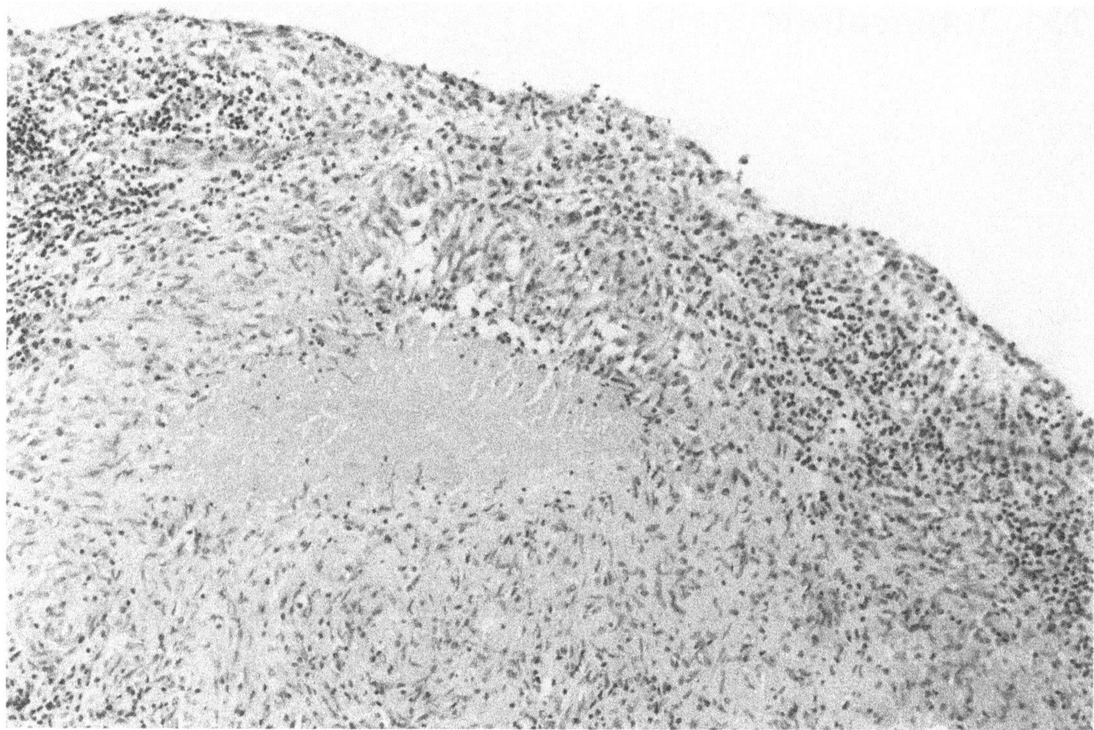

Fig. 22.1
Tuberculous arthritis

Ankle joint. "Caseous" necrotic focus in the synovial membrane, surrounded by epithelioid cells. On the outside, dense lymphocytic infiltrations (73-year-old female)

allow a clear differentiation from, for example, sarcoidosis. Small central cell necroses must cause the strongest suspicion of a tuberculous process, but here also the diagnosis "tuberculosis" should be further established clinically before the institution of tuberculostatic therapy.

2. Exudative "caseous" type:
   In contrast to the synovial processes the exudative caseous lesions are considered to be specific and are characterized by tissue necrosis surrounded by epithelioid cells (Fig. 22.1). Occasionally, there are in between giant cells of the Langhans type and a few lymphocytes. As the epithelioid cells are only loosely layered in the form of an uncohesive border, they are hard to view and often only with difficulty may be identified as such.

Differential diagnosis

The identification of the caseous necrosis can also be difficult. It must be differentiated from other phenomena which are equally anuclear, homogeneous, and eosinophile, namely fibrinous exudate, hyalinized joint capsule tissue, and necroses in rheumatoid arthritis (RA):

- Fibrinous exudate is equally homogeneous. It can, however, contain a few remnants of neutrophils or lymphocytes. At higher magnification, a fine fibrillary network can be recognized but with no tissue fragments. In contrast to this, in the tuberculous-caseous necrosis, particularly after staining the elastic fibres, indistinct structures of the destroyed tissue can still be identified.

- Hyalinized regions of the capsule tissue are equally homogeneous and eosinophile, but they show no cellular border reaction. Polarized light reveals the wave-form structure indicating the original collagenous character. In contrast, the tuberculous necrosis is granular.
- The differentiation of tuberculous necrosis from necrosis in RA can present considerable difficulties. In RA-necrosis, too, there are remnants of the original tissue structure. Old RA-necroses can disintegrate and then give a granular effect reminiscent of caseous tuberculosis. Moreover, in old necroses, the cell palisade can be discontinuous and irregular so that it is possible to confuse it with epithelioid cells. A helpful fact is that tuberculous necroses in general occur in looser tissues like lungs and synovial tissue, while RA-necroses preferentially affect collagenous structures like tendons and the fibrous section of the joint capsule. The main help in the further clarification of the diagnosis, however, is derived from the presence of epithelioid cell granulomata distributed in the wider surroundings. A final certainty in the question of a tuberculous etiology from the standpoint of morphology is the evidence of *Mycobacterium tuberculosis* in the form of acid-fast rods by means of staining by the Ziehl-Neelsen method.

Differentiation to RA-necroses

Naturally the absence of granulomata and caseation in the synovial tissue does not exclude a tuberculous origin of synovitis, as the specific process in general is accompanied by an unspecific synovitis with fibrinous exudation and lymphocytic infiltration.

Tissue material, obtained by biopsy of hip, knee, finger, wrist, and ankle joints in which a clear tuberculosis was found, according to our investigations, came almost exclusively from patients with monarthritides. They were referred to us on the suspicion of an incipient RA or another rheumatic disease. Klofkorn and Steigerwald (1976) reported two patients presenting a carpal tunnel syndrome (CTS) as an initial manifestation of tuberculosis. If there is a case of clinically clear joint tuberculosis there is in general no need for a trial biopsy, for in these cases the synovial fluid is available for a bacteriological investigation.

23 Sarcoidosis

23.1 Definition

According to the definition of the Subcommittee on Classification and Definition at the Seventh International Congress of Sarcoidosis and Other Granulomatous Diseases, sarcoidosis is a multisystemic granulomatous disorder of unknown etiology and pathogenesis which most commonly affects young adults. Its presenting manifestations most frequently involve bilateral hilar adenopathy, pulmonary infiltration, and skin or eye lesions (Hellmann and Stobo 1986).

Significance of histological diagnostics

The clinical progression and the symptoms of the disease can vary. The clinical and radiological findings are confirmed by the histological detection of widespread, non-caseating granulomata. In addition to the principal characteristic symptoms, the peripheral lymph nodes, liver, heart, kidneys, skeletal musculature, and joints may also be affected. The Kveim-test was found to be positive in 79% of 3,676 patients with sarcoidosis in a large-scale, worldwide study (Siltzbach et al. 1974). However, the specificity of this test for sarcoidosis has been questioned (Israel and Goldstein 1971). Although the tuberculin-test is always negative in patients with sarcoidosis, recent examinations show a certain resemblance to tuberculosis. In granulomata from 16 patients with sarcoidosis, Fidler and coworkers (1993) found seven cases of *Mycobacterium tuberculosis* DNA, but only one case in 16 matched controls.

23.2 Clinical Manifestations

Arthritis is the most frequent rheumatic manifestation of sarcoidosis, occurring in 5%–37% of patients. Females are two to three times more frequently affected (Maycock et al. 1963; Siltzbach and Duberstein 1968).

Rheumatic manifestations

Sarcoidosis acquires rheumatological interest because the joints and tendon sheaths are also affected in the disease process. In most cases, the arthritis starts acutely as an initial manifestation of the disease and is often associated with erythema nodosum and bilateral hilar adenopathy (Löfgren's syndrome).

Acute sarcoid arthritis

Acute sarcoid arthritis is characterized by a migrating symmetrical arthralgia, which attacks mainly the knees, ankle joints, proximal interphalangeal joints, hand joints, and elbows (Siltzbach and Duberstein 1968; Spilberg et al. 1969). The acute sarcoid arthritis starts with pain and restriction of movement. The symptoms reach their maximum intensity after about 3 days and last for between 2 weeks and 4 months. Synovial effusions are minimal, and joint deformation or destruction are not observed in acute sarcoid arthritis.

Chronic sarcoid arthritis

Chronic sarcoid arthritis can start early or late during the course of sarcoidosis and can repeatedly flare-up over the years. Mono- or oligoarticular affliction, particularly of the knee and foot joints, is typical.

Polyarticular destructive arthritis in sarcoidosis

A rare, special form of chronic sarcoid arthritis starts insiduously and is characterized by polyarticular joint destruction. This is likely to be confused with rheumatoid arthritis (RA), particularly since approximately one-third of sarcoidosis patients are rheumatoid factor-positive (Hellmann and Stobo 1986). Periarthritis and tenosynovitis can occur separately or can be found together with both forms of arthritis.

23.3 Pathology

Round granulomata without central caseation are found histologically in both acutely and chronically affected tissues.

In one of our studies, lasting from 1994 to 1999, we were able to detect 42 times the morphological picture of sarcoidosis in tissue samples sent us without any clinical suspicion for a granulomatosis. Knees, wrist joints, and juxta-articular tendons were the most affected sites but also finger joints as well as elbows were involved.

Epithelioid cellular granulomatosis

The granulomata are formed primarily from epithelioid cells and in most cases contain multinuclear giant cells of the Langhans type. The epithelioid cells derive from the macrophage lineage. Depending on the age of the cells, the nucleus is oval to spindle-shaped and the cytoplasm is weakly eosinophilic. These granulomata are surrounded by a dense coating of lymphocytes.

Differential diagnosis of granulomata

The sarcoid granulomata show no necrotizing tendency. This alone, however, is not a reliable differential diagnostic criterion since those granulomata which are induced by *Mycobacterium tuberculosis* also rarely tend to necrotize (the intrinsic caseation occurs mostly outside the granulomata). In addition, histologically similar granulomata are found not only in tuberculosis, but also in chronic berylliosis, histoplasmosis, coccidioidomycosis, foreign body reactions (with the corresponding inclusions), schistosomiasis, and syphilis.

Although the sarcoid granuloma corresponds in principle to the tuberculoid granuloma, there are further differences besides the lack of caseation: the granulomata are in general larger ("exuberant") and more similar to each other than those in tuberculosis. The giant cells are also, on average, larger. In persistent disease, they may also contain crystalline inclusions (Schaumann bodies). The giant cells are more often located in the centre, compared with those in tuberculosis granulomata, and the lymphocytic coating is, moreover, more pronounced. The diagnosis

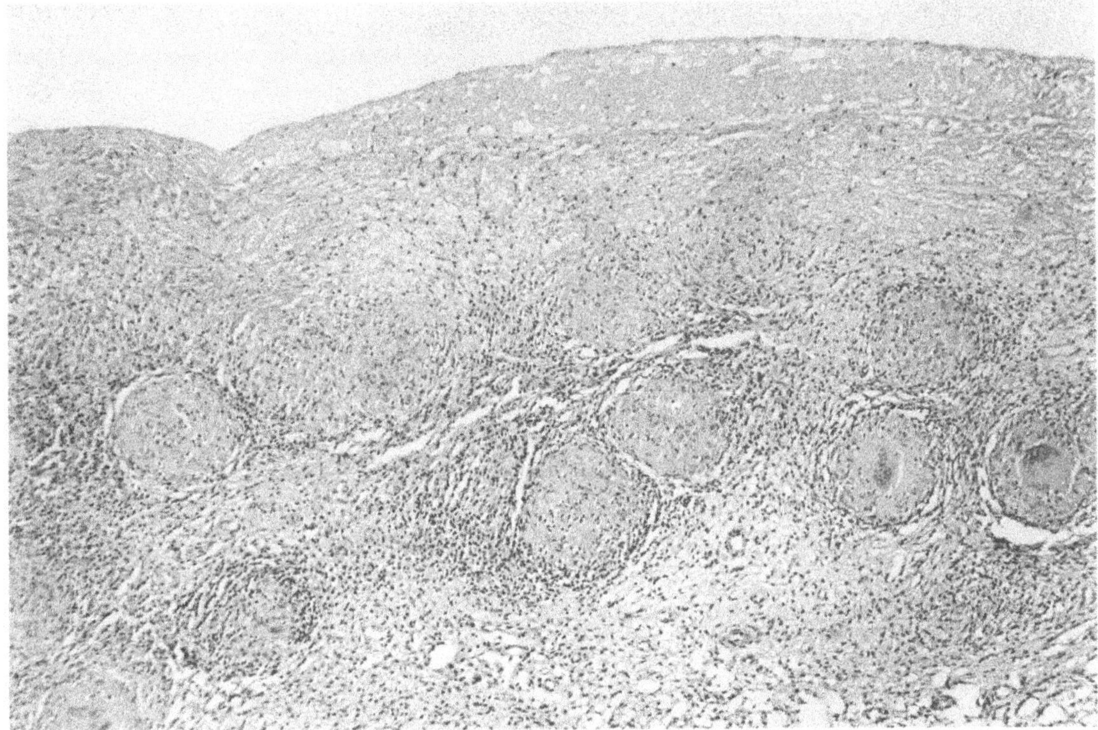

Knee. Numerous epithelioid cellular granulomata with giant cells predominantly located in the centre. Sarcoidosis has triggered a marked accompanying synovitis with high-grade infiltration by lymphocytes, macrophages, and isolated neutrophils. Superficial fibrin deposits (38-year-old male)

Fig. 23.1
Sarcoidosis

which decides upon the therapy has, however, to be confirmed by additional clinical and bacteriological evidence.

Synovitis

The clinical picture of sarcoid arthritis is mainly determined by the non-specific inflammatory process which accompanies the specific granulomatous process (Figs. 23.1–23.3). Thereby villous proliferation, fibrin exudation, and lymphocytic infiltration occur.

Regression

In the course of time, the granulomata can completely regress or leave behind a hyaline scar. In this process, the epithelioid cells disappear first whereas the giant cells are maintained for longer. The lymphocyte coating also remains longer, and, thus, one can occasionally find only the foci of lymphocytes surrounding single, multinucleated giant cells.

Skeletal musculature and tendons

The skeletal musculature and tendons in sarcoidosis are often asymptomatic but may occasionally also be painfully afflicted. In these cases, a high percentage of non-caseating granulomata can be detected by biopsy. Since the space between the fibres is narrow, the granulomata are quite often very small and can be completely overlain by the accompanying lymphocytic infiltration. Thus, under certain conditions, sarcoidosis of the skeletal musculature cannot be observed. It is recommended, therefore, to histologically examine the musculature in graded sections if sarcoidosis is suspected. Alternatively, groups of granulomata may be inserted in a string-like manner between the muscle fibres.

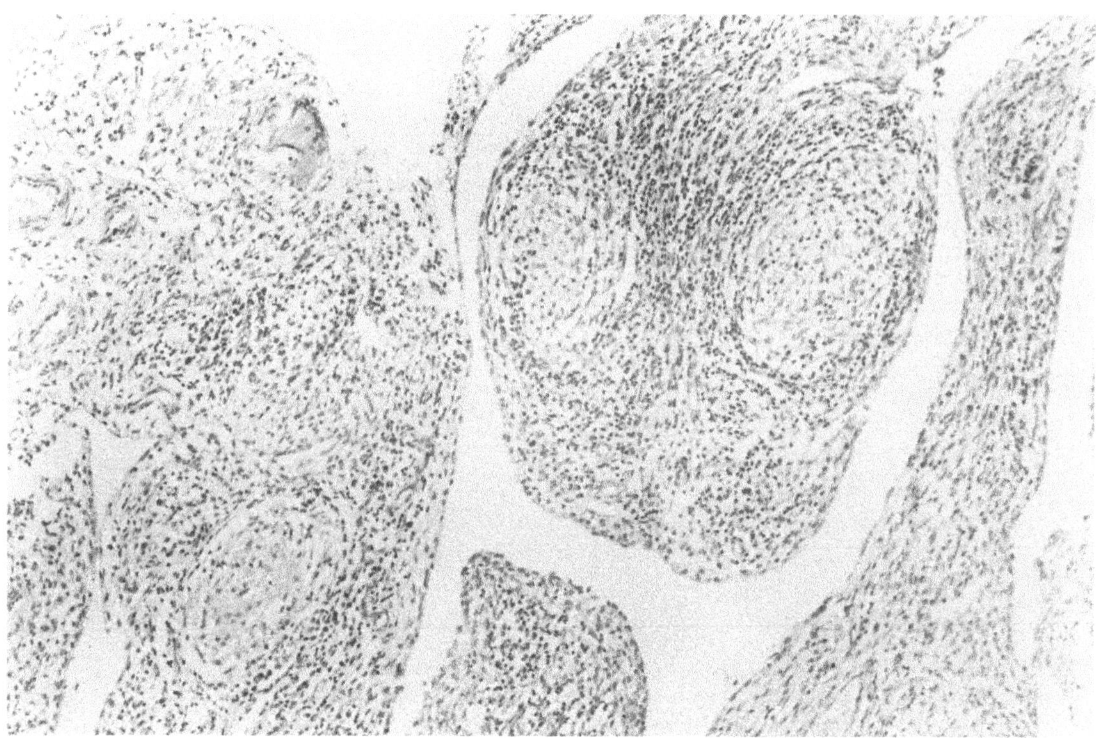

Fig. 23.2
Sarcoidosis

Knee. Synovial villi are distended by large epithelioid cellular granulomata. Only a few giant cells (9-year-old male)

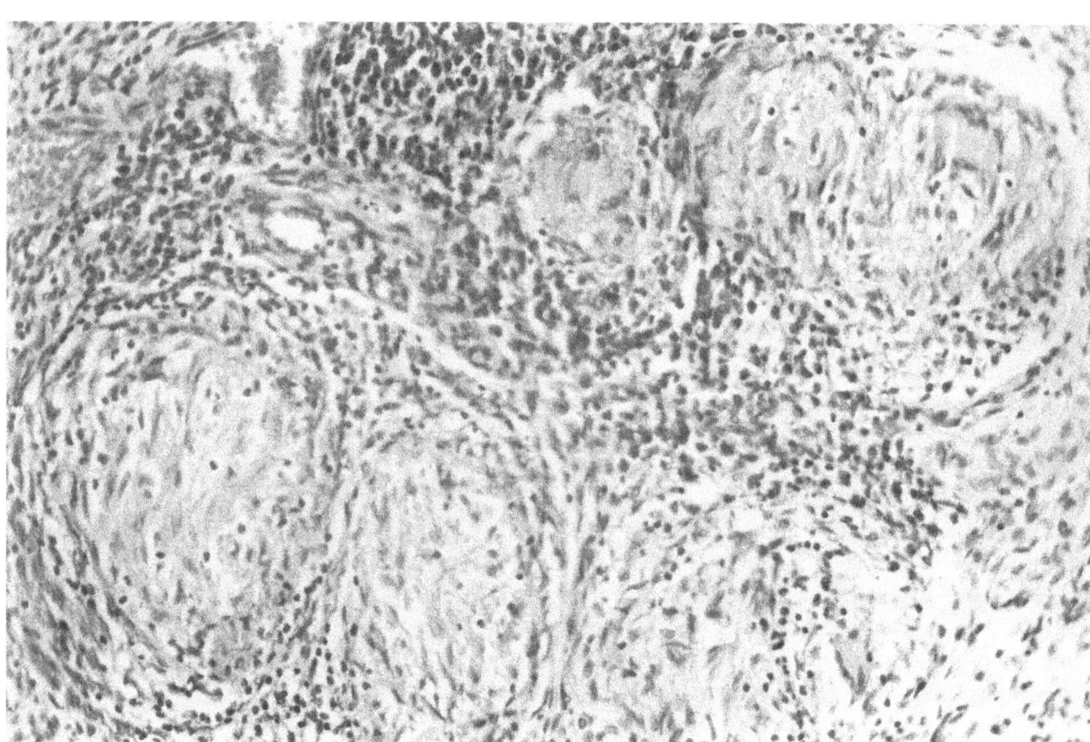

Fig. 23.3
Sarcoidosis

Knee. Peritendinous tissue with high-grade lymphocytic infiltration (9-year-old male)

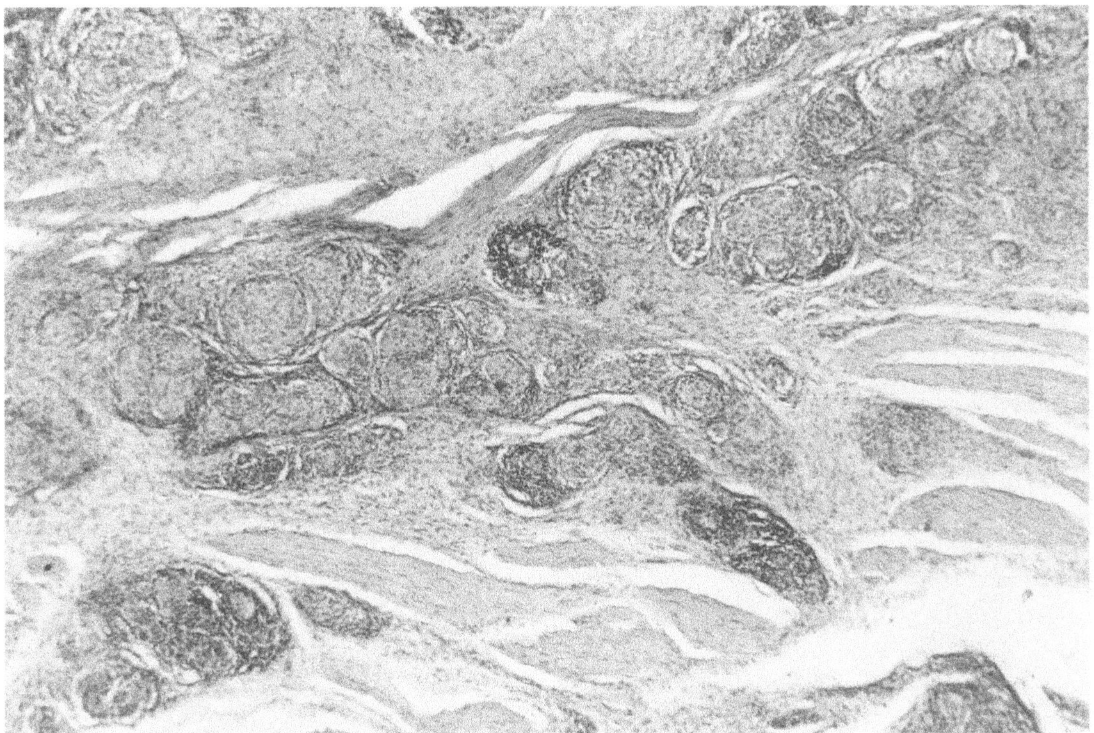

Fig. 23.4
Sarcoidosis

Wrist joint. Densely packed epithelioid cellular granulomata which destructively intervene the fibre bundles of the tendon (39-year-old female)

The sarcoid granulomata not only push the muscle fibres apart, they also destroy them. This is often recognized at the edges of the granulomata. Nevertheless, muscle weakness and an increase of muscle enzymes in serum may be absent. We found similar changes also in the adjacent tendons where the granulomata destructively intervene the fibre bundles of the tendons (Fig. 23.4).

Destructive potency of sarcoid granulomata

The destructive power of the sarcoid granulomata becomes especially evident when the skeletal system is afflicted: as well as round, focal destruction of the phalanges, metacarpals, and nasal bones, the process can "tunnel through" the cortex and shaft of the phalanx and cause high-grade destruction.

Metabolic activity

Besides the localized destructive potency there is evidence of metabolic activity of the epithelioid cells of the sarcoid granulomata in the synthesis of angiotensin I-converting enzyme and 1.25 dihydroxyvitamin D (Silverstein et al. 1976; Barbour et al. 1981; Maesaka et al. 1982; Mason et al. 1984).

HLA-B8

The fact that an increased incidence of HLA-B8 was observed in patients with sarcoid arthritis indicates a possible predisposition, but still leaves open the question of the etiology of sarcoidosis.

24 Viral-Induced Arthritides

Arthritides as occasional symptoms accompanying viral diseases are well documented. In most cases, they manifest as a transient arthralgia only, frequently associated with myalgia. Arthritides in the narrower sense with mono- or oligoarticular symptoms are present less often. These processes are characterized by effusions and are self-limiting, remission is usually within a few days, rarely within weeks. A few cases of polyarthritides, however, have been reported, accompanying rubella and resembling rheumatoid arthritis (RA; Vischer 1996). Males suffering from epidemic parotitis (mumps) may develop arthritides in large joints. Arthralgias have also been observed in the prodromal stage of hepatitis B.

To what extent these very few cases may contribute to our understanding of the pathogenesis of RA must at present remain undecided. What is important to note of though, is, that during the normal course of viral-induced arthritides no destruction of any kind has been observed.

A summary of viral illnesses associated with arthritis and of their clinical manifestations is given in Table 24.1 (Schnitzer 1985).

As these transitory articular processes do not lead to biopsies or surgical interventions, we do not - apart from some accidental findings - have the material needed for gaining knowledge about any pathological changes of the synovia.

Table 24.1. Viral-induced arthritides. Rheumatic manifestations in viral diseases (Schnitzer 1985)

Viral disease	Prevalence of rheumatic manifestations	Joint involvement[a]				Duration	Comments
		Symmetric	Asymmetric	Small	Large		
Hepatitis B	10%–25%; Male=female	++++	+	++++	++; knees	7–21 days	Onset during prodome, often coincidental with rash
Rubella	15%–30% of adult women; 1%–6% of adult men; uncommon in children	++++	+	++++	+++; knees	3–14 days	Tendinitis and carpal tunnel syndromes common, rash often precedes arthritis
Rubbella vaccine-induced	1%–5% of children; adult women >adult men	++++	+	+++	+++; knees	1–5 days	Arthralgias >arthritis Prolonged course and recurrences observed
Alphavirus infections							
Ross River	Majority of adults	+	+++	++++	+	7–28 days	Pain may persist for weeks to months
Chikungunya	Majority of adults	–	–	–	–	–	--
O'nyong-nyong	Majority of adults	+++	+	++	++	3–7 days	Joint swelling uncommon; arthralgias precede rash
Mumps	0.4%; males >females	+	+++	+	+++	7–14 days	Parotitis precedes arthritis by 1–2 weeks; high incidence of orchitis; salicylates provide little
relief							
Enterovirus infections	≥0.13%	++	++	++	++; knees	10–15 days	Diagnosis difficult to confirm because of multiple immunotypes

Smallpox	0.25%–0.5%; 2.5% of children <10 years old	++	+	+	++++	Weeks	Onset 10–30 days after rash; secondary to osteomyelitis; can be seen after vaccinia infection
Adenovirus infections	Case reports	++	+	++	++	7–35 days	–
Herpesvirus infections	Case reports	+	+++	+	++++	Variable, 7 days to 1 month	VZV: female predominance noted
Erythema infectiosum	Variable: up to 74% of adults, 5% of children	++	++	+	++++; knees	4–10 days	Infectious etiology inferred by epidemiology

[a]++++ predominant; +++ marked; ++ common; + infrequent.

25 Villo-Nodular Synovitis

25.1 Definition

Under the designation villo-nodular synovitis (VNS) a group of idiopathic proliferative processes is summarized which can progress diffusely or focally in the synovial tissue of joints and tendon sheaths.
Behind this somewhat puzzling name hides a complex disease picture which has tumour-like as well as inflammatory components. It is, thus, understandable that the character of the VNS process is interpreted controversially by different examiners. The collective designation VNS indeed prejudges an inflammatory process but there can be no doubt that the clinical/radiological behaviour, as also the morphological picture, is hallmarked predominantly by an isomorphic proliferation of synovial cells.

25.2 Clinical Manifestations

Although the microscopic picture characterizes the whole group of VNS, four different VNS types can be differentiated, however, due to their macroscopic appearance and their biological behaviour:

1. The intrinsic, widespread pigmented VNS (synonyms: synovialxanthoma, synovial fibroendothelioma, benign fibrous histiocytoma, xanthomatous giant cell tumour) is the prototype of the group. It attacks predominantly young adults, with no sexual preference. It occurs unilaterally in 80% and prefers knees, followed by hip and foot joints, elbows, finger joints and tendon sheaths. This form spreads diffusely in the synovial membrane of the joints and the tendon sheaths. The tissue is brown-red with yellow sections. The surface is rich in villi. The VNS tissue can invade the area of the cartilage-bone border along the foramina nutricia causing radiologically recognizable erosions in the bone.
2. The localized nodular synovitis (synonyms: benign giant cell synovialoma, benign synovialoma) attacks only a defined synovial section in the form of a lobed nodule. The surface is free of villi. On the cut surface the tendency of the tumour to fibrose is perceptible. Localized nodular synovitis occurs main-

ly in adults of both sexes, often as a unilateral lesion of the knee. Up till now, invasion of the bone has not been observed.

3. The localized nodular tenosynovitis (synonyms: giant cell tumour of the tendon sheath) is restricted to tendons of the hand and foot. The macroscopical and microscopical aspect does not differ from that of the localized nodular synovitis. Localized nodular tenosynovitis prefers young female adults. A typical site is the flexor surface of the middle and index finger. In a few cases the bone is eroded.
4. The fibroma of the tendon sheath is the last member which still has to be subsumed under the group notation VNS. The tendency for fibrosation towards hyalinization, which is significantly less distinctive in the other VNS forms, dominates here. The tumour grows slowly and is well defined. It occurs in every age-group with a significant predilection for the male sex. Typical sites are fingers, hand joints, and lower arms, rarely are the feet and foot joints attacked.

25.3 Pathology

Two basic forms

Microscopically, one can differentiate two basic forms of VNS:
1. The diffuse VNS
2. The localized nodular synovitis

Unspecific morphological constituents

The following morphological constituents are common to all VNS types:
1. A superficial villi formation which can, however, be absent in the nodular form
2. A widespread isomorphic proliferation of synovial cells in the stroma
3. Multinucleated giant cells without foreign contents
4. Deposits of cellularly-stored iron pigment
5. Focal accumulations of lipid-loaded macrophages

None of these elements is, however, by itself a morphological speciality of VNS.
1. The capability of an excessive formation of villi belongs to the typical, unspecific reaction forms of the synovial membrane. The normal synovial membrane reacts to different stimuli, under certain circumstances, with an excessive villi formation even in osteoarthritis (OA) or internal joint injury. An exception is bacterial synovitis because, in this case, the synovial structure is destroyed by enzymes from accumulated neutrophils (see p. 386). The villous proliferation in VNS does not overstep the scope of the new villi formation as it does in various, partly trivial joint diseases.
2. The transformation of synovial stroma cells to a polygonal cell type with unusual proliferation ability also belongs to the reaction pattern of these mesenchymal cells which, in contrast to normal connective tissue cells, possess a certain multipotency. Already in the context of rheumatoid arthritis (RA), high-grade tlp can occur in the synovial stroma (see p. 89). In the different forms of VNS, the proliferative pro-

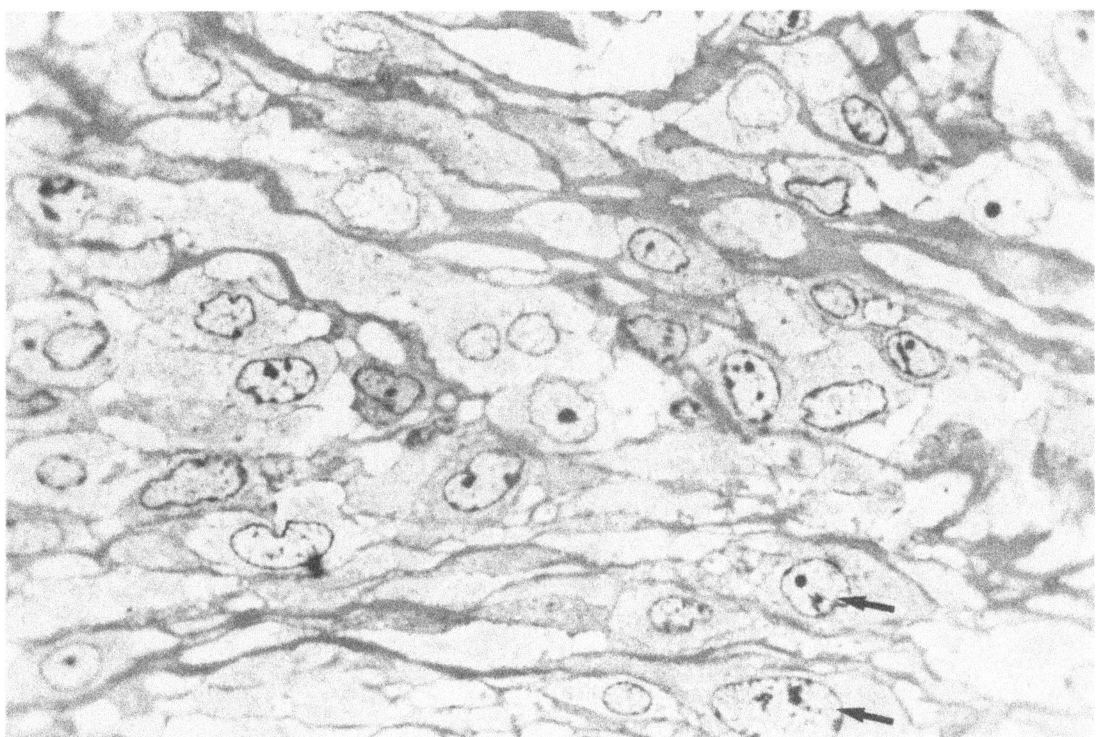

High-grade proliferation of polygonal synoviogenous cell elements. Uniform, large, vesicular nuclei with 1–2 nucleoli (*arrows*, semi-thin section)

Fig. 25.1
Villo-nodular synovitis

cess solely is quantitatively augmented to excess and dominates the morphological picture (Fig. 25.1). The designation "nodular" results from the fact that the proliferation areas are frequently localized "knot-shaped" in the synovial membrane.

3. Multinucleated giant cells without foreign bodies are also an unspecific element of the synovial reaction pattern (Fig. 25.2). They can often be found in RA, and also in other longer-lasting joint diseases.
4. The storage of iron pigment in macrophages is an almost regular finding in synovial tissue in RA.
5. Widespread areas with cellular lipid accumulation ("foamy cells") are found occasionally, also in old scarred synovial processes in RA (Fig. 25.3).

In summary, it can be said that the morphological constituents of the VNS-group consist of elements of unspecific reactions of the synovial membrane. At the same time, however, they give an insight into the varied capability of the multipotent synovial tissue. The morphological picture of the VNS-group shows, nevertheless, the following characteristics:

Morphological characteristics

- In RA, the isomorphic proliferation of the stroma cells is restricted to the superficial sections, whereas in VNS also the deeper layers can be characterized by this proliferation. The assumption that in the isomorphically proliferated cells it concerns proliferative reactions of the lining cells due to inflam-

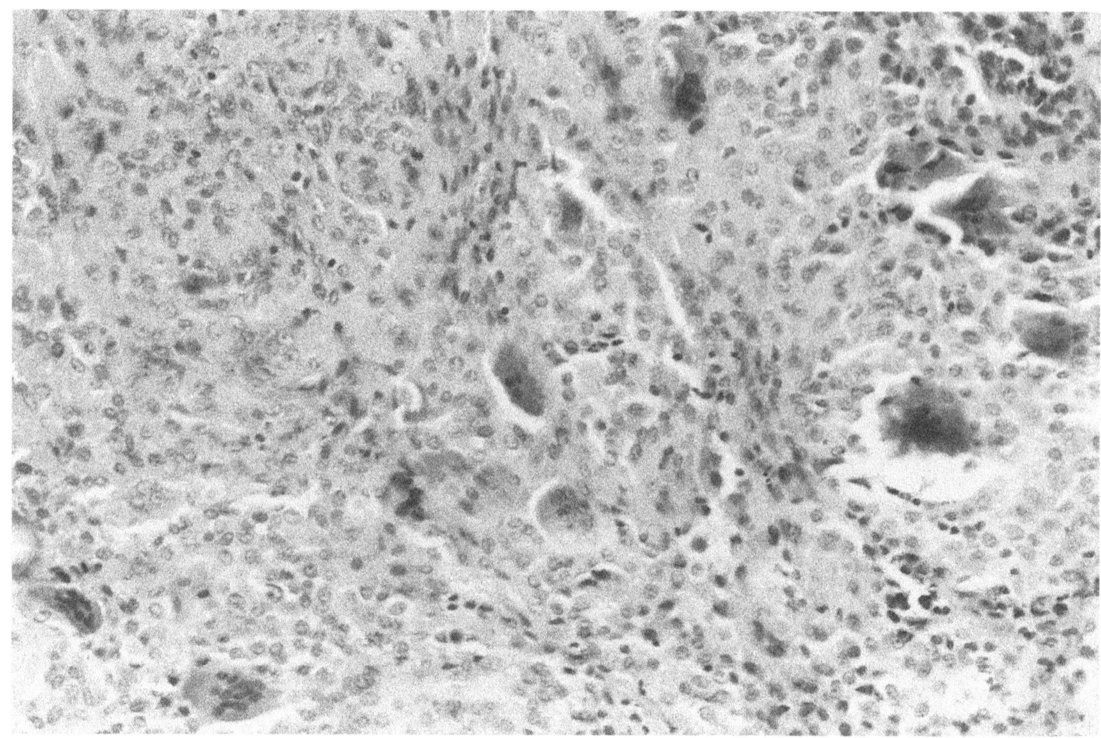

Fig. 25.2
Villo-nodular synovitis

Knee. Multinuclear giant cells, surrounded by proliferated synoviogenous cells (47-year-old female)

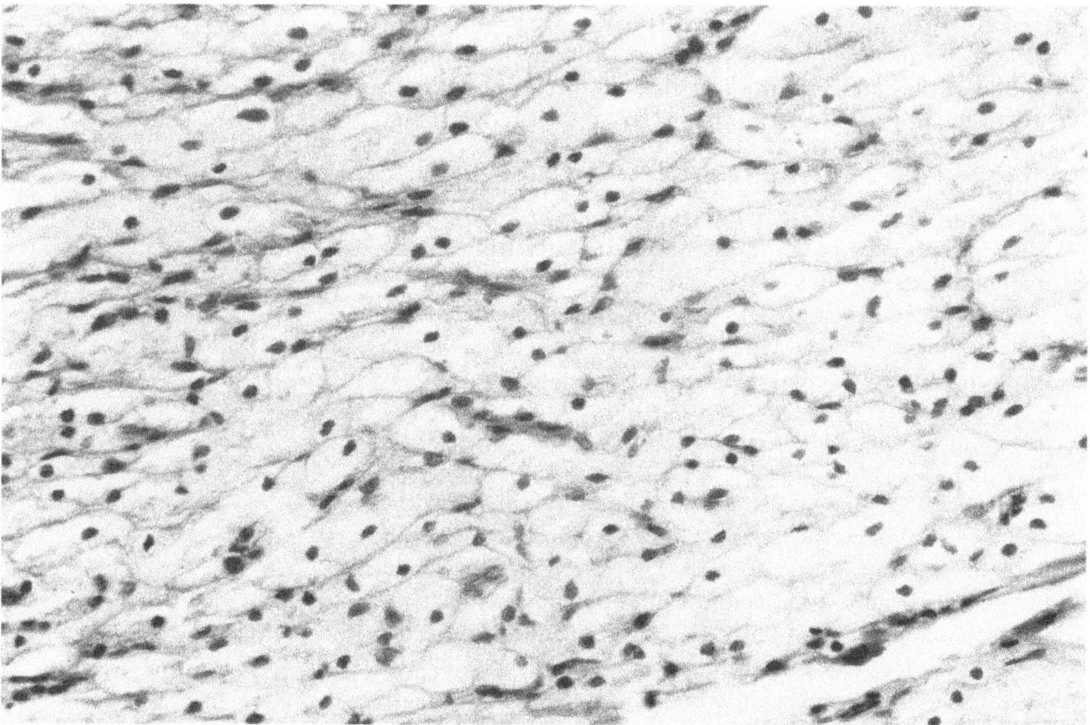

Fig. 25.3
Villo-nodular synovitis

Knee. Typical area of "foamy cells" (30-year-old male)

matory stimuli underestimates the multipotency of the synovial membrane stroma.

- The cell nuclei in tlp of RA are regular, light, and vesicular. The size of the cell nucleus in the VNS-group is, however, slightly variable. The nuclei are generally smaller and dark. Mitoses are rare in both.
- Giant cells in RA and other synovitides lie strictly in contact with the lining cells and, in general, vary little in size and form. In the VNS-group, in contrast, they are variously large and scattered across the whole proliferated stroma.
- In RA, the haemosiderin which is stored in siderophages occurs mainly at the border between the synovial membrane and the capsula fibrosa, deposited in small foci around blood vessels. In the VNS-group, in contrast, the siderophages lie irregularly distributed in the tissue.

Inflammatory components

The classification of VNS as "synovitis" is due to irregular infiltrations of lymphocytes and plasma cells. This, however, is a completely uncharacteristic finding which can be observed as an ubiquitous accompanying phenomenon in all possible synovial reactions and, thus, it participates unjustly in the naming of the VNS. We observed in a series of 14 cases of localized VNS of the knee in addition to the classical features a chronic cell infiltration in all samples in which CD8+ T cells were conspicuous. A high portion of non-phagocytotic cells resorbed iron and became CD68+. A proportion of mononuclear cells expressed collagen type I (Oehler et al. 2000).

Macroscopical aspect

The iron content gives the VNS process macroscopically a characteristic red-brown colour. In between, the lipid-loaded segments can protrude as yellow foci.

Biological dignity

Concerning the controversial question as to whether the process of the VNS-group are inflammatory or tumourous, we would like to decide ourselves in favour of the tumour-character of this group. It has, however, to be emphasized that "tumour" is a broad notation which is often unjustifiably associated with malignancy. Tumour designates firstly only a local uncontrolled overproduction of local structural elements which have escaped the control of their matrix. Such a process is clearly distinguished from a cell- or fibre hyperplasia like it follows repair at inflammatory or other tissue destruction sites, is under local control, and is limited in time by the remodelling of the tissue integrity.

In the whole VNS-group, and also in the intrinsically pigmented VNS, there exists, however, an uncontrolled but locally restricted proliferation of immature synovial stroma cells. A process of this kind cannot be explained by preceding or accompanying inflammation.

Regressive changes

The life-span of these slow-growing, benign, autonomous tissue processes is generally limited with ageing of the tumours, by regressive changes such as fibrosis, bleeding, and necroses (Fig. 25.4).

Bone destruction

The question as to which way benign tumours of the VNS-group can destroy bone structures, as demonstrated by X-ray pictures, remains to be clarified. Although, also in comparison with RA, it is only concerned with discrete, restricted erosions, an enzymat-

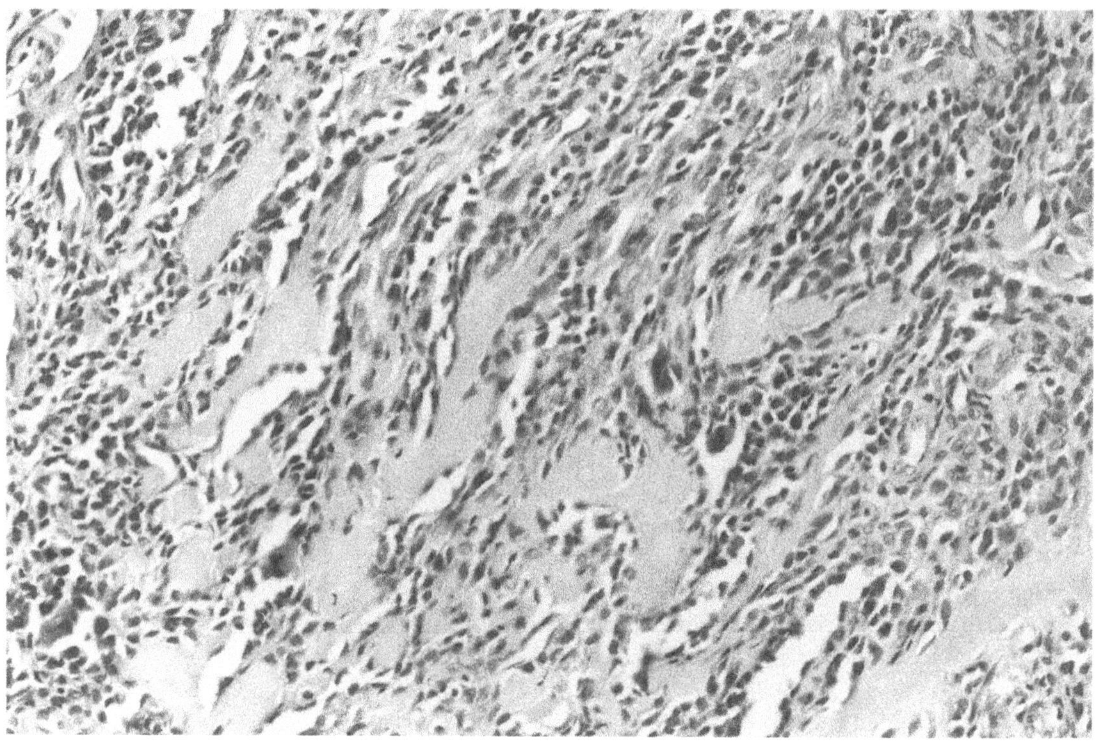

Fig. 25.4
Villo-nodular synovitis

Knee. Regressive transformation with subsiding proliferative activity. New formation of collagen fibres, in between hyaline areas (39-year-old male)

ic degradation of bone tissue has, nevertheless, taken place here. It reminds one closely of the results of the studies of Harris (1976) which showed in vitro release of proteolytic enzymes from synovial cells in different diseases. It must be assumed therefore that the proliferated synoviogenic cell elements of the VNS are also capable of a corresponding release of enzymes. For a degradative function, direct contact between cell and substrate is required under the exclusion of the synovial inhibitors. This requirement is provided for the slow, expansively growing VNS. VNS is a benign lesion that, nonetheless, possesses the capacity for local recurrence, according to investigations by Enzinger and Weiss (1983) in 10–20%. Wright (1951) reported a recurrence rate of 44% and indicated that extended follow-up data on outpatients account for the higher rate. Recurrences seem to develop more often in very cellular lesions with increased mitoses and in patients who have simple enucleations.

25.4 Synovial Sarcoma

Synonyms: malignant synovialoma, monophasic synovial sarcoma, biphasic synovial sarcoma.

Whereas the benign synovial tumours are characterized by a lively cell picture with giant cells, polyhedral stroma cells, siderophages, and "spongy cells", the sarcoma of the synovial tissue shows the unmistakably, mainly monomorphic picture of a malignant neoplasia. Nevertheless, the sarcoma of the synovial membrane also reflects the complex capability of the synovial tissue. Since although the synovial sarcoma consists only of immature cell elements, in these tumours the different morphological potencies of their original tissue can find their expression. In contrast to the sarcomas and carcinomas which originate from a defined homogeneous matrix (e.g. fibrosarcoma, chondrosarcoma, squamous epithelial carcinoma, adenocarcinoma), the variants of the synovial sarcomas reflect the morphological ambivalence of the synovial membrane. As presented in detail in the chapter RA (see p. 89), the synovial tissue has potential for an exophytic growth of the lining cells in the form of villous hyperplasia, and also for a diffuse hyperplasia of the stroma cells (tlp). Both potencies reflect themselves in the types of synovial sarcoma. Both expression forms can, alone or in combination, determine the picture of the synovial sarcoma.

Three types of synovial sarcoma

Enzinger and colleagues (1969) and Hajdu and colleagues (1977) have therefore prepared the following classification of the monophasic and biphasic types of synovial sarcoma:

1. The monophasic-epithelial-like type is characterized by epithelial-like tubular structures. Hereby, the potency of the lining cells to develop exophytic proliferations is realized.
2. The monophasic-spindle-cell type is characterized by the compact deposition of spindle-polygonal cells. In this form, the proliferative potency of the synovial stroma cells is realized.
3. In the biphasic type, both structural potencies occur combined.

Biological dignity

Geiler (1961), supported by substantial evidence, recommended that only those tumours in which at least sparse, pseudo-epithelial structures, possibly only in the form of clefted lacunae, are detectable should be recognized as synovial sarcomas. Following evaluation of 135 fatal cases, Geiler assumes the biphasic type to be the prognostically optimal form of the synovial sarcoma.

Four reaction forms of synovial membrane

If one views the multiple and unusual reaction forms of the synovial membrane retrospectively, its special position within the body tissue, especially the "embankment tissues", and its special nature cannot be overlooked. The following stepladder of morphological reaction forms of the synovial membrane can be erected:

1. Villous hyperplasia of the lining cells as an unspecific reaction form of all inflammatory stimuli.
2. Tlp of the synovial stroma cells with invasion of cartilage and bone in the context of RA.
3. VNS as a mixed cell, benign tumour formation with low invasive potency.
4. Synovial sarcoma as a malignant neoplasm with invasive and metastasizing tendency, with the capability to realize both structural potencies of the synovial membrane.

The reaction forms all together represent an oncological character of the synovial membrane and throw light on the special destruction models of RA.

Problems of assessment by biopsy

This schematic classification does, however, enable recognition of the differential diagnostic problems for the pathologists in the assessment of a sample biopsy if, for example, only the compact spindle-cell component is taken. In such cases, distinction of a simple spindle-cell sarcoma of the connective tissue is not possible.

26 Baker's Cyst*

26.1 Definition

William Morrant Baker (1839–1896) observed a cyst formation at the interior surface of the popliteal space as a synovial hernia connected with the joint cavity (Baker 1877).

26.2 Pathogenesis

Profuse effusions, through an unphysiological increase of internal pressure in the joint, can rupture the continuity of the synovial membrane. In these cases, the liquid content of the joint permeates the layers of the adjoining connective tissue and thus generates a new cavity, the size of which depends on the amount of fluid, pressure, and duration of the process. It is thus a question of joint herniae, the most well recognized and clinically striking of which is the so-called Baker's cyst.

26.3 Pathology

The inner lining of these joint herniae is formed of a granulation tissue with numerous macrophages. It never develops a regular synovial membrane, the morphological characteristic of which is the ability to form villi. Thus, the inner surface of the joint hernia is flat and smooth. An increasingly fibrous capsule, the wall of which can contain lymphoctyes and siderophages, develops over a period of time around the cystic cavity (Fig. 26.1).
Joint herniae, particularly the Baker's cysts, contain in the majority of cases old, condensed fibrin masses, occasionally interspersed with neutrophils, as remnants of past exudative attacks and probable superinfections. Cartilage and bone residues are also often found in between. In contrast to the genuine joint cavity, the fibrin masses in joint herniae are not integrated into villi. Instead, these newly formed joint cavities, most of all the Baker's cyst, form a debris dump, where the residues of past inflammatory and destructive episodes are found.

**Synonym:* popliteal cyst

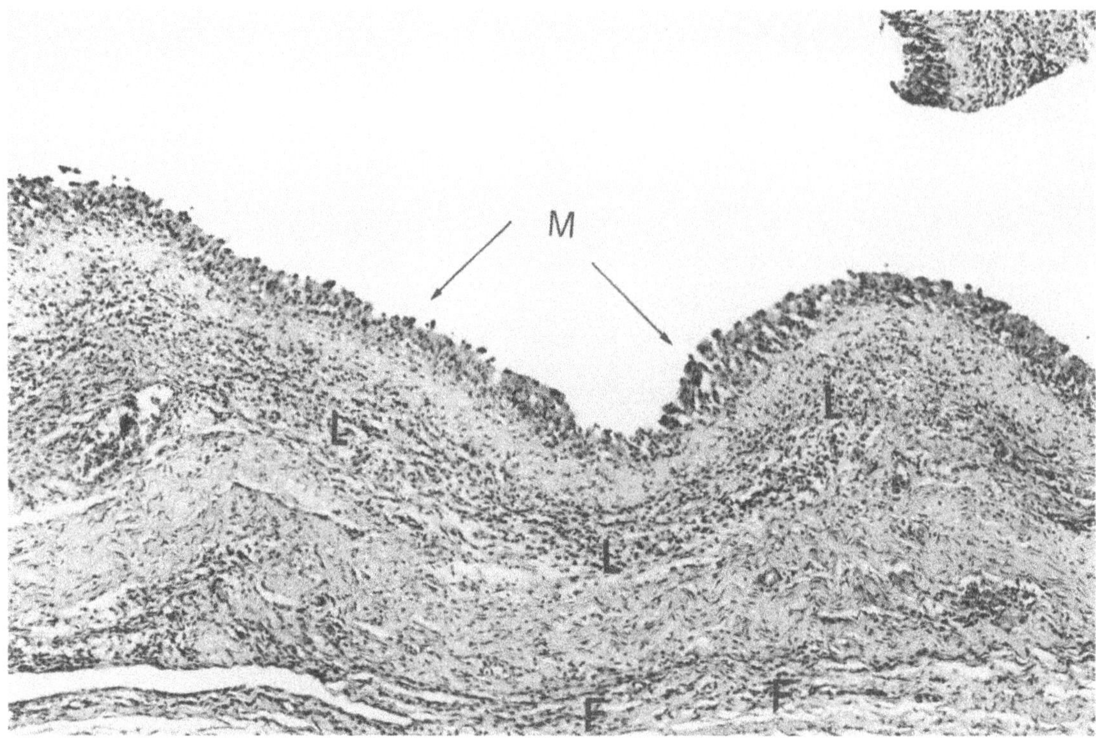

Fig. 26.1
Older Baker's cyst

Coated with a layer of macrophages (*M*). Ligamentous infiltrates with lymphocytes (*L*). Compact fibrous wall (*F*)

27 Carpal Tunnel Syndrome

27.1 Definition

Neuropathy

Carpal tunnel syndrome (CTS), characterized by a neuropathy of the nervus medianus (median nerve), is caused by an increase in pressure in the carpal tunnel, which leads to an interruption of the microcirculation and ischaemic dysfunction, until there is permanent damage to the median nerve.

27.2 Clinical Features

Leading clinical symptoms are nocturnal pain, frequently accompanied by paraesthesia in the innervation area of the median nerve. The result is an impairment of function of the fingers.

27.3 Anatomical Situation

Median nerve

Therapy

The carpal tunnel is bound laterally by the tubercle of the scaphoid bone, and the trapezoid bone, medially by the pisiform and unciform bone and ventrally by the transverse carpal ligament. This narrow channel transmits the median nerve together with the flexor tendons of the thumb and fingers surrounded by the tendon sheaths and interstitial connective tissue. In pathological conditions, each of these structures and also the transverse ligament can increase in volume, compressing the median nerve and giving rise to CTS. Therapy consists of the cutting and resection of the transverse carpal ligament.

27.4 Etiology

The causes of CTS can be local and systemic tenosynovitides as in the context of rheumatoid arthritis (RA; see p. 110), bacterial or other infections, amyloid deposits, haemorrhages as in haemophilia or a hypertrophy of the transverse carpal ligament resulting from diabetes mellitus.

27.5 Pathology

In the course of a study we have histologically investigated tissue from the carpal canal, obtained operatively from 152 patients with CTS. In 39 cases we found a RA; 113 patients with a so-called idiopathic CTS certainly suffered from the symptomatology of a CTS but did not show any systemic disorder. The patients with RA showed in 95% uncharacteristic inflammatory changes such as considerable synovial hyperplasia (49%) or dense lympho-plasmocytic infiltrates (32%), but no tumour-like proliferation or RA-necroses. In contrast, only in 47% of the 113 patients with idiopathic CTS we observed inflammatory signs, amongst them 15% considerable synovial hyperplasia and 9% dense lympho-plasmocytic infiltrates.

Uncharacteristic inflammatory changes

The inflammatory process, thus, is distinguished in both CTS-groups only quantitatively. According to our observations the proof of lympho-plasmocytic infiltrates in the peritendinous tissue of patients with CTS is certainly compatible with an inflammatory systemic disease, as RA, its diagnostic value, however, is low. In the material we have investigated, non-inflammatory, degenerative changes predominated with 53% in the specimens of patients with clinical CTS.

Diagnostic value

The already mentioned endangering of tendons and peritendinous tissue according to the infavourable anatomic conditions in the carpal canal make it understandable that chronic overstress in the region of the flexors of the hand in the course of time leaves its traces at the structures of the peritendinous tissue. If these changes trigger the clinical phenomenon of CTS depends on the fact if and to what extent this process leads to an increase in volume and, so, to compressing and irritation of the median nerve. Mainly in elderly patients, mechanical overstress of the tendon sheaths and peritendinous tissue through friction in the bony carpal canal can lead to degenerative changes in the form of swelling and fibrosis and, thus, to an increase in volume. In these cases, focal degenerations of collagen fibres and dying of fibroblasts can be found (Fig. 27.1) The surviving cells undergo a chondroid metaplasia. The mechanical irritation can cause seldom also a low-grade inflammatory irritation. In such cases, a few lymphocytes can be seen but no neutrophils in the neighbourhood of blood vessels.

Chronic overstress

Chondroid metaplasia

In approximately 10% of the cases with clinical symptoms of a CTS, we found traces of a clinically unexpected bacterial inflammation. In these cases the peritendinous connective tissue is characterized by lamellated fibrin deposits and loose granulocyte infiltrations. After subsidence of the acute infection, only nuclear debris and fibrin remnants are observable, which become increasingly organized after a few days through sprouting fibroblasts and capillaries.

In five cases (four dialysis patients and one RA patient) out of 326 cases of CTS, which reached our institute in the years 1988–1998, we detected amyloid deposits in the collagenous peritendinous tissue.

Amyloid

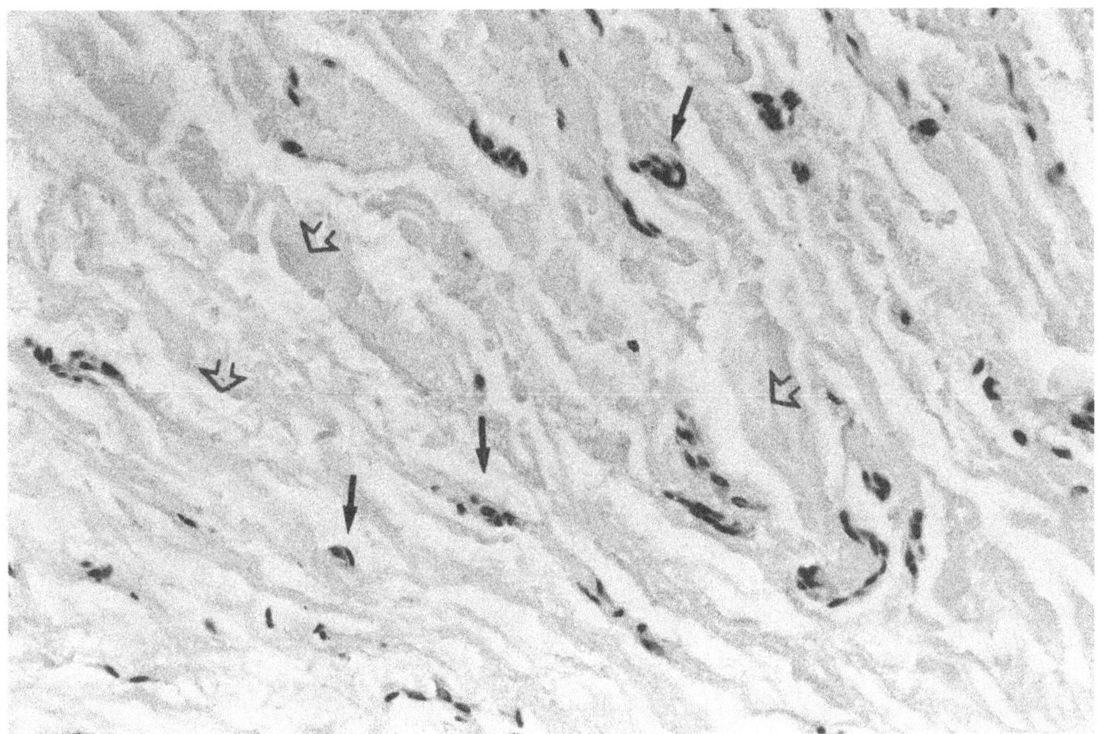

Focal degeneration of collagen fibres (*open arrows*) and remnants of dead fibroblasts (*solid arrows*)

Fig. 27.1
Carpal tunnel syndrome

28 Dupuytren's Contracture*

28.1 Definition

Dupuytren's disease is characterized by shortening of the palmar fascia, leading to progressive digital flexion deformity.

28.2 History

Dupuytren's contracture was named after the French surgeon Guillaume Dupuytren. In 1832, he gave for the first time a full description of the disease in which a multinodular cell proliferation occurs on the underside of the palmar aponeurosis.

28.3 Epidemiology

The prevalence of Dupuytren's contracture is 25% in Northern Europeans over 60 years of age, and 40% in those over 80 years. The lesion occurs less frequently in persons of Asian and African origin. According to various authors, Dupuytren's contracture affects men two to eight times more often than it does women.

28.4 Etiology

The etiology of Dupuytren's contracture is unclear. There is no evidence for an inflammatory causation. Associations with alcoholism, diabetes mellitus, smoking, manual work/microtrauma, epilepsy, and cirrhosis of the liver are known. Repeated microtraumata (e.g. by mechanical stress) are implicated as a triggering factor, but otherwise no explanation for the systemic disorder has been found.

* *Synonym:* palmar fibromatosis

28.5 Clinical Manifestations

Dupuytren's contracture starts clinically with a nodular thickening in the region of the palmar aponeurosis. Later, a contracture develops. The fact that in about 40% of patients both hands are affected (Meister 1984) and in addition a plantar fibromatosis (Ledderhose's disease 1897), a penis fibromatosis (Peyronie's disease 1743), or fibrous "knuckle pads" can occur, indicates the systemic character of the disease.

28.6 Pathology

The palmar aponeurosis divides distally into four slips which merge with the digital sheaths of the flexor tendons. The superficial layer of the aponeurosis is bound to the adjoining subcutaneous fat tissue and thus is also fixed to the skin. This explains the involvement of the palmar surface of the hand in the tendon contracture.

Macroscopic findings

Macroscopically, Dupuytren's contracture consists of vitreous, grey nodules in the tissue of the aponeurosis. As it is an underlying cellular proliferation of the palmar aponeurosis the process possesses a time sequence which is characterized in three stages (Meister 1984):

Microscopic findings

Stage of proliferation

Myofibroblasts

1. Stage of proliferation: in the proliferation stage, there occurs among the otherwise scanty cells of the tendon tissue growth clusters of spindle elements with vesicular nuclei. In the period of maximum growth, the presence of mitoses indicates proliferative activity (Fig. 28.1). Jemec and coworkers (1999) were able to establish an increased expression of c-myc. Indications suggesting an imbalance between proliferation and apoptosis were certainly found in specimens taken from fibrosarcomas, but not in those taken from the lesions in Dupuytren's contracture. The character of these proliferating cells is controversial. A number of investigators see in them myofibroblasts, which are also responsible for the excess of production of collagen type III. Whether this is caused by an increased production or whether it is due to a decreased production of collagen type I, is as yet open to debate (Kloen 1999). The contraction of the fascia would then be due to these contractile elements. Light-microscopically as well as electron-microscopically, the myofibroblasts show morphological characteristics of fibroblasts but also of smooth muscle cells. At certain sites, they are connected to the connective tissue by extracellular fibrils consisting of fibronectin of the onco-fetal type. The fibrils are believed to develop under mechanical influences, and TGF-β1 seems to play a role, too. Electron-microscopically, these cells display during the proliferation stage the characteristic features of myofibroblasts, during later stages they resemble fibroblasts (Tomasek et al. 1999). We retain doubts concerning this interpretation that implies a special cell type, as we have seen similar cell growth in other fibrous tissues like tendons and joint capsules and we were consistently convinced of the high-grade proliferation power

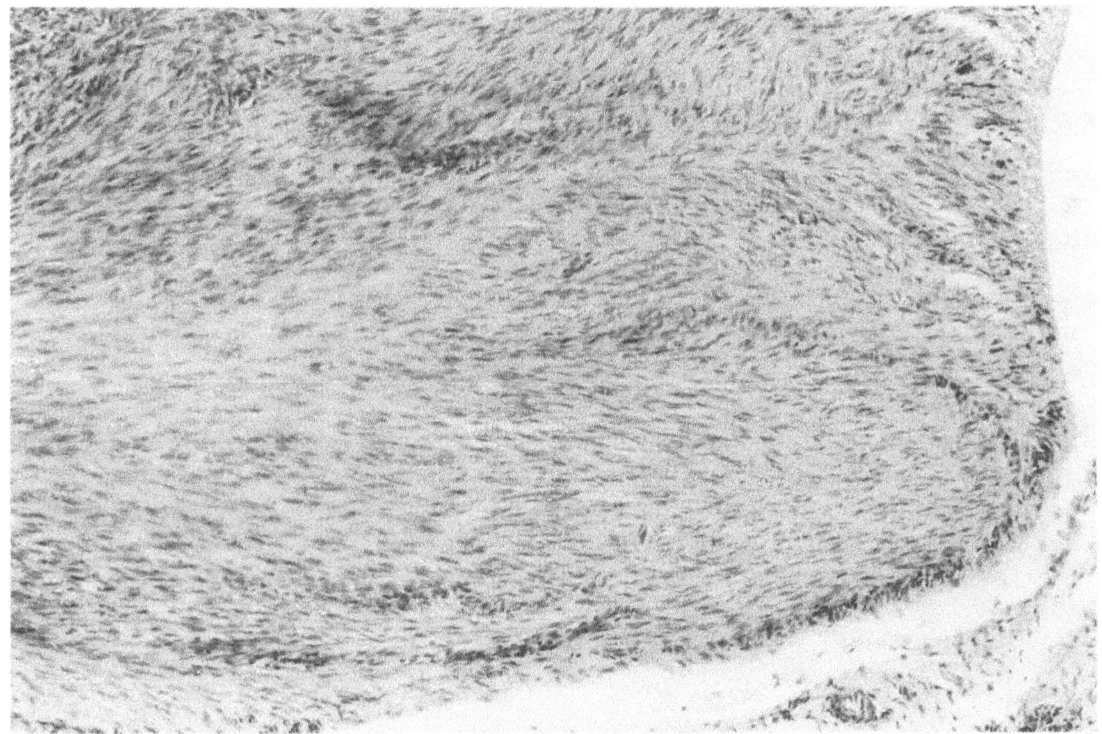

Stage of proliferation. Focal, excessive proliferation of fibroblasts (66-year-old male)

Fig. 28.1
Dupuytren's contracture

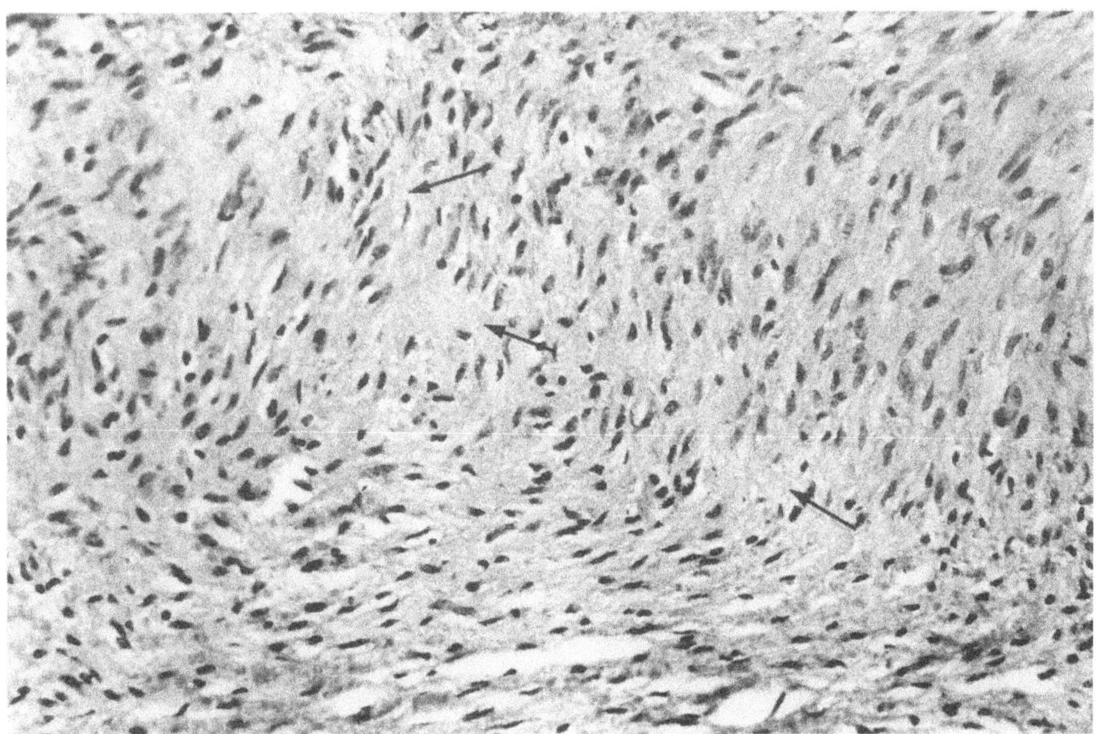

Stage of involution. Cell nuclei irregular. Beginning formation of collagen fibres (*arrows*; 49-year-old male)

Fig. 28.2
Dupuytren's contracture

and multiple adaptability of the fibroblasts. The collagen fibres are destroyed in the mass of proliferation.

Stage of involution

2. Stage of involution: after the fading of the major proliferation, there follows the involution stage. The cell thickness has decreased. The cells are now narrow, the cell nucleus dark and rod-shaped. A clear regeneration of fibres is already starting (Fig. 28.2).

Residual stage

3. Residual stage: in the residual stage, following a diminution of the proliferative processes, there remains a nodule-shaped mass with few cells and rich in fibres. In multifocal cases, all three phases of the process can take place alongside each other in the fibrous tissue.

Clinical significance

The amount of contraction seems to be determined by the degree of fibrosing and the fusion of the collagen fibres with the subcutis and the cutis. It can seriously endanger the ability to perform manual work. The proliferative process is benign, but it shows a tendency to recur after successful operation. The treatment of Dupuytren's contracture therefore consists of a full resection of the aponeurosis.

29 De Quervain's Tenosynovitis and Trigger Finger (Tendopathia Nodosa)*

29.1 Definition

De Quervain's tenosynovitis is a disorder characterized by pain on the radial (thumb) side of the wrist, impairment of thumb function, and thickening of the ligamentous structure covering the tendons in the first dorsal compartment of the wrist. It is precisely defined as stenosing tenosynovitis of the first dorsal compartment (Moore 1997).

29.2 History

De Qervain, a Swiss physician, is given credit for first describing the condition that bears his name. He reported five cases in 1895 and eight additional cases in 1912 (de Quervain 1912a,b). Finkelstein from the Hospital for Joint Diseases in New York City published a landmark article in 1930 that included a comprehensive review of the literature, 24 additional cases, and results of some animal experiments.

Finkelstein's review

29.3 Epidemiological Aspects

De Quervain's tenosynovitis primarily affects women (gender ratio approximately 10:1) between the ages of 35 and 55 years (Moore 1997).
Numerous studies were undertaken in order to establish an association between certain occupations and the occurrence of de Quervain's tenosynovitis. Moore and Garg (1994) performed a retrospective cohort morbidity study that compared the incidence and spectrum of distal upper extremity disorders associated with 37 job categories with the ergonomic task requirements of the jobs. The case definition for de Quervain's tenosynovitis was pain and tenderness localized to the radial aspect of the wrist plus a positive Finkelstein's test (see below). Of the 104 observed conditions, there were three cases of de Quervain's teno-synovitis. All

Synonyms: stenosing tenosynovitis, stenosing tenovaginitis

three jobs involved loading of the thumb combined with moderate wrist deviation. Ranney and coworkers (1995) examined 146 female workers in five industries for the presence of musculoskeletal disorders in the upper limbs. Twelve women (15% of affected subjects) had 14 diagnoses of de Quervain's tenosynovitis. Ten diagnoses involved the right side. Two cases had bilateral diagnoses. There were no detected cases in packaging, two in electronics, four in assembly, two in cashiers, and four in sewing. Moore (1997) emphasized that relationships between ergonomic exposure factors and morbidity have not yet been published.

29.4 Clinical Aspects

Mechanical impingement of tendon

The thickening of the retinaculum as well as the increase in volume of the shared tendon sheath of the abductor pollicis longus and extensor pollicis brevis inhibits gliding of the tendon through the abnormal fibro-osseous canal and can cause mechanical impingement of the tendon against the retinaculum. Consequences are pain in the area of the radial styloid, waning of grip, and limited extension of the thumb (Finkelstein's test). To perform the test, the examiner grasps the patient's thumb, then deviates the wrist to the ulnar side. Intense localized pain at the first dorsal compartment is considered a positive test (Finkelstein 1930). Pain is the most prominent symptom, but some patients report stiffness or neuralgia-like complaints (Kelly and Jacobsen 1964).

"Trigger finger"

Secondary changes may occur in the tendon with enlargement distal to the constriction. There may be a snapping sensation with movement of the enlarged segment of tendon through the changed ring: then the phenomenon "trigger finger" comes into being because of nodular swellings ("tendopathia nodosa"). Not infrequently, rheumatoid nodules (necroses in rheumatoid arthritis, RA) will develop within the tendons, and they may "lock" the finger painfully into flexion.

Analogous processes

Occasionally, analogous processes may take place in other areas of the body, e.g. in flexor carpi radialis tendon, resulting in pain at the base of the thenar eminence, the common peroneal sheath, causing pain on the lateral aspect of the ankle, and the tibialis posterior tendon, presenting with pain below and behind the medial malleolus after prolonged standing and walking.

29.5 Pathology

The term tenosynovitis implies an inflammatory process for which, however, there are no histopathological observations to support this inflammatory view. This is why the term "tendovaginitis", as indispensable as it is for general communication and understanding, is essentially confusing and incorrect. Infections and their traces, scars, however, may occasionally lead to stenoses of tendon sheaths.

Mechanical strain

As thorough studies performed by Moore (1997) prove, the basic mechanism for the development of de Quervain's tenosynovitis is excessive mechanical strain on peritendinous tissues, on struc-

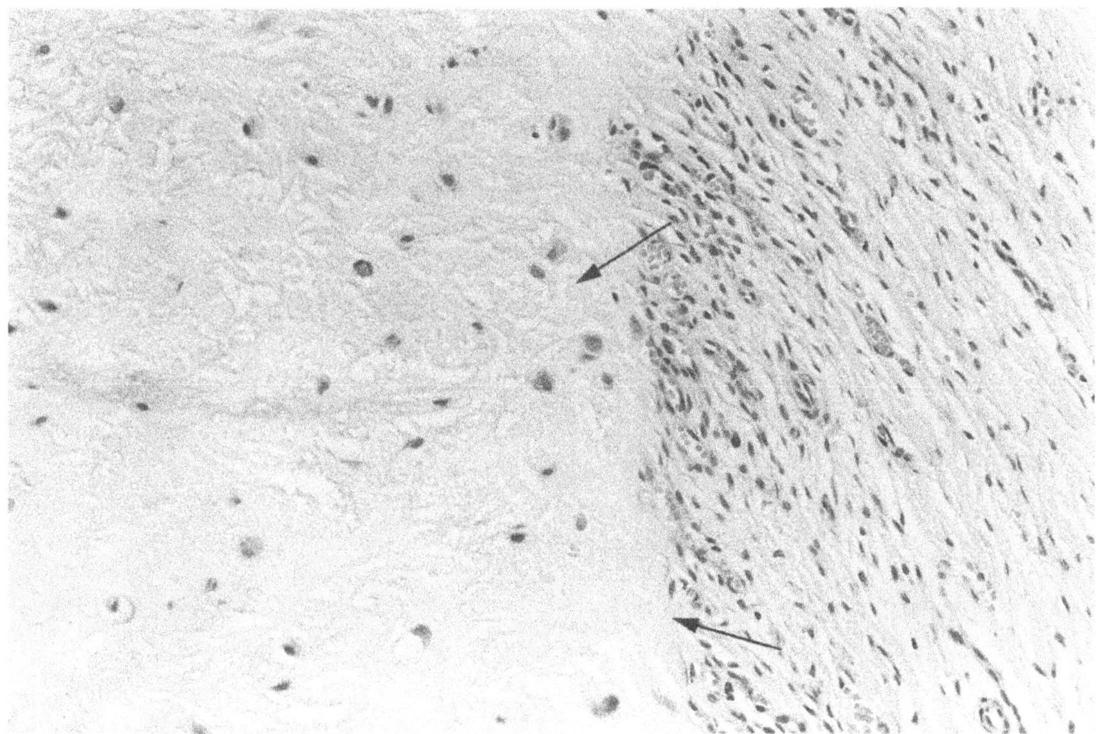

Considerable enlargement of tendon sheath (*arrows*) with chondroid metaplasia

Fig. 29.1
De Quervain's tenosynovitis

tures constructing the retinaculum, as well as on the tendon sheaths. The primary pathological change is a thickening of the extensor retinaculum that covers the first dorsal compartment of the wrist. The retinaculum fibroses, undergoes hyaline degeneration and chondroid metaplasia. All this leads to a thickening; depending on the degree of mechanical damage, the retinaculum becomes two to four times as broad as it is normally. During our studies, we found especially impressive the changes within the tissue of tendon sheaths of patients suffering from de Quervain's tenosynovitis. We agree with Clarke and coworkers (1998) who described a deposition of dense fibrous tissue within the up to five times thicker than normal tendon sheath, in which the collagen bundles were often found to be aligned perpendicular to the direction of the tendons. The most impressive feature was a striking and characteristic accumulation of mucopolysaccharides dispersed between the layers of fibrous tissue of the tendon sheaths seen on staining with alcian blue. In accordance with Clarke and coworkers (1998), we could not find any signs suggesting an inflammatory origin or an interference of inflammatory mechanisms. The electron-optical studies performed by Ippolito and coworkers (1985) also confirm the entirely degenerative character of the disease: a thickening of the collagen fibre bundle in the distal and middle third of the tendon sheath as well as myxoid degeneration and chondroid metaplasia (Fig. 29.1). From our observations, the chondroid metaplasia of collagenous tissue shows an adaptive reaction to reduced oxygen tension. While collagenous tissue after fibrosing still contains sufficient

Accumulation of mucopolysaccharides

Chondroid metaplasia

blood vessels to satisfy the reduced oxygen requirement of the few fibroblasts present, increased hyalinisation decreases the number of blood vessels until they completely perish. The collapse of the oxygen supply results in the destruction of most of the fibroblasts. The surviving cells undergo a chondroid transformation. An explanation for this phenomenon lies in the fact that the chondrocytes, thanks to their glycolytic metabolism, can exist almost without oxygen.

30 Bursae

30.1 Definition

Bursae are enclosed cavities filled with a mucoid-like fluid, which function as mechanical defence elements at exposed sites. Shock absorption and a gliding function are provided simply by a viscous fluid-filled cushion at these sites.

Genesis

Only a very few bursae are already present at birth. The vast majority develops during the first years of life under the influence of mechanical pressures. While the ganglion (see p. 441) is formed in rigid fibrous tissue through mucous coating within the collagen fibrous framework, the bursae are formed initially from a tear between the parallel tissue layers with different sheer stresses in the loose connective tissue.

30.2 Pathology

The cellular lining of the bursae can be either completely absent or be formed of a single-staged, flat cell layer, which consists of fibroblasts or macrophages depending on the degree of irritation (Fig. 30.1). This cellular lining is not a genuine synovial membrane. Thus, in a bursa, there is never any formation of villi, which are a specific characteristic of the synovial membrane.

Bursae are liable to exudative inflammation, predominantly in the region of the knee and elbow joints. Depending on the duration of the inflammation, the lumen contains different old fibrin which can remain for a long time in the bursa, as the lining has only a low propensity for organization. In the course of years, the wall of the bursa thickens. It is formed from a broad, cell-deficient collagenous capsule. Numerous newly-formed, small calibre blood vessels in the fibrosed vessel wall, often producing a densely branched effect, result from inflammatory episodes. A few lymphocytes can be present among them. Bursae can also be a site of rheumatoid arthritis-necroses (RA-necroses; see p. 116).

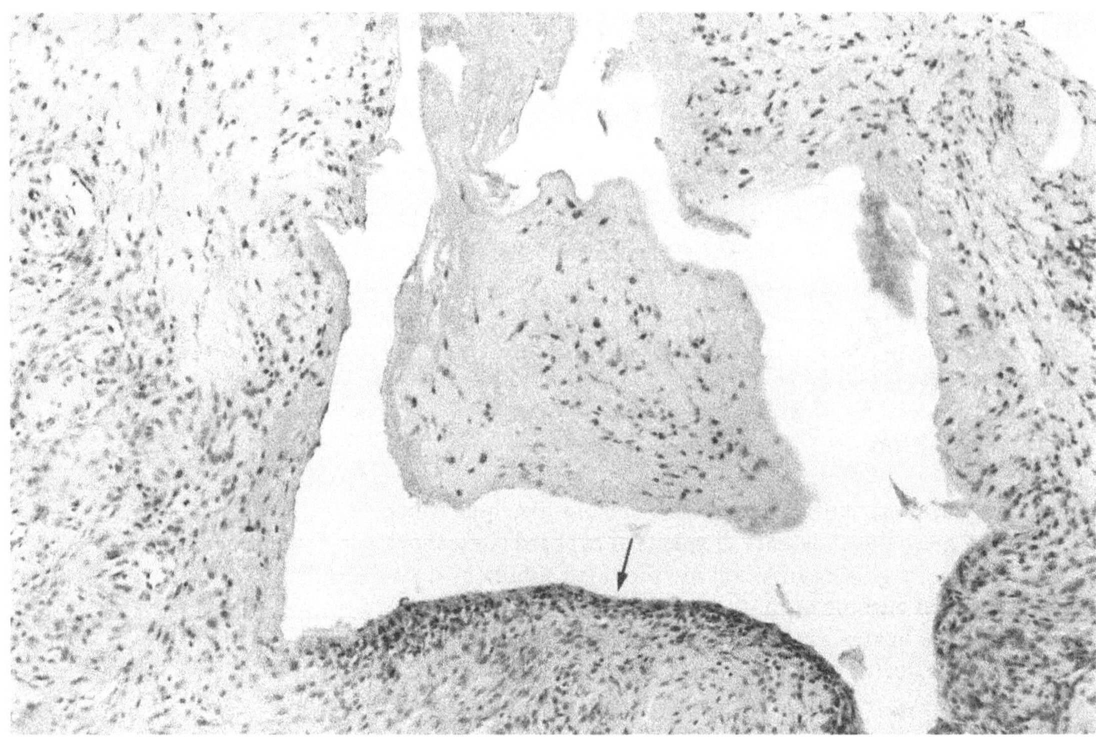

Fig. 30.1
Bursitis

Old fibrin remnant in the lumen. Partial coat of macrophages (*arrow*). Fibrous capsule wall infiltrated by lymphocytes and plasma cells

31 Ganglion

31.1 Definition

A ganglion is a cyst formation in collagenous tissues such as tendon sheaths, tendons, joint capsule tissue, and menisci. In contrast to the bursa, which occurs in loose connective tissue, the ganglion develops in the interior of rigid fibrous tissue.

31.2 Clinical Manifestation

Para- and intra-articular ganglia and cysts are frequently detected during routine examinations using ultrasound, computed tomography (CT) or magnetic resonance imaging (MRI). They are seen around various joints, such as the hip, knee, ankle, foot, shoulder, elbow, wrist, hand, spine or the temporomandibular joints, and in the periosteum. Some may not manifest clinically, others may cause pain or swelling or may impair joint function. They are often associated with underlying joint disorders such as trauma, degenerative changes or inflammation. In a group of 1,767 consecutive patients referred for an MRI examination of the knee, 23 patients (1.3%) were diagnosed with intra-articular ganglia of the knee in either Hoffa's fat pad, the anterior or the posterior cruciate ligaments (Bui-Mansfield and Youngberg 1997).

31.3 Pathology

Degenerative changes

In this bradytrophic tissue, there are probably hypoxia-induced degenerative changes which are manifest as focal mucous areas in the tissue. The resulting mucopolysaccharides merge within the spaces and these can develop into stoutly filled cysts. These cavities have no cellular lining, the mucous contents are weakly basophilic. Microscopically, the development of the ganglion can be studied from its smallest beginning as follows:

Basophilic substance

Initially, there are small, often multiple foci in which the collagen structure is disaggregated. Instead of dense fibres there is a mucoid, weakly basophilic substance in which a few stellar mesenchymal cells are deposited. Cystic cavities develop by confluence and extension from these focal mucous areas. At first, they are

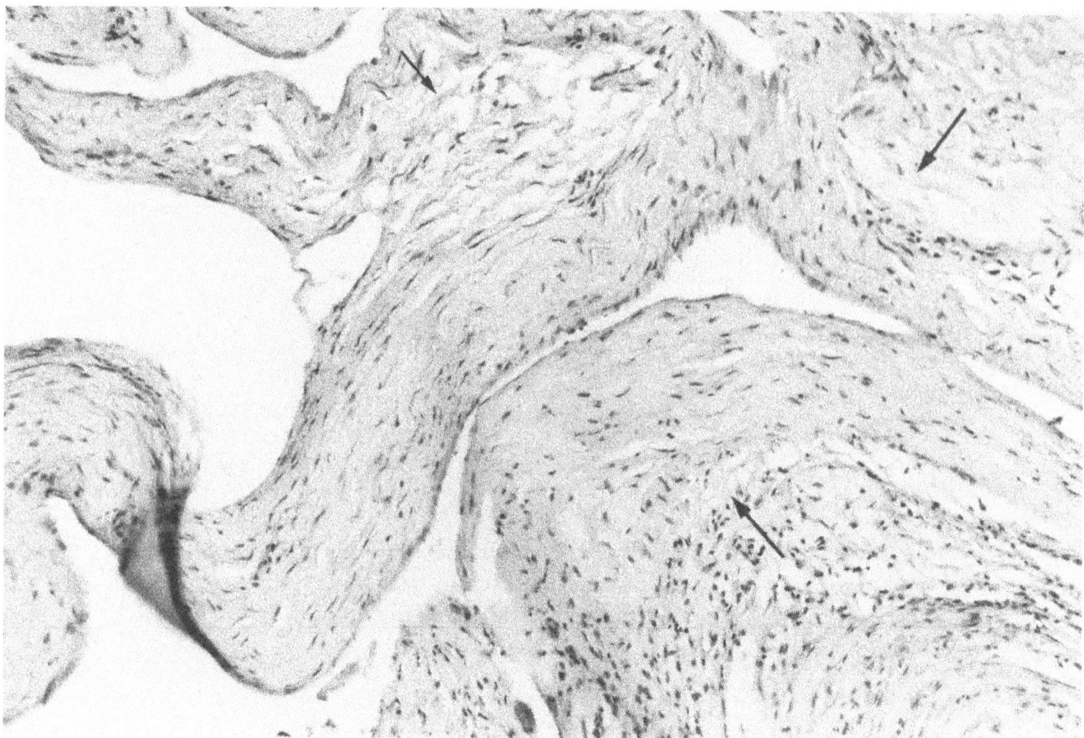

Fig. 31.1 Ganglion

Branched tissue space without cellular lining. Compact fibrous cell-deficient wall structure. Within the tissue of the wall, small focal mucous areas (*arrows*)

still partly lined with some flat cells but these disappear subsequently with increasing age of the cyst. In the course of time, the inner pressure of the cyst produces an often considerable increase in volume, so that meandering intertwined, mucous-filled cavities are formed. In addition, a progressively thick fibrous cyst capsule develops. Progression of the ganglion formation can be recognized in the fact that new mucous foci are found chiefly in the region of old cysts (Fig. 31.1).

There is no basis for postulating an inflammatory origin for ganglion formation. It attracts notice, however, that the ganglia develop exclusively in rigid collagenous tissue, i.e. in a bradytrophic tissue with scanty blood supply; thus, it seems possible that, for example, under mechanical stress the blood vessels become constricted and local hypoxia leads to mucous degeneration. Such a process does not seem unlikely, if one considers that the fibroblasts, in addition to collagen type I, secrete proteoglycans, metalloproteinases, collagenases, and their inhibitors. A hypoxia can, for example, disturb the regulation between substrate and enzymes and, thus, provide the condition for an autochtonous, non-inflammatory tissue decomposition.

32 Possibilities and Limitations of Synovial Biopsy

The diagnostic value of a synovial biopsy is generally considered to be limited for the following reasons: In contrast to organs with a well defined architecture as, for example the liver, the kidney, and the heart, the synovial membrane has no definite structure, that is to stay no defined cell composition. In organ tissue, qualitative and quantitative variations from the well-known pattern are recognized and are associated with specific pathological phenomena. In synovial tissue, however, there is no defined structure or cell composition, and therefore only a few points of orientation are available. Thus, from the structural point of view, the synovial membrane should be regarded as a plain, loose mesenchymal tissue whose surface is sealed off from a fluid-containing space by a lining cell layer. Thus, pathological changes of the synovial membrane cannot be analyzed by disturbances of the given structure, but rather from reactions of the following morphological components:

1. Hyperplasia
   The synovial membrane reacts to various stimuli with an increase in the surface area in the form of villi. Villous formation can be excessive in certain cases. The synovial membrane shares this exophytic tendency with other mesodermal surfaces (pleura, peritoneum).
2. Proliferation
   The cellular elements of synovial membrane have a marked tendency for hypertrophy, hyperplasia, and proliferation. Involved are:
   - Lining cells
     These normally flat, single-layered cells can be arranged in a cubic, cylindrical or multi-layered form.
   - Synovial stroma cells
     These, in general, loosely positioned, plain cells which are indistinguishable from normal fibroblasts have a hyperplastic and proliferative potency, ranging from considerable to excessive, forming plasma-rich cells with vesicular nuclei and scattered mitoses.
3. Infiltration
   The loose structure of the synovial tissue provides abundant space for colonization by infiltrating cells, lymphocytes, plasma cells, macrophages, and occasionally short-lived, rapidly migrating neutrophils.
4. Rheumatoid necroses ("rheumatoid nodules")
   Rheumatoid necroses develop in dense collagenous tissue (see p. 112). The loose structure of the synovial membrane is, thus, unsuitable for them, but they can be established in the fibre-dense capsula fibrosa.

A pathologist, making a diagnostic evaluation of the synovial membrane, is somewhat in the same position as a 17th century visitor to a theatre, in which a Commedia del Arte performance has already begun: the scenery of the stage is scanty, the characters, lining cells, lymphocytes, plasma cells, and synovial stroma cells, are always the same stereotypes – how could he tell what play is being performed? In the same way, the synovial membrane shows no notable differences in the various non-bacterial arthritides, and, furthermore, lymphocytes, plasma cells, and macrophages show no preference for any one of these diseases. Nevertheless, as the result of many years of experience we can distinguish certain morphological features which may contribute to a diagnostic evaluation.

From our observations, certain differences occur in the villous structure which are useful for the differential diagnosis:

Synovial membrane in OA

▸ Synovial membrane in osteoarthritis (OA) or internal joint injury: the villi are medium long and mostly plump. Fibrin is found only minimally on the surface or is absent. The lining cell layer is single-staged and flat. The villous stroma is markedly loose-structured and transparent ("glass villi"; see p. 340). The stroma is relatively poor in blood vessels. Sometimes, small clusters of lymphocytes are found surrounding a small blood vessel. Otherwise, lymphocyte or plasma cell infiltrates are rare. Neutrophils do not occur. The exception to this is the long standing coxarthrosis where the stroma is frequently more densely fibrosed. There is, however, never a proliferation of the synovial stroma cells.

Synovial membrane in PSA

▸ Synovial membrane in psoriatic arthritis (PSA) or in family of seronegative spondarthritides (SSA): the villi are medium-long to long and predominantly small. The lining cell layer is mostly single-staged, the cells are cubic. In the context of the disease process activity, however, the lining cells can proliferate and become multi-layered. In striking contrast to this, the cells of the villous stroma are completely inactive. They never show a proliferation. The villous stroma is uniformly moderately fibrosed (clearly more intensive than in OA). The lympho-plasma-cellular infiltration is diffuse and varies between low- and high-grade in which plasma cells predominate. Neutrophils are not present. The most reliable criterion is a marked new formation of thin-walled blood vessels with wide lumina which, unlike those of rheumatoid arthritis (RA), occur predominantly in the periphery of the villi. It has to be taken into consideration that subsided bacterial infections can leave numerous blood vessels which show, however, a thick wall and a wide lumen (see p. 390).

Synovial membrane in RA

▸ Synovial membrane in RA: in the literature, illustrations of tissue frequently occur with villi and lympho-plasmocytic infiltrates which are interpreted as "typical" and even as "specific" for RA and are often used as reference for animal models. This is, however, misleading because these features are not characteristic and the behaviour of individual structural components (lining cells, blood vessels, stroma proliferation, and stroma density) is not taken into consideration (see p. 62).

Time and again, critical authors have argued that the synovial membrane in RA lacks specific morphological features and have questioned the diagnostic value of a synovial biopsy.

Early RA

The exceptional interest of clinicians in an early diagnosis of RA is understandable. While in several other arthritides, such as SSA, OA or bacterial arthritis (BA), morphological features are distinct even at early stages, RA seems to lack specific, unquestionable characteristics. As early as 1955, the problems were illustrated by the classic studies of Kulka and coworkers: they examined specimens of patients who were supposed to be affected from RA by a time period of no longer than 1 year. The changes described, such as synovial hyperplasia, lymphocyte infiltrations, and slight fibrin deposits, did not supply a functional profile, even less so as it was later discovered that the patients had different forms of arthritides. The studies of Schumacher and Kitridou (1972) merit special attention. The synovial tissue they studied was taken from 24 patients with a recent onset of the respective disease, i.e. not more than 30 days prior. Among these cases were six with RA, and three with juvenile chronic arthritis (JCA). Both diagnoses were confirmed retrospectively. The histological and electron-microscopic investigations of the authors revealed lining cell proliferation with varying intensities in all specimens, up to a maximum of ten cell layers. The infiltrates were mainly perivascular, they consisted predominantly of lymphocytes, but there was no follicle formation. Plasma cells were rare in the early cases. Also Zvaifler et al. (1994) tend to attribute them to later stages. Occasionally, neutrophils in the superficial synovial membrane were observed in five of six patients. Interesting is the authors' assertion that the degree of inflammation in a 3-day-old lesion was markedly more intense than that in two 30-day-old lesions.

We think that the particular significance of this study is the light- and electron-microscopic evidence of early inflammatory changes in venules and, sporadically, in arterioles. These results also confirm our observations (see p. 67). We regard the changes that can be confirmed mainly electron-microscopically as a convincing documentation of the local manifestation of a systemic process. Any immunological process may lead to ubiquitous slight blood vessel changes, the visible manifestation of which are painful inflammations of the joints.

No specific profile of synovial membrane in RA

The studies of Lindblad and Hedfors (1985) confirm the lack of reliable morphological criteria for identifying an RA synovitis also after some duration of the disese. They examined bioptic material taken from 12 patients with different diagnoses and at different stages. They describe synovial hyperplasia and predominantly perivascular infiltrates consisting mainly of CD4+ T lymphocytes. The authors had, however, the impression of a more-than-usual presence of Ig+ lymphocytes and plasma cells in the tissue samples of RA patients. Any characteristics other than these were not found. For orthopaedic surgeons, though, who perform arthroscopies, the observation of a significant correlation between the arthroscopic and the microscopic signs indicative of synovitis, should be of special interest.

In summary, all the above-mentioned findings confirm the hesitation in validating the diagnosis of RA by lining cell hyperplasia and CD4+ T lymphocytes, both of which are found in early as well as late synovitis in other inflammatory joint diseases. This opinion has been especially emphasized by Zvaifler and coworkers (1994). The presence of B lymphocytes or plasma cells are considered to be of a certain diagnostic and prognostic value.
Even though synovitis in RA has no specific profile, the morphological process can be described as follows: on the surface, fibrin exudates only of small to moderate extent can be seen. The fibrin is compact and may contain isolated neutrophils but no nuclear debris and no cartilage sequestra. The lining cell layer can show all stages of proliferation, depending on the activity of the process. The synovial stroma cells, in contrast to the other non-bacterial arthritides, can proliferate to a greater or lesser degree, whereby the border-line to the lining cell layer disappears. Otherwise, the stroma is irregularly fibrosed. The age of the process is reflected by the increasing content of collagen fibres. The infiltration of CD4+ T lymphocytes and plasma cells is both qualitatively and quantitatively totally inconstant and unspecific: it can be minimal or excessive. True lymph follicles are rare. Neutrophils do not belong to the picture of RA (see p. 68). The formation of new blood vessels is low-grade, uncharacteristic, and without preference for the periphery of the villi (see above). While rheumatoid necroses do not occur in the structurally loose synovial membrane, they can, however, establish themselves in this scar tissue as clear "leading fossils" of seropositive RA if the synovial membrane thickens due to scar formation in the course of years of disease.

Synovial membrane: diagnosing by differentiation

Because in RA structure, cell proliferation, and cell infiltration change with regard to quantity and composition during the lifelong disease, a histological diagnosis is best achieved by differentiation. The specimen's characteristics should be delineated against ordinarily well-definable synovial processes, e.g. against PSA or other SSA by observing the behaviour of small blood vessels (see p. 181), against OA on the basis of its characteristic type of villi (see p. 340) or against BA which is characterized by destruction and reconstruction of the synovial membrane.

Synovial membrane in BA

▸ Synovial membrane in BA and bacterial superinfection: in both cases, the picture is characterized in general by extensive fibrin masses, in contrast to the rather discrete fibrin exudates in non-bacterial arthritides. In the acute stage, the fibrin contains large masses of neutrophils, the proteases of which degrade the fibrin layer by layer. In this way, the characteristic lamellation of the fibrin in BA is formed observable even months after the destruction of the neutrophils. A further characteristic of BA is the loss of the synovial architecture, i.e. the villi are destroyed and the synovial surface becomes smooth. The stroma is, depending on the time-span of the disease process, changed into granulation or scar tissue and contains at first neutrophils and lymphocytes and later only a rather large number of lymphocytes and plasma cells. Here, the absence of neutrophils can be deceptive in view of the bacterial genesis of the disease. An insight into the destructive character of BA and also bacterial superinfection is provided by the enzymatically degraded cartilage sequestra which remain for a long time after the regression of the bacterial infection. Therefore, it is evident that by careful morphological analysis of the tissue samples some important and frequently occurring arthritides can be diagnosed with certainty and true accuracy. As a matter of course, the diagnosis of joint diseases characterized by granulomata or crystal deposits presents no difficulties. In other words: a synovial biopsy makes sense because it can lead in many cases to significant diagnostic decisions.

References

Adamicek P (1998) Ausbildung synovialer Zottenvegetationen über synoviogenem Pannus. Med. Dissertation. Universität Mainz

Adams R (1875) Treatise on rheumatic gout, or chronic rheumatic arthritis, of all joints. Churchill, London, Alexander of Tralles

Adamson TC 3rd, Fox RI, Frisman DM, Howell FV (1983) Immunohistologic analysis of lymphoid infiltrates in primary Sjögren's syndrome using monoclonal antibodies. J Immunol 130:203–208

Afzelius A (1910) Verhandlungen der Dermatologischen Gesellschaft zu Stockholm, Sitzung vom 28. Oktober 1909. Arch Dermatol Syph (Berlin) 101:404

Ahern M, Lever JV, Cosh J (1983) Complete heart block in rheumatoid arthritis. Ann Rheum Dis 42:389–397

Aho K, Ahvonen P, Lassus A, Sievers K, Tiilikainen A (1976) Yersinia arthritis and related diseases: Clinical and immunogenetic implications. In: Dumonde DC (ed) Infection and immunology in the rheumatic diseases. Blackwell, Oxford, p 431–344

Ahvonen P (1972) Human yersiniosis in Finland. II. Clinical features. Ann Clin Res 4:39–48

Aicher WK, Stransky G, Gay RE, Gay S (1991) Synovial lining cells derived from patients with rheumatoid arthritis (RA) produce reverse transcriptase. Arthritis Rheum 34 (Suppl):177

Aicher WK, Heer AH, Trabandt A, et al. (1994) Overexpression of zinc-finger transcription factor Z-225/egr-1 in synoviocytes from RA patients. J Immunol 152:5940–5948

Aigner T, Stöss H, Weseloh G, et al. (1992) Activation of collagen type II expression in osteoarthritic and rheumatoid cartilage. Virchows Archiv B Cell Pathol 62 (6): 337–345

Aigner T, Bertling W, Stöss H, et al. (1993) Independent expression of fibril-forming collagens I, II and III in chondrocytes of human osteoarthritic cartilage. J Clin Invest 91:829–837

Akkoc N, Geiler T, State M, Hieronymus T, Lorenz H-M, Kalden JR (1997) FAS antigen stimulation of human fibroblasts leads to proliferation rather than to apoptosis. Arthritis Rheum 40:131

Alarcón AS (1986) Rheumatoid arthritis: Overview, epidemiology, etiology, pathogenesis, and pathology. In: Cohen AS, Bennett JC (eds) Rheumatology and Immmunology, 2nd edn. Grune & Stratton, Orlando, pp 196–214

Alarcón-Segovia D, Ibanez G, Velazquez-Forero F, Hernandez-Ortiz J Gomzalez-Jimenez Y (1974a) Sjögren's syndrome in systemic lupus erythematosus: Clinical and subclinical manifestations. Ann Intern Med 81:577

Alarcón-Segovia D, Ibanez G, Hernandez-Ortiz J, Cetina JA, Gomzalez-Jimenez Y, Diaz-Jouanen E (1974b) Salivary gland involvement in diseases associated with Sjögren's syndrome: I. Radionuclide and roentgenographic studies. J Rheumatol 1:159

Albertini von A (1953) Zur Pathogenese des rheumatischen Granuloms. Schweiz med Wschr 83 (34):772

Alibert JL (1810) Précis théorique et pratique sur les maladies de la peau. De l'imprimerie de doublet, Paris, p 65

Alibert JL (1818) Précis théorique et pratique sur les maladies de la peau. 1st edn., vol. 1, Caille et Ravier, Paris, p 21

Altmeyer P, Holzmann H (1984) Zur Kenntnis einer Osteoarthropathie bei der Pustulosis palmaris et plantaris. Vortrag auf dem 1. Frankfurter Gespräch "Dermatologie und Nuklearmedizin", September 1978

Amor B, Toubert AA (1993) Reactive arthropathy, Reiter's syndrome and enteric arthropathy in adults. In: Maddison PJ, Isenberg DA, Woo P, Glass DN (eds) Oxford Textbook of Rheumatology, vol. 2. University Press, Oxford New York Tokyo, pp 699–709

Amor B, Dougados M, Mijiyawa M (1990) Critères de classification des spondylarthropathies. Revue du Rhumatisme et des Maladies ostéoarticulaires 57:85–89

Anaya J-M, Liu GT, D'Souza E, Ogawa N, Luan X, Talal N (1995) Primary Sjögren's syndrome in men. Ann Rheum Dis 54:748–751

Ansar Ahmed S, Penhale WJ, Talal N (1985) Sex hormones, immune responses, and autoimmune diseases: Mechanisms of sex hormone action. Am J Pathol 121:531–551

Arahata K, Engel AG (1984) Monoclonal antibody analysis of mononuclear cells in myopathies. I: Quantitation of subsets according to diagnosis and sites of accumulation and demonstration and counts of muscle fibers invaded by T cells. Ann Neurol 16:193–208

Arapakis G, Tribe CR (1963) Amyloidosis in rheumatoid arthritis investigated by means of rectal biopsy. Ann Rheum Dis 22:256

Aretaeus (1856) The extant works of Aretaeus, the Cappadocian. Sydenham Society, London

Arend WP, Dayer JM (1990) Cytokines and cytokine inhibitors or antagonists in rheumatoid arthritis. Arthritis Rheum 33 (3):305–315

Arnett FC (1984) HLA and the spondylarthropathies. In: Calin A (ed) Spondylarthropathies. Grune & Stratton, Orlando, pp 297–321

Arnett FC (1986) Seronegative Polyarthritis. In: Cohen AS, Bennett JC (eds) Rheumatology and Immunology, 2nd edn. Grune & Stratton, Orlando, pp 221–228

Arnett FC (1987) Seronegative spondylarthropathies. Bull Rheum Dis 37:1–12

Arnett FC (1989) Seronegative Spondarthritiden. EULAR Bull 3:85–94

Arnett FC, Edworthy SM, Block DA, McShane DJ, Fries JF, Cooper NS, Healey LA, Kaplan SR, Liang MH, Luthra HS, Medsger TA, Mitchell DM, Neustadt DH, Pinals RS, Schaller JG, Scharp JT, Wilder RL, Hunder GG (1988) The American Rheumatism Association 1987 revised criteria for the classification of rheumatoid arthritis. Arthritis Rheum 31:315–324

Asbrink E, Olsson I, Novmark A (1986) Erythema chronicum migrans Afzelius in Sweden: A study on 231 patients. Zbl Bakt Hyg A 263:229–236

Aschoff L (1904) Zur Myokarditisfrage. Verh dtsch Ges Path 8:46

Assoian RK, Fleurdelys BE, Stevenson HC, Miller PJ, Madtes DK, Raines EW, Ross R, Sporn MB (1987) Expression and secretion of type beta transforming growth factor by activated human macrophages. Proc Natl Acad Sci 84:6020–6024

Atkins CJ, Kondon JJ, Quismorio FP, Frion GJ (1972) The choroid plexus in systemic lupus erythematosus. Ann Intern Med 76:56

Aufdermaur M (1953) Spondylitis ankylopoetica. Pathologische Anatomie. Documenta Geigy H 2, Basel

Aufdermaur M (1989) Pathogenesis of square bodies in ankylosing spondylitis. Ann Rheum Dis 48:628–631

Aydelotte MB, Kuettner KE (1988) Differences between subpopulations of cultured bovine articular chondrocytes. I. Morphology and cartilage matrix production. Connect Tissue Res 18:205–222

Aydelotte MB, Kuettner KE (1992) Heterogeneity of articular chondrocytes and cartilage matrix. In: Woessner Jr JF, Howell DS (eds) Joint Cartilage Degradation: Basic and Clinical Aspects. Marcel Dekker Inc., New York Basel Hong Kong, pp 37–65

Aydelotte MB, Schleyerbach R, Zeck BJ, Kuettner KE (1986) Articular chondrocytes cultured in agarose gel for study of chondrocytic chondrolysis. In: Kuettner KE, Schleyerbach R, Hascall VC (eds) Articular Cartilage Biochemistry. Raven Press, New York, pp 235–256

Aydelotte MB, Schumacher BL, Kuettner KE (1992) Heterogeneity of articular chondrocytes. In: Kuettner KE, Schleyerbach R, Peyron JG, Hascall VC (eds) Articular Cartilage and Osteoarthritis. Raven Press, New York, pp 237–249

Baggenstoss AH, Rosenberg EF (1941) Cardiac lesions associated with chronic infectious arthritis. Arch Intern Med 67:241

Baillou de G (1643) Liber de Rheumatismo. Opuscula Media. J Quesnet, Paris

Baker WM (1877) On the formation of synovial cysts in the leg in connection with disease of the knee joint. Saint Bartholomew's Hosp Report 13:245

Ball GV (1993) Ankylosing spondylitis. In: McCarty DJ, Koopman WJ (eds) Arthritis and Allied Conditions, 12th edn. Lea & Febiger, Philadelphia London (A Textbook of Rheumatology, vol 1) pp 1051–1060)

Ball J (1971) Enthesopathy of rheumatoid and ankylosing spondylitis. Ann Rheum Dis 30:213–223

Ball J (1979) Articular pathology of ankylosing spondylitis. Clin Orthop 143:30–37

Ball J (1983) The enthesopathy of ankylosing spondylitis. Br J Rheumatol 22 (Suppl 2):25–28

Banker BQ, Engel AG (1986) The polymyositis and dermatomyositis syndromes. In: Engel AG, Banker BQ (eds) Myology. McGraw-Hill, New York, pp 1385–1422

Bannatyne GA (1896) Rheumatoid arthritis: Its pathology, morbid anatomy and treatment, 1st edn, Bristol

Bannwarth A (1941) Chronisch lymphozytäre Meningitis, entzündliche Polyneuritis und "Rheumatismus". Arch Psychiatr Nervenkr 113:284–376

Barber HS (1957) Myalgic syndrome with constitutional effects: Polymyalgia rheumatica. Ann Rheum Dis 16:230

Barbour G, Coburn J, Slatopulsky E, et al. (1981) Hypercalcemia in an anephric patient with sarcoidosis: Evidence for extrarenal generation of 1,25-dihydroxyvitamin D. N Engl J Med 305:404

Barland P, Novikoff AB, Hamerman D (1964) Fine structure and cytochemistry of the rheumatoid synovial membrane with the special reference to lysosomes. Am J Pathol 44:853–859

Barnes L, Rodnan GP, Medsger TA, Short D (1979) Eosinophilic fasciitis; a pathologic study of twenty cases. Am J Pathol 96:493–518

Barrera P, Boerbooms AMT, Janssen EM, Sauerwein RW, Gallati H, Mulder J, de Boo T, Demacker PNM, van de Putte LBA, van der Meer JWM (1993) Circulating soluble tumor necrosis factor receptors, interleukin-2 receptors, tumor necrosis factor alpha, and interleukin-6 levels in rheumatoid arthritis: a longitudinal evaluation during methotrexate and azathioprine therapy. Arthritis Rheum 36:1070–1079

Bartels EM, Danneskiold-Samsoe B (1986) Histological abnormalities in muscle from patients with certain types of fibrositis. Lancet 1:755–757

Bauer W, Bennet GA, Zeller JW (1941) Pathology of joint lesions in patients with psoriasis and arthritis. Trans Ass Am Phys 56:349

Baumann H, Gauldie J (1994) The acute phase response. Immunol Today 15:74–80

Bayliss MT (1990) Proteoglycan structure and metabolism during maturation and aging of human articular cartilage. Biochem Soc Trans 18:799–802

Bayliss MT (1992) Metabolism of animal and human osteoarthritic cartilage. In: Kuettner KE, Schleyerbach R, Peyron JG, Hascall VC (eds) Articular Cartilage and Osteoarthritis. Raven Press, New York, pp 487–500

Bazin P (1860) Lécons théoriques et cliniques sur les affections cutanées de nature arthritique et arthreuse. Delahaye, Paris

Bechterew von W (1893) Steifigkeit der Wirbelsäule und ihre Verkrümmung als besondere Erkrankungsform. Neurol Zbl 12:633

Bechterew von W (1899a) Über ankylosierende Entzündung der Wirbelsäule und der großen Extremitätengelenke. Dtsch Z Nervenheilk 15:37

Bechterew von W (1899b) Neue Beobachtungen und pathologisch-anatomische Untersuchungen über Steifigkeit der Wirbelsäule. Dtsch Z Nervenheilk 15:45

Behçet H (1937) Über rezidivierende Aphtose, durch ein Virus verursachte Geschwüre am Mund, am Auge und an den Genitalien. Derm Wochenschr 105:1152–1157

Belmont HM, Abramson SB, Lie JT (1996) Pathology and pathogenesis of vascular injury in systemic lupus erythematosus. Arthritis Rheum 39 (1):9–22

Bely M (1990) Sekundäre Amyloidose bei chronischer Polyarthritis. Zentralbl Pathol Jena 136:337–355

Bely M, Apathy A (1991a) Herzveränderungen bei chronischer Polyarthritis. Zentralbl Pathol Jena 137:325–336

Bely M, Apathy A (1991b) Clinopathology of the lung. In: Bely M, Apathy A (eds) Organ Manifestations of Rheumatoid Arthritis. Globo, Budapest

Benach JL, Bosler EM, Hanrahan JP, et al. (1983) Spirochetes isolated from the blood of two patients with Lyme disease. N Engl J Med 308:740–742

Bengtsson A, Hénriksson KG, Larsson J (1986) Muscle biopsy in primary fibromyalgia. Scand J Rheumatol 15:1–6

Bennett GA, Zeller JW, Bauer W (1940) Subcutaneous nodules of rheumatoid arthritis and rheumatic fever. Arch Pathol 30:70

Benninghoff A (1939) Allgemeine Anatomie und Bewegungsapparat. In: Lehmanns JF (ed) Lehrbuch der Anatomie des Menschen, vol I. München Berlin

Berman A, Espinoza LR, Diaz JD, et al. (1988) Rheumatic manifestations of human immunodeficiency virus infection. Am J Med 85:59–64

Berry CL (1993) Of faddism, toxic oil, and skleroderma. J Pathol 170:419–420

Bessen DE, Jones KF, Fischetti VA (1989) Evidence for two distinct classes of streptococcal M-protein and their relationship to rheumatic fever. J Exp Med 169:269–283

Bierther MF, Wegner KW (1971) Elektronenmikroskopische Untersuchungen synovialer Gefäßveränderungen bei chronischer Polyarthritis. Z Rheumaforsch 30:214

Biesecker G, Katz S, Koffler D (1981) Renal localization of the membrane attack complex in systemic lupus erythematosus – nephritis. J Exp Med 154:1779

Bijlsma JW, Derksen RW, Huber-Bruning O, Borleffs JC (1988) Does Aids "cure" rheumatoid arthritis? Ann Rheum Dis 47:350–351

Biondi Oriente C, Scarpa R, Pucino A, Oriente P (1989) Psoriasis and psoriatic arthritis: Dermatological and rheumatological co-operative clinical report. Acta Derm Venereol (Suppl) 146:69–71

Bjelle A (1979) Pyrophosphate arthropathy. Scand J Rheumatol 8:145–153

Bluestein HG (1978) Antineuronal factors in the serum of patients with systemic lupus erythematosus. Proc Natl Acad Sci 75:9365

Bluestein HG (1979) Heterogeneous neurotoxic antibodies in systemic lupus erythematosus. Clin Exp Immunol 35:210

Bluestein HG, Zvaifler NJ (1976) Brain-reactive lymphocytotoxic antibodies in the serum of patients with systemic lupus erythematosus. J Clin Invest 57:509
Bluestone R (1985) Ankylosing spondylitis. In: McCarty DS (ed) Arthritis and Allied Conditions, 10th edn. Lea & Febiger, Philadelphia (A Textbook of Rheumatology)
Bodeutsch C, Wilde de PCM, Kater L, Houwelingen van JC, Hoogen van den FHJ, Kruize AA, Hené RJ, Putte van de LBA, Vooijs GP (1992) Quantitative immunohistologic criteria are superior to the lymphocytic focus score criterion for the diagnosis of Sjögren's syndrome. Arthritis Rheum 35 (9):1075
Boedeker CW (1859) Über das Alkapton. Zschr rat Med 7:130–145
Böni A, Kaganas G (1954) Spondylitis ankylopoetica II Klinik und Therapie. Documenta Rheumatologica 3:50. Geigy, Basel
Bohemen van CG, Rumet FC, Zanen HC (1984) Identification of HLA-B27 M1 and M2 cross-reactive antigens in Klebsiella, Shigella and Yersinia. Immunology 52:607–610
Bolten W (1991) Das Cricoarytenoid-Gelenk bei der chronischen Polyarthritis. Z Rheumatol 50:1–5
Bonfa E, Golombek SJ, Kaufman LD, et al. (1987) Association between lupus psychosis and anti-ribosomal p protein antibodies. N Engl J Med 317:265–271
Botstein GR, Sherer GK, LeRoy EC (1982) Fibroblast selection in scleroderma: an alternative model of fibrosis. Arthritis Rheum 25:189–195
Botzenhardt C (1975) Fibroblastäre Proliferation und lymphozytäre Infiltration des Stratum synoviale bei chronischer Polyarthritis in Beziehung zur klinischen Aktivität der Erkrankung. Med. Dissertation. Universität Mainz
Bouillaud JB (1836) Nouvelles recherches sur le rhumatisme articulaire aigu et sur la loi decoincidence de la pericardite avec cette maladie. Paris
Bourdillon C (1888) Psoriasis et arthropathies. A. Parent Imprimeur de la Faculté de Médicine. A Davy, Paris
Boyer RS, Sun NCY, Verity A, Nies KM, Louie JS (1980) Immunperoxidase staining of the choroid plexus in systemic lupus erythematosus. J Rheum 7:645-650
Brandt KD (1985a) Pathogenesis of osteoarthritis. In: Kelley WN, Harris Jr ED, Ruddy S, Sledge CB (eds) Textbook of Rheumatology, vol 2, 2nd edn. WB Saunders Company, Philadelphia London Toronto Mexico City Rio de Janeiro Sydney Tokyo, pp 1417–1431
Brandt KD (1985b) Osteoarthritis: Clinical patterns and pathology. In: Kelley WN, Harris Jr ED, Ruddy S, Sledge CB (eds) Textbook of Rheumatology, vol 2, 2nd edn. WB Saunders Company, Philadelphia London Toronto Mexico City Rio de Janeiro Sydney Tokyo, pp 1432–1448
Braun J, Bollow M, Remlinger G, Eggens U, Rudwaleit M, Distler A, Sieper Y (1998) Prevalence of spondylarthropathies in HLA-B27 positive and negative blood donors. Arthritis Rheum 41:58–67
Breutjens JR, Sepulevda M, Balish T (1976) Interstitial immune complex nephritis in patients with systemic lupus erythematosus. Kidney Int 7:342
Brewerton DA, Hard FD, Nicholls A, Caffrey M, James DC, Sturrock RD (1973) Ankylosing spondylitis and HLA-27. Lancet 1:904-907
Briem H, Evengard B, Jonsson M (1978) Reiter's syndrome complicating Salmonella enteritis infection. Lancet 2:112
Briem H, Norberg R, Jonsson M, et al. (1980) Circulating immune complexes in patients with intestinal infections. J Infect 2:215–220
Brodie BC (1813) Pathological researches respecting the diseases of joints. Medico-chir Trans 4:207–277
Bromley M, Woolley DE (1984) Histopathology of the rheumatoid lesion – identification of cell types at sites of cartilage erosion. Arthritis Rheum 27 (8):857–863

Brown MA, Pile KD, Kennedy LG, Calin A, Darke C, Bell J, Wordsworth BP, Cornelis F (1996) HLA class I associations of ankylosing spondylitis in the white population in the United Kingdom. Ann Rheum Dis 55:268–270

Brown MA, Kennedy LG, MacGregor AJ, Darke C, Duncan E, Shatford JL, Taylor A, Calin A, Wordsworth P (1997) Susceptibility to ankylosing spondylitis in twins. Arthritis Rheum 49 (10):1823–1828

Brückle M, Suckfüll M, Fleckenstein W, Weiss C, Müller W (1990) Gewebe-pO_2-Messung in der verspannten Rückenmuskulatur (m. erector spinae). Z Rheumatol 49:208–216

Büchner F (1975) Allgemeine Pathologie und Ätiologie, 6th edn. Urban und Schwarzenberg, München Berlin Wien

Buckingham RB, Prince RK, Rodnan GP, Taylor F (1978) Increased collagen accumulation in dermal fibroblast cultures from patients with progressive sclerosis (scleroderma). J Lab Clin Med 92:5

Bui-Mansfield LT, Youngberg RA (1997) Intraarticular ganglia of the knee: prevalence, presentation, etiology, and management. Am J Roentgenol 168 (1):123–127

Bulkley BH, Roberts WC (1975) The heart in systemic lupus erythematosus and the changes induced in it by corticosteroid therapy: A study of 36 necropsy patients. Am J Med 58:243

Bulpitt KJ, Verity MA, Clements PJ, Paulus HE (1990) Association of L-tryptophan and an illness resembling eosinophilic fasciitis: Clinical and histopathologic findings in four patients with eosinophilia myalgia syndrome. Arthritis Rheum 33:918–929

Burgdorfer W, Barbour AG, Hayes SF, Benach JL, Grunwald E, Davis JP (1982) Lyme disease – a tick borne spirochetosis? Science 216:1317–1319

Burmester GR, Stuhlmüller B, Keyszer G, Kinne RW (1997) Mononuclear phagozytes and rheumatoid arthritis. Mastermind or workhorse in arthritis? Arthritis Rheum 40:5–18

Butler WT, Sharp JT, Rossen RD, Lindskey MD, Mittal KK, Gard DA (1972) Relationship of the clinical course of systemic lupus erythematosus to the presence of circulating lymphocytotoxic antibodies. Arthritis Rheum 15:231

Bywaters EGL (1950) The relation between heart and joint disease including "rheumatoid heart disease" and chronic post-rheumatic arthritis (type Jaccoud). Brit Heart J 12:101

Bywaters EGL (1968) Diagnostic criteria for Still's disease. In: Bennett P, Wood P (eds) Population Studies of the Rheumatic Diseases. New York

Bywaters EGL (1970) Juvenile chronische Polyarthritis (Stillsche Krankheit). In: Schoen R, Böni A, Miehlke K (eds) Klinik der rheumatischen Erkrankungen. Springer, Berlin Heidelberg New York

Bywaters EGL (1976) The pathology of Still's disease. In: Jayson MJV (ed) Still's Disease: Juvenile Chronic Polyarthritis. Academic Press, London

Bywaters EGL (1977) Pathologic aspects of juvenile chronic polyarthritis. Arthritis Rheum 20 (Suppl):271–276

Bywaters EGL, Ansell BM (1965) Monoarticular arthritis in children. Ann Rheum Dis 24:116–122

Calabrese LH, Kelley DM, Myers A, et al. (1991) Rheumatic symptoms and human immunodeficiency virus infection: The influence of clinical and laboratory variable in a longitudinal cohort study. Arthritis Rheum 34:257–263

Calamia KT, Moore SB, Elveback LR, Hunder GG (1981) HLA-DR locus antigens in polymyalgia rheumatica and giant cell arteritis. J Rheumatol 8:993-996

Calin A (1984) Reiter's syndrome. In: Calin A (ed) Spondylarthropathies. Grune & Stratton, Orlando, pp 119–149

Calin A (1992) Update on the spondylarthropathies: from genes to gender, B27 to burn out. Current Rheumatol 3:4–6
Calin A, Fries JF (1975) The striking prevalence of ankylosing spondylitis in "healthy" W 27 positive males and females: A controlled study. N Engl J Med 293:835
Calin A, Elswood J, Klonda PT (1989) Destructive arthritis, rheumatoid factor, and HLA-DR4. Susceptibility versus severity, a case-control study. Arthritis Rheum 32:1221–1225
Calkins E, Cohen AS (1960) Diagnosis of amyloidosis. Bull Rheum Dis 10:215
Canoso JJ, Saini M, Hermos JA (1978) Whipple's disease and ankylosing spondylitis. Simultaneous occurrence in HLA-B27 positive males. J Rheumatol 5:79–84
Caplan A (1953) Certain unusual radiological appearances in the chests of coalminers suffering from rheumatoid arthritis. Thorax 8:29
Caroit M, Rouaud JP, Nicolas-Vullierene S (1987) Le diagnostic de la pseudopolyarthrite rhizomélique. Rhumatologie 39:215–222
Carpenter A, Karpati G, Heller I, Eisen A (1978) Inclusion body myositis: a distinct variety of idiopathic inflammatory myopathy. Neurology 28:8–17
Carpenter S (1988) Resin histology and electron microscopy in inflammatory myopathies. In: Dalakas MC (ed) Polymyositis and dermatomyositis. Butterworths, Boston, pp 195–215
Carroll MC (1998) The role of complement and complement receptors in induction and regulation of immunity. Annu Rev Immunol 16:545–568
Cassidy JT (1985) Juvenile rheumatoid arthritis.In: Kelley WN, Harris Jr ED, Ruddy S, Sledge CB (eds) Textbook of Rheumatology, vol 2, 2nd edn. WB Saunders Company, Philadelphia London Toronto Mexico City Rio de Janeiro Sydney Tokyo, pp 1247–1277
Cassidy JT, Nelson AM (1988) The frequency of juvenile arthritis (editorial). J Rheumatol 15:535–536
Cassidy JT, Levinson JE, Brewer Jr EJ (1989) The development of classification criteria for children with juvenile rheumatoid arthritis. Bull Rheum Dis 38:1-7
Castleman B, McNeely BU (1967) Case records of the Massachusetts General Hospital. New Engl J Med 76:1079
Caterson B, Hughes CE, Johnstone B, Mort JS (1992) Immunological markers of cartilage proteoglycan metabolism in animal and human osteoarthritis. In: Kuettner KE, Schleyerbach R, Peyron JG, Hascall VC (eds) Articular cartilage and Osteoarthritis. Raven Press, New York, pp 415–427
Cella M, Sallusto F, Lanzavecchia A (1997) Origin, maturation and antigen presenting function of dendritic cells. Curr Opin Immunol 9:10–16
Charcot J-M (1889) Maladies des vieillards. Goutte et rhumatisme. Lecrosnier et Babe, Paris
Chatham WW, Swaim R, Frohsin H, Heck LW, Miller EJ, Blackburn WD (1993) Degradation of human articular cartilage by neutrophils in synovial fluid. Arthritis Rheum 36:51–58
Chikanza IC, Roux-Lombard P, Dayer J-M, Panayi GS (1993) Tumour necrosis factor soluble receptors behave as acute phase reactants following surgery in patients with rheumatoid arthritis, chronic osteomyelitis and osteoarthritis. Clin Exp Immunol 92:19–22
Chu CQ, Field M, Feldmann M, Maini RN (1991) Localization of tumor necrosis factor 2 in synovial tissues and at the cartilage-pannus junction in patients with rheumatoid arthritis. Arthritis Rheum 34:1125–1132
Chuang TY, Hunder GG, Jestrup DM, Kurland LT (1982) Polymyalgia rheumatica. A ten-year epidemiologic and clinical study. Ann Intern Med 97:672-680

Chudwin DS, Daniels TE, Wara DW, et al. (1981) Spectrum of Sjögren's syndrome in children. J Pediatr 98:213–217
Churg J, Sobin LH (1982) Renal Disease. Classification and atlas of glomerular diseases. Igaku-Shoin, Tokio New York, pp 127–149
Churg J, Strauss L (1951) Allergic granulomatosis, allergic angiitis, and periarteritis nodosa. Am J Pathol 27:277
Cid MC, Font C, Coll-Vinent B, Grau JM (1998) Large vessel vasculitides. Curr Opin Rheumatol 10:18–28
Cipoletti JF, Buckingham RB, Barnes EL, Peel RL, Mahmood K, Cignetti FE, Pierce JM, Rabin BS, Rodman GP (1977) Sjögren's syndrome in progressive systemic sclerosis. Ann Intern Med 87:535
Clark JM (1991) Variation of collagen fiber alignment in a joint surface: a scanning electron microscope study of the tibial plateau in dog, rabbit and man. J Orthop Res 9:246–257
Clarke MT, Lyall HA, Grant JW, Matthewson MH (1998) The histopathology of de Quervain's disease. J Hand Surg 23B (6):732–734
Clauw DJ, Nashel PJ, Umhau A, Katz P (1990) Tryptophan-associated eosinophilic connective-tissue disease. JAMA 263:1502
Coburn AF (1931) The factor infection in the rheumatic state. Williams & Wilkins, Baltimore
Cochrane W, Davies DV, Dorling J, Bywaters EGL (1964) Ultramicroscopic structure of the rheumatoid nodule. Ann Rheum Dis 23:345–363
Cohen AS (1991) Amyloidosis. Bull Rheum Dis 40 (2):1–12
Cohen AS, Skinner M (1986) Amyloidosis. In: Cohen AS, Bennett JC (eds) Rheumatology and Immunology, 2nd edn. Grune & Stratton, Orlando, pp 294–301
Cohen JM (1983) Pseudorheumatoid nodules in an adult. J Foot Surg 22:203
Cohen RD, Conn DL, Ilstrup DM (1980) Clinical features, prognosis and response to treatment in polyarteritis. Mayo Clin Proc 55:146
Collins DH (1937) The subcutaneous nodule of rheumatoid arthritis. J Path Bact 45:97–115
Conn DL, Hunder GG (1985) Necrotizing vasculitis. In: Kelley WN, Harris Jr ED, Ruddy S, Sledge CB (eds) Textbook of Rheumatology, vol 2, 2nd edn. WB Saunders Company, Philadelphia London Toronto Mexico City Rio de Janeiro Sydney Tokyo, pp 1137–1166
Conn DL, McDuffie FC, Holley KE, Schroeter AL (1976) Immunologic mechanisms in systemic vasculitis. Mayo Clin Proc 51:511
Connor B (1695) The bones of a skeleton united without jointing or cartilage. Phil Trans B 29:21
Constantopoulos SH, Papadimitriou CS, Moutsopoulos HM (1985) Respiratory manifestations in primary Sjögren's syndrome. A clinical, functional, and histologic study. Chest 88:226–229
Cooke TD, Hurd ER, Jasin HE, Bienenstock J, Ziff M (1975) Identification of immunoglobulins and complement in rheumatoid articular collagenous tissues. Arthritis Rheum 18:541–551
Cope AP, Aderka D, Doherty M, Engelmann H, Gibbons D, Jones AC, Brennan FM, Maini RN, Wallach D, Feldmann M (1992) Increased levels of soluble tumor necrosis factor receptors in the sera and synovial fluid of patients with rheumatic diseases. Arthritis Rheum 35:1160–1169
Copeman WSC (1964) A short history of the gout. University of California Press, Los Angeles, p 35
Cornil MV (1864) Mémoire sur les coincidences pathologiques du rhumatisme articulaire chronique. CR Mem Soc Biol Series 4 (3)
Corrigan AB, Robinson RG, Terenty TR, Dick-Smith JB, Walters D (1974) Benign rheumatoid arthritis of the aged. Br Med J 9:444–445
Coste F, Forestier I (1935) Remarques sur le rheumatisme psoriasique. Rev Rhum 2:554

Crain DC (1961) Interphalangeal osteoarthritis characterized by painful, inflammatory episodes, resulting in deformity of the proximal and distal articulations. JAMA 175:1949
Crohn BB (1949) Regional ileitis. Grune & Stratton, New York
Crohn BB, Ginzburg L, Oppenheimer GD (1932) Regional ileitis - a pathological and clinical entity. JAMA 99:1323–1329
Cruickshank B (1951) Histopathology of diarthrodial joints in ankylosing spondylitis. Ann Rheum Dis 10:393
Cruickshank B (1954) The arteritis of rheumatoid arthritis. Ann Rheum Dis 13:136–146
Cruickshank B (1956) Lesions of cartilaginous joints in ankylosing spondylitis. J Path Bact 71:73
Cruickshank B (1960) Pathology of ankylosing spondylitis. Bull Rheum Dis 10:211–214
Cunnane G, Fitzgerald O, Hummel KM, Yousset P, Kane D, Gay RE, Gay S, Bresnihan B (1997) Detection of collagenase, cathepsin B and cathepsin L messenger RNA expression in synovial tissue of patients with early inflammatory arthritis. Arthritis Rheum 40:131
Cush JJ, Lipsky PE (1993) Reiter's syndrome and reactive arthritis. In: McCarty DJ, Koopman WJ (eds) Arthritis and Allied Conditions, 12th edn. Lea & Febiger, Philadelphia London (A Textbook of Rheumatology, vol 1) pp 1061–1078
Dalakas MC (1991) Polymyositis, dermatomyositis, and inclusion-body myositis. N Engl J Med 325:1487–1498
Dale JB, Chiang EC (1995) Intranasal immunization with recombinant group A streptococcal M fragment fused to the B subunit of Escherichia coli labile toxin protects mice against systemic challenge infections. J Infect Dis 171:1038–1041
Danning CL, Illei GG, Lee EG, Boumpas DT, McInnes IB (1998a) Characterization of psoriatic arthritis synovial membrane (PsA SM): Cytokine and cell activation marker expression. Arthritis Rheum 41 (9):1806
Danning CL, Illei GG, Lee EG Boumpas DT, McInnes IB (1998b) $\alpha_V\beta_3$ integrin expression in psoriatic arthritis (PsA) synovial membrane. Arthritis Rheum 41 (Suppl 9):1883
Davidson PT, Horowitz I (1970) Skeletal tuberculosis. Am J Med 48:77–84
Davies JD (1973) Behçet's syndrome with haemoptysis and pulmonary lesions. J Pathol 109:351
Davis JA, Weisman MH, Dail DH (1978) Vascular disease in infective endocarditis. Arch Int Med 138:480
Dayal AK, Kammer GM (1996) The T cell enigma in lupus. Arthritis Rheum 39 (1):23–33
Deesmochok U, Tumrasvin T (1990) Clinical study of culture-proven cases of non-gonococcal arthritis. J Med Ass Thailand 73 (11):615–623
Dequekker J, Ryckewaert A, Debeyre N, Kahn M-F, de Sèze S (1966) La polyarthrite rhumatoide débutant chez le sujet âgé. Rev Rhumatol 33:550–554
Deutsche Gesellschaft für Rheumatologie (ed) (1999) Qualitätssicherung in der Rheumatologie. Steinkopff Verlag, Darmstadt
Diamantberger S (1890) Du rhumatise noueux (polyarthrite déformante) chez les enfants. Paris
Dieppe PA, Crocker P, Huskisson EC, Willoughby DA (1976) Apatite deposition disease. A new arthropathy. Lancet 1:266-269
DiFranco M, Coari G, Bonucci E (2000) A morphological study of bone and articular cartilage in ochronosis. Virchows Arch 436 (1):74–81
Dihlmann W (1979) Current radiodiagnostic concept of ankylosing spondylitis. Skeletal Radiol 4:179–188
Dihlmann W, Delling G (1983) Disco-vertebral destructive lesions (so-called Andersson lesions) associated with ankylosing spondylitis. Skeletal Radiol 3:10–16

Dingle JT, Tyler JA (1986) Role of intercellular messengers in the control of cartilage matrix dynamics. In: Kuettner KE, Schleyerbach R, Hascall VC (eds) Articular cartilage biochemistry. Raven Press, New York, pp 181–210

Dingle JT, Saklatvala J, Hembry R, Tyler J, Fell HB, Jubb R (1979) A cartilage catabolic factor from synovium. Biochem J 184:177–180

Dixon ASJ, Ball J (1957) Honeycomb lung and chronic rheumatoid arthritis: A case report. Ann Rheum Dis 16:241

Dobbins WO (1987) HLA antigens in Whipple's disease. Arthritis Rheum 30:102–105

Doherty M, Bradfield JWB (1981) Polyarteritis nodosa associated with acute cytomegalovirus infection. Ann Rheum Dis 40:419

Doherty M, Chuck A, Hosking D, Hamilton E (1991) Inorganic pyrophosphate in metabolic diseases predisposing to calcium pyrophosphate dihydrate crystal deposition. Arthritis Rheum 34:1297–1303

Donath K, Seifert G (1972) Ultrastruktur und Pathogenese der myoepithelialen Sialadenitis. Über das Vorkommen von Myoepithelialzellen bei benignen lymphoepithelialen Läsionen. Virchows Archiv path Anat 356:315

Drosos AA, Andonopoulos AP, et al. (1988) Prevalence of primary Sjögren's syndrome in elderly population. Br J Rheumatol 27:123–127

Dubowitz V, Brooke MH (1973) Muscle biopsy: A modern approach, vol 2 in the series. Saunders, London Philadelphia Toronto (Major problems in neurology, vol 2)

Dunne JV, Carson DA, Spiegelberg HL, Alspaugh MA, Vaughn JH (1979) IgA rheumatoid factor in the sera and saliva of patients with rheumatoid arthritis and Sjögren's syndrome. Ann Rheum Dis 38:161

Dupuytren G (1832) Lécons orales de clinique chirurgicale faites a l' Hôtel-Dieu de Paris, vol 1. Paris

Duvic M, Johnson TM, Rapini RP, et al. (1987) Acquired immunodeficiency syndrome – associated psoriasis and Reiter's syndrome. Arch Dermatol 123:1622–1632

Eastmond CJ, Rennie JAN, Reid TMS (1982) Campylobacter reactive arthritis – an epidemiological study. Ann Rheum Dis 41:312

Ebringer A (1983) The cross tolerance hypothesis, HLA-B 27 and ankylosing spondylitis. Br J Rheum 22 (Suppl 2):53–66

Edwards JCW, Wilkinson LS, Pitsillides AA (1993) Palisading cells of rheumatoid nodules: comparison with synovial intimal cells. Ann Rheum Dis 52:801–805

Egelius N, Göhle O, Jonsson E, Wahlgren F (1955) Cardiac changes in rheumatoid arthritis. Ann Rheum Dis 14:11

Eisen A, Berry K, Gibson G (1983) Inclusion body myositis: myopathy or neuropathy? Neurology 33:1109–1114

Ellis SG, Verity MA (1979) Central nervous system involvement in systemic lupus erythematosus: A review of neuropathologic findings in 57 cases, 1955–1977. Sem Arthritis Rheum 8:212–221

Emery AEH, Lawrence SS (1967) Genetics of ankylosing spondylitis. J Med Genet 4:239-244

Empey DW, Hale JE (1972) Rectal and colonic ulceration in Behçet's disease. Proc Roy Soc Med 65:163-164

Engel AG, Arahata K (1986) Mononuclear cells in myopathies: quantitation of functionally distinct subsets, recognition of antigen-specific cell-mediated cytotoxicity in some diseases and implications for the pathogenesis of the different inflammatory myopathies. Hum Pathol 17:704–721

Engel AG, Emslie-Smith AM (1989) Inflammatory myopathies. Curr Opin Neurol Neurosurg 2:695–700

Engel AG, Franzini-Armstrong C (1994) Myology: Basic and Clinical, 2nd edn. McGraw-Hill, New York

Engleman EP, Bombardier C, Hochberg MC (eds) (1983) Conference on epidemiology of rheumatic diseases. Specific needs of developing countries. J Rheumatol 10 (Suppl):1–107
Enzinger FM, Weiss SW (1983) Soft tissue tumors. The CV Mosby Company, St. Louis Toronto London
Enzinger FM, Lattes R, Tolorini H (1969) Histological typing of soft tissue tumors. International histological classification of tumors, no 3, WHO, Geneva
Epstein WV (1986) The eye and connective tissue diseases. In: Cohen AS, Bennett JC (eds) Rheumatology and Immunology, 2nd edn. Grune & Stratton, Orlando, pp 179–185
Espinoza LR, Vasey FB, Oh JH, Wilkinson R, Osterland CK (1978) Association between HLA-B 38 and peripheral psoriatric arthritis. Arthritis Rheum 21:72-75
Esterhai Jr JL, Gelb I (1991) Adult septic arthritis. Orthop Clin North Am 22 (3):503–514
Eyre DR (1991) The collagens of articular cartilage. Semin Arthritis Rheumatol 3 (Suppl 2):2–11
Eyre DR, Wu J-J, Apone S (1987) A growing family of collagens in articular cartilage: Identification of 5 genetically different types. J Rheumatol Spec No 14:25-27
Eyre DR, Wu J-J, Woods PE (1992) Cartilage-specific collagens: Structural studies. In: Kuettner KE, Schleyerbach R, Peyron JG, Hascall VC (eds) Articular Cartilage and Osteoarthritis. Raven Press, New York, pp 119–131
Fagge H (1877) A case of simple synovitis of the ribs to the vertebrae, and of the arches and articular processes of the vertebrae themselves, and also of one hipjoint. Transact path Soc London 28:201
Fahr T (1918) Zur Frage des Rheumatismus nodosus. Zbl Path 29:625–630
Fairfax AJ, Haslam PL, Pavia D, et al. (1981) Pulmonary disorders associated with Sjögren's syndrome. Am J Med 199:279–295
Fam AG, Paton TW, Shamess CJ, Lewis AJ (1980) Fulminant colitis complicating gold-therapy. J Rheumatol 7:479
Fassbender HG (1963) Nosologische Typen des rheumatischen Granuloms und ihre biologische Bedeutung. Frankf Zschr Path 72:586–604
Fassbender HG (1967a) Die Bedeutung viszeraler Prozesse für Pathogenese und Nosologie der primär chronischen Polyarthritis. Frankf Zschr Path 76:243–269
Fassbender HG (1967b) L'amyloidose myocardique dans la polyarthrite rhumatoide. Médicine et Hygiène 25:456-458
Fassbender HG (1972) Konzept einer Pathosystematik der chronischen Polyarthritis. Zschr Rheumaforsch 31:129–136
Fassbender HG (1975) Pathologie rheumatischer Erkrankungen. Springer, Berlin Heidelberg New York
Fassbender HG (1979) Extra-articular processes in osteoarthropathia psoriatica. Arch Orthop Traumat Surg 95:37–46
Fassbender HG (1980) Pathological aspects and findings of Bechterew's syndrome and osteoarthropathia psoriatica. Scand J Rheumatol (Suppl) 32:50–58
Fassbender HG (1983) Histomorphological basis of articular cartilage destruction in rheumatoid arthritis. Collagen Rel Res 3:141–155
Fassbender HG (1986a) Joint destruction in various arthritic diseases. In: Kuettner KE, Schleyerbach R, Hascall VC (eds) Articular cartilage biochemistry. Raven Press, New York, pp 371–389
Fassbender HG (1986b) Strukturelle Grundlagen der Osteoarthropathia psoriatica. In: Schilling F (ed) Arthritis und Spondylitis psoriatica. Steinkopff, Darmstadt, pp 31–44
Fassbender HG (1988) Interaction between cartilage metabolism and inflammation. In: Schumacher HR (ed) Osteoarthritis - Diagnosis and Therapy. Springer, Berlin Heidelberg New York, pp 11–13

Fassbender HG (1994) Inflammatory reactions in arthritis. In: Davies ME, Dingle JT (eds) Handbook of Immunopharmacology: Immunopharmacology of joints and connective tissue. Academic Press, London San Diego New York Boston Sidney Tokyo Toronto, pp 165–198

Fassbender HG, Fassbender R (1992) Synovial characteristics of seronegative spondarthritides (Rapid communication). Clin Investig 70:706

Fassbender HG, Gay S (1988) Synovial processes in rheumatoid Arthritis. Scand J Rheumatol (Suppl) 76:1–7

Fassbender HG, Wegner K (1973) Morphologie und Pathogenese des Weichteilrheumatismus. Z Rheumaforsch 32:355–374

Fassbender HG, Zwick JC (1995) Neue Forschungsergebnisse auf dem Gebiet der Osteoarthrose. Wien Med Wschr 145:96-98

Fassbender HG, Simmling-Annefeld M, Stofft E (1980) Transformation der Synovialzellen bei rheumatoider Arthritis. Verh Dtsch Ges Path 64:193–212

Fassbender HG, Hebert TD, Seibel M (1992) Pathways of joint destruction in MTP- and MCP-joints in rheumatoid arthritis. Scand J Rheumatol 21:10–16

Fassbender R, Annefeld M (1986) Ultrastrukturelle Veränderungen in der Skelettmuskulatur bei Polymyalgia rheumatica. Dtsch Med Wochenschr 11/47:1799–1804

Fauci AS, Harley JB, Roberts WC, Ferrans VJ, Gralnick HR, Bjornson BH (1982) The idiopathic hypereosinophilic syndrome: clinical, pathophysiologic, and therapeutic considerations. Ann Intern Med 97:78–92

Fearon U, Reece R, Smith J, Emery P, Veale DJ (1998) Differential cytokines and growth factor expression: Basis for different pathogenesis of psoriatic and rheumatoid arthritis. Arthritis Rheum 41 (Suppl 9):334

Feigenbaum A (1956) Description of Behçet's syndrome in the Hippocratic third book of endemic diseases. Br J Ophtalmol 40:355

Feinglass EJ, Arnett FC, Dorsch CA, Zizic RM, Stevens MC (1976) Neuropsychiatric manifestations of systemic lupus erythematosus: Diagnosis, clinical spectrum and relationship to other features of the disease. Medicine 55:323

Felty AR (1924) Chronic arthritis in the adult, associated with splenomegaly and leucopenia. Johns Hopkins Hosp Bull 35:16

Fessel JW (1979) Renal outcomes of gout and hyperuricemia. Am J Med 67:74–82

Feurle GE (1985) Association of Whipple's disease with HLA-B27. Lancet 1:1336

Fidler HM, Rook GA, Johnson N, McFadden J (1993) Mycobacterium tuberculosis DNA in tissue affected by sarcoidosis. Br Med J 306:546–549

Fidler IJ, Gersten DM, Hart IR (1978) The biology of cancer invasion and metastasis. Advance Cancer Res 28:149–250

Fiessinger N, Leroy E (1916) Contribution a l'étude d'une epidémie de dysenterie dans la Somme. Bull Mem Soc Med Hop Paris 40:2030–2069

Fine LG (1996) Systemic sclerosis: Current pathogenetic concepts and future prospects for targeted therapy. In: Fine LG (chairman) Systemic sclerosis: Current pathogenetic concepts and future prospects for targeted therapy (Report of a meeting of physicians and scientists, London). Lancet 347:1453–1458

Finkelstein H (1930) Stenosing tendovaginitis at the radial styloid process. Am J Bone Joint Surg 12:509–540

Firestein GS, Manning AM (1999) Signal transduction and transscription factors in rheumatic disease. Arthritis Rheum 42:609–621

Firestein GS, Paine MM (1992) Stromelysin and tissue inhibitor of metalloproteinases gene expression in rheumatoid arthritis synovium. Am J Pathol 140 (6):1309–1314

Firestein GS, Yeo M, Zvaifler NJ (1995) Apoptosis in rheumatoid synovium. J Clin Invest 96:1631–1638

Fitzek JG, Schlegl J, Wessinghage D (1989) Frakturen bei chronischer Polyarthritis. Orth Praxis 5:292–306

Fleischmajer R, Gay S, Perlish JS, Cesarini J-P (1980) Immunoelectron microscopy of type III collagen in normal and scleroderma skin. J Invest Dermatol 75:189

Forestier J, Charmant P (1950) La polyarthrite chronique évolutive chez le vieillard. Concours med 21:1691

Forestier J, Robert P (1934) Ostéophytes et syndesmophytes. Gaz med Fr (Suppl Radiol) 192

Fournié A, Bouvier M, Fournié B, Colson F, Ayrolles Ch, Larbre J-P (1989) Hyperostose-ostéite-périostite, triade radiologique des enthésopathies. Remarques à propos de deux localisations fémorales inhabituelles. Rev Rhum Mal Ostéoartic 56:763–766

Fournié B (1993) Le territoire enthésique et le syndrome d'hyperostose-ostéite-périostite (HOP). Une approche nosologique radioclinique des spondylarthropathies inflammatoires. Rev Rhum Mal Ostéoartic 60:485–488

Fournié B (1998) Klinisch-anatomische Besonderheiten der Psoriasisarthritis. Rheumatol Eur 27/4:133–135

Fournié B, Granel J, Bonnet M, et al. (1992) Fréquence des signes évocateurs d'un rhumatisme psoriasique dans l'atteinte radiologique des doigts et des orteils. A propos de 193 cas. Rev Rhum Mal Ostéoartic 59:117–180

Fox RA, Isenberg DA (1997) Human immunodeficiency virus infection in systemic lupus erythematosus. Arthritis Rheum 40 (6):1168–1172

Fox RI, Carstens SA, Fong S, Robinson CA, Howell SA, Vaughan JH (1982) Use of monoclonal antibodies to analyze peripheral blood and salivary gland lymphocyte subsets in Sjögren's syndrome. Arthritis Rheum 25:419

Fox RI, Bumol T, Fantozzi R, et al. (1986) Expression of histocompatibility antigen HLA-DR by salivary gland epithelial cells in Sjögren's syndrome. Arthritis Rheum 29:1105–1111

Franceschetti A, Bischler V (1950) La sclérité nodulaire nécrosante et ses rapports avec la scléromalacie. Ann Oculist 183:737

Françon F (1957) Rhumatismes inflammatoires des sujés âgés. Rhumatologie 9:51

Fraya R, Stevens MB, Bayless TM (1975) Destructive monarthritis and granulomatous synovitis as the presenting manifestations of Crohn's disease. Johns Hopkins Med J 137:151

Fujimoto T, Kato H, Ichiose E, Sasaguri Y (1982) Immune complex and mite antigen in Kawasaki disease. Lancet 2:980-981

Furie R, Kaell A, Petrucci R, Faber B, Kaplan M (1988) Systemic lupus erythematosus complicated by infection with human immunodeficiency virus. Arthritis Rheum 31 (Suppl):56

Gadher SJ, Eyre DR, Duance VC, Wotton SF, Heck LW, Shmid TM, Woolley DE (1988) Susceptibility of cartilage collagens type II, IX, X, and XI to human synovial collagenase and neutrophil elastase. Eur J Biochem 175:1–7

Galen Zit. n. Moll W

Gärtner J (1959) Skleritis nodulosa necroticans als Folge einer riesenzellhaltigen granulomatösen Angiits. Klin Mbl Augenheilk 134 (4):505

Garin C, Bujadoux C (1922) Paralysie par les tiques. J Med Lyon 71:765–767

Garrod AB (1892) Cullings from the treaties on gout and rheumatic gout. St Lewis

Gaucher A, et al. (1977) HLA antigens and alkaptonuria. J Rheumatol 3 (Suppl):97–100
Gauger M, Mohr W (1995) Neutrophile Granulozyten bei der rheumatischen Gewebsdestruktion. Akt Rheumatol 20:49–54
Gay S, Tanaka A, Tarkowski A, Gay RE, Fassbender HG (1988) Expression of oncogenes RAS and MYC in proliferating synovial lining cells in RA. Arthritis Rheum 31:R40
Gay S, Huang G, Ziegler B, Fassbender HG, Gay RE (1989) Expression of MYB, MYC, RAS, and FOS oncogenes in synovial cells of patients with rheumatoid arthritis (RA) or osteoarthritis (OA). Arthritis Rheum 32 (Suppl 4):59
Gay S, Trabandt A, Moreland LW, Gay RE (1992) Growth factors, extracellular matrix, and oncogenes in scleroderma. Arthritis Rheum 35:304–310
Gay S, Gay RE, Koopman WJ (1993) Molecular and cellular mechanisms of joint destruction in rheumatoid arthritis: two cellular mechanisms explain joint destruction? Ann Rheum Dis 52:39–47
Geczy AF, Prendergast JK, Sullivan JS, Upfold LJ, Edmonds JP, Bashir HV (1985) Possible role of enteric organisms in the pathogenesis of the seronegative arthropathies. In: Ziff M, Cohen SB (eds) Advances in Inflammation Research, vol 9. The Spondylarthropathies, pp 129–137
Geiler G (1961) Die Synovialome-Morphologie und Pathogenese. Springer, Berlin Göttingen Heidelberg
Geipel P (1906) Untersuchungen über rheumatische Myocarditis. Dtsch Arch Klin Med 85:74
Gerber MA, Shapiro ED, Burke GS, et al. (1996) Lyme disease in children in southeastern Connecticut. N Engl J Med 335:1270–1274
Gerber NJ (1989) Polymyalgia rheumatica und andere Varianten der Riesenzellarteriitis. In: Fehr K, et al. (eds) Rheumatologie in Praxis und Klinik. Thieme, New York Stuttgart, pp 1181–1196
Gershwin ME, Hyman LR, Steinberg AD (1974) The choroid plexus in CNS involvement of systemic lupus erythematosus. J Pediatr 85:385
Gewanter HL, Baum J (1989) The frequency of juvenile arthritis. J Rheumatol 16:556–557
Ghadially FN, Roy S (1967) Ultrastructure of synovial membrane in rheumatoid arthritis. Ann Rheum Dis 26:426–443
Gieseking R (1969) Feinstrukturelle Befunde am Gichtknoten. In: Verhandlungen der Deutschen Gesellschaft für Pathologie, 53. Tagung, Mainz. Fischer, Stuttgart, p 356
Gilbertson EMM (1975) Development of periarticular osteophytes in experimentally induced osteoarthritis in the dog. Ann Rheum Dis 34:12-25
Gladman DD (1992) Psoriatic arthritis: recent advances in pathogenesis and treatment. Rheum Dis Clin North Am 18:247–256
Gocke DJ, Hsu K, Morgan C, Bombardieri S, Lockshin M, Christian CL (1970) Association between polyarteritis and Australian antigen. Lancet 2:1149-1153
Goebel HH (1999) Diagnostischer Stellenwert morphologischer Untersuchungsverfahren in der Myopathologie. In: Hopf HC, Deuschl G, Diener HC, Reichmann H (eds) Neurologie in Praxis und Klinik, Bd II. Georg Thieme Verlag, Stuttgart New York, pp 467–471
Goldenberg DL, Reed JI (1985) Bacterial arthritis. N Engl J Med 21:764–771
Goldring SR, Stephenson ML, Downie E, Krane SM, Korn JH (1990) Heterogeneity in hormone responses and patterns of collagen synthesis in cloned dermal fibroblasts. J Clin Invest 85:798–803
Gonzalez S, Martinez-Borra J, Torre-Alonso JC, Gonzalez-Roces S, Sanchez del Rio J, Rodriguez PA, et al. (1999a) The MICA-A9 triplet repeat polymorphism in the transmembrane region confers additional susceptibility to the development of psoriatic arthritis and is independent of the association of Cw*0602 in psoriasis. Arthritis Rheum 42:1010–1016

Gonzalez S, Martinez-Borra J, Lopez-Larrea C (1999b) Immunogenetics, HLA-B27 and spondyloarthropathies. Curr Opin Rheumatol 11:257–264
Gordon DA, Stein JL, Broder I (1973) The extraarticular features of rheumatoid arthritis. A systematic analysis of 127 cases. Am J Med 54:445–452
Gougerot H (1925) Insuffisance progressive et atrophie des glandes salivaires et muqueuses de la bouche, des conjonctives (et parfois des muqueuses nasales, laryngées, vulvaires) "sécheresse" de la bouche, des conjonctives. Bull Soc Franç Derm Syph 32:376
Gowers WR (1904) Lumbago: its lesions and analogues. Br Med J 1:117–121
Graf M, Baici A, Sträuli P (1981) Histochemical localization of cathepsin B at the invasion front of the rabbit V2 carcinoma. Lab Invest 45 (6):587–596
Gran JT, Husby G, Thorsby E (1983) The association between rheumatoid arthritis and the HLA antigen DR 4. Ann Rheum Dis 42:292–296
Gran JT, Husby G, Hordvik M (1985) Prevalence of ankylosing spondylitis in males and females in a young middle-aged population of Tromsø, northern Norway. Ann Rheum Dis 44:359–367
Granfors K, Jalkanen S, Essen von R, et al. (1989) Yersinia antigens in synovial fluid cells from patients with reactive arthritis. N Engl J Med 320:216–221
Green L, Myers OL, Gordon W, Briggs B (1981) Arthritis in psoriasis. Ann Rheum Dis 40:366–369
Greenwald CA, Peebles CL, Nakamura RM (1978) Laboratory tests for antinuclear antibody (ANA) in rheumatic diseases. Lab Med 9 (4):19
Greif G, Bandilla K, Schilling F (1985) Psoriasisarthritis. Internist Welt 10:275–278
Grenier P, Bletry O, Cornud F, Godeau P, Nahum H (1981) Pulmonary involvement in Behçet's disease. Am J Radiol 137:565
Grimley PM, Sokoloff L (1966) Synovial giant cells in rheumatoid arthritis. Am J Pathol 49:931–954
Gross WL (1991) Neue Aspekte bei der Wegenerschen Granulomatose. Dt Ärztebl 88 (1/2):24–30
Güntz E (1933) Beitrag zur pathologischen Anatomie der Spondylarthritis ankylopoetica. Fortschr Röntgenstr 47:683
Hahn K, Thiers G, Eißner D (1985) Knochen- und gelenkszintigraphische Befunde bei Psoriasis. In: Holzmann H, Altmeyer P, Hör G, Hahn K (eds) Dermatologie und Nuklearmedizin. Springer, Berlin Heidelberg New York, pp 26–35
Hajdu SI, Shiu MH, Fortner JG (1977) Tendosynovial sarcoma. A clinicopathologic study of 136 cases. Cancer 39:1201
Hamashima Y, Tasaka K, Hoshino T, Nagata N, Furukawa F, Kao T, Tanaka H (1982) Mite-associated particles in Kawasaki disease. Lancet 2:266
Hamerman D (1989) The biology of osteoarthritis. N Engl J Med 320:1322–1330
Hamuryudan V, Yurdakul S, Yazici H (1997) Morbus Behçet. Rheumatol Eur 26/1:31–33
Hanly JG, Pledger D, Parkhill W, Roberts M, Gross M (1990) Phenotypic characteristics of dissociated mononuclear cells from rheumatoid synovial membrane. J Rheumatol 17:1274–1279
Hanly JG, Walsh NM, Sangalang V (1992) Brain pathology in systemic lupus erythematosus. J Rheumatol 19:732–741
Hanly JG, Walsh NM, Fisk JD, et al. (1993) Cognitive impairment and autoantibodies in systemic lupus erythematosus. Br J Rheumatol 32:291–299
Hardin JA, Steere AC, Malawista SE (1979a) Immune complexes and the evolution of Lyme arthritis – Dissemination and localization of abnormal C1q binding activity. N Engl J Med 301:1358-1363

Hardin JA, Walker LC, Steere AC, Trumble TC, Tung KSK, Williams Jr RC, Ruddy S, Malawista SE (1979b) Circulating immune complexes in Lyme arthritis - Detection by the 125 I-$C1_q$ binding, $C1_q$ solid phase and Raji cell assays. J Clin Invest 63:468-477
Hardin JG, Halla JT (1993) Cervical spine syndromes. In: McCarty DJ, Koopman WJ (eds) Arthritis and Allied Conditions, 12th edn. Lea & Febiger, Philadelphia London (A Textbook of Rheumatology, vol 2) pp 1563–1571
Hardingham T, Bayliss M (1990) Proteoglycans of articular cartilage: Changes in aging and joint disease. Semin Arthritis Rheum 20 (Suppl 1):12–33
Hardingham TE, Fosang AJ, Dudhia J (1992) Aggrecan: the chondroitin sulphate/keratan sulphate proteoglycan from cartilage. In: Kuettner KE, Schleyerbach R, Peyron JG, Hascall VC (eds) Articular Cartilage and Osteoarthritis. Raven Press, New York, pp 5–20
Harris Jr ED (1972) A collagenolytic system produced by primary cultures of rheumatoid nodule tissue. J Clin Invest 51:2973
Harris Jr ED (1976) Recent insights into the pathogenesis of the proliferative lesion in rheumatoid arthritis. Arthritis Rheum 19 (1):68–72
Harris Jr ED, Cohen GL, Krane SM (1969) Synovial collagenase: Its presence in culture from joint disease of diverse etiology. Arthritis Rheum 12:92–102
Harris Jr ED, Di Bona DR, Krane SM (1970) A mechanism for cartilage destruction in rheumatoid arthritis. Trans Assoc Am Phys 83:267–276
Harris Jr ED, Faulkner CS II, Brown FE (1975) Collagenolytic systems in rheumatoid arthritis. Clin Orth Rel Res 110:303–315
Hart FD (1953) Ankylosing spondylitis. Schweiz med Wschr 83:786
Hart FD (1966) Lesions learnt in a twenty-year study of ankylosing spondylitis. Proc Roy Soc Med 59:456
Harten P (1996) Neuropsychiatrischer systemischer Lupus erythematodes. Akt Rheumatol 21:77–88
Harth M, Robinson CEG (1962) Gouty arthritis in a D.V.A. Hospital: A retrospective study. Med Serv J Canada 18:671–674
Harvey AM, Shulman LE, Tumulty PA, et al. (1954) Systemic lupus erythematosus: Review of the literature and clinical analysis of 138 cases. Medicine 33:291
Haupt HM, Moore GW, Hutchins GM (1981) The lung in systemic lupus erythematosus - Analysis of the pathologic changes in 120 patients. Am J Med 71:791-798
Haydl H, Petershofer H, Ellegast HH, Prohaska E (1984) Zur Diagnose der Osteoarthropathia psoriatrica - Gegenüberstellung von klinischen, radiologischen und szintigraphischen Befunden. Wien Klin Wschr 96:337–343
Hayreh SS (1997) Anterior ischemic optic neuropathy. Clin Neurosci 4:251–263
Hayward WS, Neel BG, Astrin SM (1981) Activation of a cellular oncogene by promotor insertion in ALV-induced lymphoid leukosis. Nature 290:475–480
Healey LA (1986) Rheumatoid arthritis in the elderly. Clin Rheum Dis 12 (1):173–179
Healey LA, Wilske KR (1978) The systemic manifestations of temporal arteritis. Grune & Stratton, New York
Heberden W (1802) Commentaries on the history and cure of disease. T Payne, London
Hebert TD, Siebert G, Fassbender HG (1990) Bakterielle Superinfektion (BSI) bei chronischen Gelenkerkrankungen. Z Rheumatol 49 (Suppl 1):V-28
Hedfors E, Klareskog L, Lindblad S, Forsum U, Lindahl G (1983) Phenotypic characterization of cells within subcutaneous rheumatoid nodules. Arthritis Rheum 26:1333–1339

Heinegard D, Sommarin Y (1987) Proteoglycans: An overview. In: Cunningham LW (ed) Methods of Enzymology, Structural and Contractile Proteins, part D Extracellular Matrix, vol 144. Academic Press, Orlando, pp 305–319
Heinegard D, Lorenzo P, Sommarin Y (1995) Articular cartilage matrix proteins. In: Kuettner KE, Goldberg VM (eds) Osteoarthritic disorders. Rosemont: American Academy of Orthopedic Surgeons, pp 229–237
Hellmann DB, Stobo JD (1986) Sarcoidosis. In: Cohen AS, Bennett JC (eds) Rheumatology and Immunology, 2nd edn. Grune & Stratton, Orlando, pp 301–309
Helmchen U (1996) Nierenpathologie bei systemischem Lupus erythematodes. Akt Rheumatol 21:72–76
Hembry RM, Murphy G, Reynolds JJ (1985) Immunolocalization of tissue inhibitor of metalloproteinases (TIMP) in human cells: Characterization and use of a specific antiserum. J Cell Sci 73:105–119
Henderson DRF, Tribe CR, Dixon ASJ (1975) Synovitis in polymyalgia rheumatica. Rheumatol Rehabil 14:244
Henriksson KG, Bengtsson A, Larsson J, Lindström F, Thornell L-E (1982) Muscle biopsy findings of possible diagnostic importance in primary Fibromyalgia (Fibrositis, Myofascial Syndrome) Lancet 2:1395
Hermans PJ, Fievez ML, Descamps CL, Aupaix MA (1984) Granulomatous synovitis and Crohn's disease. J Rheumatol 11:710–712
Herzer P (1990) Lyme-Borreliose, 2nd edn. Steinkopff, Darmstadt
Herzer P, Wilske B, Preac-Mursic V, Schierz G, Schattenkirchner M, Zöllner N (1986) Lyme Arthritis: Clinical features, serological and radiographic findings of cases in Germany. Klin Wschr 64:206–215
Hibbs MS, Postlewhite AE, Mainardi CL, Seyer JM, Kang AH (1983) Alterations in collagen production in mixed mononuclear leukocyte-fibroblast cultures. J Exp Med 157:47
Hiepe F, Riemekasten G, Dörner Th (1996) Autoantikörperdiagnostik beim systemischen Lupus erythematodes (SLE). Akt Rheumatol 21:62–71
Hill GS, Hingoais N, Tron F, Bach JF (1978) Systemic lupus erythematosus: Morphologic correlations with immunologic and clinical data at the time of biopsy. Am J Med 64:61
Hippokrates: (460-377 BC) De epidemiis
Hirohata T, Kuratsume M, Nomura A, Jimi S (1975) Prevalence of Behçet's syndrome in Hawaii with particular reference to the comparison of the Japanese in Hawaii and Japan. Hawaii Med J 34:244
Hoffman GS, Specks U (1998) Antineutrophil cytoplasmic antibodies. Arthritis Rheum 41:1521–1537
Holzmann H, Hoede N, Eißner D, Hahn K (1978) Knochenbefunde bei Psoriasis. Arch Dermatol Res 262:191–196
Holzmann H, Eißner D, Hahn K, Thiers G, Böhm G (1982) Die psoriatische Osteopathie. Z Hautkr 57 (15):1144–1150
Houwer AWM (1927) Keratitis filamentosa and chronic arthritis. Transact Ophth Soc Unit Kingdom 47:88
Howell DS (1985) Diseases due to the deposition of calcium pyrophosphate and hydroxyapatite. In: Kelley WN, Harris Jr ED, Ruddy S, Sledge CB (eds) Textbook of Rheumatology, vol 2, 2nd edn. WB Saunders Company, Philadelphia London Toronto Mexico City Rio de Janeiro Sydney Tokyo, pp 1398–1416
Howell DS, Martell-Pelletier J, Pelletier J-P, Morales S, Muniz O (1984) NTP pyrophosphohydrolase in human chondrocalcinotic and osteoarthritic cartilage. II. Further studies on histologic and subcellular distribution. Arthritis Rheum 27:193–199
Hüttl S (1970) Synovial effusion. A nosographic and diagnostic study, part I. Acta Rheum Baln Pistiniana 5:1–100

Hummel KM, Neidhart M, Vilim V, Hauser N, Aicher WK, Gay RE, Gay S, Häuselmann JH (1998) Analysis of cartilage oligomeric matrix protein (COMP) in synovial fibroblasts and synovial fluids. Br J Rheumatol 37:721–728
Hunder GG (1996) Vasculitis: Diagnosis and therapy. Am J Med 100 (Suppl 2A):37S-45S
Hunder GG, Lie JT (1986) Systemic vasculitis and related disorders. In: Cohen AS, Bennett JC (eds) Rheumatology and Immunology, 2nd edn. Grune & Stratton, Orlando, pp 279–288
Hunder GG, Disney TF, Ward LE (1969) Polymyalgia rheumatica. MAYO Clin Proc 44:849
Hunter T, Gordon DA, Ogryzlo MA (1974) The ground pepper sign of synovial fluid: A new diagnostic feature of ochronosis. J Rheumatol 1:45–53
Hunziker EB (1992) Articular cartilage structure in humans and experimental animals. In: Kuettner KE, Schleyerbach R, Peyron JG, Hascall VC (eds) Articular Cartilage and Osteoarthritis. Raven Press, New York, pp 183–199
Husby G (1977) Genetic Aspects of amyloidosis. Tidssk Nor Laegeforen 97 (1):13–15
Husby G (1985) Amyloidosis and rheumatoid arthritis. Clin Exp Rheumatol 3:173–180
Husby G, Williams Jr RC, Wedege E (1979) Huntington's disease, antineuronal antibodies, brain antigens, and receptors for IgG in human choroid plexus. Adv Neurol 23:435
Huston KA, Hunder GG, Lie JT, Kennedy RH, Elveback LR (1978) Temporal arteritis: A 25-year epidemiologic, clinical and pathologic study. Ann Intern Med 88:162
International study group for Behçet's disease (1990) Criteria for diagnosis of Behçet's disease. Lancet 335:1078–1080
Ippolito E, Postacchini F, Scola E, Bellocci M, Martino de C (1985) De Quervain's disease. An ultrastructural study. Int Orthop 9 (1):41–47
Ishiguro N, Ito T, Obata K, Fujimoto N, Iwata H (1996) Determination of stromelysin-1, 72 and 92 KDa type IV collagenase, tissue inhibitor of metalloproteinase-1 (TIMP-1), and TIMP-2 in synovial fluid and serum from patients with rheumatoid arthritis. J Rheumatol 23:1599–1604
Israel HL, Goldstein RA (1971) Relation of Kveim-antigen reaction to lymphadenopathy. N Engl J Med 284:345
Jaffee BD, Claman HN (1983) Chronic graft versus host disease as a model for scleroderma, 1st description of the model systems. Cell Immunol 77:1–12
Jasin HE (1987) Intra-articular antigen-antibody reactions. Rheum Dis Clin of North Am 13 (2):179–189
Jemec B, Grobbelaar AO, Wilson GD, Smith PJ, Sanders R, McGrouther DA (1999) Is Dupuytren's disease caused by an imbalance between proliferation and cell death? J Hand Surg 24B (5):511–514
Jennette CH (1994) Nomenclature of systemic vasculitides. Proposal of an international consensus conference. Arthritis Rheum 37:187–192
Johnell O, Hulth A, Henricson A (1985) T-lymphocyte subsets and HLA-DR-expressing cells in the osteoarthritic synovialis. Scand J Rheum 14:259–264
Johnson RT, Richardson EP (1968) The neurological manifestations of systemic lupus erythematosus. Medicine 47:337
Johnston YE, Duray PH, Steere AC, Kashgarian M, Buza J, Malawista SE, Askenase PW (1985) Lyme Arthritis: Spirochetes found in synovial microangiopathic lesions. Am J Pathol 118 (1):26–34
Jurik AG, Pedersen U, Norgard A (1985) Rheumatoid arthritis of the cricoarytenoid joints: a case of laryngeal obstruction due to acute and chronic joint changes. Laryngoscope 95:846–848
Kaiser H (1969) Le traitement de la polyarthrite rhumatoide débutant chez le sujet âgé. Med et Hyg 27:1312–1314

Kaiser H (1989) Chronische Polyarthritis im Alter. In: Schattenkirchner M (ed) Rheumatische Krankheiten im Alter. Werk-Verlag Dr. Edmund Banaschewski, München-Gräfelfing (Colloquia rheumatologica 44, pp 12–18)
Kahaleh MB, LeRoy EC (1983) Endothelial injury in scleroderma: A protease mechanism. J Lab Clin Med 101:533
Kahaleh MB, Sherer GK, LeRoy EC (1979) Endothelial injury in scleroderma. J Exp Med 149:1326
Kalliomäki JL, Leino R (1979) Follow-up studies of joint complications in Yersiniosis. Acta Med Scand 205:521–525
Kaplan MH (1963) Immunologic relation of streptococcal and tissue antigens. I. Properties of an antigen in certain strains of group A streptococci exhibiting an immunologic cross reaction with human heart tissue. J Immunol 90:595–606
Kaplan MH, Suchy ML (1964) Immunologic relation of streptococcal and tissue antigens. II. Common reactions of antisera to mammalian heart-tissue with a cell wall constituent of certain strains of group A streptococci. J Exp Med 119:643–650
Kassan SS, Hoover R, Kimberly RP (1977) Increased incidence of malignancy in Sjögren's syndrome. Abstract. Arthritis Rheum 20:123
Kato S, Kimura M, Tsuji K (1978) HLA antigens in Kawasaki disease. Pediatr 61:252
Kawakami A, Eguchi K, Matsuoka N, Tsuboi M, Kawabe Y, Aoyagi T, Nagataki S (1996) Inhibition of Fas antigen-mediated apoptosis of rheumatoid synovial cells in vitro by transforming growth factor beta1. Arthritis Rheum 39:1267–1276
Kawasaki T (1967) MCLL: clinical observation of 50 cases. Jap J Allergy 16:178
Keat AC (1983) Reiter's syndrome and reactive arthritis in perspective. N Engl J Med 309:1606–1615
Keat AC, Maini RN, Nkwazi GC, et al. (1978) Role of Chlamydia trachomatis and HLA-B 27 in sexually acquired reactive arthritis. Br Med J 1:605-607
Keat AC, Thomas BJ, Taylor-Robinson D (1983) Chlamydial infection in the etiology of arthritis. Br Med Bull 39:168–174
Kellgren JH, Moore R (1952) Generalized osteoarthritis and Heberden's nodes. Br Med J 1:181–187
Kellgren JH, O'Brien WM (1962) On the natural history of rheumatoid arthritis in relation to the sheep cell agglutination test. Abstract. Arthritis Rheum 5:115
Kellgren JH, Ball J, Fairbrother RW, Barnes KL (1958) Suppurative arthritis complicating rheumatoid arthritis. Br Med J 1:1193
Kelly AP, Jacobsen HS (1964) Hand disability due to tenosynovitis. Ind Med Surg 33:570–574
Kelly PJ, Martin WJ, Coventry MB (1970) Bacterial (suppurative) arthritis in the adult. J Bone Surg Am 52:1595–1602
Kemp A (1977) Monozygotic twins with temporal arteritis and ophthalmic arteritis. Acta Ophth K'hvn 55:183
Kennedy M, Felson DT (1996) A prospective long-term study of fibromyalgia syndrome. Arthritis Rheum 39:682–685
Khan MA (1982) Axial arthropathy in Whipple's disease. J Rheumatol 9:928–929
Kimura JH, Kuettner KE (1986) Studies on the synthesis and assembly of cartilage proteoglycans. In: Kuettner KE, Schleyerbach R, Hascall VC (eds) Articular Cartilage Biochemistry. Raven Press, New York, pp 257–272
Kirkland KB, Klimko TB, Meriwether RA, et al. (1997) Erythema migrans-like rash illness at a camp in North Carolina: a new tick-borne disease? Arch Intern Med 157:2635–2641
Kitsis E, Weissmann G (1991) The role of the neutrophil in rheumatoid arthritis. Clin Orthop 265:63–72

Klein R, Bänsch M, Berg PA (1992) Clinical relevance of antibodies against serotonin and gangliosides in patients with primary fibromyalgia syndrome. Psychoneuroendocrinology 6:593–598

Klein RG, Hunder GG, Stanson AW, Sheps SG (1975) Large artery involvement in giant cell (temporal) arteritis. Ann Intern Med 83:806–812

Klemperer P, Pollack AD, Baehr G (1941) Pathology of disseminated lupus erythematosus. Arch Path 32:569

Klemperer P, Pollack AD, Baehr G (1942) Diffuse collagene disease; acute disseminated lupus erythematosus and diffuse skleroderma. J Am Med Ass 119:331

Klimiuk PA, Goronzy JJ, Björnsson J, Beckenbaugh RD, Weyand CM (1997) Tissue cytokine patterns distinguish variants of rheumatoid synovitis. Am J Pathol 151:1311–1319

Klinge F (1927) Die Eiweißüberempfindlichkeit (Gewebsanaphylaxie) des Gelenks. Experimentelle pathologisch-anatomische Studie zur Pathogenese des Gelenkrheumatismus. Beitr path Anat 83:183

Klinge F (1930) Das Gewebsbild des fieberhaften Rheumatismus. I.-III. Mitt.: Das rheumatische Frühinfiltrat (akutes-degeneratives-exsudatives Stadium). Das Granulom und die Narbe. Virchows Arch path Anat 279:438

Klinge F (1933) Der Rheumatismus. Pathologisch-anatomische und experimentell pathologische Tatsachen und ihre Auswertung für das ärztliche Rheumaproblem. In: Hueck W, Frei W (eds) Ergebnisse der allgemeinen Pathologie und pathologischen Anatomie, vol 27. Bergmann, München

Kloen P (1999) New insights in the development of Dupuytren's contracture: a review. Br J of Plastic Surgery 52:629–635

Klofkorn RW, Steigerwald JC (1976) Carpal tunnel syndrome as the initial manifestation of tuberculosis. Am J Med 60 (4):583–586

Knox WE (1958) Sir Archibald Garrod's inborn errors of metabolism. II. Alkaptonuria. Am J Hum Genet 10:95–124

Knudson W, Subbaiah S, Pauli B (1990) Proteoglycan synthesis by normal and neoplastic human transitional epithelial cells. J Cell Biochem 43:265–279

Köhler H, Uehlinger E, Kutzner J, Weihrauch TR, Wilbert L, Schuster R (1975) Sternokostoklavikuläre Hyperostose. Dtsch Med Wschr 100:1519-1523

Kölle G (1970) Klinisches Bild und Verlauf der juvenilen rheumatoiden Arthritis und des Still-Syndroms. Mschr Kinderhk 118:488

Kölle G (1975) Juvenile rheumatoide Arthritis (juvenile chronische Polyarthritis) und das Still-Syndrom. Eine klinische und katamnestische Dokumentation. Rheumaforum 4. Braun, Karlsruhe

Kohn NN, Hughes RE, McCarthy DJ, Faires JS (1962) The significance of phosphate crystals in the synovial fluid of arthritic patients: The pseudogout syndrome. II. Identification of crystals. Am Intern Med 56:738

Kong L, Ogawa N, Nakabayashi T, Liu GT, D'Souza E, McGuff HS, Guerrero D, Talal N, Dang H (1997) FAS and FAS ligand expression in the salivary glands of patients with primary Sjögren's syndrome. Arthritis Rheum 40 (1):87–97

Korn JH (1996) Immunological pathogenetic mechanisms. In: Fine LG (chairman) Systemic sclerosis: Current pathogenetic concepts and future prospects for targeted therapy (Report of a meeting of physicians and scientists, London). Lancet 347:1453–1458

Kovacs EJ (1991) Fibrogenic cytokines: the role of immune mediators in the development of scar tissue. Review. Immunol today 1 (12):17–23

Krensky AM, Berenberg W, Shanley K, Yunis E (1981) HLA antigens in mucocutaneous lymph node syndrome in New England. Pediatr 67:741

Kriegsmann J, Bräner R, Petrow PK, Gaumann A, Klein C, Kirkpatrick CJ, Gay RE, Gay S (1997) Hyperplasia of the synovial lining layer - increased proliferation or reduced apoptosis? Arthritis Rheum 40 (Suppl 9):293
Kruize AA, Hené RJ, Heide van der A, Bodeutsch C, Wilde de PCM, Bijsterveld van OP, Jong de J, Feltkamp TEW, Kater L, Bijlsma JWJ (1996) Long-term followup of patients with Sjögren's syndrome. Arthritis Rheum 39 (2):297-303
Kuettner KE, Goldberg V (eds) (1995) Osteoarthritic disorders. Am Acad of Orthop Surgeon Press, Rosemont, Il, p XXI
Kulka JP, Bocking D, Ropes MW, et al. (1955) Early joint lesions of rheumatoid arthritis. Arch Pathol 59:129-150
Kurki P, Aho K, Palosuo T, Heliövaara M (1992) Immunopathology of rheumatoid arthritis. Antikeratin antibodies precede the clinical disease. Arthritis Rheum 35:914-917
Kussmaul A, Maier R (1866) Über eine bisher nicht beschriebene eigenthümliche Arterienverkalkung (Periarteriitis nodosa), die mit Morbus Brightii und rapid fortschreitender allgemeiner Muskellähmung einhergeht. Dtsch Arch Klin Med 1:184
Labowitz R, Schumacher HR (1971) Articular manifestations of systemic lupus erythematosus. Ann Intern Med 74:911-921
LaDu BN, Zannoni VG, Laster L, Seegmiller JE (1958) The nature of the defect in tyrosine metabolism in alcaptonuria. J Biol Chem 230:251-260
Lagier R (1980) The concept of osteoarthrotic remodeling as illustrated by ochronotic arthropathy of the hip: An anatomicoradiological approach. Virchows Arch (A) 385:293-298
Lambert JR, Wright V (1977) Psoriatic spondylitis: A clinical and radiological description of the spine in psoriatic arthritis. Quart J Med 46:411-425
Lancefield RC (1933) A serological differentiation of human and other groups of hemolytic streptococci. J Exp Med 57:577
Landré-Beauvais A (1800) Doit-on admettre une nouvelle espèce de goutte sous la dénomination de goutte asthènique primitive? JA Brosson, Paris
Lark MW, Bayne EK, Lohmander LS (1995) Aggrecan degradation in osteoarthritis and rheumatoid arthritis. Acta Orthop Scand 6 (Suppl 26):92-97
Lasègue C (1864) Considerations sur la sciatique. Archives gen Med 2:558
Lawrence JS (1960) Heritable disorders of connective tissue. Proc R Soc Med 53:522-526
Lawrence JS (1969) Generalized osteo-arthrosis in a population sample. J Epidemiol 90:381-389
Lawrence RC, Shulman LE (eds) (1984) Epidemiology of the rheumatic Diseases. Proceedings of the Fourth International Conference, National Institute of Health. Gower Medical Publisher Ltd, New York
Lawrence RC, Helmick CG, Arnett FC, Deyo RA, Felson DT, Giannini EH, Heyse SP, Hirsch R, Hochberg MC, Hunder GG, Liang MH, Pillemer SR, Steen VD, Wolfe F (1998) Estimates of the prevalence of arthritis and selected musculoskeletal disorders in the United States. Arthritis Rheum 41:778-799
Lebowitz WB (1963) Heart in rheumatoid arthritis (rheumatoid disease): Clinical and pathological study of 62 cases. Ann Intern Med 58:102
Ledderhose G (1897) Zur Pathologie der Aponeurose des Fusses und der Hand. Arch Klin Chir 55:694
Leicht MJ, Harrington TM, Davis DE (1987) Cricoarytenoid arthritis: a cause of laryngeal obstruction. Ann Emerg Med 16:885-888
Leirisalo M, Skylv G, Kousa M, Voipio-Pulki LM, Suoronta H, Nissilä M, Hvidman L, Nielsen ED, Sveijgaard A, Tiilikainen A, Laitinen O (1982)

Follow-up study on patients with Reiter's disease and reactive arthritis with special reference to HLA-B27. Arthritis Rheum 25:249–256

Leisen JC, Duncan H, Riddle JM, Pitchford WC (1988) The erosive front: A topographic study of the junction between the pannus and the subchondral plate in the macerated rheumatoid metacarpal head. J Rheumatol 15:17–22

Lennert K (1961) Cytologie und Lymphadenitis. In: Uehlinger E (ed) Handbuch der speziellen pathologischen Anatomie und Histologie, vol 1. Springer, Berlin Göttingen Heidelberg

Leri A (1899) La spondylose rhizomélique. Rev Med 19:597, 691, 801

LeRoy EC (1972) Connective tissue synthesis by scleroderma skin fibroblasts in cell culture. J Exp Med 135:1351–1362

LeRoy EC (1985) Scleroderma (Systemic sclerosis). In: Kelley WN, Harris Jr ED, Ruddy S, Sledge CB (eds) Textbook of Rheumatology, vol 2, 2nd edn. WB Saunders Company, Philadelphia London Toronto Mexico City Rio de Janeiro Sydney Tokyo, pp 1183–1205

LeRoy EC (1994) The control of fibrosis in systemic sclerosis: a strategy involving extracellular matrix, cytokines, and growth factors. J Dermatol 21:1–4

LeRoy EC, Mercurio SM, Sherer GK (1982) Replication and phenotypic expression of control and scleroderma human fibroblasts: Responses to growth factors. Proc Nat Acad Sci USA 79:1286

LeRoy EC, Kahaleh MB, Mercurio S (1983) A fibroblast mitogen present in scleroderma but not in control sera: Inhibition by proteinase inhibitors. Rheumatol Int 3:35

Leung DYM, Schlievert PM, Meissner HC (1998) The immunopathogenesis and management of Kawasaki syndrom. Arthritis Rheum 41:1538–1547

Leventhal LH, Naides SJ, Freundlich B (1991) Fibromyalgia and parvovirus infection. Arthritis Rheum 34:1319–1324

Li F, Nanagara R, Rothfuss S, et al. (1994) Demonstration of peptidoglycan in synovial fluid cells as a possible arthritogenic factor in psoriatic arthritis. Arthritis Rheum 37:204

Liang GC, Simkin PA, Hunder GG, Wilske KR, Healey LA (1974a) Familial aggregation of polymyalgia rheumatica and giant cell arteritis. Arthritis Rheum 17:19-24

Liang GC, Simkin PA, Mannik M (1974b) Immunoglobulins in temporal arteries: An immunofluorescent study. Ann Intern Med 81:19-24

Lichtenstein L, Scott HW, Levin MH (1956) Pathologic changes in gout: Survey of 11 necropsied cases. Am J Pathol 32:871–895

Lindahl G, Hedfors E, Klareskog L, Forsum U (1985) Epithelial HLA-DR expression and T lymphocyte subsets in salivary glands in Sjögren's syndrome. Clin Exp Immunol 61:475–482

Lindblad S, Hedfors E (1985) Intra-articular variation in synovitis. Local macroscopic and microscopic signs of inflammatory activity are significantly correlated. Arthritis Rheum 28:977–986

Linde van der MR, Ballmer PE (1993) Lyme carditis. In: Weber K, Burgdorfer W, Schierz G (eds) Aspects of Lyme borreliosis. Springer, Berlin, pp 131–145

Linden van der SM, Valkenburg HA, Cats A (1984a) Evaluation of diagnostic criteria for ankylosing spondylitis: a proposal for modification of the New York criteria. Arthritis Rheum 27:361–368

Linden van der SM, Valkenburg HA, Jongh de BM, Cats A (1984b) The risk of developing ankylosing spondylitis in HLA-B27 positive individuals: a comparison of relatives of spondylitis patients with the general population. Arthritis Rheum 27:241–249

Lindstrom C, Wramsby H, Ostberg G (1972) Granulomatous arthritis in Crohn's disease. Gut 13:257

Löffler W, Koller F (1955) Die Gicht. In: Bergman von G, Frey W, Schwiegle H (eds) Handbuch der Inneren Medizin, vol VII/2. Springer, Berlin Göttingen Heidelberg, p 435

Lohmander LS (1990) Osteoarthritis: Man, models and molecular markers. In: Maroudas A, Kuettner KE (eds) Methods in Cartilage Research. Academic Press, London, pp 337–362
Lohmander LS (1992) Molecular markers of cartilage turnover: A role in monitoring and diagnosis of osteoarthritis? In: Kuettner KE, Schleyerbach R, Peyron J, Hascall VC (eds) Articular Cartilage and Osteoarthritis. Raven Press, New York, pp 653–667
Lospalluto J, Dorward B, Miller Jr W, Ziff M (1962) Cryoglobulinemia based on interaction between a gamma macroglobulin and 7S gamma globulin. Am J Med 32:142
Lotz BP, Engel AG, Nishino H, Stevens JC, Litcy WJ (1989) Inclusion body myositis. Brain 112:727–742
Lüders CJ, Klemens F (1963) Die rheumatoiden granulomatös-nekrotisierenden Skleritiden und Episkleritiden. Albrecht v Graefes Arch klin exp Ophth 165:545
Lühr T (1997) Ablagerung von Immunkomplexen im humanen Gelenkknorpel bei vier Erkrankungen des rheumatischen Formenkreises. Med Dissertation. Universität Mainz
Maciewicz RA, Wotton SF, Etherington DJ, Duance VC (1990) Susceptibility of the cartilage collagens type II, IX and XI to degradation by the cysteine proteinases, cathepsin B and L. FEBS Lett 269:189–193
Mäkela AL, Mäkinen E, Lorenz K, Rikalainen H (1979) Veränderungen der Halswirbelsäule bei juveniler rheumatoider Arthritis. Fortschr Geb Roentgenstr Nuklearmed 131:420
Märker-Hermann E, Fassbender HG, Kessler S, Thomssen S, Meyer zum Büschenfelde KH, Blessing M (1997) Transgenic mice with an epidermal overexpression of bone morphogenic protein-6 (BMP-6) present with psoriatic skin lesions and osteoarthropathy. Arthritis Rheum 40 (Suppl 9):S 261
Maesaka J, Bautman V, Shakamuri S (1982) Elevated 1,25-dihydroxyvitamin D levels - occurrence with sarcoidosis with end-stage renal disease. Arch Intern Med 142:1206
Malawista SE, Steere AC, Harding JA (1984) Lyme disease: a unique human model for an infectious etiology of rheumatic disease. Yale J Biol Mcd 57:473 477
Malemud CJ, Goldberg VM, Moskowitz RW, Getzy LL, Papay RS, Norby DP (1982) Biosynthesis of proteoglycan in vitro by cartilage from human osteochondrophytic spurs. Biochem J 206:329
Mandel NS (1976) The structural basis of crystal-induced membranolysis. Arthritis Rheum 19:439
Mandel NS, Mandel GS (1982) Structures of crystals that provide inflammation. In: Weissmann (ed) Advances in Inflammation Research, vol 4. Raven Press, New York, p 73
Mankin H (1974) Discussion of paper by Sokoloff L. In: Ali SY, Elves MW, Leaback DG (eds) Normal and osteoarthrotic articular cartilage. Institute of Orthopaedics, London, p 123
Mankin HJ, Brandt KD, Shulman LE (1985) Workshop on etiopathogenesis of osteoarthritis: Proceedings and recommendations. J Rheumatol 13:1126–1160
Mannik M, Person RE (1994) Deep penetration of antibodies into the articular cartilage of patients with rheumatoid arthritis. Rheumatol Int 14:95–102
Maricq HR, Spencer-Green G, LeRoy EC (1976) Skin capillary abnormalities as indicators of organ involvement in scleroderma (systemic sclerosis), Raynaud's syndrome, and dermatomyositis. Am J Med 61:862–870
Marie P, Astie C (1897) Sur un cas de cyphose hérédo-traumatique. Presse méd 205
Mark von der K, Kirsch T, Aigner T, et al. (1992) The fate of chondrocytes in osteoarthritis cartilage: Regeneration, dedifferentiation or hypertrophy. In: Kuettner KE, Schleyerbach R, Peyron JG, Hascall VC (eds)

Articular cartilage and Osteoarthritis. Raven Press, New York, pp 221–234
Maroudas A, Grushko G (1990) Measurement of swelling pressure of cartilage. In: Maroudas A, Kuettner KE (eds) Methods in cartilage research. Academic Press, London, pp 298–301
Maroudas A, Katz EP, Wachtel EJ, Mizrahi J, Soudry M (1986) Physiochemical properties and functional behaviour of normal and osteoarthritic human cartilage. In: Kuettner KE, Schleyerbach R, Hascall VC (eds) Articular Cartilage Biochemistry. Raven Press, New York, pp 311–330
Maroudas A, Schneiderman R, Popper O (1992) The role of water, proteoglycan and collagen in solute transport in cartilage. In: Kuettner KE, Schleyerbach R, Peyron JG, Hascall VC (eds) Articular cartilage and Osteoarthritis. Raven Press, New York, pp 355–371
Marsal L, Windblad S, Wollheim FA (1981) Yersinia enterocolitica arthritis in southern Sweden: A four-year follow up study. Br Med J 283:101–103
Marshall JL, Olsson SE (1971) Instability of the knee: A long term study in dogs. J Bone Surg 53A:1561
Martel-Pelletier J, Alaaeddine N, Pelletier JP (1999) Cytokines and their role in the pathophysiology of osteoarthritis. Front Biosci 4:694–703
Martinet Y, Bitterman PB, Mornex J-F, Grotendorst GR, Martin GR, Crystal RG (1986) Activated human monocytes express the c-sis protooncogene and release a mediator showing PDGF-like activity. Nature 319:158–160
Martinez-Lavin M, Hermosillo AG, Rosas M, Soto M-E (1998) Circadian studies of autonomic nervous balance in patients with fibromyalgia. A heart rate variability analysis. Arthritis Rheum 41:1966–1971
Mason RS, Frankel T, Chan Y, et al. (1984) Vitamin D conversion by sarcoid lymph node homogenate. Ann Intern Med 100:59
Matthay RA, Schwartz MI, Petty TL, Stanford RE, Gupta RC, Sahn SA, Steigerwald JC (1974) Pulmonary manifestations of systemic lupus erythematosus: Review of twelve cases of acute lupus pneumonitis. Medicine 54:397
Maurer K (1979) Basic data on arthritis of knee, hip, and sacroiliac joints in adult ages 25–74 years: United States 1971–1975. Vital and Health Statistics, Series 11, No 213, DHEW publication No (PHS) 79–1661. Hyattsville, MD. National Center for Health Statistics
Mauviel A (1993) Cytokine regulation of metalloproteinase gene expression. J Cell Biochem 53:288–295
Maycock RL, Bertrand P, Morrison CE, Scott JH (1963) Manifestations of sarcoidosis. Am J Med 35:67
Mayne R (1989) Cartilage collagens: What is their function, and are they involved in articular disease ? Arthritis Rheum 32:241–246
Mayne R, Burgeson R (eds) (1987) Structure and function of collagen types. Academic Press, Orlando
McBeth J, Macfarlane GJ, Benjamin S, Morris S, Silman AJ (1999) The association between tender points, psychological distress, and adverse childhood experiences. Arthritis Rheum 42:1397–1404
McCarty DJ (1986) Crystal deposition diseases: Calcium pyrophosphate dihydrate (pseudogout) and basic calcium phosphate. In: Cohen AS, Bennett JC (eds) Rheumatology and Immunology, 2nd edn. Grune & Stratton, Orlando, pp 338–345
McCarty DJ, Hollander JL (1961) Identification of urate crystals in gouty synovial fluid. Ann Intern Med 54:452
McCarty DJ, Kohn NN, Faires JS (1962a) The significance of calcium phosphate crystals in the synovial fluid of arthritis patients: The "pseudogout syndrome". I. Clinical aspects. Ann Intern Med 56:711
McCarty DJ, Brill JM, Harrop D (1962b) Aplastic anaemia secondary to gold-salt therapy: Report of a fatal case and a review of the literature. JAMA 179:655

McCarty DJ, Halverson PB, Carrera GF, Brewer BJ, Kozin F (1981) "Milwaukee shoulder": Association of microspheroids containing hydroxyapatite crystals, active collagenase, and neutral protease with rotator cuff defects. I. Clinical aspects. Arthritis Rheum 24:464–473
McDowell A, Engel A, Massey JT, et al. (1981) Plan and operation of the 2nd National Health and Examination Survey 1976–1980. Vital and Health Statistics, Series 1, No 15. Hyattsville, MD. National Center of Health Statistics
McDuffie FC, Sams Jr WM, Maldonado JE, Andreini PH, Conn DL, Samayoa EA (1978) Hypocomplementemia with cutaneous vasculitis and arthritis: Possible immune complex syndrome. Mayo Clin Proc 48:340
McMenemey WH, Lawrence BJ (1957) Encephalomyelopathy in Behçet's disease. Report of necropsy findings in two cases. Lancet 2:353
Meachim G, Brooke G (1984) The pathology of osteoarthritis. In: Moskowitz RW, Howell DS, Goldberg VM, Mankin JH (eds) Osteoarthritis: Diagnosis and Management. WB Saunders Company, Philadelphia, pp 29–42
Medsger Jr TA (1986) Behçet's disease. In: Cohen AS, Bennett JC (eds) Rheumatology and Immunology, 2nd edn. Grune & Stratton, Orlando, pp 245–247
Medsger Jr TA (1986) Pulmonary manifestations of connective tissue diseases. In: Cohen AS, Bennett JC (eds) Rheumatology and Immunology, 2nd edn. Grune & Stratton, Orlando, pp 191–195
Medsger Jr TA, Dawson WN, Masi AT (1979) The epidemiology of polymyositis. Am J Med 48:715–723
Meier-Willersen HJ, Maiwald M, Herbay von A (1993) Morbus Whipple in Assoziation mit opportunistischen Infektionen. Dtsch Med Wschr 118:854–860
Meister HP (1984) Tumoren und tumorförmige Veränderungen des Weichgewebes. In: Doerr W, Uehlinger E (begr) Doerr W, Seifert G (eds) Spezielle pathologische Anatomie, vol 18/II. Springer, Berlin Heidelberg New York Tokyo, pp 1237–1413
Mendler M, Eich-Bender SG, Vaughan L, Winterhalter KH, Bruckner P (1989) Cartilage contains mixed fibrils of collagen types II, IX, and XI. J Cell Biol 108:191–197
Menninger H, Lambusch L, Mohr W, Wessinghage D (1983) Immunkomplexe: Mediatoren für die Bildung von entzündlichem Granulationsgewebe? Z Rheumatol 42:7–15
Mertz PD (1990) Geschichte der Gicht. Kultur- und medizinhistorische Betrachtungen. Thieme, Stuttgart New York
Méry JP, Morel-Maroger L, Boelaert J, Richet G (1973) Evolution anatome-clinique des glomérulites diffuses et focales au cours du lupus érythémateux dissémine. Nephrol J Urol 79:321
Mesara BW, Brody GL, Oberman HA (1966) "Pseudorheumatoid" subcutaneous nodules. Am J Clin Path 45:684–691
Mikulicz J (1937–1938) Concerning peculiar symmetrical disease of lacrimal and salivary glands. Med Classics 2:165
Mills JA (1994) Systemic lupus erythematosus. N Engl J Med 330 (26):1871–1879
Missen GAK, Tailor JD (1956) Amyloidosis in rheumatoid arthritis. J Pathol Bacteriol 71:179
Misskampf HJ (1984) Zusammenhang zwischen Synovialstromazellproliferation bei chronische Polyarthritis – und Arthrose-Patienten und klinischen Daten unter besonderer Berücksichtigung der Rheumafaktoren. Med. Dissertation, Universität Mainz
Missmahl HP (1965) Diagnose der generalisierten Amyloidosen. Dtsch med Wschr 90:394
Missmahl HP (1972) Amyloid. In: Bock HE, Hartmann F (eds) Klinik der Gegenwart. Urban und Schwarzenberg, München Berlin Wien

Mitchell DM, Spitz PW, Young DY, Bloch DA, McShane DJ, Fries JF (1986) Survival, prognosis, and causes of death in rheumatoid arthritis. Arthritis Rheum 29 (6):706–714

Mitrovic DR, Stankovic A, Iriarte-Borda O, et al. (1988) The prevalence of chondrocalcinosis in the human knee joint. An autopsy survey. J Rheumatol 15:633–641

Mohr W (1984) Arthropathien. In: Doerr W, Seifert G (eds) Spezielle pathologische Anatomie. Pathologie der Gelenke und Weichteiltumoren I. Springer, Berlin Heidelberg New York Tokyo, pp 373–547

Mohr W (1991) Kalziumpyrophosphat-Dihydrat-Ablagerungen im Knorpel von Femurköpfen nach Schenkelhalsfraktur. Akt Rheumatol 16:210–213

Mohr W, Hummler N (1986) Zerstört das Pannusgewebe bei der chronischen Polyarthritis einen Knorpel mit vitalen Chondrozyten? Akt Rheumatol 11:162–168

Mohr W, Menninger H (1979) Neutrophile Granulozyten bei der entzündlich-rheumatischen Knorpeldestruktion. Bull Schweiz Akad Med Wiss 35:443–451

Mojcik CF, Shevach EM (1997) Adhesion molecules. A rheumatologic perspective. Arthritis Rheum 40:991–1004

Molina R, Provost TT, Arnett FC, et al. (1986) Primary Sjögren's syndrome in men. Clinical, serologic, and immunogenetic features. Am J Med 80:23–31

Moll JMH (1985) Inflammatory bowel disease. In: Clinics in Rheumatic Diseases, vol 11, No 1. WB Saunders Company, London Philadelphia Toronto, pp 87–111

Moll JMH, Wright V (1973) Psoriatic arthritis. Arthritis Rheum Semin 3:55–78

Moore JS (1997) De Quervain's tenosynovitis. Stenosing tenosynovitis of the first dorsal compartment. J Occup Environ Med 10 (39):990–1002

Moore JS, Garg A (1994) Upper extremity disorders in a pork processing plant: relationships between job risk factors and morbidity. Am Ind Hyg Assoc J 55:703–715

Morales TJ, Kuettner KE (1982) The properties of the neutral proteinase released by primary chondrocyte cultures and its action on proteoglycan aggregate. Biochem Biophys Acta 705:92–101

Morgan WS, Castleman BA (1953) Clinicopathologic study of Mikulicz's disease. Am J Pathol 29:471

Movat HZ, Moore RH (1957) The nature and origin of fibrinoid. Am J Clin Pathol 28:331–353

Müller von F (1913) Differentiation of the diseases included under chronic arthritis. 17th International Congress of Medicine, London

Müller W, Schilling F (1982) Differentialdiagnose rheumatischer Erkrankungen, 2nd edn. Aesopus, Basel Wiesbaden

Müller-Ladner U (1995) T cell-independent cellular pathways of rheumatoid joint destruction. Curr Opin Rheumatol 7:222–228

Müller-Ladner U, Kriegsmann J, Gay RE, Koopman WJ, Gay S, Chatham WW (1995) Progressive joint destruction in a human immunodeficiency virus-infected patient with rheumatoid arthritis. Arthritis Rheum 38:1328–1332

Müller-Ladner U, Kriegsmann J, Gay RE, Gay S (1995) Oncogenes in rheumatoid arthritis. Rheum Dis Clin North Am 21:675–690

Mulherin D, Fitzgerald O, Bresnihan B (1996) Synovial tissue macrophage populations and articular damage in rheumatoid arthritis. Arthritis Rheum 39:115–124

Munthe E (1972) Anti-IgG and antinuclear antibodies in juvenile rheumatoid arthritis. Scand J Rheumatol 1:161-170

Murphy G (1995) Matrix metalloproteinases and their inhibitors. Acta Orthop Scand 66 (Suppl 266):55–60

Murphy G, McGuire MB, Russell RGG, Reynolds JJ (1981) Characterization of collagenase, other metallo-proteinases and an inhibitor

(TIMP) produced by human synovium and cartilage in culture. Clin Sci Lond 61:711–716
Murphy G, Hembry RM, Hughes CE, Fosang AJ, Hardingham TE (1990) Role and regulation of metalloproteinases in connective tissue turnover. Biochem Soc Trans 18:812–815
Murray RO (1965) The aetiology of primary osteoarthritis of the hip. Br J Radiol 38:810
Mutru O, Laasko M, Isomäki H, Koota K (1985) Ten year mortality and causes of death in patients with rheumatoid arthritis. Br Med J 290:1797–1799
Nadelman RB, Wormser GP (1998) Lyme borreliosis. Lancet 352:557–565
Nadelman RB, Horowitz HW, Hsieh T-C, et al. (1997) Simultaneous human ehrlichiosis and Lyme borreliosis. N Engl J Med 337:27–30
Nakayama DA, et al. (1984) Tophaceous gout: A clinical and radiographic assessment. Arthritis Rheum 27:468–471
Nanagara R, Li F, Beutler A, Hudson A, Schumacher Jr HR (1995) Alteration of Chlamydia trachomatis biologic behaviour in synovial membranes. Arthritis Rheum 38 (10):1410–1417
Nasu T (1975) Takayasu's truncoarteritis in Japan: A statistical observation of 76 autopsy cases. Pathol Microbiol 43:140
Natvig JB, Førre Ø, Randen I, Steinitz M, Thompson K, Waalen K (1988) B lymphocytes, B cell clones and rheumatoid factor antibodies in rheumatoid inflammation. Scand J Rheumatol (Suppl) 76:217–227
Needleman BW, Wigley FM, Stair RW (1992) IL-1, IL-2, IL-4, IL-6, TNF alpha and IFN-gamma levels in sera from patients with scleroderma. Arthritis Rheum 35:67–72
Niepel GA, Sitaj S (1979) Enthesopathy. Clin Rheum Dis 5 (3):857–872
Niepel GA, Kostka D, Kopecky S, Manca S (1966) Enthesopathy. Acta rheumat balneol Pistiniana 1, Piestany
Nikkari ST, Hoyhtya M, Isola J, Nikkari T (1996) Macrophages contain 92-kd gelatinase (MMP-9) at the site of degenerated internal elastic lamina in temporal arteritis. Am J Pathol 149:1427–1433
Nimni ME (1997) Collagen, structure and function. Encyclopedia of Human Biology, 2nd edn, vol 2, pp 877–895
O'Duffy JD (1990) Vasculitis in Behçet's disease. Rheum Dis Clin North Am 16:423–431
O'Duffy JD, Goldstein NP (1976) Neurologic involvement in seven patients with Behçet's disease. Am J Med 61:170–178
Oegema TR, Thompson RC (1990) Cartilage-bone interface (tidemark). In: Brandt KD (ed) Cartilage Changes in Osteoarthritis. Indiana University School of Medicine, Indianapolis, pp 43–52
Oegema TR, Thompson RC (1992) The zone of calcified cartilage. Its role in osteoarthritis. In: Kuettner KE, Schleyerbach R, Peyron JG, Hascall VC (eds) Articular cartilage and Osteoarthritis. Raven Press, New York, pp 319–331
Oehler S, Fassbender HG, Neureiter D, Meyer-Scholten C, Kirchner T, Aigner T (2000) Cell populations involved in pigmented villonodular synovitis of the knee. J Rheumatol 27:463–70
Ohno S, Aoki K, Sugiura S, Nakayama E, Itakura K (1973) HLA-B and Behçet's disease. Lancet 2:1383–1384
Olsen BR (1992) Molecular biology of cartilage collagens. In: Kuettner KE, Schleyerbach R, Peyron JG, Hascall VC (eds) Articular cartilage and Osteoarthritis. Raven Press, New York, pp 151–165
Oppenheimer A (1943) Development, clinical manifestations, and treatment of rheumatoid arthritis of the apophyseal intervertebral joints. Am J Roentgenol 49:49
Ornstein MH, Dubin Kerr L, Spiera H (1995) A reexamination of the relationship between active rheumatoid arthritis and the acquired immunodeficiency syndrome. Arthritis Rheum 38 (11):1701–1706
Orringer MB, Dabich L, Zarafonetis CJD, Sloan H (1976) Gastroesophageal reflux in esophageal scleroderma: Diagnosis and implications. Ann Thorac Surg 22:120

Osung OA, Chandra M, Holborow EJ (1982) Antibodies to intermediate filaments of the cytoskeleton in rheumatoid arthritis. Ann Rheum Dis 41:69–73

Ott VR, Wurm H (1957) Spondylitis ankylopoetica. Steinkopff, Darmstadt

Otto HF, Remmele W (1996) Kolon und Rektum. In: Remmele W (ed) Pathologie, Bd 2. Springer, Berlin Heidelberg New York, pp 533–675

Otto HF, Wanke M, Zeitlhofer J (1976) Darm und Peritoneum. In: Doerr W, Seifert G, Uehlinger E (eds) Spezielle pathologische Anatomie, Bd II/2. Springer, Berlin Heidelberg

Palmosky MJ, Brandt KD (1982) Immobilization of the knee prevents osteoarthritis after anterior cruciate ligament transection. Arthritis Rheum 25:1201

Pamir NM, Kansu T, Erbengi A, Zileli T (1981) Papilledema in Behçet's syndrome. Arch Neurol 38:643

Papaioannou CC, Gupta RC, Hunder GG, McDuffie FC (1980) Circulating immune complexes in giant cell arteritis and polymyalgia rheumatica. Arthritis Rheum 23:1021-1025

Parrott DP, Goldberg RL, Kaplan SR, Fuller GC (1982) The effect of lymphokines on proliferation and collagen synthesis of cultured human synovial cells. Eur J Clin Invest 12:407

Partridge REH (1986) Low back pain. In: Cohen AS, Bennett JC (eds) Rheumatology and Immunology, 2nd edn. Grune & Stratton, Orlando, pp 156–164

Pauli BU, Schwartz DE, Thonar EJ-MA, Kuettner KE (1983) Tumor invasion and host extracellular matrix. Cancer Metast Rev 2:129–152

Payne GS, Bishop JM, Varmus HE (1982) Multiple arrangements of viral DNA and an activated host oncogene in bursal lymphomas. Nature 295:209–215

Pease CT, Shattles W, Charles PJ, Venables PJW, Maini RN (1989) Clinical, serological, and HLA phenotype subsets in Sjögren's syndrome. Clin Exp Rheumatol 7:185–190

Perez HD, Kramer N (1981) Pulmonary hypertension in systemic lupus erythematosus. Semin Arthritis Rheum 11:177-181

Perlish JS, Bashey RI, Stephens RE, Fleischmajer R (1976) Connective tissue synthesis by cultured scleroderma fibroblasts. I. In vitro collagen synthesis by normal and scleroderma dermal fibroblasts. Arthritis Rheum 19:891

Peters MS, Gleich GJ, Dunnette SL, Fukuda T (1988) Ultrastructural study of eosinophils from patients with the hypereosinophilic syndrome: a morphological basis of hypodense eosinophils. Blood 71:780–785

Petrow PK, Theis B, Eckard A, Karbowski A, Eysel P, Salzmann G, Gaumann A, Gay RE, Gay S, Klein C, Kirkpatrick CJ, Kriegsmann J (1997) Determination of proliferating cells at the sites of cartilage invasion in patients with rheumatoid arthritis. Arthritis Rheum 40 (Suppl 9):251

Peyronie F (1743) Sur quelques obstacles qui s'opposent a l'éjaculation naturelle de la semence. Mémoires Acad Roy Chir Paris 1:425

Philipps PE (1988) The role of infectious agents in the spondylarthropathies. Scand J Rheumatol 17:435–443

Picken RN, Strle F, Ruzic-Sabljic E, et al. (1997) Molecular subtyping of Borrelia burgdorferi sensu lato isolates from five patients with solitary lymphocytoma. J Invest Dermatol 108:92–97

Pillemer SR, Bradley LA, Crofford LJ, Moldofsky H, Chrousos GP (1997) The neuroscience and endocrinology of fibromyalgia. Arthritis Rheum 40:1928–1939

Plaas AHK, Sandy JD (1995) Proteoglycan anabolism and catabolism in articular cartilage. In: Kuettner KE, Goldberg VM (eds) Osteoarthritic disorders. American Academy of Orthopedic Surgeons, Rosemont, pp 103–116

Plotz PH, Rider LG, Targoff IN, Raben N, O'Hanlon TP, Miller FW (1995) Myositis: Immunologic contributions to understanding cause, pathogenesis, and therapy. Ann Intern Med 122:715–724
Pomerance A (1975) Cardiac involvement in rheumatic and "collagen" diseases. In: Pomerance A, Davies MJ (eds) The pathology of the heart. Blackwell, Oxford, pp 279–306
Poole AR (1995) Imbalances of anabolism and catabolism of cartilage matrix components in osteoarthritis. In: Kuettner KE, Goldberg VM (eds) Osteoarthritic disorders. American Academy of Orthopedic Surgeons, Rosemont, pp 247–260
Poole CA, Ayad S, Schofield JR (1988) Chondrons from articular cartilage: (1) Immunolocalization of type VI collagen in the pericellular capsule of isolated canine chondrons. J Cell Sci 90:635–643
Poole CA, Gilbert RT, Ayad S, Plaas AHK (1993) Immunolocalisation of type VI collagen, decorin, and fibromodulin in articular cartilage and isolated chondrons. Trans Orthop Res Soc 18:644
Prescott RJ, Freemont AJ, Jones CJ, Hoyland J, Fielding P (1992) Sequential dermal microvascular and perivascular changes in the development of scleroderma. J Pathol 166:255–263
Přibram (1901) Der akute Gelenkrheumatismus. In: Nothnagels spezielle Pathologie und Therapie, Bd 5, p 2
Pritzker KPH, Renlund RC, Cheng P-T (1980) Calcium pyrophosphate crystal arthropathy in femoral heads. Lab Invest 42:144
Pritzker KPH, Renlund RC, Cheng P-T (1983) Which comes first – osteoarthritis or crystals? A study of surgically removed femoral heads. J Rheumatol 10 (9):38–39
Prockop DJ, Kivirikko KL (1995) Collagens: Molecular biology, diseases, and potentials for therapy. Ann Rev Biochem 64:403–434
Proud D, Kaplan AP (1988) Kinin formation: Mechanisms and role in inflammatory disorders. Ann Rev Immunol 6:49–83
Quervain de F (1895) Über eine Form von chronischer Tendovaginitis. Cor-Bl f schweiz Aerzte 25:389–394
Quervain de F (1912a) Über das Wesen und die Behandlung der stenosierenden Tendovaginitis am Processus styloideus radii. München Med Wschr 1:5
Quervain de F (1912b) Stenosierende Tendovaginitis am Handgelenk. Cor-Bl f schweiz Aerzte 42:355
Radin EL (1972–1973) The physiology and degeneration of joints. Semin Arthritis Rheum 2:245
Rahmann MU, Ahmed S, Schumacher AR, Zeiger AR (1990) High levels of antipeptidoglycan antibodies in psoriatic and other seronegative arthritides. J Rheumatol 17:621–625
Rahn DW, Malawista SE (1993) Lyme disease. In: McCarty DJ, Koopman WJ (eds) Arthritis and Allied Conditions, 12th edn. Lea & Febiger, Philadelphia London (A Textbook of Rheumatology, vol 2) pp 2067–2079
Ranney D, Wells R, Moore A (1995) Upper limb musculoskeletal disorders in highly repetitive industries: precise anatomical physical findings. Ergonomics 38:1408–1423
Redler I, Mow VC, Zimny ML, Mansell J (1975) The ultrastructure and biomechanical significance of the tidemark of articular cartilage. Clin Orthop 112:357–362
Reginato AJ, Schumacher HR, Martinez VA (1973) Ochronotic arthropathy with calcium pyrophosphate crystal deposition. Arthritis Rheum 16:705–714
Reif MC, Constantiner A, Levitt MF (1981) Chronic gouty nephropathy: A vanishing syndrome? N Engl J Med 304:535–536
Reinhold-Keller E, Kekow J, Schnabel A, Schmitt WH, Heller M, Beigel A, Duncker G, Gross WL (1994) Influence of disease manifestation and antineutrophil cytoplasmic antibody titer on the response to pulse cyclophosphamide therapy in patients with Wegener's granulomatosis. Arthritis Rheum 37 (6):919–924

Reiter H (1916) Über eine bisher unerkannte Spirochäteninfektion (Spirochaetosis arthritica). Dtsch med Wschr 42:1535–1538

Relman DA, Schmidt ThM, MacDermott RP, Falkow St (1992) Identification of the uncultured bacillus of Whipple's disease. N Engl J Med 327:293–301

Remky H (1972) Augenbeteiligung bei rheumatischen Erkrankungen. In: Mathies H (ed) Organmanifestationen. Aktuelle Rheumaprobleme. Banaschewski, München

Rest van der M, Mayne R (1988) Type IX collagen proteoglycan from cartilage is covalently cross-limited to type II collagen. J Biol Chem 263:1615–1618

Reveille JD (1993) The interplay of nature versus nurture in predisposition to the rheumatic diseases. Rheum Dis Clin North Am 19:15–27

Rider LG, Gurley RC, Pandey JP, Torre de la IG, Kalovidouris AE, O'Hanlon TP, Love LA, Hennekam RCM, Baumbach LL, Neville HE, Garcia CA, Klingmann J, Gibbs M, Weisman MH, Targoff IN, Miller FW (1998) Clinical, serologic, and immunogenetic features of familial idiopathic inflammatory myopathy. Arthritis Rheum 41:710–719

Riemann J, Riemann F, Schilling F (1974) Lungenbeteiligung bei der Spondylitis ankylopoetica. Kasuistik zur "Bechterew-Lunge". Prax Pneumol 28:148

Ringel SP, Carry MR, Aquilera AJ, Starcevich JM (1986) Quantitative histopathology of the inflammatory myopathies. Arch Neurol 43:1004–1009

Roberts J, Burch TA (1966) Prevalence of osteoarthritis in adults by age, sex, race, and geographic area: United States 1960–1962. Vital Health and Statistics, Series 11, No 15, publication No (PHS) 1000. Washington, DC. National Center for Health Statistics

Roberts WC (1968) Cardiac valvular lesions in rheumatoid arthritis. Arch intern Med 122

Robertson MDJ, et al. (1968) Rheumatoid lymphadenopathy. Ann Rheum Dis 27:253–260

Rodnan GP (1972) Progressive systemic sclerosis (scleroderma). In: Hollander JL, McCarty Jr DJ (eds) Arthritis and Allied Conditions, 8th edn, Lea & Febiger, Philadelphia, pp 962–1005

Roggendorf W (1995) Kreislaufstörungen des zentralen Nervensystems. In: Remmele W, Peiffer J, Schröder JM (eds) Pathologie. Springer, Berlin Heidelberg New York (Neuropathologie, Muskulatur, Sinnesorgane, 2. neubearb Aufl, Bd 6, pp 62–106)

Ronzière M-C, Ricard-Blum S, Tiollier J, Hartmann DJ, Garrone R, Herbage D (1990) Comparative analysis of collagens solubilized from human foetal, and normal and osteoarthritic adult articular cartilage, with emphasis on type VI collagen. Biochim Biophys Acta 1038:222–230

Ropes MW (1976) Systemic lupus erythematosus. Harvard University Press, Cambridge

Rose HM, Ragan C, Pearce E, Lipman MO (1948) Differential agglutination of normal and sensitized sheep erythrocytes by sera of patients with rheumatoid arthritis. Proc Soc exp Biol 68:1–16

Rose JH, Belsky MR (1989) Psoriatic arthritis in the hand. Hand Clin 5:137–144

Rosenberg L (1992) Structure and function of dermatan sulfate proteoglycans in articular cartilage. In: Kuettner KE, Schleyerbach R, Peyron JG, Hascall VC (eds) Articular cartilage and Osteoarthritis. Raven Press, New York, pp 45–63

Rosenberg LC, Buckwalter JA (1986) Cartilage proteoglycans. In: Kuettner KE, Schleyerbach R, Hascall VC (eds) Articular Cartilage Biochemistry. Raven Press, New York, pp 39–58

Rosenthal J, Bole GG, Robinson WD (1980) Acute non-gonococcal infectious arthritis. Arthritis Rheum 23:889–897

Rothfield NF (1985) Clinical features of systemic lupus erythematosus. In: Kelley WN, Harris Jr ED, Ruddy S, Sledge CB (eds) Textbook of Rheumatology, vol 2, 2nd edn. WB Saunders Company, Philadelphia London Toronto Mexico City Rio de Janeiro Sydney Tokyo, pp 1070–1097
Rothfield NF (1993) Systemic lupus erythematosus: Clinical aspects and treatment. In: McCarty DJ, Koopman WJ (eds) Arthritis and Allied Conditions, 12th edn. Lea & Febiger, Philadelphia London (A Textbook of Rheumatology, vol 2) pp 1155–1177
Roy EP, Gutmann L (1988) Muscle disease. Neurol Clin 6 (3):621–636
Rubinow A (1986) Whipple's disease. In: Cohen AS, Bennett JC (eds) Rheumatology and Immunology, 2nd edn. Grune & Stratton, Orlando, pp 242–245
Rubinow A, Canoso JJ, Goldenberg DL, Cohen AS, Shirahama T (1981) The arthritis of Whipple's disease. Isr J Med Sci 17:445–451
Ruffer MA, Rietti A (1911–1912) On osseous lesions in ancient egyptians. J Path Bact 16:439
Ruggieri A, LeRoy EC (1986) Scleroderma (systemic sclerosis). In: Cohen AS, Bennett JC (eds) Rheumatology and Immunology, 2nd edn. Grune & Stratton, Orlando, pp 257–268
Russell AS, Davis P, Percy JS, et al (1977) The sacroiliitis of acute Reiter's syndrome. J Rheumatol 4:293
Sack U, Stiehl P, Geiler G (1994) Distribution of macrophages in rheumatoid synovial membrane and its association with basic activity. Rheumatol Int 13:181–186
Sah RL, Kim YJ, Grodzinsky AJ, Plaas AHK, Sandy JD (1992) Effects of static and dynamic compression on matrix metabolism in cartilage explants. In: Kuettner KE, Schleyerbach R, Peyron JG, Hascall VC (eds) Articular cartilage and Osteoarthritis. Raven Press, New York, pp 373–392
Sairanen E, Tiilikainen A (1975) HL-A27 in Reiter's disease following shigellosis. Scand J Rheumatol 8 (Suppl):30–31
Sairanen E, Paronen I, Mähönen H (1969) Reiter's syndrome: A follow-up study. Acta Med Scand 185:57–63
Salisbury AK, Duke O, Paulter LW (1987) Macrophage-like cells of the pannus area in rheumatoid arthritis joints. Scand J Rheumatol 16 (4):263–272
Saxne T, Heinegard D (1992) Cartilage oligomeric matrix protein: a novel marker turnover detectable in synovial fluid and blood. Br J Rheumatol 31:583–591
Scarpa R, Oriente P, Pucino A, et al. (1984) Psoriatic arthritis in psoriatic patients. Br J Rheumatol 23:246–250
Schacherl M, Schilling F (1967) Röntgenbefunde an den Gliedmaßengelenken bei Polyarthritis psoriatica. Zschr Rheumaforsch 26:442–450
Schaller JG (1977) Juvenile rheumatoid arthritis. Series 1. Arthritis Rheum (Suppl) 20:165–170
Schenk RK, Eggli PS, Hunziker EB (1986) Articular cartilage morphology. In: Kuettner KE, Schleyerbach R, Hascall VC (eds) Articular Cartilage Biochemistry. Raven Press, New York, pp 3–22
Schilling F (1967) Gicht-Diagnose, Differentialdiagnose und Therapie. Ärztl Fortbildung 16:36
Schilling F (1974) Spondylitis ankylopoetica – Die sogenannte Bechterewsche Krankheit und ihre Differentialdiagnose (einschließlich Spondylosis hyperostotica, Spondylitis psoriatica und chronisches Reiter-Syndrom). In: Diethelm L (ed) Handbuch der Medizinischen Radiologie, vol VI/2. Springer, Berlin Heidelberg New York, pp 452–689
Schilling F (1984) Chronische Polyarthritis: Röntgendiagnostik. In: Mathies H (ed) Handbuch der inneren Medizin, vol VI/2. Springer, Berlin Heidelberg, pp 128–176

Schilling F (1987) Rheumatologische Befunde bei seronegativen Spondarthritiden. In: Holzmann H, Altmeyer P, Marsch WCh, Vogel HG (eds) Dermatologie und Rheuma. Springer, Berlin Heidelberg New York London Paris Tokyo, pp 182–201

Schilling F, Schacherl M (1967) Röntgenbefunde an der Wirbelsäule bei Polyarthritis psoriatica und Reiter-Dermatose: Spondylitis psoriatica. Zschr Rheumaforsch 26:450–459

Schilling F, Stadelmann M-L (1986) Definition und Nosologie, Typeneinteilung und klinisches Bild der Arthritis und Spondylitis psoriatica. In: Schilling F (ed) Arthritis und Spondylitis psoriatica. Steinkopff, Darmstadt, pp 1–21

Schilling F, Schacherl M, Bopp A, Gamp A, Haas JP (1963) Veränderungen der Halswirbelsäule (Spondylitis cervicalis) bei der chronischen Polyarthritis und bei der Spondylitis ankylopoetica. Der Radiologe 12:483–501

Schilling F, Fassbender HG, Stiehler T (1986) Spondarthritis hyperostotica pustulo-psoriatica. In: Schilling F (ed) Arthritis und Spondylitis psoriatica. Steinkopff, Darmstadt, pp 289–296

Schlosstein L, Terasaki PI, Bluestone R, et al. (1973) High association of an HL-A antigen W 27 with ankylosing spondylitis. N Engl J Med 288:704–706

Schmid TM, Linsenmayer TF (1987) Type X collagen. In: Mayne R, Burgeson RE (eds) Structure and Function of Collagen Types. Academic Press, Orlando

Schmidli J, Hunziker T, Moesli P, Schaad UB (1988) Cultivation of Borrelia burgdorferi from joint fluid three months after treatment of facial palsy due to Lyme borreliosis. J Infect Dis 158:905–906

Schneider M, Specker Ch (1996) Lupus und Butterfly. Akt Rheumatol 21:48–61

Schnitzer TJ (1985) Viral arthritis. In: Kelley WN, Harris Jr ED, Ruddy S, Sledge CB (eds) Textbook of Rheumatology, vol 2, 2nd edn. WB Saunders Company, Philadelphia London Toronto Mexico City Rio de Janeiro Sydney Tokyo, pp 1540–1556

Schnitzer TJ, Ansell BM (1977) Amyloidosis in juvenile chronic polyarthritis. Arthritis Rheum (Suppl) 20:245

Schoen RT (1988) Lyme disease diagnosis can be troublesome. In: Rheumatol Consultant, vol 2, 1:1–7

Schönlein JL (1837) Allgemeine und spezielle Pathologie und Therapie. Zürich

Schönthal A, Herrlich P, Rahmsdorf HJ, et al. (1988) Requirement for fos gene expression in the transcriptional activation of collagenase by other oncogenes and phorbol esters. Cell 54:325–344

Schröder JM (1982) Pathologie der Muskulatur. Springer, Berlin Heidelberg New York (Spezielle pathologische Anatomie, Bd 15)

Schröder JM (1995a) Pathologie des peripheren Nervensystems. In: Remmele W, Peiffer J, Schröder JM (eds) Pathologie. Springer, Berlin Heidelberg New York (Neuropathologie, Muskulatur, Sinnesorgane, 2. neubearb Aufl, Bd 6) pp 349–402)

Schröder JM (1995b) Pathologie der Skelettmuskulatur. In: Remmele W, Peiffer J, Schröder JM (eds) Pathologie. Springer, Berlin Heidelberg New York (Neuropathologie, Muskulatur, Sinnesorgane, 2. neubearb Aufl, Bd 6) pp 405–469)

Schumacher HR (1973) Joint involvement in progressive systemic sclerosis (scleroderma): a light and electron microscopic study of synovial membrane and fluid. Am J Clin Pathol 60:593–600

Schumacher HR (1976) Ultrastructural findings in chondrocalcinosis and pseudogout. Arthritis Rheum 19:413

Schumacher HR (1985) Synovial fluid analysis. In: Kelley WN, Harris Jr ED, Ruddy S, Sledge CB (eds) Textbook of Rheumatology, vol 1, 2nd edn. WB Saunders Company, Philadelphia London Toronto Mexico City Rio de Janeiro Sydney Tokyo, pp 561–568

Schumacher HR (1993) Ochronosis, hemochromatosis, and Wilson's disease. In: McCarty DJ, Koopman WJ (eds) Arthritis and Allied Conditions, 12th edn. Lea & Febiger, Philadelphia London (A Textbook of Rheumatology, vol 2) pp 1913–1925
Schumacher HR, Holdsworth DE (1977) Ochronotic arthropathy. 2. Clinicopathologic studies. Semin Arthritis Rheum 6:207–246
Schumacher HR, Kitridou RC (1972) Synovitis of recent onset. A clinicopathologic study during the first month of disease. Arthritis Rheum 15:465–485
Schumacher HR, Fishbein P, Phelps P, et al. (1975) Comparison of sodium urate and calcium pyrophosphate crystal phagocytosis by polymorphonuclear leukocytes. Effects of crystal size and other factors. Arthritis Rheum 18:783
Schumacher HR, Tse R, Reginato A, Miller J, Maurer K (1976) Hydroxyapatite-like crystals in synovial fluid cell vacuoles: A suspected new cause for crystal-induced arthritis. Arthritis Rheum 19:821
Schumacher HR, Gibilisco P, Reginato A, Cherian V, Gordon G (1983) Implication of crystal deposition in osteoarthritis. J Rheumatol (Spec Issue) 9:40–41
Schur PH (1986) Systemic lupus erythematosus. In: Cohen AS, Bennett JC (eds) Rheumatology and Immunology, 2nd edn. Grune & Stratton, Orlando, pp 247–257
Schur PH (1994) Arthritis and autoimmunity. Arthritis Rheum 37 (12):1818–1825
Scott JE (1990) Proteoglycan-collagen interactions and subfibrillar structure in collagen fibrils. Implications in the development and aging of connective tissues. J Anat 169:223–235
Scribonius WA (1584) Idea medicinae secundum logicas theses, acc. de inspectione urinarum contra eos, qui ex qualibet urina de quolibet morbo judicare volunt. Lemgo
Segal I, Fink G, Machtey I, et al. (1981) Pulmonary function abnormalities in Sjögren's syndrome and the sicca complex. Thorax 36:286–289
Seibel MJ, Duncan A, Robins SP (1989) Urinary hydroxy-pyridinium crosslinks provide indices of cartilage and bone involvement in arthritic diseases. J Rheumatol 16:964–970
Seifert G (1966) Mundhöhle, Mundspeicheldrüsen, Tonsillen und Rachen. In: Doerr W, Uehlinger E (eds) Spezielle pathologische Anatomie, vol 1. Springer, Berlin Heidelberg New York
Seifert G (1971) Die Pathologie der Speicheldrüsen im Rahmen der Kollagenkrankheiten. HNO 19:193
Sharp J (1957) Differential diagnosis of ankylosing spondylitis. Br Med J 1:975
Sharp J (1965) Ankylosing spondylitis. A review. In: Dixon ASJ (ed) Progress in clinical rheumatology. Churchill, London, p 180
Shikano S (1966) Ocular pathology of Behçet's syndrome. In: Monacelli M, Nazarro P (eds) International Symposium of Behçet's Disease. Rome. Karger, Basel, pp 111–136
Shimizu T, Ehrlich GE, Inaba G, Hiyashi K (1979) Behçet's disease (Behçet's syndrome). Sem Arthritis Rheum 4:223
Shiozawa K, Tanaka Y, Imura S, Shiozawa S (1997) Elderly-onset rheumatoid arthritis: Ageing as an independent marker for better joint prognosis. Arthritis Rheum 40 (9):151
Shiozawa S, Jasin HE, Ziff M (1980) Absence of immunoglobulins in rheumatoid cartilage-pannus junctions. Arthritis Rheum 23:816–821
Shore A, Ansell BM (1982) Juvenile psoriatic arthritis – an analysis of 60 cases. J Pediatr 100:529–535
Shulman LE (1974) Diffuse fasciitis with hypergammaglobulinemia and eosinophilia: A new syndrome? J Rheumatol 1 (Suppl 1):46
Shulman LE (1990) The eosinophilia-myalgia syndrome associated with ingestion of L-Tryptophan. Arthritis Rheum 33 (7):913–917

Sieper J, Braun J (1995) Pathogenesis of spondylarthropathies. Persistent bacterial antigen, autoimmunity, or both? Arthritis Rheum 38 (11):1547–1554
Siltzbach LE, Duberstein JL (1968) Arthritis in sarcoidosis. Clin Orthop Rel Res 57:31-50
Siltzbach LE, James DG, Neville E, et al. (1974) Course and prognosis of sarcoidosis around the world. Am J Med 57:847-852
Silverstein E, Friendland J, Lyons HA, Gourin A (1976) Markedly elevated angiotensin converting enzyme in lymph nodes containing nonnecrotizing granulomas in sarcoidosis. Proc Natl Acad Sci USA 73:2137
Simmling-Annefeld M, Fassbender HG (1979) Transformation of the capillary wall elements in synovial tissue in rheumatoid arthritis. Z Rheumatol 38:153–156
Singer JM, Plotz CM (1956) The latex fixation test. I. Application of the serologic diagnosis of rheumatoid arthritis. Am J Med 21:888–892
Sjögren H (1933) Zur Kenntnis der Keratokonjunktivitis sicca. Acta Ophth 11:1–151
Sloane BF, Dunn JR, Honn KV (1981) Lysosomal cathepsin B with metastatic potential. Science 212:1151–1153
Smiley JD (1995) Psoriatic arthritis. Publication of arthritis foundation. Bull Rheum Dis 44 (4)
Smith ME, Bywaters EGL (1968) Mortality and prognosis related to the amyloidosis of Still's disease. Ann Rheum Dis 27:137
Smythe HA, Sheon RP (1990) Fibrositis/fibromyalgia: A difference of opinion. Bull Rheum Dis 39 (3):1–8
Sobao Y, Tsuchiya N, Takiguchi M, Tokunaga K (1999) Overlapping peptide-binding specificities of HLA-B27 and B39: evidence for a role of peptide supermotif in the pathogenesis of spondylarthropathies. Arthritis Rheum 42 (1):175–181
Sokoloff L (1963) The pathophysiology of peripheral blood vessels in collagen disease. In: Orbinson JH, Smith DE (eds) The Peripheral Blood Vessels. Williams & Wilkins, Baltimore, pp 297
Sokoloff L (1964) Cardiac involvement in rheumatoid arthritis and allied disorders: current concepts. Med Concepts Cardiovasc Dis 33:847
Sokoloff L, Varma AA (1988) Chondrocalcinosis in surgically resected joints. Arthritis Rheum 31:750–756
Solomon L (1976) Patterns of osteoarthritis of the hip. J Bone Joint Surg 58B:176-183
Sonozaki H, et al. (1981) Incidence of arthro-osteitis in patients with pustulosis palmaris et plantaris. Ann Rheum Dis 40:554
Southwood TR, Petty RE, Malleson PN, et al. (1989) Psoriatic arthritis in children. Arthritis Rheum 32:1007–1013
Spilberg I, Siltzbach LE, McEwen CE (1969) The arthritis of sarcoidosis. Arthritis Rheum 12:126-137
Spilberg I, Gallacher A, Mandell B (1977) Calcium pyrophosphate dihydrate (CPPD) crystal-induced chemotactic factor: Subcellular localization role of protein synthesis and phagocytosis. J Lab Clin Med 89:817-822
Spilberg I, Mandell B, Mehta J, Simchowitz L, Rosenberg D (1979) Mechanism of action of colchinine in acute urate crystal-induced arthritis. J Clin Invest 64:775-780
Spilberg I, McLain D, Simchowitz L, Berney S (1980) Colchinine and pseudogout. Arthritis Rheum 23:1062-1063
Stanek G, Klein J, Bittner R, Dietmar G (1990) Isolation of Borrelia burgdorferi from the myocardium of a patient with longstanding cardiomyopathy. N Engl J Med 322:249–252
Stanek G, O'Connell S, Cimmino M, et al. (1996) European Union concerted action on risk assessment in Lyme borreliosis: clinical case definition for Lyme borreliosis. Wien Klin Wschr 108:741–747

Stark TW, Hirokawa RH (1982) Gout and its manifestations in the head and neck. Otolaryngol Clin North Am 15:659–664
State of Connecticut Department of Public Health (1993) Lyme disease update. Conn Epidemiol 13:9
Stecher RM, Ausenbachs A (1955) Vererbungen bei Erkrankungen der Gelenke. Z Rheumaforsch 14:209
Steere AC (1989) Lyme Disease. N Engl J Med 321:586–596
Steere AC, Malawista SE (1985) Lyme Disease. In: Kelley WN, Harris Jr ED, Ruddy S, Sledge CB (eds) Textbook of Rheumatology, vol 2, 2nd edn. WB Saunders Company, Philadelphia London Toronto Mexico City Rio de Janeiro Sydney Tokyo, pp 1557–1563
Steere AC, Malawista SE, Snydman DR, Andiman WA (1976) A cluster of arthritis in children and adults in Lyme, Connecticut. Arthritis Rheum 19:824
Steere AC, Malawista SE, Snydman DR, Shope RE, Andiman WA, Ross MR, Steele FM (1977a) Lyme arthritis: An epidemic of oligoarticular arthritis in children and adults in three Connecticut communities. Arthritis Rheum 20:7–17
Steere AC, Hardin JA, Malawista SE (1977b) Erythema chronicum migrans and Lyme arthritis. Cryoimmunoglobulins and clinical activitiy of skin and joints. Science 196:1121
Steere AC, Malawista SE, Hardin JA, Ruddy S, Askenase PW, Andiman WA (1977c) Erythema chronicum migrans and Lyme arthritis: The enlarging clinical spectrum. Ann Intern Med 86:685–698
Steere AC, Hardin JA, Ruddy S, Mummaw JG, Malawista SE (1979a) Lyme arthritis: Correlation of serum and cryoglobulin IgM with activity and serum IgG with remission. Arthritis Rheum 22:471-483
Steere AC, Gibofsky A, Patarroyo ME, Winchester RJ, Hardin JA, Malawista SE (1979b) Chronic Lyme arthritis: Clinical and immunogenetic differentiation from rheumatoid arthritis. Ann Intern Med 90:286–291
Steere AC, Gibofsky A, Hardin JA, Winchester RJ, Malawista SE (1979c) Lyme arthritis: Immunologic and immunogenetic markers. Abstract. Arthritis Rheum 22:662
Steere AC, Brinckerhoff CE, Miller DJ, Drinker H, Harris Jr ED, Malawista SE (1980) Elevated levels of collagenase and prostaglandin E2 from synovium associated with erosion of cartilage and bone in a patient with chronic Lyme arthritis. Arthritis Rheum 23:591–599
Steere AC, Grodzicki RL, Kornblatt AN, Craft JE, Barbour AG, Burgdorfer W, Schmid GP, Johnson E, Malawista SE (1983) The spirochetal etiology of Lyme disease. N Engl J Med 308:733–740
Stein HB, Urowitz MB (1976) Gold-induced enterocolitis. J Rheumatol 3:21
Stiehl P, Kluger K-M (1994) Gelenkerguß-Befunde bei alkaptonurischer Arthropathie (Ochronose). Z Rheumatol 53:150–154
Still GF (1897) On a form of chronic joint disease in children. Med Chir Trans 80:47 (reprinted (1941) in Arch Dis Child 16:156)
Stockmann R (1920) Rheumatism and Arthritis. Green & Sons, Edinburgh
Stockwell RA (1979) Biology of cartilage cells. In: Harrison RJ, Mc Minn RMH (eds) Biological Structure and Function, vol 7. Cambridge University Press, Cambridge, pp 67–69
Stofft E, Zschäbitz A, Pöttgen K, Kunt T, Nissen A (1988) Zur Morphologie und Morphometrie der Synovialiszellen bei Arthrose und rheumatoider Arthritis. Abstract. Z Rheumatol 47:271
Stollermann GH (1997) Rheumatic fever. Lancet 349:935–942
Strand V, Talal N (1980) Advances in the diagnosis and concept of Sjögren's syndrome (autoimmune exocrinopathy). Bull Rheum Dis 30:1046–1052
Strauer BE, Brune I, Schenk H, Knoll D, Perings E (1975) Lupus-Kardiomyopathie bei unkompliziertem Lupus erythematodes. Dtsch Med Wschr 100:2138–2144

Strle F, Nadelman RB, Cimperman J, et al. (1999) Comparison of culture-confirmed erythema migrans caused by Borrelia burgdorferi sensu stricto in New York State and by Borrelia afzelii in Slovenia. Ann Intern Med 130 (1):32–36

Strümpell A (1884) Lehrbuch der spec. Pathologie und Therapie der Inneren Krankheiten, vol 2, 8th edn. Vogel, Leipzig

Stuart JM, Postlethwaite AE, Kang AH (1983) Evidence of cell-mediated immunity to collagen in patients with progressive systemic sclerosis. Abstract. Arthritis Rheum 26:170

Subcommittee for scleroderma criteria of the American Rheumatism Association diagnostic and therapeutic criteria committee (1980) Preliminary criteria for the classification of systemic sclerosis (scleroderma). Arthritis Rheum 23:581–590

Sundy JS, Haynes BF (1995) Pathogenic mechanisms of vessel damage in vasculitis syndromes. Rheum Dis Clin North Am 21:861–881

Swaay van H (1950) Spondylitis ankylopoetica. Een pathogenetische studie. Med. Dissertation. Leyden

Swann DA, Slayter HS, Silver FH (1981) The molecular structure of lubricating glycoprotein-I, the boundary lubricant for articular cartilage. J Biol Chem 256:5921–5925

Swanson SAV, Freeman MAR (1970) The mechanics of synovial joints. In: Simpson DC (ed) Modern Trends in Biomechanics, vol 1. Butterworth, London, p 239

Sweet MBE, Thonar EJ-MA, Immelman AR, Solomon L (1977) Biochemical changes in progressive osteoarthrosis. Ann Rheum Dis 36:387–398

Swift HF (1924) Die Pathogenese des Rheumatismus. J Exp Med 39:497

Swygert LA, Maes EF, Sewell L, Falk H, Kilbourne EM (1990) Eosinophilia-myalgia syndrome; results of national surveillance. J Am Med Assoc 264:1698–1703

Sydenham T (1683) Tractatus de podagra et hydrope. G Kittilby, London

Sydenham T (1701) Of a Rheumatism. The whole works of that excellent practical physician Dr. Thomas Sydenham. Übersetzt aus dem Lateinischen von John Pechey, London

Symmons DPM (1988) Mortality in rheumatoid arthritis. Br J Rheumatol 27 (Suppl I):44–54

Symmons DPM, Salmon M, Bacon PA (1985) A study of lymph node lymphocytes in rheumatoid arthritis. Adv Exp Med Biol 186:1027

Symmons DPM, Salmon M, Bacon PA (1987) The significance of lymphadenopathy in rheumatoid arthritis. Q J Med 65:873–874

Talal N (1986) Sjögren's syndrome. In: Cohen AS, Bennett JC (eds) Rheumatology and Immunology, 2nd edn. Grune & Stratton, Orlando, pp 290–294

Talal N (1993) Sjögren's syndrome and connective tissue diseases associated with other immunologic disorders. In: McCarty DJ, Koopman WJ (eds) Arthritis and Allied Conditions, 12th edn. Lea & Febiger, Philadelphia London (A Textbook of Rheumatology, vol 2) pp 1343–1356

Talal N, Bunim JJ (1964) The development of malignant lymphoma in Sjögren's syndrome. Am J Med 36:529

Talal N, Moutsopoulos HM, Kassan SS (eds) (1987) Sjögren's syndrome: Clinical and immunologic aspects. Springer, New York

Talalajew WT (1924) Weitere Beiträge zur Frage der pathologischen Anatomie des akuten Rheumatismus. In: 1. allruss path Kongr Petrograd. Ref in Zbl Path 35

Tan EML, Uitto J, Bauer EA, Eisen AZ (1981) Human skin fibroblasts in culture: Procollagen synthesis in the presence of sera from normal human subjects and from patients with dermal fibroses. J Invest Dermatol 76:462

Taylor-Robinson D, Thomas BJ, Dixey J, Osborn MF, Furr PM, Keat AC (1988) Evidence that Chlamydia trachomatis causes seronegative arthritis in women. Ann Rheum Dis 47:295–299

Tengnér P, Halse A-K, Haga H-J, Jonsson R, Wahren-Herlenius M (1998) Detection of anti-Ro/SSA and anti-La/SSB autoantibody-producing cells in salivary glands from patients with Sjögren's syndrome. Arthritis Rheum 41 (12):2238–2248

Thomas AF, Solomon L, Rabson A (1975) Polyarthritis associated with Yersinia enterocolitica infection. S Afr Med J 49:18–20

Thonar EJ-MA, Kuettner KE (1987) Biochemical basis of agerelated changes in proteoglycans. In: Wight TN, Mecham RP (eds) The Biology of extracellular matrix: Proteoglycans. Academic Press, New York, pp 211–246

Thonar EJ-MA, Williams JM, Maldonado BA, Lenz ME, Schnitzer TJ, Campion GV, Kuettner KE, Sweet MBE (1991) Serum keratan sulfate concentration as a measure of the catabolism of cartilage proteoglycans. In: Kresina TF (ed) Monoclonal Antibodies, Cytokines, and Arthritis: Mediators of Inflammation and Therapy. Marcel Dekker Inc, New York Basel Hongkong, pp 373–397

Thorel Ch (1915) Pathologie der Kreislauforgane des Menschen. Erg allg Path path Anat 17 (II):90

Todd RC, Freeman MAR, Pirie CJ (1972) Isolated trabeculae fatigue fractures in the femoral head. J Bone Surg 54B:723-782

Tomasek JJ, Vaughan MB, Haaksma CJ (1999) Cellular structure and biology of Dupuytren's disease. Hand Clinics 15 (1):21–34

Tourtellotte WW (1970) On cerebrospinal fluid IgG quotients in multiple sclerosis and other diseases. J Neurol Sci 10:279

Trabandt A, Aicher WK, Gay RE, Sukhatme VP, Nilson-Hamilton M, Hamilton RT, McGhee JR, Fassbender HG, Gay S (1990) Expression of the collagenolytic and ras-induced cysteine proteinase Cathepsin L and proliferation-associated oncogenes in synovial cells of MRL/L mice and patients with rheumatoid arthritis. Matrix 10:349–361

Trabandt A, Gay RE, Fassbender HG, Gay S (1991) Cathepsin B in synovial cells at the site of joint destruction in rheumatoid arthritis. Arthritis Rheum 34 (11):1444–1451

Trabandt A, Aicher WK, Gay RE, et al. (1992) Spontaneous expression of immediately-early response genes c-fos and egr-1 in collagenase-producing rheumatoid synovial fibroblasts. Rheumatol Int 12:53–59

Trepo CG, Zuckerman AJ, Bird RC, Prince AM (1974) The role of circulating hepatitis B antigen/antibody immune complexes in the pathogenesis of vascular and hepatic manifestations in polyarteritis nodosa. J Clin Pathol 27:863-868

Tsuboi M, Eguchi K, Kawakami A, Matsuoka N, Kawabe Y, Aoyagi T, Maeda K, Nagataki S (1996) Fas antigen expression on synovial cells was downregulated by interleukin 1. Biochem Biophys Res Comm 218:280–285

Tugwell P, Dennis DT, Weinstein A, et al. (1997) Clinical guideline 2: Laboratory evaluation in the diagnosis of Lyme disease. Ann Intern Med 127:1109–1123

Turner RE, Frank MJ, VanAusdal D, Bollet AJ (1960) Some aspects of the epidemiology of gout: Sex and race incidence. Arch Intern Med 106:400–406

Tyler JA, Bolis S, Dingle JT, Middleton JFS (1992) Mediators of matrix metabolism. In: Kuettner KE, Schleyerbach R, Peyron JG, Hascall VC (eds) Articular cartilage and Osteoarthritis. Raven Press, New York, pp 251–264

Ueda H, Saito Y, Ito I, Yamaguchi H, Takeda T, Morooka S (1971) Further immunological studies of aortitis syndrome. Jpn Heart J 12:1

Uehlinger E (1973) Knochenveränderungen bei entzündlich-rheumatischen Erkrankungen vom pathologisch-anatomischen Standpunkt. Verh Ges Rheumatol. Steinkopff, Darmstadt

Urban JPG (1990) Solute transport between tissue and environment. In: Maroudas A, Kuettner K (eds) Methods in cartilage research. Academic Press, London, pp 241–273

Urban JPG (1994) The chondrocyte: A cell under pressure. Br J Rheumatol 33:901–908

Urrows S, Affleck G, Tennen H, Higgins P (1994) Unique clinical and psychological correlates of fibromyalgia tender points and joint tenderness in rheumatoid arthritis. Arthritis Rheum 37:1513–1520

Utsinger PD (1976) Relationship of lymphocytotoxic antibodies to lymphopenia and parameters of disease activity in systemic lupus erythematosus. J Rheumatol 3:175-185

Vainio K (1967) Synovectomies of the hand and wrist in rheumatoid arthritis. In: Groupe d'Etude de la Main (eds) La Main Rhumatismale - Expansion Scientifique Française. Paris

Valesova M, Trnavsky K, Hulinska D, Alusik S, Janousek J, Jirons J (1989) Detection of borrelia in the tissue from a patient with Lyme borreliosis by electron microscopy. J Rheumatol 16:1502–1505

Vaughan L, Mendler M, Huter S, Bruckner P, Winterhalter KH, Irwin M, Mayne R (1988) D-periodic distribution of collagen type IX along the cartilage fibrils. J Cell Biol 106:991–997

Vecchi De (1910) Contributo sperimentale alla conosensa di miocardite reumatica. In: Pathologica, vol II, no 47. Genova

Venables PJW (1988) Epstein-Barr virus infection and autoimmunity in rheumatoid arthritis. Ann Rheum Dis 47:265–269

Venables PJW, Shattles W, Pease CT, Ellis JE, Charles PJ, Maini RN (1989) Anti-La (SS-B): a diagnostic criterion for Sjögren's syndrome? Clin Exp Rheumatol 7:181–184

Vignon E, Arlot M, Vignon G (1977) Etude de la cellularité du cartilage articulaire fissuré. Comparisons des lésions liées et de l'âge des lésions arthrosiques de la tête femorale humaine. Pathol Biol 25:29–32

Vischer TL (1996) Virale Arthritis mit Ausnahme von Aids. Rheumatol Eur 25 (3):109–110

Vitali C, Tavoni A, Viegi G, et al. (1985) Lung involvement in Sjögren's syndrome: A comparison between patients with primary and with secondary syndrome. Ann Rheum Dis 44:455–461

Vuorio T, Kähäri V-M, Black C, Vuorio E (1991) Expression of osteonectin, decorin, and transforming growth factor-beta 1 genes in fibroblasts cultured from patients with systemic sclerosis and morphea. J Rheumatol 18:247–251

Waaler E (1940) On occurrence of a factor in human serum activating the specific agglutination of sheep blood corpuscles. Acta Path Microbiol Scand 17:172–188

Waaler E, Tonder O, Milde E-J (1976) Immunological histological studies of temporal arteries from patients with temporal arteritis and/or polymyalgia rheumatica. Acta Pathol Microbiol Scand 84:55-63

Wagenhäuser FJ (1969) Die Rheumamorbidität. Huber, Bern Stuttgart Wien

Waterhouse JP, Doniach I (1966) Post-mortem prevalence of focal lymphocytic adenitis of the submandibular salivary gland. J Pathol Bact 91:53

Wegener F (1939) Über eine eigenartige rhinogene Granulomatose mit besonderer Beteiligung des Arteriensytems und der Nieren. Beitr Pathol Anat Allg Pathol 102:36

Weiss L, Ward PM (1983) Cell detachment and metastasis. Cancer Metast Rev 2:111–127

Weiss SJ (1989) Tissue destruction by neutrophils. N Engl J Med 320:365–376

Weissmann G (1971) Lysosomes and the mediation of tissue injury in arthritis. In: Müller W, Harwerth H-G, Fehr K (eds) Rheumatoid Arthritis. London New York, pp 141–154

Werb Z (1992) The biologic role of metalloproteinases and their inhibitors. In: Kuettner KE, Schleyerbach R, Peyron JG, Hascall VC (eds) Articular cartilage and Osteoarthritis. Raven Press, New York, pp 295–304

Werb Z, Burleigh MC (1974) A specific collagenase from rabbit fibroblasts in monolayer culture. Biochem J 137:373–385

Weyand CM, Goronzy JJ (1999) Arterial wall injury in giant cell arteritis. Arthritis Rheum 42 (5):844–853

Weyand CM, Hicok KC, Hunder GG, Goronzy JJ (1994) Tissue cytokine patterns in patients with polymyalgia rheumatica and giant cell arteritis. Ann Intern Med 121:484–491

Weyand CM, Wagner AG, Björnsson J, Goronzy JJ (1996) Correlation of the topographical arrangement and the functional pattern of tissue-infiltrating macrophages in giant cell arteritis. J Clin Invest 98:1642–1649

Whaley K, Alspaugh MA (1985) Sjögren's syndrome. In: Kelley WN, Harris Jr ED, Ruddy S, Sledge CB (eds) Textbook of Rheumatology, vol 1, 2nd edn. WB Saunders Company, Philadelphia London Toronto Mexico City Rio de Janeiro Sydney Tokyo, pp 956–978

Whipple GH (1907) A hitherto undescribed disease characterised anatomically by fat and fatty acids in the intestinal and mesenteric lymphatic tissues. Bull John Hopk Hosp 18:382

White MH (1895) Colitis. Lancet i:538

Wikaningrum R, Highton J, Parker A, Coleman M, Hessian PA, Roberts-Thomson PJ, Ahern MJ, Smith MD (1998) Pathogenic mechanisms in the rheumatoid nodule. Arthritis Rheum 41 (10):1783–1797

Wilkinson IM, Russell RWR (1972) Arteries of the head and neck in giant cell arteritis: A pathological study to show the pattern of arterial involvement. Arch Neurol 27:378-391

Wilkinson M, Bywaters EGL (1957) Clinical features and course of ankylosing spondylitis. Ann Rheum Dis 17:209

Willan R (1808) Cutanous diseases. J Johnson, London

Williams HJ, Biddulph EC, Coleman SS, Ward JR (1977) Isolated subcutaneous nodules (pseudorheumatoid). J Bone Joint Surg 59A:73–76

Williams JA, Thonar EJ-MA (1989) Early osteophyte formation after chemically induced articular cartilage injury. Am J Sports Med 1:7–15

Williams Jr RC (1986) Rheumatic fever. In: Cohen AS, Bennett JC (eds) Rheumatology and Immunology, 2nd edn. Grune & Stratton, Orlando, pp 214–221

Willkens RF, Arnett FC, Bitter T, et al. (1981) Reiter's syndrome: Evaluation of preliminary criteria for definite disease. Arthritis Rheum 24:844–849

Wilson KH, Blitchington R, Frothingham R, Wilson JAP (1991) Phylogeny of the Whipple's disease-associated bacterium. Lancet 338:474–475

Winchester R (1990) AIDS and the rheumatic diseases. Bull Rheum Dis 39:1–10

Winfield JB, Winchester RJ, Kunkel HG (1976) Association of cold-reactive antilymphocyte antibodies with lymphopenia in systemic lupus erythematosus. Arthritis Rheum 18:587

Witmer R (1970) Rheumatische Augenerkrankungen. In: Schoen R, Böni A, Miehlke K (eds) Klinik der rheumatischen Erkrankungen. Springer, Berlin Heidelberg New York, p 268

Witter J, Roughley P, Webber C, Roberts N, Keystone E, Poole AR (1987) The immunologic detection and characterization of cartilage proteoglycan degradation products in synovial fluids of patients with arthritis. Arthritis Rheum 30:519–29

Woessner JF (1991) Matrix metalloproteinases and their inhibitors in connective tissue remodeling. Faseb J 5:2145–2154

Woldorf NM, Pastore PN, Terz J (1971) Rheumatoid arthritis of the cricoarytenoid joint. Arch Otolaryng 93:623–627

Wolfe F (1988) Fibrositis, fibromyalgia, and musculoskeletal disease: The current status of the fibrositis syndrome. Arch Phys Med Rehabil 69:527–531

Wolfe F, Smythe HA, Yunus MB, Bennett RM, Bombardier C, Goldenberg DL, et al. (1990) The American College of Rheumatoloy 1990 criteria for the classification of fibromyalgia: report of the multicenter criteria committee. Arthritis Rheum 33:160–172
Wolfe F, Ross K, Anderson J, Russell IJ, Hebert L (1995) The prevalence and characteristics of fibromyalgia in the general population. Arthritis Rheum 38:19–28
Wolfe F, Russell IJ, Vipraio G, Ross K, Anderson J (1997) Serotonin levels, pain treshold, and fibromyalgia symptoms in the general population. J Rheumatol 24:555–559
Wolman L, Darke CS, Young A (1965) The larynx in rheumatoid arthritis. J Laryng 79:403–434
Woodrow JC (1988) Genetics of the spondarthropathies. In: Greenan DM (ed) Bailliere's Clinical Rheumatology, vol 2, no 3: Genetics of Rheumatoid Diseases. Bailliere Tindall, London Philadelphia Sydney Tokyo Toronto, pp 603–622
Wooley DE (1984) Proteolytic enzymes of invasive cells. In: Mareel MM, Calman KC (eds) Invasion. Experimental and Clinical Implications. Oxford University Press, Oxford New York Tokyo, pp 228–251
Wortmann RL (1994) Searching for the cause of fibromyalgia. Is there a defect in energy metabolism? Arthritis Rheum 37:790–793
Wright CJE (1951) Benign giant cell synovioma. Br J Surg 38:257
Wright V (1985) Psoriatic arthritis. In: Kelley WN, Harris Jr ED, Ruddy S, Sledge CB (eds) Textbook of Rheumatology, vol 2, 2nd edn. WB Saunders Company, Philadelphia London Toronto Mexico City Rio de Janeiro Sydney Tokyo, pp 1021–1031
Wright V, Moll JMH (1976) Seronegative Polyarthritis. North-Holland Publishing Company, Amsterdam New York Oxford
Wurm H (1957) Zur pathologischen Anatomie und Pathologie der entzündlichen Wirbelsäulenversteifung (Bechterew-Marie-Strümpell). Z Rheumaforsch 14:337–364
Wyngaarden JB (1960) Gout. In: Stanbury JB, Fredrickson DS, Wyngaarden JB (eds) The Metabolic Basis of Inherited Diseases. McGraw-Hill, New York, pp 679–760
Yanni G, Whelan A, Feighery C, Bresnihan B (1994) Synovial tissue macrophages and joint erosion in rheumatoid arthritis. Ann Rheum Dis 53:39–44
Yazici H, Chamberlain MA, Schreuder I, D'Amaro J, Muftuoglu M (1980) HLA antigens in Behçet's disease. A reappraisal by a comparative study of Turkish and British patients. Ann Rheum Dis 39:344-348
Yazici H, Yurdakul S, Hamuryudan V (1999) Behçet's syndrome. Curr Opin Rheumatol 11:53–57
Youinou P (1995) Genetik der antinukleären Antikörperproduktion beim primären Sjögren-Syndrom. Rheumatol Eur 24/2:60–62
Young D, Schwedel JB (1944) The heart in rheumatoid arthritis. A study of 38 autopsy cases. Am Heart J 28:1
Yunus M, Masi AT, Calabro JJ, Miller KA, Feigenbaum SC (1981) Primary fibromyalgia (fibrositis), clinical study of 50 patients with matched normal controls. Sem Arthr Rheum 11:151–171
Yurdakul S, et al. (1983) The arthritis of Behçet's disease: a prospective study. Ann Rheum Dis 42:505–515
Yurdakul S, et al. (1988) The prevalence of Behçet's syndrome in a rural area in Northern Turkey. J Rheumatol 15:820–822
Zalokar J, Lellouch J, Claude JR (1981) Goutte et uricemia dans une population de 4663 hommes jeunes actifs. Semin Hop Paris 13–14:664–670
Zeek PM, Smith CC, Weeter JC (1948) Studies on periarteritis nodosa. III. The differentiation between the vascular lesions of periarteritis nodosa and of hypersensitivity. Am J Pathol 24:889
Zellner E (1928) Zur Kenntnis der Arthropathia psoriatica. Münch Med Wschr 75:903

Zhang Y, Gripenberg-Lerche C, Söderström K-O, Toivanen A, Toivanen P (1996) Antibiotic prophylaxis and treatment of reactive arthritis. Arthritis and Rheum 39 (7):1238–1243

Ziegler B, Gay RE, Huang G-Q, Fassbender HG, Gay S (1989) Immunohistochemical localisation of HTLV-I p19- and p24-related antigens in synovial joints of patients with rheumatoid arthritis. Am J Pathol 1:1–5

Ziff M (1991) Role of the endothelium in chronic inflammatory synovitis. Arthritis Rheum 34:1345–1352

Ziff M, Kantor T, Bien E, Smith A (1953) Studies on the composition of the fibrinoid material of the subcutaneous nodule of rheumatoid arthritis. J Clin Invest 32:1253–1259

Zitnan D, Sitaj S (1958) Mnohoprocentua familiarna kalcifikacia ortikularnych chrupich. Bratisl Lek Listy 38:217

Zschäbitz A, Stofft E (1988) The lectin binding pattern of normal and pathologically altered synovial tissue. Histol Histopathol 3:419–424

Zufferey P, Meyer OC, Grossin M, Kahn MF (1995) Primary Sjögren's syndrome (SS) and malignant lymphoma. Scand J Rheumatol 24:342–345

Zvaifler NJ, Woods Jr VL (1985) Etiology and pathogenesis of systemic lupus erythematosus. In: Kelley WN, Harris Jr ED, Ruddy S, Sledge CB (eds) Textbook of Rheumatology, vol 2, 2nd edn. WB Saunders Company, Philadelphia London Toronto Mexico City Rio de Janeiro Sydney Tokyo, pp 1042–1070

Zvaifler NJ, Boyle D, Firestein GS (1994) Early synovitis - Synoviocytes and mononuclear cell. Sem Arthritis Rheum 23 (6):11–16

Subject Index

GPSR Compliance
The European Union's (EU) General Product Safety Regulation (GPSR) is a set of rules that requires consumer products to be safe and our obligations to ensure this.

If you have any concerns about our products, you can contact us on

ProductSafety@springernature.com

In case Publisher is established outside the EU, the EU authorized representative is:

Springer Nature Customer Service Center GmbH
Europaplatz 3
69115 Heidelberg, Germany

www.ingramcontent.com/pod-product-compliance
Ingram Content Group UK Ltd.
Pitfield, Milton Keynes, MK11 3LW, UK
UKHW061705190726
13853UKWH00008B/2412
* 9 7 8 3 6 6 2 0 4 8 2 0 7 *